Anatomy and Physiology of Hearing for Audiologists

Anatomy and Physiology
of Hearing for Audiologists

WILLIAM W. CLARK, Ph.D.
Professor of Otolaryngology
Director, Program in Audiology and Communication Sciences
Washington University School of Medicine
St. Louis, Missouri

KEVIN K. OHLEMILLER, Ph.D.
Associate Professor of Otolaryngology
Washington University School of Medicine
St. Louis, Missouri

THOMSON
DELMAR LEARNING

Australia • Brazil • Canada • Mexico • Singapore • Spain • United Kingdom • United States

MW

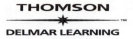

Anatomy and Physiology of Hearing for Audiologists
by William W. Clark and Kevin K. Ohlemiller

Vice President, Health Care Business Unit: William Brottmiller
Director of Learning Solutions: Matthew Kane
Senior Acquisitions Editor: Sherry Dickinson
Product Manager: Juliet Steiner
Editorial Assistant: Angela Doolin
Marketing Director: Jennifer McAvey

Marketing Manager: Chris Manion
Marketing Coordinator: Vanessa Carlson
Production Director: Carolyn Miller
Senior Content Project Manager: James Zayicek
Art Director: Jack Pendleton

Printed in the United States of America
1 2 3 4 5 6 7 8 XXX 11 10 09 08 07

Library of Congress Cataloging-in-Publication Data
Application submitted.
ISBN 1-4018-1444-1

For more information, contact
Thomson Delmar Learning
5 Maxwell Drive
Clifton Park, NY 12065

Or find us on the World Wide Web at
http://www.delmarlearning.com

For permission to use material from this text or product, contact us by
Tel (800) 730-2214
Fax (800) 730-2215
www.thomsonrights.com

Notice to the Reader

5/5/09

KKO Dedication: To Mary E. (Jerry) Ohlemiller

Contents

Preface

In the Preface to Volume 1 of his 1970 textbook *Foundations of Modern Auditory Theory* (New York: Academic Press, 1970), Jerry Tobias relates a story about a little girl who was interested in rabbits. She went to the library and checked out a book recommended by the helpful librarian. It was an excellent book, well written, with many illustrations. When the little girl brought it back a few weeks later, the librarian asked her how she enjoyed the book. "Not much," she replied. "It told me more about rabbits than I wanted to know."

The editors of this textbook are scientists who currently teach basic science courses in an Au.D. program. This work grew from our conviction that no other textbook currently in print meets the needs of the current generation of audiologists. Stated simply, books currently available are either written by scientists for their colleagues and tell the student "too much about rabbits," or they are targeted for undergraduates or master's degree audiology students and are even less useful. Our attempts to rely on current textbooks have forced us to either supplement generously the content of our courses or serve as "interpreters" for the texts aimed at the scientific community. A major goal of the editors was to produce a textbook that provides a strong foundation in anatomy and physiology of hearing for audiologists that is both comprehensive and palatable.

Recent years have seen both the expanse of the duties of audiologists and the sophistication of their equipment grow almost beyond recognition. Today, audiologists must understand at an intuitive level how specific ear pathologies present in the clinic. They must understand why prescribed diagnostic tests allow the inference of specific inner ear pathology. They must understand how the current limitations of hearing aids and cochlear implants arise both from how the inner ear functions and the physical limitations of hardware and circuitry. Audiologists must be able to communicate in the language of otologists the nature of patient needs. However, they must also communicate in language just as precise to their patients, so that complex biologic and physical concepts are understood, permitting decisions that are both highly informed and highly personal. As "biological fixes"—for example, gene therapy, stem cell therapy, and other strategies to promote repair and regeneration in the inner ear—become a reality, it will be tremendously important for audiologists to track both the relevant technology and the ethical issues, reminding both physicians and basic scientists whom it is they serve.

The arrival of the Au.D. as the entry-level degree confirms that audiologists today cannot serve well if they are reluctant to embrace basic science or are content to conduct clinical tests. They must be conversant in both clinical and basic hearing science literature, and they must be prepared to engage in research when new questions confront them. It is our experience, however, that many undergraduate programs that feed audiology graduate programs are somewhat lax in teaching basic science. Somehow, Au.D. programs must, in a few short years, bring students from often sparse science backgrounds to ease in discussing concepts such as bandwidth, distortion, and nonlinearity. An effective textbook to cover this span in such a short time has not, in our collective experience, ever existed. This book represents our earnest attempt to bring such a book into existence.

ORGANIZATION OF THE BOOK
Part I: Foundation

This book focuses on a basic understanding of hearing and begins appropriately with topics that are the foundation to any consideration of the auditory system. A key to understanding the anatomy and physiology of the auditory system begins with a basic knowledge about sound, acoustics, and how sounds are processed. Chapters 1 and 2 deal with understanding the physics of sound production, transmission, and absorption by the ear. We begin with descriptions of the physical bases of sound including discussions about sound measurement, propagation and absorption, hearing sensitivity, and classes of sounds. Audiologists also need to have an understanding of the basic characteristics of filters and spectral processing and the nature of sound transmission through the ear and how that limits or explains normal hearing sensitivity. Consideration is given to how sound transmission changes through an earplug, a hearing aid, a conductive hearing loss, or a cochlear implant. To close our discussion on foundations, we move from physical and engineering concepts to fundamental biologic concepts of the auditory system. To appreciate how the ear works and how disease processes affect hearing, we provide a basic description of cellular and subcellular anatomy and physiology of the cell and some of its basic functions. We also give a general overview of the structure and function of nerve cells and provide a foundation for the more comprehensive information about the auditory nervous system that is detailed in later chapters.

Part II: Anatomy and Physiology

Part II of this textbook introduces the anatomy and physiology of auditory system. These chapters start by exploring the structural, developmental, and physiologic complexity of the peripheral portions of the organ of hearing and conclude with details on the central nervous and vestibular systems. The development of the ear is covered first (Chapter 6), and it is one of the more remarkable examples of engineering in the vertebrate body. In the fetus, the ear starts to function as the auditory system matures, and by birth, it is fully capable of analyzing sounds in the environment.

The anatomy and physiology of the outer and middle ear is described next (Chapter 7), followed by a detailed chapter on cochlear anatomy (Chapter 8). From these elementary considerations of the peripheral auditory system, we introduce a series of chapters (Chapters 9 through 13) that explore the mechanics and neurobiology of cochlear function in more detail. We begin with a classic view of mechanical tuning of the basilar membrane (Chapter 9), then consider recent theories about how active processes sharpen mechanical tuning (Chapter 10). Chapters 11 and 12 cover cochlear afferent and efferent anatomy and function. The frequency tuning of the healthy basilar membrane is sufficiently sharp to account for normal perceptual ability to distinguish between sound frequencies. Therefore, cochlear hair cells need to retain this sharpness of tuning in transmitting excitation to afferent neurons. Although afferent neurons transmit only stimulus information passed on by hair cells, they also "re-encode" the stimulus in a way that virtually replaces the original stimulus waveform. One of our major goals in these chapters is to show the similarities in the shape of input-output curves of the basilar membrane, inner hair cells, and afferent fibers. Unfortunately, hearing usually occurs in a noisy environment. Afferent fiber responses are less well distinguished in noise, thus making hearing more difficult. Current studies of the efferent olivocochlear system are clarifying how the efferent system works to adapt the afferent system to background noise and provide protection to the ear from exposure to loud sounds.

Related to efferent fiber function is also the discovery of audiofrequency sounds or echoes in response to sounds and, in some cases, spontaneously as well. Chapter 13 addresses current knowledge regarding otoacoustic emissions. We know that metabolic energy is required for the generation of otoacoustic emissions. These emissions provide evidence for the presence of an active amplification mechanism within the inner ear and can be used to test the robustness of the efferent system. We conclude this section on anatomy and physiology with chapters describing the human brain (Chapter 14), the auditory CNS (Chapter 15), and the vestibular system (Chapter 16). Our brains analyze and store information about the external and internal environments and guide our behavior. We hope you will come to understand that a combination of anatomic, functional, and developmental views is necessary to understand the way the brain and especially the auditory central nervous system work, as well as some of the pathologies that you will see as audiologists and educators. We also provide greater detail on how the auditory central nervous system encodes and represents the spectral and temporal aspects of sounds, as well as the location of their source.

Part III: Pathology of Hearing

The third and final part of this textbook concerns how sensory cells of the inner ear can be destroyed by excessive exposure to noise, certain drugs, infections in the inner ear, genetic mutations, and aging. We discuss not only some ear-related symptoms and descriptions of ear diseases (Chapter 17), but also recent advances in our understanding of the mechanisms behind these disease processes. Nearly every person has experienced at least one time a hearing loss caused by excessive noise exposure. Chapter 18 provides a summary of the behavioral effects of noise on hearing, and Chapter 19 provides a detailed discussion of ototoxicity. Ototoxicity is the capacity of a drug or chemical agent to cause damage to the structure and or function of the inner ear. Many agents can cause ototoxicity. These compounds may affect hearing, balance, or a combination of both.

Chapter 20 covers genetic aspects of hearing loss. About half of congenital (present at birth) hearing loss results from genetic mutations. If impaired hearing is not due to drugs or noise, then it is likely caused by some hereditary mechanism. An unknown proportion of adult-onset hearing loss has an explicitly genetic cause or is strongly influenced by genetics. The ongoing revolution in molecular techniques and genetic manipulation virtually guarantees that audiologists will take part in discussions centered on diagnosing, managing, and eventually treating hearing loss associated with specific genetic defects.

The most common form of sensorineural hearing loss treated by audiologists is presbycusis. Chapter 21 contains an exposition of the combination of genetic and environmental factors that contribute to this most common form of neurodegenerative disorder related to aging. It will increasingly preoccupy most audiologists as our population ages. This final section concludes with a discussion of future therapies that may either prevent or "cure" hearing loss by rescuing hair cells after injury or by inducing hair cell regeneration (Chapter 22). Studies of hair cell regeneration in nonmammalian species have raised the hope that it might be possible to induce similar forms of regeneration in the human ear. For this goal to be realized, however, we need to understand the basic biology of the regenerative process.

About the Authors

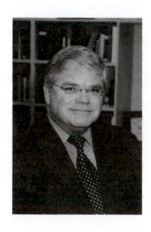

Dr. William W. Clark is the Director of the Program in Audiology and Communication Sciences (PACS) at Washington University School of Medicine in St. Louis, Missouri, where he also holds the rank of Professor in the Department of Otolaryngology and Department of Education. The PACS program trains teachers of the deaf, audiologists, and research scientists. Before his appointment in the School of Medicine, Dr. Clark was a Senior Research Scientist at Central Institute for the Deaf and served as the Chairman of the Department of Speech and Hearing at Washington University. He has taught basic and advanced courses in acoustics, anatomy, research methods, and hearing disorders for many years. His work on noise-induced hearing loss encompasses laboratory studies of exposure in animal subjects and field surveys of exposure and hearing loss both within and outside the workplace. Dr. Clark has published more than 80 articles on the effects of noise on hearing and cochlear anatomy, physiology, and bioacoustics.

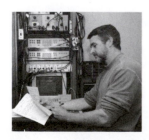

Dr. Kevin K. Ohlemiller received his B.S. in Biology from Indiana University in 1983 and Ph.D. in Neuroscience from Northwestern University in 1990 under the direction of Dr. Jonathan Siegel. He performed postdoctoral studies under Dr. Nobuo Suga of Washington University in St. Louis, Missouri, from 1990 to 1993, then joined the research staff of the Central Institute for the Deaf, also in St. Louis. Dr. Ohlemiller joined the faculty of Washington University Medical

School in 2003 and is presently a Research Associate Professor in the Department of Otolaryngology and a member of the faculty of the Washington University Program in Audiology and Communication Sciences. Dr. Ohlemiller has taught basic hearing science to students in audiology and deaf education since 1995. He has authored more than 50 articles and book chapters on topics covering basic cochlear function, neuroethology of the central auditory system, genetic hearing and vision loss, noise-induced hearing loss, and age-related hearing loss. He resides in Olivette, Missouri, with his wife, Melinda; his sons, Jacob and Dillon; four cats; and a lizard.

Acknowledgments

This book would not have been completed without the support of many people. The editors are particularly grateful to the contributors who accepted our invitation to participate by writing chapters for the book. All are accomplished scientists and physician-scientists who teach in educational programs, and their unique expertise has contributed significantly to the depth and quality of the information in the book.

Two other individuals were instrumental in moving the book from concept to reality. René Miller, our graduate program assistant, managed all the details of the preparation, obtaining permissions, editing text, working with the publisher, and serving as the central clearinghouse for the project. This was an "extra" responsibility for René, and we greatly appreciate her support and assistance. Juliet Steiner, Product Manager at Thomson Learning was amazing. Her interest, her dedication and perseverance, and, most importantly, her unwavering enthusiasm for the project kept the editors motivated during challenging times. The editors offer our sincere thanks to Juliet for all her support.

Finally, Kevin Ohlemiller extends his heartfelt thanks to his wife, Melinda, and sons, Jacob and Dillon, for their patience and encouragement during the writing and editing of this book. Bill Clark offers his personal thanks to his wife, Chris, fellow educator and Director of the Family Center at the Central Institute for the Deaf, for her continued support and for always reminding him that there is a person on the other end of every experiment. He is also grateful for having the opportunity to work with and learn from Hallowell Davis and Ira Hirsh during his career at the Central Institute for the Deaf. It was an honor for him to become friends with these two great men, and this book is dedicated to their legacy.

Contributors

Barbara A. Bohne, Ph.D.
Professor of Otolaryngology
Washington University School of Medicine
St. Louis, Missouri

J. David Dickman, Ph.D.
Professor of Neurobiology
Washington University School of Medicine
St. Louis, Missouri

Brian T. Faddis, Ph.D.
Assistant Professor of Otolaryngology
Washington University School of Medicine
St. Louis, Missouri

Asim Haque, Ph.D.
Washington University School of Medicine
St. Louis, Missouri
University of Mississippi School of Medicine
Jackson, Mississippi

Gary W. Harding, M.S.E.
Associate Professor of Otolaryngology
Washington University School of Medicine
St. Louis, Missouri

Leonard P. Rybak, M.D., Ph.D.
Professor of Surgery
Division of Otolaryngology
Southern Illinois University School of Medicine
Springfield, Illinois

Dwayne D. Simmons, Ph.D.
Associate Professor of Otolaryngology
Washington University School of Medicine
St. Louis, Missouri

Mark E. Warchol, Ph.D.
Professor of Otolaryngology
Washington University School of Medicine
St. Louis, Missouri

Part

I

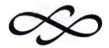

Foundation

Chapter

1

Introduction

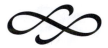

Dwayne D. Simmons, Ph.D.
Associate Professor of Otolaryngology
Washington University School of Medicine
St. Louis, Missouri

William W. Clark, Ph.D.
Director, Program in Audiology and Communication Sciences
Washington University School of Medicine
St. Louis, Missouri

Audiology is a branch of science that is devoted to the study of hearing and balance and their disorders. Although other health care providers, including physicians, occupational and physical therapists, speech-language pathologists, and counselors, may assess, diagnose, treat, and rehabilitate individuals with hearing- and balance-related problems and disabilities, the audiologist is the primary practitioner who assesses the nature and extent of the disorder and recommends treatment options. Audiologists are licensed professionals who have received clinical and educational training to allow them to conduct diagnostic testing, fit assistive devices, including hearing aids and cochlear implants, provide rehabilitative and counseling services, conduct intraoperative neurophysiologic monitoring, and dispense hearing aids.

The term *audiology* was coined at the end of World War II and was intended to describe newly established aural rehabilitation programs for soldiers returning from battle with hearing deficits (Canfield, 1949). According to Davis (1991), the practitioners of this new field were psychologists, physiologists, and otologists with special knowledge about hearing and hearing disorders. The term was suggested because the military had referred to their efforts as "auricular training," which implied teaching soldiers to wiggle their ears! Davis and his colleagues believed that the term *aural rehabilitation* was too narrow, so they settled on *audiology* despite its derivation from Greek and Latin roots. The term was intended to represent the basic and applied science foundation of the profession that comprised the disciplines of psychology, physiology, and acoustics, as well as the delivery of state-of-the art clinical care for patients and clients.

The profession has grown significantly since those early beginnings. There were approximately 1,500 audiologists in the United States in 1969 (Katz, 1978). These professionals received their academic and clinical training in master's degree graduate programs. Currently, the Bureau of Labor Statistics estimates there are approximately 10,000 jobs for audiologists in the United States (Bureau of Labor Statistics, 2006). More than half of these individuals work in medical settings, including physicians' or other healthcare practitioners' offices, in hospitals, or in outpatient health centers. Others work in educational settings or private practice. Over the same period, the scope of practice of audiology has grown even more, creating increasing pressure on academic programs to expand their curriculum. The result has been the transition of the entry-level degree requirement to a doctoral degree, the **Au.D.,** which is now offered by more than 70 programs in the United States (American Speech-Language-Hearing Association [ASHA], 2006a).

Another outcome of this growth has been a shift in emphasis away from basic sciences and toward clinical practice. This shift is largely due to the expansion of the clinical scope of practice in audiology and a growing shortage in the ranks of faculty with basic and applied science backgrounds teaching in Au.D. programs.

The expansion of the scope of practice of the field has been impressive. A popular textbook used in audiology programs in the late 1960s and early 1970s was the second edition of *Audiology,* by Hayes Newby (Newby, 1964). The well-informed audiologist of that era was required to know about air- and bone-conduction hearing testing, about basic speech tests and masking, and about some special tests, such as the Stenger or Doerfler–Stewart tests for malingering, and tests for loudness recruitment, the SISI (short increment sensitivity index) and the ABLB (alternate binaural loudness balance test). The section of *Audiology* devoted to testing the hearing of infants and toddlers emphasized observing the child's behavior and using some play audiometry techniques for toddlers. At the time, audiologists did not prescribe, fit, or sell hearing aids; as a result, audiology programs emphasized diagnostics and rehabilitation exclusively.

Although the book was excellent and widely used in its day, consider just a short list of the knowledge and skills required of the audiologist of today that were not covered in the 1964 textbook. There was no mention of objective tests, such as acoustic reflex measures or tympanometry, both based on physiologic measures of middle ear impedance. This is not surprising, because clinical development of acoustic immittance measures did not occur until the 1970s. Otoacoustic emissions were not covered because they were not discovered until the late 1970s (Kemp, 1978), although they had been predicted since the

1940s (Gold, 1948). Similarly, although electrophysiologic measures of brain activity (e.g., electroencephalogram [EEG]) had been developed, specialized versions appropriate for assessing the auditory system, such as the auditory brainstem response (ABR), were not available to audiologists of the 1960s. Arguably, the two biggest technologic developments for treating patients with impaired hearing, cochlear implants and digital hearing aids, had yet to be invented. And if they had been available, they may have fallen into the domain of the hearing aid dispenser, rather than the audiologist. Finally, tests of balance and balance disorders have only recently been included in the scope of practice for audiologists.

Given the rather dramatic expansion of the practice of audiology, it is not surprising that graduate education programs are placing enhanced emphasis on the clinical training of audiologists, and consequently finding less time to address the basic and applied scientific foundations of the profession. An additional pressure is the "graying" of the ranks of Ph.D.-trained scientists among the faculty of training programs, and a shortage of younger scientists to replace them, further challenging the future of the profession. Both professional organizations that represent audiologists, the American Speech-Language-Hearing Association (ASHA) and the American Academy of Audiology, have responded to the challenge by implementing plans and initiatives to preserve and enhance the science bases of the profession (ASHA, 2006b).

The contributing authors of this textbook are all scientists and physician-scientists who teach in clinical programs; they collectively believe in the value of the basic sciences in clinical audiology and offer their work in this book as a foundation for future clinicians.

WHY DOES AN AUDIOLOGY STUDENT NEED TO KNOW ABOUT THE ANATOMY AND PHYSIOLOGY OF HEARING?

If this were a class discussion, one might anticipate a question of this type: "Why does an audiologist need to know so much about the anatomy and physiology of hearing? Isn't it sufficient to be able to conduct and interpret the tests we do, and explain them to patients?"

An obvious response is that you cannot understand any clinical test only by knowing how to give it and score it. Sound interpretation of the results requires an understanding of the underlying principles that contribute to your findings. Simply stated, this is the "professional" part of audiology, as opposed to the "technical" part. A technician can be trained to administer nearly all the tests used by audiologists, but integrating them into a clinical evaluation and providing recommendations for rehabilitation requires far more knowledge and skills.

Furthermore, a clear understanding of the scientific foundation for the practice is a necessary prerequisite for developing new and better tests for assessment and rehabilitation. If our expertise was limited to getting better and better at the tests already in practice, we'd still be doing the SISI and ABLB tests taught in the 1970s! The expansion of the scope of practice is directly related to new knowledge and understanding created by scientific study of hearing and balance that has occurred with the growth of the profession. The incredible advances in cochlear implant technology and in digital signal processing for hearing aids would not have happened without a partnership between clinicians and scientists, both with separate expertise, but focused on using the science to develop better tools for assessment and rehabilitation. And although the scientists have extensive skills related to their own field of interest, they need the input of clinicians to help them convert their laboratory or "bench" work to clinical practice.

The process of converting bench science to clinical practice has been called **translational research,** and it has been targeted by the National Institutes of Health (NIH) as a priority (NIH, 2006). Part of the rationale for supporting this kind of partnership is an understanding that the process is bidirectional; that is, it is a two-way street. As scientists develop new findings and tools, the clinicians explore ways to implement the knowledge at the patient's bedside. Their experiences then guide the bench scientists' work to better develop useful interventions. The success of translational research depends on good communication between the scientist and clinician, and the best way to guarantee that communication is to educate the scientist about clinical practice and the audiologist about basic science. Armed with a shared knowledge base, the partnership can be used to develop new tools effectively. One of the goals in writing this book was to improve the shared knowledge base for such a partnership.

The audience for this book is primarily in the early stages of an audiology training program. If you are an audiology student, you probably have already heard that today's modern digital hearing aid is a sophisticated instrument. One of the features of many digital hearing aids is called **wide dynamic range compression (WDRC).** WDRC algorithms apply more amplification or gain to soft sounds and less or no gain to loud sounds. Some instruments allow dividing the spectrum into channels and applying differential amounts of compression through each channel, a feature particularly useful to patients with steeply sloping audiograms.

Why do patients need WDRC in their hearing aids? A basic and correct answer is that individuals with sensorineural hearing losses often have difficulty perceiving soft sounds, but louder sounds present less difficulty, and in some cases, very loud sounds are more bothersome to the individual with a sensorineural hearing loss than a patient with normal hearing. This phenomenon is called **loudness recruitment,** and the hearing aid technology is designed to capture the wide dynamic range of sounds in the environment and to "compress" them into a range that fits the patient's reduced dynamic range, by amplifying very soft sounds more than mid-level or loud ones.

This response is a clinical explanation. We learned what the patient could not do and devised a treatment strategy designed to overcome the patient's loss. In this example, the strategy is effective, and WDRC is a useful component of today's hearing aid. But more can be learned by asking additional basic questions about the patient's hearing problems. Why does he/she have difficulty hearing soft sounds? How can loud sounds be even louder in the damaged ear than in the normal ear? How does the normal ear handle incoming sound over such a large range of in-

tensities or pressures that can be as much as 140 decibels (dB)? And finally, what is wrong with the patient's ear that prevents it from functioning normally?

An understanding of the basic anatomy and physiology of normal hearing can help us understand both the patient's problem and the goal of the technology used in intervention (i.e., the WDRC aid). Therefore, a logical first question is: How does the normal inner ear hear over such a large dynamic range? After you finish studying this book, you will know that the "main" sensory receptor for hearing is the inner hair cell (IHC). All the other cell types in the inner ear are members of the "supporting cast"; although they are important for maintaining the energy for transduction, for providing the chemical and molecular stimuli for hearing, only the IHCs appear to be the sensory transducers.

Unfortunately, the IHC has a fundamental problem: it can respond electrically over a range of only about 60 dB. Practically, then, if we were hearing only with our IHCs, we would not hear any sounds softer than about 30 to 40 dB sound pressure level (SPL), and our ears would be saturated by any sounds louder than about 90 to 100 dB SPL. This is shown schematically in the middle panel of Figure 1–1. So how is the dynamic range problem solved by the inner ear? The answer is that the mammalian inner ear uses WDRC itself. The active movement of outer hair cells (OHCs), recordable as otoacoustic emissions, provides about 30 dB of gain for very low level signals that are not strong enough to excite the IHCs directly. This amplification process has been called the **cochlear amplifier,** and the movement added by the OHC activity raises the input to the IHCs to a sufficient level to excite them. Greater than about 30 dB SPL, the mechanical response of the basilar membrane, driven directly by energy incoming sound wave, swamps the active process, and the response is more linear. At high levels, two different mechanisms serve to limit input to the IHCs. The **acoustic reflex,** activated by sound input and mediated through the 5th and 7th cranial nerves, causes contraction of the **stapedius** and **tensor tympani muscles** of the middle ear, which alters its impedance and reduces sound transmission by up to 20 dB for intense sound input. A second inhibitory mecha-

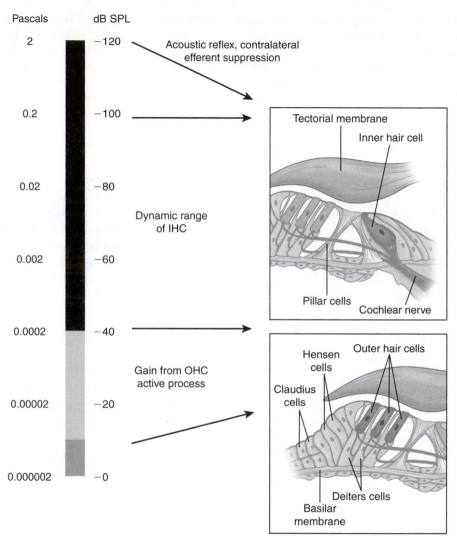

FIGURE 1-1 Cartoon showing physiologic mechanisms involved in compressing the 120-dB range of hearing into the 60-dB range of sensitivity of the inner hair cells. Low-level signals are amplified by the outer hair cell (OHCs) active motility, increasing the level of the input signal by up to 30 dB. The inner hair cell (IHC) is stimulated mechanically by the energy from external sounds louder than about 30 to 40 dB sound pressure level (SPL), but its electrical response saturates at about 100 dB SPL. At very high input sound levels, the acoustic reflex and the efferent system limit input to the IHCs. All values are approximate.

nism is mediated by the efferent pathways. These are also activated by sound input, and they inhibit both the cochlear amplifier and the response of the IHCs by different mechanisms. Stated simply, the efferent pathways can serve as a "volume" control on the IHC-OHC complex, allowing the cochlear ampli-

fier to operate at full volume for low-level inputs, but turning it down or off at higher levels, and to inhibit the IHCs at levels where their output is saturated.

In other words, the normal ear is also a wide dynamic range compressor. When a patient has a sensorineural hearing loss, he or she loses some of the ability to hear wide dynamic range compress sounds, and the hearing aid that can restore this process is more successful and tolerated by the patient. In fact, armed with knowledge about normal physiology, as an audiology student, you could predict that a patient with nonfunctional OHCs would have a hearing loss of up to about 30 dB. At levels greater than 30 dB, hearing would depend on the functional integrity of the IHCs, but if they were still working, the patient would respond rather normally. At high levels of input, however, both the acoustic reflex threshold and the efferent pathways might be affected because they are both driven by afferent input from the IHCs, and this might be damaged. Accordingly, you would predict that a patient with a sensorineural hearing loss, compared with normal hearing, would have a reduced dynamic range, would not be able to hear soft sounds, but would hear progressively louder sound closer to "natural," and in some cases, would report very high level sounds as louder than normal. This is precisely what is seen clinically. Some patients with recruiting ears do show abnormal sensitivity to loud sounds, and this has been called **hyper-recruitment.**

The point of this exercise is to demonstrate the inter-relations between the clinical presentation of hearing disorders and the underlying principles explaining their bases and approaches to rehabilitating them. By understanding the foundations, the audiologist can better assess hearing problems, apply the appropriate rehabilitative strategies, and develop new methods for evaluating and treating individuals afflicted with hearing or balance problems. This book provides some of that foundation.

WHO BENEFITS FROM THIS TECHNOLOGY?

Biomedical, behavioral, and clinical sciences have made astounding leaps forward since the late 1990s alone, making this an exciting time for anyone embarking on a health-related career. Because of advances in technology and research, health-care professionals have an amazing repertoire of tools at their disposal. The knowledge gained through applied and basic research also makes possible an unprecedented level of clinical service and care. For the audiologist and those interested in hearing, balance, and communication disorders, there has been an explosion in knowledge about the biology of the ear, as well as human communication. In addition, the technologies used to test and treat hearing loss have expanded greatly. Although hearing impairment and deafness can occur at any age, increasingly the focus of audiologic assessment and care is split between very young or more senior populations. We now know that it is important to detect hearing loss as early as possible so that a child can develop appropriate communication and learning skills. Universal screening of newborn babies is now the norm in most states. Universal screening involves a simple, painless hearing test given to all infants to determine whether they can hear sound. Without newborn hearing screening, hearing losses might not be noticed until the child begins to have difficulties speaking and learning. At the other end of the spectrum, an aging population with most people living longer, more active lives has presented particular challenges for all health-care professions and, in particular, has created a demand for highly trained audiologists. New technologies such as digital hearing aids and cochlear implants, as well as aural rehabilitation programs are helping more and more people to live normal and active lives well into their seventh, eighth, and ninth decades. Given such a rich environment and integration of knowledge, it is essential that students of audiology are familiar with the development, anatomy, physiology, and pathology of the auditory and vestibular systems, as well as the evaluation, rehabilitation, and psychology of hearing and balance. This textbook provides the basic science foundation of hearing for students of audiology and provides a balance between depth of coverage and understandability for the student without a strong science background.

PART I: FOUNDATION

This book focuses on a basic understanding of hearing and begins appropriately with topics that are the foundation to any consideration of the auditory system. A key to understanding the anatomy and physiology of the auditory system begins with a basic knowledge about sound, acoustics, and how sounds are processed. Chapters 2 and 3 deal with understanding the physics of sound production, transmission, and absorption by the ear. We begin with descriptions of the physical bases of sound, including discussions about sound measurement, propagation and absorption, hearing sensitivity, and classes of sounds. Audiologists also need to have an understanding of the basic characteristics of filters and spectral processing, the nature of sound transmission through the ear, and how that limits or explains normal hearing sensitivity. Consideration is given to how sound transmission changes through an earplug, a hearing aid, a conductive hearing loss, or a cochlear implant. To close our discussion on foundations, we move from physical and engineering concepts to fundamental biological concepts of the auditory system. We give you a basic understanding of cellular and subcellular anatomy and physiology of the cell and some of its basic functions to help you appreciate how the ear works and how disease processes affect hearing. We also give a general overview of the structure and function of nerve cells and provide a foundation for the more comprehensive information about the auditory nervous system found in later chapters.

PART II: ANATOMY AND PHYSIOLOGY

Part II of this textbook introduces the anatomy and physiology of auditory system. These chapters start by exploring the structural, developmental, and physiologic complexity of the peripheral portions of the organ of hearing and conclude with details on the central nervous system (CNS) and the vestibular system. The anatomic relations of the peripheral auditory system are shown in Figure 1-2.

The outer and middle ears develop to enhance the collection of auditory signals before they reach the inner ear, where the sensory organs are located. No other sensory system, except perhaps the eye, has adapted such an intricate mechanism to ensure that proper perceptual information is extracted

from a stimulus. The inner ear is divided into distinct auditory and vestibular organs (see Figure 1-1). The cochlea contains the sensory cells responsible for converting mechanical waves into electrical activity that is transmitted to the brain and perceived as sound. The development of the ear is one of the more remarkable examples of engineering in the vertebrate body. In the fetus, the ear starts to function as the auditory system matures, and by birth, it is fully capable of analyzing sounds in the environment. From these elementary considerations of the peripheral auditory system, we introduce a series of chapters that explore the mechanics and neurobiology of cochlear function in more detail. We begin with descriptions of the classical view of mechanical tuning of the basilar membrane and then consider recent theories about how active processes sharpen mechanical tuning. The frequency tuning of the healthy basilar membrane is sufficiently sharp to account for normal perceptual ability to distinguish between sound frequencies. Therefore, cochlear hair cells need to retain this sharpness of tuning in transmitting excitation to afferent neurons. Although afferent neurons only transmit stimulus information passed on by hair cells, they also "re-encode" the stimulus in a way that virtually replaces the original stimulus waveform. One of our major goals in the chapters in Part II is to show the similarities in the shape of input-output curves of the basilar membrane, IHCs, and afferent fibers. Unfortunately, hearing usually occurs in a noisy environment. Afferent fiber responses are less well distinguished in noise, thus making hearing more difficult. Current studies of the efferent olivocochlear system are clarifying how the efferent system works to adapt the afferent system to background noise and provides protection to the ear from exposures to loud sounds. Related to efferent fiber function is also the discovery of audiofrequency sounds or echoes in response to sounds and, in some cases, spontaneously as well. We know that metabolic energy is required for the generation of echoes called *otoacoustic emissions.* These emissions provide evidence for the presence of an active amplification mecha-

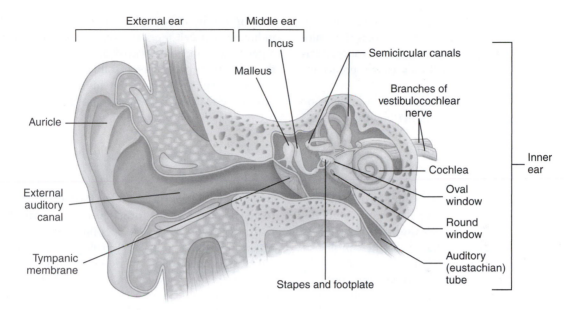

FIGURE 1-2 Anatomy of the ear.

nism within the inner ear and can be used to test the robustness of the efferent system. We conclude this section on anatomy and physiology with a consideration of human brain, the auditory CNS, and the vestibular system. Our brains analyze and store information about the external and internal environment and guide our behavior. We hope you will come to understand that a combination of anatomic, functional, and developmental views is necessary to understand the way the brain and especially the auditory CNS work, as well as some of the pathologies that you will see as audiologists and educators. We also provide greater detail on how the auditory CNS encodes and represents the spectral and temporal aspects of sounds, as well as the location of their source.

PART III: PATHOLOGY OF HEARING

Permanent loss of sensory cells is manifested as a sensorineural hearing loss. The third and final part of the book concerns how sensory cells of the inner ear can be destroyed by excessive exposure to

noise, certain drugs, infections in the inner ear, genetic mutations, and aging. We discuss not only some ear-related symptoms and descriptions of ear diseases, but some recent advances in our understanding of the mechanisms behind these disease processes. At one time or another, nearly everyone has experienced a hearing loss caused by excessive noise exposure. Ototoxicity is the capacity of a drug or chemical agent to cause damage to the structure, function, or both of the inner ear. Many agents can cause ototoxicity. These compounds may affect hearing, balance, or a combination of both. About half of congenital (present at birth) hearing loss results from genetic mutations. If impaired hearing is not due to drugs or noise, then it is likely caused by some hereditary mechanism. An unknown proportion of adult-onset hearing loss has an explicitly genetic cause, or is strongly influenced by genetics. The ongoing revolution in molecular techniques and genetic manipulation virtually guarantees that audiologists will take part in discussions centered on diagnosing, managing, and eventually treating hearing loss associated with specific genetic defects. A combination of genetic and environmental factors, age-related hearing loss, or presbycusis, is the major form of hearing loss and the major neurodegenerative disease of aging. It will increasingly preoccupy most audiologists.

We conclude this final section with a discussion of future therapies that may either prevent or "cure" hearing loss by rescuing hair cells after injury or by inducing hair cell regeneration. Studies of hair cell regeneration in nonmammalian species have raised the hope that it might be possible to induce similar forms of regeneration in the human ear. For this goal to be realized, however, we need to understand the basic biology of the regenerative process.

⤳ SUMMARY ⤳

Clinical audiologists need a sound understanding of the basic and applied scientific principles underlying the tests and assessments they use every day to treat patients with hearing or balance problems. Their expertise not only helps the patients who benefit from their clinical intervention, but also helps basic scientists design experiments that can ultimately lead to treatment, cure, or prevention of illnesses, injuries, and diseases that affect the more than 30 million people in the United States who have significant hearing or balance problems. This synergistic interaction between discovery and treatment depends on scientists learning about how their endeavors can help people with impaired function and on clinicians learning from their patients what treatments work, what treatments do not work, and what treatments are needed to mediate the effects of hearing or balance problems. The audiologist plays a key role in carrying treatments from bench to practice, and this book is intended to provide some of the tools necessary for the journey.

⤳ KEY TERMS ⤳

Acoustic reflex
Au.D.
Audiology

Cochlear amplifier
Hyper-recruitment
Loudness recruitment

Stapedius muscle
Tensor tympani muscle
Translational research

Wide dynamic range compression

⤳ STUDY QUESTIONS ⤳

1. What is an audiologist and what does an audiologist do?

2. Why does an audiologist need a sound background in the basic and applied sciences?

3. What is meant by the term *translational research*? How is it relevant to audiology?

4. Identify two ways the normal ear can expand the dynamic range of hearing.

5. Name three areas of the scope of practice of audiology that have been introduced since the early 1970s.

⚘REFERENCES⚘

American Speech-Language-Hearing Association [ASHA]. (2006a). *Guide to graduate programs.* Retrieved October 22, 2006, from http://www.asha.org/gradguide.

ASHA. (2006b). *Focused initiative on the critical shortage of doctoral students.* Retrieved October 22, 2006, from http://www.asha.org/about/leadership-projects/national-office/focused-initiatives/04-archive/doctoral04.htm

Bureau of Labor Statistics, U.S. Department of Labor. (2006). *Occupational outlook handbook, 2006-07 edition: Audiologists.* Retrieved October 22, 2006, from http://www.bls.gov/oco/ocos085.htm.

Canfield, N. (1949). *Audiology, the science of hearing, a developing professional specialty.* Springfield, IL: C.C. Thomas.

Davis, H. (1991). *The professional memoirs of Hallowell Davis.* St. Louis, MO: The Central Institute for the Deaf.

Gold, T. (1948). Hearing II. The physical basis of the action of the cochlea. *Proceedings of the Royal Society of Britain, 135,* 492–498.

Katz, J. (1978). *Handbook of clinical audiology.* Baltimore: Williams & Wilkins.

Kemp, D. T. (1978). Stimulated acoustic emissions from within the human auditory system. *Journal of the Acoustical Society of America, 64,* 1386–1391.

Newby, H. (1964). *Audiology* (2nd ed.). New York: Meredith Publishing Company.

National Institutes of Health. (2006). *National Institutes of Health roadmap.* Retrieved October 22, 2006, from http://nihroadmap.nih.gov/clinicalresearch/overview-translational.asp.

Chapter

Basic Acoustics and Noise

William W. Clark, Ph.D.
Director, Program in Audiology
and Communication Sciences
Washington University School of Medicine
St. Louis, Missouri

Akey to understanding the anatomy and physiology of the auditory system for audiologists and other related professionals is a basic knowledge about sound and its engineering cousin, acoustics. After all, the primary function of the auditory system for mammals is to serve as a receptor for sound. Although it is true that the large pinnae of some mammals such as rabbits and elephants serve as temperature regulators, the primary function of these appendages is to funnel sound into the ear canal. You will learn in other chapters about how the auditory system converts acoustic, or mechanical, energy into electrical signals that are decoded by the brain. However, before the signal becomes electrical, every step in the process—from production of the sound, its transmission through air or other media to the ear, and the effects of the pinna, the outer and middle ears, and the mechanical response of the inner ear—is a mechanical, physical, acoustic response. To understand how the ear processes sounds, we need to understand the physics of sound production, transmission, and absorption by the ear. This chapter provides descriptions of the physical bases of sound in non-engineering terms. We start with a definition, then follow with discussions about sound measurement, propagation and absorption, hearing sensitivity, and finally, we consider a special class of sounds: noise. This chapter presents material at an introductory level, and it is designed specifically to provide a foundation for understanding principles described in later chapters. Acquisition of more comprehensive information about the important role of acoustics in audiology can be obtained from other program coursework, or from the texts listed at the end of the chapter.

A WORLD OF SOUND

What is sound? **Sound** is defined acoustically as a particle disturbance in an elastic medium, which is propagated through the medium. For a sound to occur, a medium must have density and elasticity. Although sound can occur in any medium with those characteristics, including most solids, liquids, and gasses, we usually think about sound transmission in "our" medium, air. Air is composed of particles (air molecules) that have weight and elasticity. In fact, one cubic meter (m^3) of air weighs about 1.3 kilograms (kg), and it is quite elastic; that is, it can easily be compressed into a volume much smaller than 1 m^3. This is a useful fact for scuba divers who can squeeze 1 hour's worth of breathing air (about 1,500 L) in a 20-L tank.

The information provided earlier allows us to answer one of the questions all of us were asked in elementary school: If a tree falls in the forest and no one is there to hear it, does it make a sound? The answer, from an acoustic point of view, is a *resounding* "YES!" But audiologists, speech pathologists, teachers, and other professionals are concerned about the sense of hearing; that is, the perception of an acoustic event by a human listener. Adding a perceptual requirement to the definition then produces another definition: "Sound is a compression wave propagated through a medium that is capable of producing a sensation in the human ear" (Albers, 1970). Now, when the tree question is asked again, the answer is "NO."

This discussion highlights an important distinction between two different ways of considering sound. Engineers and scientists are concerned with sound as energy that can be measured and quantified; no consideration is usually given to whether the sound can be perceived by human listeners. However, hearing health professionals are usually concerned about the *effects* of sound on humans: what and how we hear, what sounds please us, what sounds annoy us, what sounds interfere with our ability to communicate with each other, and what sounds can be damaging to our hearing. These definitions are necessarily more complex than "simple" quantitative descriptions of acoustic energy, and they often are expressed in perceptual terms such as *loudness* or *pitch*.

MEASUREMENT OF SOUND

A general description of a sound should include a description of *what* the sound is, and *how much* of it is present. A **metathetic continuum** is used to describe the "what" quantity, and a **prothetic continuum** is used to describe the "how much" quantity. In acoustics and audiology, **frequency** of the sound is the metathetic variable, and the **(acoustic) intensity** or **sound pressure level (SPL)** of the sound is the prothetic variable.

First, let us consider frequency. *Frequency* is defined as the number of periodic repetitions of a sound in 1 second, that is, the number of cycles per second of that sound. By convention, the term *Hertz,* or Hz, is used to label the frequency of a sound. A sound of 1,000 Hz contains 1,000 cycles in 1 second. Similarly, a sound of 20 Hz repeats 20 times per second. As the frequency of a sound changes from "low" to "high," the perception associated with frequency (known as the pitch) also changes from "low" to "high." Note that the perceptual attribute, the pitch, does not get *bigger* as the frequency goes from low to high; it simply *changes* from one attribute, low pitch, to a different attribute, high pitch. This is what is meant by a metathetic continuum. The frequency of a sound is determined by the characteristics of the sound source. A tuba and a piccolo produce different frequency sounds because they differ in size.

The second dimension is the "how much" dimension. By this, we are referring to the amount of energy present in the sound, expressed commonly as its intensity. In acoustics, energy or *intensity* is defined as the acoustic power flowing through a unit of area, and the units of measurement are watts per meter squared (W/m^2). In practice, engineers usually measure the pressure variations produced by the acoustic power in units of Newtons per meter squared (N/m^2), or other equivalent measures expressed in dynes or Pascals. These units are metric equivalents to a unit more familiar to us: pounds per square inch (psi). Therefore, the energy (or intensity) continuum is a prothetic continuum: As intensity increases, the perceptual attribute, the loudness of a sound, also increases; it is not different, there is just more of it.

Frequency and Period

As mentioned earlier, the frequency of a sound is the number of periodic oscillations per second (expressed in Hertz [Hz]). The **period** of a sound is

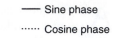
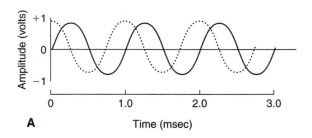
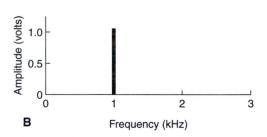

FIGURE 2-1   Sinusoid at 1 kHz in time (A) and frequency (B) domain.

defined as the amount of time required to complete one cycle, and it is the reciprocal of the frequency:

$$F = 1/P \text{ and } P = 1/F$$

Therefore, the period of a 1,000-Hz tone is 1 millisecond (0.001 second), and the frequency of a tone whose period is 0.05 second is 20 Hz. The relation between period and frequency of a sound can be seen easily in graphic form (Figure 2-1).

Figure 2-1 shows a single tone oscillating sinusoidally, shown in the time (see Figure 2-1A) and frequency domains (see Figure 2-1B). Using this simple illustration helps point out the different information available in each panel. From Figure 2-1A, one can observe that the period of the signal is 1.0 millisecond, and the maximum, or peak amplitude, is 1.0 volt (V). Given the reciprocal relation between period and frequency, this signal has a frequency of 1.0 kilohertz (kHz). Furthermore, because it is a single sinusoid, no energy is present at any other frequency. This is shown graphically in Fig-

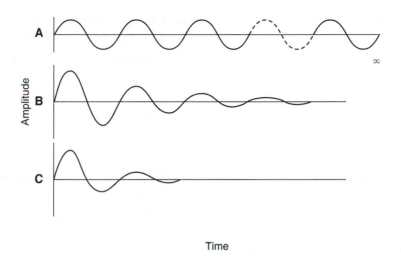

FIGURE 2-2 Damping of a sine wave. Undamped (A), moderately damped (B), highly damped (C).

ure 2-1B as a single line at 1.0 kHz, with an amplitude of 1.0 V. But there is more information in Figure 2-1A than is shown in Figure 2-1B. From Figure 2-1A, we can deduce that the amplitude of the sinusoid that has a frequency of 1.0 kHz has amplitude of 0 V at time = 0 millisecond. Thereafter, the signal "ebbs" and "flows" sinusoidally between the maximum and minimum amplitudes, and repeats one complete cycle every millisecond. However, because the axis of Figure 2-1B does not contain specific information about the amplitude in the time domain, identical plots for Figure 2-1B would be obtained regardless of whether the 1,000–Hz sinusoid started at time 0 with any amplitude (within the range of −1 to +1 volts, of course). The specific relation between the amplitude of the sine wave and the period is referred to as the **phase** of the signal. Phase is measured in degrees or radians. Recall a circle is 360 degrees, or 2 pi radians. For signal A (Figure 2-2), we would say it was in "sine phase," meaning its amplitude followed the sine of the amplitudes as the signal traveled through one complete cycle. In contrast, if we started measuring the signal when the amplitude was +1 V, at time = 0 millisecond (sine wave in dotted lines in Figure 2-2), it would have the same frequency and period, but its amplitude would be "displaced" from the original signal by 90 degrees, or

2 pi radians. Therefore, we would say that the phase shift of the latter signal was 90 degrees, or 2 pi radians, and, furthermore, that the signal "leads" the original signal.

Another important characteristic of sound propagation that is not shown in Figure 2-1 is **damping.** Damping is a reduction in amplitude with successive oscillations determined by the frictional resistance in a system. An example of damping exhibited by a tuning fork after it is struck is shown in Figure 2-2.

It can be seen that the amplitude of the oscillations exhibits a progressive reduction with time. Damping is caused by the internal friction of the tuning fork and the resistance of the air molecules. Common experience tells us that there is an inverse relation between the sharpness of tuning of a physical system and the amount of damping. Consider, for example, what happens if you use a mallet to strike an object that has low internal friction, such as a wind chime. You will hear a sharply tuned tone that continues to "ring" long after the impact. In contrast, if you strike a metal garbage can lid (which has high internal friction) with the same mallet, you will hear only a short-duration "thunk." In summary, the wind chime produces a sharply tuned "note" after being struck, but it does not follow the input (the hammer strike) well at all in the time domain, unless you "damp" the chime by grabbing it with your hand. In contrast, the garbage can lid follows the hammer strike well in the time domain, but produces a broadly tuned "thunk." Later in this textbook you will learn how the mammalian auditory system manages to preserve sounds in the time and frequency domains at the same time.

Speed of Sound

Although the frequency of a sound is dependent on the characteristics of the source, the **speed of sound** is dependent on the characteristics of the medium, namely, the elasticity, density, and temperature of the medium. Sound travels faster in water than in air because water has a higher density and it is much less compressible than air. The speed of sound is also faster at higher temperatures. In air, sound travels at approximately 340 m/sec (1,125 feet/sec) at a temperature of 72°F. We understand from common experience that some amount of time is required for sound to reach our ears. From the outfield bleachers, the crack of the bat is heard after the batter is observed hitting the ball. And traveling at about 0.2 mile/sec, we hear the sound of distant thunder some time after seeing the flash of lightning, the number of seconds telling us how far away the lightning struck (5 seconds = about 1 mile). In water at a temperature of 20°C, sound travels at a speed of approximately 4,850 feet/sec, or about 4 times faster than it does in air.

Wavelength

Knowledge about the speed of sound allows us to calculate the other important variable of sound: its **wavelength.** Wavelength, abbreviated by the Greek symbol lambda (λ), is the distance between two identical points on a periodic signal. It is equal to the speed divided by the frequency:

$$\lambda = C/F$$

At 340 m/sec, the wavelength of a 1,000-Hz tone is:

$$\frac{340 \text{ m}}{1,000 \text{ Hz}} = 0.034 \text{ m/cycle} = 13.4 \text{ inches/cycle}$$

TABLE 2-1   Relation between Frequency (in Hertz) and Wavelength (in Feet)

Frequency (Hz)	Wavelength
125	8'
250	4'
500	2'
1,000	1'
2,000	6"
4,000	3"
8,000	1.5"
16,000	0.75"

Considering that a 1,000-Hz tone has a wavelength of (about) 1 foot, wavelengths of other audible frequencies can easily be estimated by remembering that doubling the frequency causes the wavelength to decrease by half and halving the frequency increases the wavelength by a factor of 2. Using this rubric, Table 2-1 can be constructed.

Remember that these wavelengths apply only to sounds in air. Because wavelength is defined as the speed of sound divided by the frequency, the wavelengths in other solids, liquids, or gases are related to those in air by the ratio of their speeds of transmission. In water, the wavelength of a 1-kHz sound is about 4 feet.

HEARING SENSITIVITY
Frequency Domain

Humans cannot hear sounds of all frequencies. The range of human hearing extends from a low-frequency limit of about 20 Hz to a high-frequency limit of about 20 kHz for excellent, young ears. Signals less than 20 Hz are not perceived as sound, and sounds in this range are described as **infrasound.** If they are loud enough, sounds in the infrasonic range can be felt, rather than heard. Most of us are familiar with "boom box" automobiles. Equipped with powerful subwoofer speakers, the audio output includes significant infrasonic energy that adds a sense of feeling to the listening experience and can rattle the windows in neighboring cars and houses. It can be said that boom box automobiles add a new meaning to the phrase *touched by the music!*

Sounds with frequencies greater than 20 kHz are also not usually perceived, and these sounds are called **ultrasound.** Although ultrasonic signals are useful for cleaning jewelry, producing fetal images, and operating motion detectors, they cannot be perceived and, therefore, are not sounds by Albers's definition.

Intensity or Sound Pressure

The strength or power of a sound is described by its intensity, or the power per unit area the source imposes on the medium. A tuning fork, for example, does work as it vibrates and pushes air molecules back and forth. Each oscillation of the fork causes the air molecules next to it to be alternatively squeezed together and pulled apart. These "local pressure" disturbances are then propagated through the medium. Because it is much easier to measure pressure than intensity, sound level meters are designed to measure the atmospheric pressure variations caused by the sound, rather than the actual intensity of the sound.

The human ear is sensitive over a tremendous range of intensities. At threshold, a good, young, normal human can detect an acoustic intensity as weak as 10^{-12} W/m^2. That same young ear can be exposed to an intensity of 10^2 W/m^2 for a brief period without sustaining damage. The range from threshold to maximum tolerable level is called the *dynamic range* of the ear, and the ratio is 10^{14} : 1, that is, 100 thousand billion to 1. Expressed as a ratio of pressure variations, the range is 10^7 to 1.

These large pressure variations can best be understood by an analogy. Imagine a giant eardrum, which moves back and forth from its position of rest by 1 foot at threshold. How far would that eardrum move at the maximum tolerable level? When asked that question, most elementary school children respond with guesses of 100 to 500 feet; a few adventuresome souls may hazard a 1-mile estimate. However, the answer is 1,894 miles! An eardrum in St. Louis that moves back and forth 1 foot at threshold would move from St. Louis to San Francisco to New York to St. Louis for a very loud sound.

Because these large ratios were difficult to deal with, scientists and engineers invented a shorthand method to describe the strength of sound: the **decibel scale (dB).** A complete description of the derivation of the decibel scale is beyond the scope of this chapter. However, decibels are commonly used to express the SPL of a given sound and the ratio of intensities, or pressures, of two sounds to each other. Three characteristics of the decibel scale are relevant to the discussion:

1. The scale is logarithmic.

2. It requires a stated reference value.

3. Zero decibel does not mean there is no sound; rather, it means the measured quantity is equivalent to the reference value.

In hearing science, the decibel scale is referenced to the threshold of human hearing (10^{-12} W/m^2 for intensity and the equivalent pressure of 2×10^{-5} Pascals), and the strength of sound is referred to as the SPL in decibels. The formulas for decibels are given below for informational purposes only.

$$\text{Intensity level: dB IL} = 10 \log (I \text{ measured}/ I \text{ reference}),$$
$$\text{where } I \text{ reference} = 10^{-12} \text{ W/m}^2$$

$$\text{SPL} = 10 \log (P \text{ measured})^2/(P \text{ reference})^2,$$
$$\text{where } P \text{ reference} = 2 \times 10^{-5} \text{ Pascals}$$

In decibels, therefore, the range of human hearing extends from 0 dB SPL to about 140 dB SPL. A chart showing the decibel scale is provided in Table 2-2.

Table 2-2 presents the acoustic intensities (measured in W/m^2) and pressures (measured in N/m^2, or Pascals) that correspond to SPLs from -10 to 140 dB SPL. Note that a 20-dB increase in the sound level represents a 10-fold increase in the pressure and a 100-fold increase in intensity. This is because the intensity of a sound wave in a medium is proportional to the square of the pressure. An increase in intensity of 100-fold increases the pressure squared by 100; therefore, the pressure change is the square root of 100, or 10. This relation is confusing to many audiologists, and a good rule of thumb to remember is "A dB is a dB!" Thus, a 10-dB increase in intensity rep-

TABLE 2-2   Decibel Scale

Intensity (W/m²)	Decibels	Pressure (N/m²)
100	140	200
10	130	632
1	20	20
0.1	110	6.32
0.01	100	2.0
0.001	90	0.63
0.0001	80	0.2
0.00001	70	0.063
0.000001	60	0.02
0.0000001	50	0.0063
0.00000001	40	0.002
0.000000001	30	0.00063
0.0000000001	20	0.0002
0.00000000001	10	0.000063
0.000000000001	0	0.00002
0.0000000000001	−10	0.0000063

resents a 10-dB increase in pressure as well. You cannot "double the pressure" *and* "double the intensity" of a sound at the same time. If you double the pressure, you will "automatically" increase the intensity by fourfold (i.e., pressure squared).

A further complication of the decibel scale is that the measures as stated earlier give no consideration to whether a sound is audible to a human listener. An ultrasonic jewelry cleaner may produce 140 dB SPL at 30 kHz, but it would be inaudible. Therefore, sound level meters include a filter network that approximates the human response to sound at moderate intensities. This network is called the **A-weighted filter network,** and SPLs determined with the A-weighting network in place are noted as "sound pressure level, dBA."

SOUND PROPAGATION

Another area that requires our attention is determining what happens to a sound as it travels through the medium from a source to a receiver. In our case, the "receiver" is the ear, and the "medium" is air. We need to understand how sound travels in a medium, and what happens to it when it encounters objects that have different physical characteristics. Imagine for a moment that sound could travel only in straight lines, and that the walls of rooms could not reflect any sound. You would not be able to hear around corners! Experience tells us that sound does not travel in straight lines. If I walk out into the hall and speak to you, you most likely would still be able to hear me. The sound would be different, to be sure, but you could still hear it. Most likely, you would sense that the sound seemed "dull" or "muffled." This sensation is produced because not all sounds bend around objects equally. The amount of bending depends on the size of the object and the wavelength of the sound passing by. Consider the example mentioned here. Sounds with wavelengths that are longer than the opening of the doorway will bend around the corner; higher frequency sounds tend to be directional and will carry in a more straight-line fashion down the hall.

The principle that needs to be remembered is that when the wavelength of a sound is long with respect to the object, the sound wave tends to bend around it. Conversely, when the wavelength of a sound is short with respect to the dimensions of the object, the object casts a *sound shadow,* and the SPL is reduced behind the object. In many parts of the United States, busy roads that traverse residential neighborhoods are built with so-called noise berms, or barriers along the sides of the roadway. Similar types of barriers are commonly constructed near the ends of runways at commercial airports. Although popular, these barriers really do not work very well because the low-frequency sounds bend around the barrier. The major acoustic advantage provided by the berm is that sound has to travel a longer distance from the source to the receiver and is, therefore, at a lower SPL because it is farther away from the source. But what does this mean in a practical sense? We will refer back to this question later in this section.

Although audiologists are sometimes called on to consult or provide expertise concerning environmental acoustics, most of their work is done on a smaller scale, usually within arm's reach of the ear. So let us consider acoustic propagation near the human

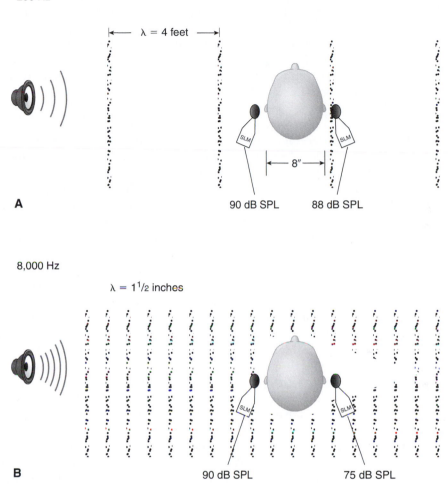

250 Hz

λ = 4 feet

8"

A

90 dB SPL   88 dB SPL

8,000 Hz

λ = 1^1/$_2$ inches

B

90 dB SPL   75 dB SPL

FIGURE 2-3   Head in a sound field at 250 Hz (A) and 8,000 Hz (B).

head. Because we're hard-headed creatures, our heads have density and elasticity that differs considerably from that of air. The average human head has a diameter of about 8 inches. Now, remembering our rule of wavelengths, we can see that signals with frequencies greater than 2 kHz have wavelengths that are smaller than the head; signals less than 1,000 Hz have wavelengths longer than the diameter of the head. Therefore, low-frequency signals bend around the head, but the head casts an appreciable signal for signals of high frequencies. Figure 2-3 shows the results of an experiment that you can easily conduct, assuming you have an anechoic chamber!

The experiment in Figure 2-3 is performed as follows: Place an average human head in a sound field with no significant reflections and position a loudspeaker directly opposite one ear. Play pure tone signals from the loudspeaker and measure the SPL at the ear pointing toward the loudspeaker and the ear pointing away from the loudspeaker. At 250 Hz (see Figure 2-3A), you observe that the SPL is about 90 dB SPL at the closer ear, and about 88 dB SPL at the ear within the head shadow. Even though the farther ear is completely within the shadow of the head, the sound is nearly the same because the long wavelength of the 250-Hz signal bends around the head. Now repeat the experiment but use a signal of 8 kHz (see Figure 2–3B). Now you observe that the SPL is still 90 dB at the nearer ear, but sound level at the farther ear is only about 73 dB SPL. This is because the wavelength of the 8-kHz signal is small in comparison with the head diameter, and the head casts an appreciable shadow on the acoustic signal. The "take home" message here is that even if the sound comes from only one direction in a sound field, the sound level at the two ears is approximately the same for low-frequency sounds. In more typical environments that include reflective surfaces, the differences between the two ears are usually even smaller. In the high frequencies, it is possible to get interaural differences of up to about 17 dB, but it is impossible for one ear to receive more than about 17 dB more sound than the other ear in field conditions.

The preceding examples point out one of the four scenarios that can happen to a sound when it encounters a barrier: It can be *diffracted*. The other things that can happen are: It can be absorbed, reflected, or transmitted. An easy way to remember these four characteristics is to consider that sound **DARTs** around: It is diffracted, absorbed, reflected, or transmitted. We have already discussed diffraction. Now let us consider the other three scenarios.

Absorption occurs when the vibratory energy in a signal is lost from the system in the form of heat. Acoustic ceiling panels are a good example of a "sound absorber"; they actually trap the sound within the panel, and because the fibers are soft and not elastic, their friction serves to absorb some of the incoming sound and convert the movement into heat. When sound travels in any medium, including air, a little of the energy is absorbed, but the panels do a much better job than air.

Reflection and its complement, transmission, occur when sound travels from one medium to another with different physical (and acoustic) characteristics. A good example is the transmission of sound from air into seawater. In the ear, the cochlea is filled with endolymph and perilymph, fluids that have similar densities and elasticities as seawater. When sound travels from one medium to another,

the amount of energy transmitted is dependent on the ratio of the **characteristic impedances** of the media. The characteristic impedance represents the density and elasticity of each of the media. If the term r represents the ratio of these quantities in two media, the fraction of the energy transmitted is represented by:

$$T = 4r/(r + 1)^2$$

and the energy reflected is represented by the remainder, $1 - T$. It can be seen from the formula that transmission is perfect if the specific acoustic resistances of the media are the same. If, however, the properties of the two media are significantly different, then r becomes large and T becomes very small. In this case, the barrier between the media acts like a "sound mirror," and most of the incident energy is reflected. In the case of air and seawater, 99.9% of the incident sound energy striking the interface between air and seawater is reflected; only 0.1% is transmitted. Remembering the rules for decibels stated earlier, if only 1/1,000 of the energy is transmitted, the loss in decibels is 10 times the logarithm of 0.001, or 30 dB. This presents a particular problem for human hearing. Chapter 7 describes how the middle ear serves as an "impedance matching transformer" to help overcome the disadvantage posed to the auditory system that "hears" sounds in air but "processes" them in fluids.

In fact, the characteristics of sound-encountering barriers are central to all our discussions about the anatomy and physiology of hearing. The pinna "funnels" sound into the ear canal because its acoustic impedance differs from air. The ear canal acts like an acoustic resonator (see discussion in Chapter 3) and "funnels" energy to the tympanic membrane. The middle ear is a mechanical structure with its own characteristics—mass and elasticity—that determine its mechanical response to acoustic input. And finally, the cochlea itself is a finely tuned mechanical analyzer that behaves in ways dictated by the laws of (acoustic) physics. The physical attributes of each of these mechanical structures are covered in other chapters in this textbook. Additional information about complex signals and filters is provided in Chapter 3.

Finally, we need to consider how the strength of a sound decreases as one moves away from the source. It should come as no surprise that if you move your ear farther away from the source of a sound, the SPL decreases. You can talk quietly to a colleague if he or she is close to you, but you will need to raise your voice if they are 200 feet away. This is because the source power, measured in watts, "spreads out" over a larger and larger area as the sound wave disperses into the medium. Now, physicists like to give examples that can never exist in the real world because they are easier to understand than the horribly complex "real-world" state; for example, consider that the source of a sound (like my voice if I were lecturing to you) is coming from a small, spherical balloon that is expanding and contracting to produce the pressure disturbances in air. As the disturbance created by the balloon propagates throughout the medium, the size of the sphere over which the power is distributed gets larger and larger. But because there is only a finite amount of power, the amount of power per unit of area (i.e., the intensity) goes down as the sound wave propagates away from the source. Imagine that someone gave you two gallons of paint and asked you to paint a doll house with one gallon and a real house with the second. The thickness of the paint on the dollhouse would undoubtedly be much greater than the thickness of the paint on the house; both houses have the same amount of paint on them, but the real house has the paint spread over a much larger area. Now, if you read the previous sentence and substitute the word *power* for *paint,* you understand the physical principle. In acoustic terms, the "intensity" is the thickness of the paint, or the "power per unit area." For a sound source propagating in a sphere, the acoustic intensity falls off with the square of the distance from the source; this is called the **inverse square law.** In practical terms, it means that for each doubling of distance from the source of a sound, the acoustic intensity and the resultant SPL will fall by 6 dB. In the "real world," the distribution of sounds does not follow the inverse square law precisely because reflections from the ground and other objects alter the spherical path of the incident sound wave; thus, the level usually falls

off at a lower rate, say 5 dB per doubling. In our earlier example, assume that I am 6.25 feet from you and my voice level is 68 dB SPL at your ear. Therefore, the SPL would be 63 dB at 12.5 feet; 58 dB at 25 feet; 53 dB at 50 feet; 48 dB at 100 feet; and 43 dB at 200 feet. If I were lecturing in a classroom that had a background noise level of 55 dB SPL, any student more than 25 feet from me would have a signal-to-noise ratio of less than 3 dB at their ear, hardly an acceptable situation for listening.

Finally, let us return to our noise berm example. We are going to repeat the same measurements we just made, only this time a barrier that is 15 feet tall is inserted midway between the speaker and listener. Without the berm, the SPL at a distance of 50 feet is 53 dB SPL, as earlier. With the noise barrier in place, the source sound has to travel up and over the barrier to reach the ear of the listener, a distance of about 58.3 feet as opposed to the 50-foot direct-line distance. Using the real-world 5 dB per doubling rule, the sound level at the listener's ear would be 51.9 dB SPL, only a little more than 1 dB less than the level without the berm in place. If the source is kept in the same place (25 feet from the speaker) and the listener moves away from the berm, the effect of the berm height becomes less and less, and is less than 0.2 dB at a speaker-to-listener distance of 200 feet. So why do communities build noise berms if they work so poorly? In the opinion of many, noise barriers prevent individuals from seeing the source of offending noise, and eliminating the sight of the offending noise source appears to make people more tolerant of it.

As audiologists, we must be concerned with more than just the acoustic descriptors of sounds. A complete understanding of the effects of sounds on people requires knowledge of the physical characteristics of sound, the anatomic and physiologic substrates that govern its transduction by listeners with normal and impaired hearing, and the psychological and social implications of sounds and noise. This text considers the anatomic and physiologic foundations of normal and impaired hearing. We conclude our discussion of the physical characteristics of sound by considering the measurement and effects of *unwanted* sound, usually called **noise.**

WHEN IS A SOUND A NOISE?

The definition of *noise* is actually rather complex. In acoustics, *noise* refers to any signal that is aperiodic. In engineering, *noise* usually means a signal that interferes with the quality or detection of another signal. In psychoacoustics, noise is usually defined as "unwanted sound." Although this definition is probably the most useful for our purposes, even it can be problematic. Is rock music noise? The answer depends on who is hearing it. Similarly, although a loud rattle coming from the engine of a car is most assuredly a noise to the owner, it may carry useful information to the mechanic whose job it is to repair the engine, and would not be considered noise.

Noise also differs in the way it affects people. In low doses, noise can be soothing and can be wanted sound. Patrons of libraries are less distracted by footsteps, whispers, or page-turning when an air conditioner or ventilator produces a soft sound that masks the irregular noises. In moderate doses, noise can annoy us. It makes communication difficult, affects task performance, increases blood pressure, and causes stress. In high doses, noise can cause temporary or permanent hearing losses.

Perhaps the most general and most useful definition of noise was proposed by Kryter (1996), who described noise as an "acoustic signal which can negatively affect the physiological or psychological well-being of an individual." This definition covers all of the effects listed in this section. This chapter limits the discussion to one aspect of annoyance caused by noise, interference with speech communication, and more generally to the risk for permanent hearing loss posed by excessive exposure to occupational or recreational noise.

COMMUNICATION IN NOISE

Background noise affects the ability of people to communicate orally. Figure 2-4 provides a graph showing the relation among background noise level, talker-to-listener distance, and vocal effort required for effective speech communication. The vertical axis is the A-weighted sound level of background noise measured in decibels. The horizontal axis is the distance between the talker and listener in feet. The regions below the contours are those combinations of distance, background noise levels, and vocal outputs wherein speech communication is practical between adults who speak similar dialects of American English. The four contours represent increasing vocal effort ranging from normal voice (area of normal speech communication), raised vocal effort (communication possible), shouting (communication difficult), and levels at which communication is impossible even with maximum vocal effort.

Consider a situation where the background level is 50 dBA. Normal speech communication can occur at talker-to-listener distances of about 20 feet; at distances greater than 20 feet, communication is still possible, but it is necessary to raise one's voice level. In a background level of 60 dBA, the normal communication range is reduced to about 8 feet; at greater distances, communication is possible, but only with increased vocal effort. For higher background levels (e.g., 80 dBA), it is necessary to shout at distances greater than 5 feet, and communication is difficult. In many industrial settings, the background noise level is at or more than 80 dBA; in these settings, communication is difficult for distances greater than 5 feet without shouting, and for levels greater than 90 dBA, communication is impossible at distances more than 10 to 15 feet. Clearly, speech communication is difficult or impossible for individuals in environments where the background noise levels are greater than 80 dBA.

HOW MUCH NOISE IS TOO MUCH?

If the human ear is exposed to noise of sufficient strength or of sufficient duration, or both, a sensorineural hearing loss can occur. As stated earlier, the hazard associated with a particular noise exposure depends not only on the strength or level of the sound, but also its spectral characteristics, its temporal pattern, the number or repetitions, and the duration of the exposure. Further complicating the attempt to provide a simple descriptor for hearing hazard is that individuals vary widely in their susceptibility to noise exposure; therefore, it is impossible to specify an exposure limit that is guaranteed to

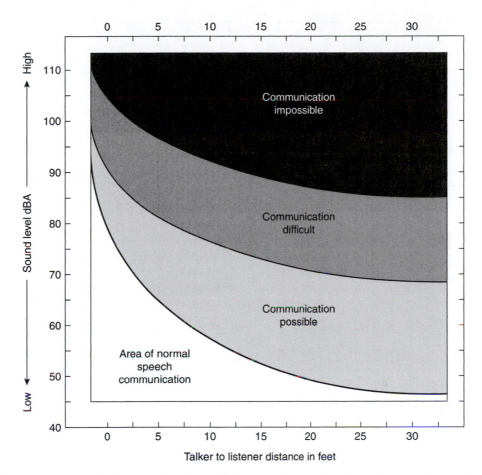

FIGURE 2-4 Speech communication as a function of background level and talker-to-listener distance in feet. (Adapted from Environmental Protection Agency [EPA], 1972.)

protect everyone. An additional complication is that because the effects of noise often go unnoticed by the patient, precise exposure histories are nearly impossible to obtain.

One way of thinking about hazard to hearing from sound exposure is to consider the dynamic range of the human ear. This range is shown in Figure 2-5. The bottom curve in Figure 2-5 represents auditory sensitivity for healthy young human ears. Signals presented at levels below the bottom graph are inaudible and obviously pose no risk for producing hearing loss. At the other extreme is the threshold of

pain, about 140 dB SPL. Sounds presented in excess of the pain threshold could present a risk for noise-induced hearing loss for just one short exposure; however, a precise estimate of the threshold for injury from a single brief exposure cannot be made at this time (Committee on Hearing and Bioacoustics [CHABA], 1993). Although considerable evidence suggests the ear can be injured by impulsive sounds with peak levels greater than 160 dB SPL (CHABA, 1993a; Clark, 1991), several studies have failed to document permanent injuries for brief continuous exposures at levels of up to 140 dB SPL (CHABA, 1993b;

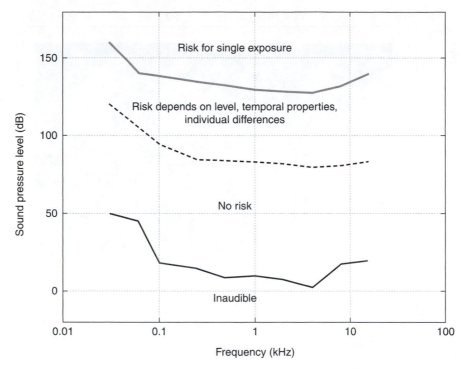

FIGURE 2-5 Categorization of the range of human hearing with respect to the risk for hearing loss. *Closed circles* denote audibility, *open circles* denote risk for temporary threshold shift, and *closed circles* denote permanent injury.

David et al., 1950; Ward, 1962). The federal noise standard, Occupational Safety and Health Administration (OSHA) 1910.95 (U.S. Department of Labor, 1983), prohibits single exposures greater than 140 dBA. In light of the scientific evidence, this exposure limit is reasonable.

Between the extremes of the threshold of pain and the threshold of audibility are two categories: risk and no risk. The "no risk" category can be called "effective quiet" or safe levels of exposure. Exposures in this range present no risk for acoustic injury, regardless of the duration of the exposure, the number of exposures, or the temporal spacing of the exposures. The "no risk" category is bounded on the upper side by levels that will not produce a measurable temporary threshold shift (TTS). These levels are also consistent with exposure limits specified by the relatively new American National Standard Institute (ANSI) S3.44 (1996). At 4.0 kHz, the frequency

most affected by noise, ANSI S3.44 specifies a level of 75 dB SPL as the lower limit of permanent threshold shift (PTS). That is, exposure centered at 4.0 kHz for nearly a lifetime (8 hours/day) will produce no PTS in any percentile of the population.

When the ear is exposed continuously between 75 and 140 dBA for long periods, permanent hearing losses can occur. These exposures occur commonly in the workplace and in the leisure environment. Chapter 18 provides further discussion of noise-induced hearing losses.

MEASUREMENT OF NOISE EXPOSURE

Noise exposure associated with the workplace has been known to produce hearing loss for centuries. In fact, "boilermakers' deafness" was the term coined to describe the now-familiar bilateral sensorineural

TABLE 2-3 Occupational Safety and Health Administration Maximum Daily Noise Exposure Limit

Duration per Day (hours)	Sound Level (dBA)
16	85
8	90
6	92
4	95
3	97
2	100
1.5	102
1	105
0.5	110
≤0.25	115

Adapted from U.S. Department of Labor CFR 29, 1910.95. Occupational noise exposure standard. Code of Federal Regulations, Title 29, Chapter XVII part 1910, Subpart G, 48FR9776, March 8, 1983.

hearing loss associated with excessive exposure to occupational noise. Largely from knowledge gained through field studies of hearing loss in industrial workers and military personnel, the U.S. Department of Labor (1983) promulgated regulations in the 1970s and 1980s designed to protect the hearing of employees who work in noisy environments. The regulations specified that employees be protected against the hazardous effects of noise when daily sound levels exceed those listed in Table 2-3.

The levels stated in Table 2-3 represent the maximum allowable daily noise exposure, or the **permissible exposure limit** (PEL), as specified by OSHA and other federal agencies. The PEL for an 8-hour exposure is referred to as the *criterion;* it reflects the sound level in dBA that reaches the PEL after 8 hours of exposure. Note that for exposures of other durations, the allowable daily exposure level is increased or decreased by 5 dB for each halving or doubling of exposure duration. Ninety decibels is allowed for 8 hours daily, 95 decibels for 4 hours daily, and so on. Each of the exposures listed in Table 2-3 represents an equivalent "time-weighted average" (TWA) exposure of 90 dBA for 8 hours. By definition, an 8-hour TWA of 90 dB represents 100% of the allowable "dose."

When the daily noise exposure is composed of two or more periods of noise exposure of different levels, their effects are combined by the following rule:

$$C_1/T_1 + C_2/T_2 + \ldots C_n/T_n,$$

where C is exposure duration at a given level, and T is allowable duration at that level.

"Percentage allowable dose" is then calculated by multiplying the result by 100%. That is,

$$D = 100 \star (C_1/T_1 + C_2/T_2 + \ldots C_n/T_n)$$

All exposures between 80 and 130 dBA are required to be integrated into the dose calculation. Exposures below the so-called threshold are not counted in the calculation of daily exposure; threshold values range from 80 to 90 dBA among various regulations.

The preceding calculations are most easily understood by considering a real-world example. During a typical 8-hour workday, a sheet metal worker might be engaged in the following activities: grinding, buffing, cutting, and packaging metal products. Of course, he or she would most likely also have some breaks, including lunch. A study of the actual noise levels experienced by the worker and the amount of time spent on each activity is shown in Table 2-4.

To determine the total daily dose (in percent) for the worker, one simply calculates the contribution of each exposure and adds them up. This is accomplished by dividing, for each exposure level, the duration of the exposure (*C* in the formula) by the allowable duration *(T)* and multiplying the result by 100 to calculate the percentage. A worker exposed to grinding noise at 92 dBA for 2 hours would reach 100% of the allowable dose in 6 hours (from Table 2-1). Therefore, after 2 hours, he or she would have accumulated 33.3% of the allowable dose (2 hours/6 hours allowed × 100%). Note that exposures less than 80 dBA do not contribute to the dose (i.e., *T* is infinite). Calculation of the total dose for the worker is made in Table 2-5.

Therefore, this employee's exposure would not exceed OSHA's PEL. The dose could also be expressed as a TWA level in decibels by calculating

TABLE 2-4   Distribution of Noise Level and Duration for a Hypothetical Worker during an 8-Hour Workday

Activity	Level (dBA)	Duration (hours)
Grinding	92	2.0
Buffing	85	2.5
Cutting	100	0.5
Packaging	75	2.0
Lunch, other breaks	79	1.0

TABLE 2-5   Contribution of Early Noise Activity to Overall Daily Noise Dose

Activity	C/T	Dose (%)
Grinding	2/6	33
Buffing	2.5/16	16
Cutting	0.5/2	25
Packaging	2/∞	0
Lunch, other breaks	1/∞	0
Total	0.74	74

the 8-hour exposure level that would result in the same dose:

$$TWA = 16.61 * \log 10 \ (dose/100) + 90,$$

or 87.8 dBA. It is important to remember that "dose" and "TWA" actually refer to the same measurement: the 8-hour equivalent exposure for any measured duration or combination of levels and durations, expressed as percentage or decibels.

As amended in 1983, the current U.S. occupational noise exposure standard identifies a TWA of 85 dBA, or 50% dose, as an "action level." Workers covered by the standard and who are exposed above the action level must be provided an effective hearing conservation program, including annual audiometric evaluations, personal hearing protection if desired, and education programs. With a daily noise exposure of 74%, or a TWA above 85 dBA, the sheet metal worker described earlier should be in a company hearing conservation program.

The exposure limits set by OSHA were empirically determined from epidemiologic and laboratory data concerning hearing damage from noise exposure and were designed to protect employees against sustaining a material impairment in hearing after a working lifetime. They were derived by subtracting the percentage of workers sustaining a material impairment in hearing as a function of exposure level from a control population without occupational exposure. The resultant percentage is the "percent risk" or "percent additional risk" of a material impairment in hearing after, for example, 40 years of exposure above that expected from presbycusis and sociocusis alone. Estimates of percent risk vary depending on which criteria and databases are used; from evaluation of all data, it can be concluded that the PEL of 90 dBA, with the 85 dBA action level, if enforced, would protect virtually the entire working population from sustaining an occupational noise-induced hearing loss (ANSI, 1996).

The OSHA noise standards are useful to the physician in arriving at a diagnosis, and for the audiologist in determining whether a recommendation about hearing protection should be made. First, because workers exposed to excessive occupational noise should be in a hearing conservation program, evidence of exposure history and prior company-obtained audiograms may be available for consideration. If the worker is not in a hearing conservation program, he or she may not work in significant occupational noise. Unfortunately, because not all workers are covered by OSHA standards and because enforcement has been weak, lack of participation in a hearing conservation program by a worker does not guarantee he or she has not been exposed to excessive occupational noise. However, in evaluating a patient, if it is determined that exposure to occupational noise did not exceed a TWA of 85 dBA, or a dose of 50%, then exposure to occupational noise should be ruled out as a causative factor.

The American Conference of Government Industrial Hygienists (ACGIH) has also listed guidelines for occupational exposure to noise (ACGIH, 2005). These limits are specified as "threshold limit values" (TLVs), and they differ from the OSHA standards in several important ways. First, they specify the criterion level as a daily exposure of 85 dBA, rather than the 90 dBA TWA specified by OSHA. Second, an exchange rate of 3 dB is used rather than the 5-dB exchange rate used by OSHA. These two differences make the ACGIH TLV more conservative than the OSHA PEL for most exposures, particularly when the exposure level fluctuates during the work shift. However, the TLV is specified by ACGIH as the minimum exposure at which one should consider implementing a hearing conservation program; it does not imply an upper limit of tolerable exposure. Viewed in this way, no conflict exists between the ACGIH TLV and the OSHA PEL.

⌁ SUMMARY ⌁

This chapter has reviewed the basic physical attributes of sound: how it is measured, and how human hearing sensitivity is characterized in physical terms. It is expected that most readers will have already been exposed to these concepts in their coursework in acoustics and psychoacoustics; this chapter is presented only as a basic review of the fundamental concepts we think are important to the understanding of anatomy and physiology of hearing.

A second goal was to summarize some general information about the effects of noise on hearing and human communication. This information, particularly the methods for calculating hazardous occupational noise exposures pursuant to federal regulations, is covered in more detail because it is not generally available to audiologists in traditional textbooks. A clear understanding of how one may assess noise exposures quantitatively can help the hearing professional assess the relative contributions of the many pathologic processes that contribute to sensorineural hearing loss and that are covered in Section III.

⌁ KEY TERMS ⌁

Acoustic intensity
A-weighting filter
Characteristic
    impedance
Damping
DART

Decibel
Frequency
Infrasound, ultrasound
Inverse square law
Metathetic continuum
Noise

Period
Permissible exposure
    limit
Phase
Prothetic continuum
Sound

Sound pressure
Sound pressure level
    (SPL)
Speed of sound
Wavelength

⌁ STUDY QUESTIONS ⌁

1. Audiologists often use the term *dynamic range* to express the boundary conditions of human hearing. In the frequency domain, the range is 20 Hz to about 20,000 Hz; in the intensity domain, the range is from about 0 to about 120 dB SPL. In linear terms, which of the ranges, frequency or intensity, is larger, and by how much?

2. Explain how noise berms positioned alongside highways reduce complaints from nearby residents.

3. Why do sound level meters incorporate an A-weighted filter network?

4. A rock band produces an average sound pressure level of 100 dBA measured at the ear of a listener 200 feet from the stage. What would the level be at the listener's ear if he or she moved to a distance of 50 feet from the stage?

⚛REFERENCES⚛

Albers V. M. (1970). *The world of sound.* New York: A.S. Barnes and Company.

American Conference of Governmental Industrial Hygienists (ACGIH). (2005). *2005-2006 threshold limit values (TLVs) for chemical substances and physical agents and biological exposure indices (BEIs).* Cincinnati, OH: ACHIG.

American National Standards Institute, Inc. (ANSI). (1996). *American National Standard: determination of occupational noise exposure and estimation of noise-induced hearing impairment* (ANSI S3.44-1996). New York: American National Standards Institute, Inc.

CHABA (Committee on Hearing and Bioacoustics). (1993a). *Hazardous exposure to steady-state and intermittent noise* (Report of Working Group 101, Committee on Hearing, Bioacoustics, and Biomechanics, Commission on Behavioral and Social Sciences and Education). Washington, DC: National Research Council, National Academy Press.

CHABA (Committee on Hearing and Bioacoustics). (1993b). *Hazardous exposure to impulsive noise* (Report of Working Group 102, Committee on Hearing, Bioacoustics, and Biomechanics, Commission on Behavioral and Social Sciences and Education). Washington, DC: National Research Council, National Academy Press.

Clark, W. W. (1991). Noise exposure from leisure activities: A review. *Journal of the Acoustical Society of America, 90,* 175–181.

Davis, H., Morgan, C. T., Hawkins, J. E. Jr., et al. (1950). Temporary deafness following exposure to loud tones and noise. *Acta Otolaryngologica Supplements, 88,* 1–57.

Environmental Protection Agency (EPA). (1972). *Effects of noise on people* (EPA Report No. NTID 300.7,50). Washington, DC: EPA.

Kryter, K. D. (1996). *Handbook of hearing and the effects of noise.* New York: Academic Press.

U.S. Department of Labor. (1983, March 8). CFR 29, 1910.95: Occupational noise exposure standard. Code of Federal Regulations, Title 29, Chapter XVII part 1910, Subpart G, 48FR9776.

Ward, W. D. (1962). Damage risk criteria for line spectra. *Journal of the Acoustical Society of America, 34,* 1610–1619.

⚛SUGGESTED READING⚛

Acoustics

Hartmann, W. M. (1997). *Signals, sound, and sensation.* New York: American Institute of Physics Press. (A comprehensive treatment of the physics of sound and psychoacoustics.)

Haughton, P. (2002). *Acoustics for audiologists.* San Diego: Academic Press. (Presents a more comprehensive assessment of acoustics, but assumes some background in mathematics, basic physics, and electric circuit theory.)

Speaks, C. E., Zobits, M. R., & Carney E. (1999). *Introduction to sound: Acoustics for the speech and hearing sciences.* New York: Singular Publishing. (This is a good general overview, presented [intentionally] without complex mathematics.)

Noise Measurement and Hazard Assessment

Berger, E. H., Royster, L. H., Royster, J. D., Driscoll, D. P., & Layne, M.P. (Eds.). (2000). *The noise manual* (5th ed.). Fairfax, VA: American Industrial Hygiene Association. (Covers virtually all aspects of noise and hearing conservation, including the responsibilities of audiologists involved in hearing conservation programs, and contains particularly strong chapters on hearing protector use.)

Dobie, R. A. (1993). *Medical-legal evaluation of hearing loss.* New York: Van Nostrand Reinhold. (Valuable reference for the audiologist when considering the relative roles of aging [presbycusis], occupational and nonoccupational noise exposures, and other medical pathologies on the hearing levels of patients.)

Chapter 3

Filters and Spectra

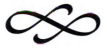

William W. Clark, Ph.D.
Director, Program in Audiology
and Communication Sciences
Washington University School of Medicine
St. Louis, Missouri

Although the principles are based on the "rigorous" sciences of physics and mathematics, an understanding of the basic characteristics of **filters** and spectral processing are crucial for the audiologist. Consider for a moment something that appears to be quite simple: the passage of sound energy into the cochlea for transduction. We learned in Chapter 2 how to quantify and measure the intensity and frequency of a sound wave in air, and if the presence of an observer (usually a person) had no effect on that process, our quest to understand how sound energy leads to hearing would be finished. Fortunately, however (or perhaps unfortunately for the student), inserting a person into a sound field creates a real disturbance. Because the density and elasticity of our bodies differ appreciably from air, when a sound wave traveling in a field encounters the body, it is altered in complex but predictable ways. And, of course, to sense sounds, acoustic energy must reach the sensory receptor cells in the cochlea. The route is complex, but the first stage is reached when a propagating sound wave encounters an object, in this case, a person.

One of our most unusual-looking appendages is the pinna, or auricle, that sits on either side of our head. You may have wondered why on earth you were fitted with such complicated devices, and you probably know that the pinnae can "funnel" sound down into the ear canal. "Funneling" happens because the impedance of the cartilaginous processes of the pinna is much different than air, and sound waves striking the pinna are reflected downward and into the ear canal. As a result, sound is reflected before being directed down into the ear canal. And the reflection is far from simple: The complex shape of the pinna, with its torturous ridges and recesses, affects sounds of different wavelengths differently. Sound complicated? It certainly is; but in reality, it is just the start of the journey of sound into the inner ear.

This chapter considers the characteristics of filters and spectral (or frequency) processing, and develops a description of what happens to sound in air as it is transmitted through the auditory system to the hair cells of the cochlea. At the end of this chapter, you should have an understanding of the nature of sound transmission into the sensory receptors

and how that limits or explains normal hearing sensitivity. Finally, this chapter considers the effect of wearing a hearing aid on sound transmission to the inner ear.

The first order of business is to acquire a few tools, borrowed from engineering and acoustics, to aid in our understanding. Knowledge about spectral processing and filters also is necessary.

SPECTRAL PROCESSING

Chapter 2 discusses how frequency, period, and phase characteristics of an acoustic signal are related by considering the simplest form of sound, a sine wave. In fact, by the time most audiology students encounter this textbook in their graduate careers, they have already been introduced to the ubiquitous sine wave. It might be surprising to learn, therefore, that sine waves are actually quite rare, and thus are seldom encountered in real life. The reason is that the physical characteristics of sound sources limit their ability to move precisely in sinusoidal fashion. For example, a pure-tone audiometer is an electroacoustic device that generates "pure" tones at discrete frequencies, from 125 Hz to 8 kHz. It contains electronic circuitry that delivers sinusoidally varying voltages to an earphone or loudspeaker at different frequencies. The earphone or loudspeaker is a mechanical device that contains a permanent magnet surrounding a coil attached to a stiff diaphragm. The purpose of the earphone is to convert an electrical signal into an acoustic sound wave. Voltage changes in the coil alter the magnetic field and cause the diaphragm to vibrate back and forth with a velocity that is proportional to the voltage change. Because the system is mechanical and has mass and stiffness, the resulting vibration does not follow the voltage input precisely in time; the result is a generated waveform that is "almost, but not quite" sinusoidal; that is, the waveform is distorted slightly. In fact, the American National Standard Specification for Audiometers (ANSI S 3.6, 1996) allows up to 2.5% total distortion in the pure tone signal for an audiometer.

Because "true" sinusoidal signals are so rare, what should we call all the "other" sounds of nature? All sounds that are not sinusoidal are called **complex** waves. You can imagine that categorizing complex waves must be extraordinarily complex, and it is. Examples of complex waves commonly encountered by audiologists include music, speech, and noise. Complex waves can be further differentiated by their temporal characteristics. If the waveform repeats itself in the time domain, it is called a **periodic** complex wave. If there is no regular or periodic repetition in the time domain, the wave is called an **aperiodic** signal. Music and speech are good examples of periodic complex signals, although sometimes the waves are only approximately periodic, and are called *quasiperiodic*. Noise, in contrast, is characterized by random *amplitude* fluctuations, and is appropriately called an *aperiodic signal;* that is, it does not repeat periodically in time, and unlike periodic signals, its future cannot be predicted by its past. A graph depicting the amplitude distribution of noise is shown in Figure 3-1.

Figure 3-1 shows only the **waveform,** a description of how the amplitude of the noise is distributed in the time dimension. It is also possible to describe the **spectrum** of the noise. *Spectrum* is a way of describing how energy is distributed across frequency. An *amplitude spectrum* is a graph that shows the amplitude (usually the sound pressure level [SPL]) of each frequency represented in the signal. Considered as a whole, the human auditory system can respond to a range of frequencies that extends from about 20 Hz to about 20 kHz. A convenient way of describing this range, and which makes sense for the way humans perceive sound, is to divide the spectrum into separate bands with constant ratios of the upper (f_u) and lower (f_l) frequencies. A ratio of 2:1 is called an **octave,** and expressed this way the range of human hearing extends over approximately 10 octaves. The frequency scale, like the decibel scale, is logarithmic, but it is expressed as a logarithm to the base 2, rather than 10.

Because the amplitude deviations of the noise shown in Figure 3-1 are random in level and time and present at all frequencies, it follows that a representation of this noise in the frequency domain, averaged over a long period, would return a horizontal, flat line. That is, all frequencies would be present and, on the average, would be of equal am-

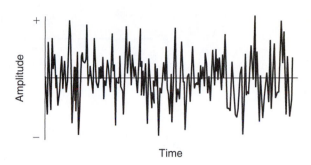

FIGURE 3-1 Amplitude spectrum of an aperiodic signal (noise). Notice that the signal displays no periodicities in the time domain.

plitude. This particular "brand" of noise is called **white noise,** indicating that all spectral components have, on the average, equal amplitude. Another way of saying this is that white noise contains equal energy per cycle. White noise is not always useful for the audiologist. For example, an octave band of noise centered at 500 Hz has 353.5 cycles in it (353.5–707.0 Hz). If the sound level of 1 cycle of that noise is 35.5 dB SPL, then the overall level ($L_{overall}$) is:

$$L_{overall} = \text{level per cycle} + 10^* \log$$
$$(\text{bandwidth, in Hertz})$$
$$= 35.5 + 10^* \log (353.5)$$
$$= 35.5 + 25.5$$
$$= 60 \text{ dB SPL}$$

Another octave band of noise, this time centered at 4,000 Hz instead of 500 Hz, but presented at the same level per cycle, would have a higher overall SPL, because there are more cycles in the 4,000-Hz octave band (2,828) than in the 500-Hz octave band. Specifically, the overall level would be:

$$L_{overall} = 35.5 + 10 \log (2,828)$$
$$= 35.5 + 34.5$$
$$= 69 \text{ dB SPL}$$

or 9 dB greater than the octave band centered at 500 Hz. The preceding calculations demonstrate an important rule for white noise: Because the bandwidth of successive octaves represents a doubling of the number of cycles, the overall level of white noise

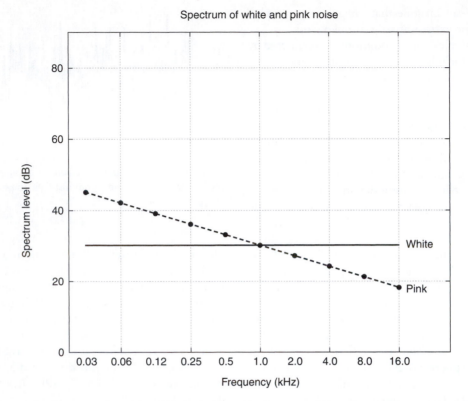

Spectrum of white and pink noise

FIGURE 3-2   Amplitude spectra for white noise and pink noise. Because white noise contains equal energy per cycle, the amplitudes of all frequency components occur at the same level. Pink noise, in contrast, is equal energy per octave; the spectral density decreases by 3 dB for each doubling in frequency.

increases by 3 dB for every octave band. The 4-kHz octave band noise (OBN) above is 3 octaves above the 500-Hz OBN; therefore, the overall level is 3 octaves times 3 dB, or 9 dB greater than the lower band, no matter what the spectrum level of the noise is.

Because audiologists often want to present bands of masking noise at the same overall level, the spectrum of white noise can be "tilted" to compensate for the increasing bandwidth of successive octaves. By adjusting the amplitude spectrum in the frequency domain to a slope of −3 dB per doubling, that is, the spectrum level by frequency decreases by 3 dB per doubling, the 3–dB/octave increase for white noise caused by bandwidth doubling can be offset, and the result is a noise than has equal energy per octave. This type of noise is still aperiodic and is called **pink noise.** Plots of the am-

plitude spectrum for white and pink noise are shown in Figure 3-2.

A slightly more complicated example of a complex waveform and its associated amplitude spectrum is shown in Figure 3-3. The complex waveform is shown at the bottom left of Figure 3-3A. Notice that the waveform is a little complicated; in fact, it looks like a ski slope with a number of "bumps" in it. The graph shows two complete cycles of this waveform, each with a period of T milliseconds. It can also be seen that the amplitude crosses zero at times that correspond to 0.5 T and T, and again at 1.5 and 2 T, but repeats itself with a period of T (in milliseconds). This "basic" waveform creates the **fundamental frequency,** and it is displayed on the right panel of Figure 3-3A as the lowest frequency, or left-hand component. Other

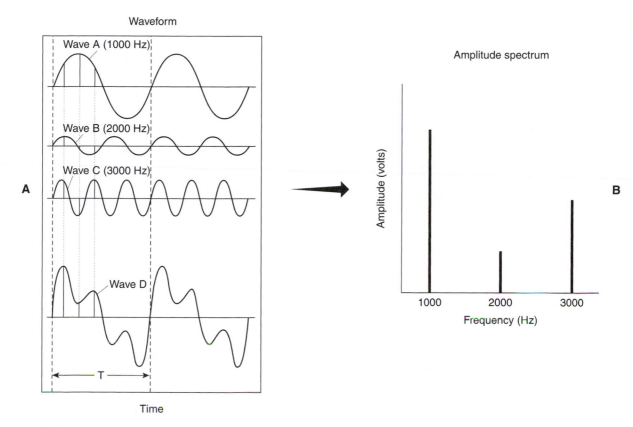

FIGURE 3-3 (A) Complex waveform created by the addition of three sinusoidal signals of different frequencies and amplitudes, but all starting at 0 degrees phase. The complex waveform at the bottom is the sum of the instantaneous amplitudes of each of the components. (B) The amplitude spectrum of the complex signal. Note that the amplitudes and frequencies of the components can be discerned in the graph, but not their phases.

components with different periods are also shown on the right panel of Figure 3-3A, with their position on the abscissa indicating the frequency of the component and the amplitudes of each component shown in the ordinate. A sound that is composed of discrete frequencies is called a *periodic signal,* and lines on the line spectrum that appear at integral multiples of the lowest frequency are called *harmonics,* or *overtones.* The sounds of musical instruments are good examples of "periodic" and "complex" signals. Human speech is also an example of a complex, periodic sound.

One of the characteristics of periodic signals that can be seen in Figure 3-3 is that all the harmonics of the signal share one "common" feature: when they

are added together, the total waveform has a period that is equal to the period of the fundamental. Therefore, the waveform of the sum of the three sinusoidal signals repeats at the frequency of the fundamental, and the signals add up without interfering with each other; that is, the oscillation at 1,000 Hz is undisturbed by the oscillation at 2,000 or 3,000 Hz. The resultant amplitude of the complex signal is the simple sum of each of the instantaneous amplitudes of the source signals. This general principle is called the principle of **superposition,** and it is a characteristic of sound waves traveling in any medium that behaves linearly, like air.

The other "take-home message" is that the complex signal shown at the bottom of the figure

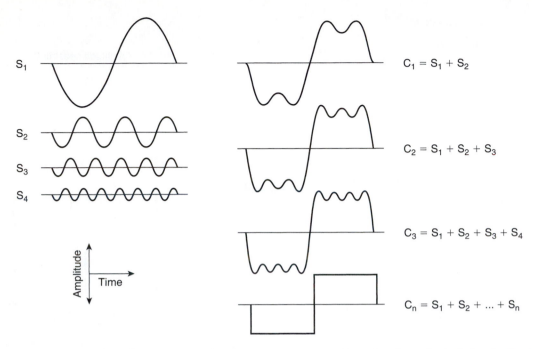

FIGURE 3-4   Decomposition of a square wave into its component parts. Note that the series includes the fundamental frequency and the odd harmonics.

can be decomposed into a series of sinusoidal signals that make it up. That is, any periodic signal, no matter how complex, can be represented by a series of sinusoidal signals with appropriate amplitudes and starting phases. This fundamental principle is called **Ohm's acoustic law.** It was originally proposed to describe the perception of sounds of musical instruments, but it can be used generally to describe the composition of any complex periodic signal.

Let's take an example here: a square wave (shown in the bottom right portion of Figure 3-4). We are sure you will agree that this wave looks anything but sinusoidal! However, this square wave can be constructed by adding together a series of sinusoids (see Figure 3-4, left). Notice that the series of sinusoids does not include every harmonic. With respect to the fundamental signal (S_1), the second, third, and fourth components (or harmonics) are odd integral multiples of the fundamental and have lower amplitudes. That is, signal S_2 is the third harmonic ($3S_1$), S_3 is the fifth harmonic ($5S_1$), and so on. As successive odd

harmonics are added, the combined waveform approaches a true square wave.

The amplitude spectrum of the complex signal in Figure 3-3A is shown in Figure 3-3B. It displays the amplitudes and frequencies that are present in the complex wave we observed initially. You can verify the information in the amplitude spectrum by studying the "source" sinusoids for the complex signals. For example, in Figure 3-3, the three components exist at frequencies of 1,000, 2,000, and 3,000 Hz, and their peak amplitudes are represented by the vertical excursions of the waveforms for each.

The physical principles discussed earlier are important to the audiologist. That any periodic complex sound can be decomposed into a series of signals of appropriate amplitude and phase, and represented in the time and frequency domain, is a key concept. The most common sounds in the environment, such as speech, music, or the sound of a passing truck, are all complex acoustic signals. They most likely would not be totally random but would have discernible peaks and valleys in them. The process of "decoding" these complex signals into their component parts was solved in the early nineteenth century by mathematician J. B. J. Fourier, who had previously served as the Governor of Lower Egypt under Napoleon. Fourier developed his theory to help describe the process of transfer of heat. The essence of the **Fourier transform** is that it takes the value of any function and converts it to another, related function. Although the details of the mathematics are beyond the scope of this text, the important thing for audiologists is that the transform can be used to describe the response of any physical system in the time or frequency domain. The functions are $f(t)$ and $F(\omega)$, where t is time and ω is called the "angular frequency" $(2\pi f)$. When $F(\omega)$ is obtained from $f(t)$, we say $F(\omega)$ is the Fourier transform of $f(t)$. The transform can also be applied in the opposite direction, that is, from the frequency domain to the time domain, and this process is called an **inverse Fourier transform.** Audiologists, engineers, and auditory physiologists often use a "shorthand" method to approximate the Fourier series. Basically, it involves sampling a signal over a discrete period of time and estimating the frequency components. This technique is called a **fast Fourier transform (FFT),** and it is often implemented in computer programs to extract frequency information from a complex signal recorded in the time domain. For example, instruments that are used to measure distortion product otoacoustic emissions (DPOAEs) use an FFT analysis to extract the DPOAE response from the complex waveform measured in the ear canal (see Chapter 13 for details).

FILTERS

In general terms, a *filter* is any device that modifies the spectrum of its input and passes only a portion of the spectrum to the output. The **transfer function** of a filter describes precisely the way the filter modifies the output both in the amplitude and the time domain. Filters are usually characterized by their performance in the frequency domain. A **low-pass filter** allows low frequencies to pass through to the output but attenuates the high frequencies. A **high-pass filter** attenuates low frequencies and al-

lows high frequencies to pass. A **band–pass filter** passes only frequencies in a restricted region and attenuates frequencies above and below the band. Finally, a **band-reject filter,** sometimes called a *notch filter,* passes all frequencies except those within the band, which are attenuated. Figure 3-5 shows the frequency spectrum of each of these types of filters. These types of plots are often referred to as Bode plots. Both ordinates are drawn logarithmically, with the abscissa, frequency, expressed in octaves, and the filter gain displayed on the ordinate in decibels. The cutoff frequency of the filter is defined as the half-power point, or the frequency at which the amplitude of the signal is reduced by 3 dB below the passband. The filter slope is the rate (in decibels) that the output of the filter is reduced as the signal moves outside the passband. For first-order filters, the slope is -6 dB per octave; second and higher order filters can be designed that have sharper (steeper) slopes, and the slopes increase by -6 dB per order.

Although our focus is on the frequency response of filters, it is important to realize that all filters affect the phase response of the output, as well as the amplitude. In practice, most filters exhibit a phase delay outside the filter bandwidth that has a slope (in the time domain) that is related to the amplitude response. That is, the further the amplitude of the signal is shifted, the more it is delayed. For complex signals (e.g., those shown in Figure 3-3), passing through a filter will increasingly delay the higher harmonic components, resulting in a different complex waveform. That is, the principle of superposition still holds, but the relative positions (in the time domain) of the components are changed.

Filter Characteristics

The filters described in Figure 3-5 are all passive, meaning that there is no amplification of the incoming signal by the filter. This is reflected on the y-axis of the graph, which displays a gain of 0 dB within the passband. The bandwidth of the filter is usually characterized by the range of frequencies that are at least half the power of those in the center of the passband. This bandwidth is sometimes

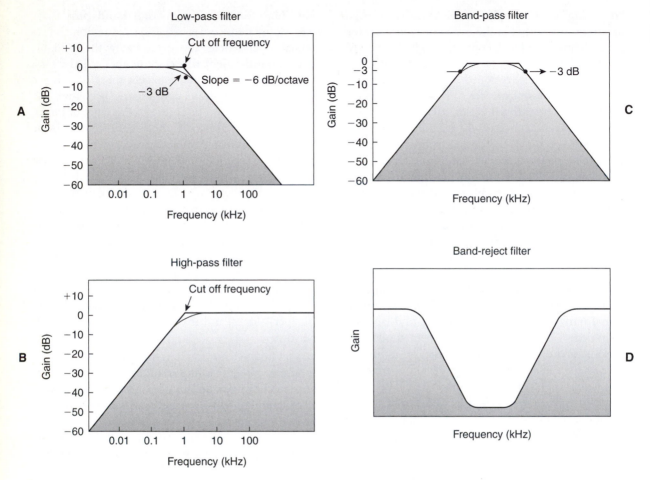

FIGURE 3-5 Examples of (A) low-pass, (B) high-pass, (C) band-pass, and (D) band-reject filters.

called the *3-dB bandwidth,* and as shown in Figure 3-5, it is slightly wider than the frequencies that exist at the maximum level.

Another characteristic that can be seen in Figure 3-5 is the slope of the filter function. This slope is expressed as the ratio of the decrement in sound intensity with frequency. Because the plots are logarithmic (decibels on ordinate, and log frequency on the abscissa), the slope is expressed in units of decibels per frequency ratio. For the first-order filters shown in Figure 3-5, the slope is −6 dB per octave, or −20 dB per decade. Higher order filters can also be designed that have steeper slopes (i.e., second order, −12 dB per octave; third order, −18 dB per octave, and so forth). Digital filters, created by fast computers, can be designed to have steep filter slopes and are limited only by the speed of the processor.

Although electronic filter characteristics are extremely important to electrical engineers and the designers of hearing aids, this book limits the discussion of filters to the effects of the mechanics and biomechanics of the ear on the incoming acoustic signal, and the ways we characterize the nature of auditory nerve fiber responses. Furthermore, because the frequency scale in Figure 3-5 is logarithmic, it is more

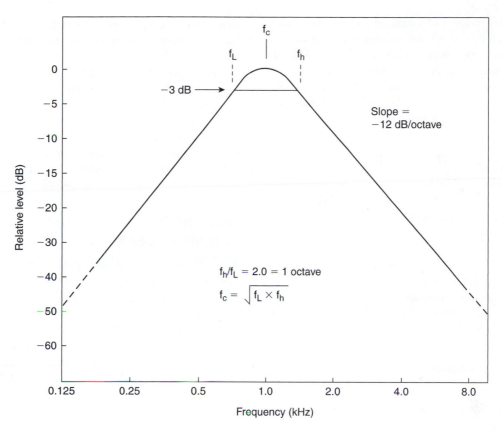

FIGURE 3-6   Idealized band-pass filter.

common to describe the bandwidth of a filter in logarithmic rather than linear terms. A constant percentage bandwidth filter is, as its name implies, designed to pass signals within a band that is a constant percentage of the center frequency (CF) of the filter. A 10% filter would have a bandwidth of 10 Hz at 100 Hz, 100 Hz at 1,000 Hz, and so on.

In practice, constant bandwidth filters are often described using octave notation. An octave band filter, for example, would extend over a frequency range of one octave; that is, the ratio of the upper and lower cutoff frequencies is 2:1. An idealized octave band filter, centered at 1,000 Hz, is shown in Figure 3-6. The lower cutoff frequency (f_l) is 0.707 kHz; the upper cutoff frequency (f_u) fulfills the octave requirement ratio of 2:1.

Because the scale is logarithmic, the CF is:

$$\text{Center frequency} = \sqrt{fl * fu}$$
$$= \sqrt{(.707)2 * (1.414)2}$$
$$= 1.000 \text{ kHz}$$

This formula is appropriate for calculating the geometric CF of any filter, if you know the lower and upper cutoff frequencies. Now that we know quite a bit about this particular octave band of noise, let us consider generalities that will allow us to describe filters of any bandwidth. First, notice that the CF is not spaced linearly between the upper and lower cutoff frequencies. In fact, as shown in Figure 3-6, the CF, expressed in log frequency, breaks the octave band into two equal parts, each a half octave wide and extending above and below the CF. Thus, if you want to create a band of noise that is one octave wide, and centered at 1.0 kHz, the lower cutoff must be a half octave below the CF, and the upper cutoff a half octave above the CF. Because the frequency scale is logarithmic, with a base of 2, the following simple formula makes this calculation easy:

$$F^n = 2^n * F_o$$

The frequency (F^n) that is a half octave greater than 1.0 kHz (F_o) is $F_o * 2^{-1/2}$, or 1.414 kHz. The frequency that is a half octave less than 1.0 kHz (F_o) is $F_o * 2^{1/2-}$, or 0.707 kHz.

Using the preceding formulas, the overall bandwidth and the upper and lower cutoff frequencies can be determined for any frequency. It is left to the reader to ascertain that a $1/3$ octave band of masking noise, centered at 3.0 kHz, extends from 2.673 to 3.367 kHz.

The "Q" of a Filter

Acousticians commonly use the letter "Q" to describe the selectivity of a filter in the frequency domain. The term "Q" stands for "quality," and it is used in physics to describe how much energy of a signal that is "put in" to a filter "comes out" unaltered, compared with how much is lost to resistive forces, that is, heat. In auditory physiology and in acoustics, the "Q" of a filter is defined as the ratio of its CF divided by its bandwidth:

$$Q = CF/bandwidth$$

In the examples presented in Figure 3-5, the Q of a one-octave band of noise, with the bandwidth measured between the half-power points, would be 1.414. In fact, for all octave bands of noise, the Q value is 1.414, because the CF of an octave band is always the bandwidth times the square root of 2.

Notice also that we have defined the bandwidth as the frequency range encompassed by the half-power (−3 dB) points. Therefore, we would say that the filter described earlier had a Q_{3dB} of 1.414. Narrower band filters, expressed the same way, will have higher Q_{3dB} values: $1/3$ octave band = 4.32; $1/10$ octave band = 14.5. The higher the Q, the more sharply tuned is the system.

Auditory physiologists also use the Q measure to describe the filter characteristics of nerve fibers. Because the slopes of auditory nerve fibers are very steep, as much as 90 to 100 dB per octave, it is more convenient and precise to measure the bandwidth for all signals within 10 dB of the peak; this ratio is called the Q_{10dB} bandwidth. The calculations are the same as the examples presented earlier.

FILTERING BY THE EXTERNAL AND MIDDLE EAR

Armed with a basic understanding of acoustics, we now can consider, in relatively simple terms, the filter effects of the outer and middle ear. (See Chapter 7 for a more complete description of the anatomy and physiology of the pinna, external canal, and middle ear.) It has already been suggested that the presence of a head and torso in an acoustic field creates a disturbance in the field. Of course, this occurs because the impedance of the head and cartilaginous portions of the auricle are quite different from air, and most of the energy of incident sound waves bounces off the surface. The sound wave that ultimately reaches the cochlear fluids and the hair cells takes a complicated journey from the free field in air to the movement of the stapes. In addition to knowing the detail of the anatomy of the ear, the audiologist also needs to know its "acoustic" anatomy and physiology.

Using acoustic terminology, we describe the head and torso as acoustic reflectors. When a person is inserted into a sound field, sound may enter the ear canal from a direct path (technically, you could see the source if you stood just outside the tympanic membrane and looked out the ear canal) or from a myriad of reflected paths. Sounds that strike the shoulder, for example, will bounce off the top of the shoulder and can reflect up into the ear canal. Sound waves that are reflected will arrive at the ear canal a little later than the direct source, because they have to travel farther, and the relative spectrum may be changed slightly. Another important object that is in the way of the sound path is the pinna, or auricle. Anatomically, the pinna is characterized by a number of tortuous ridges and furrows. Furthermore, it is not symmetric around the ear canal. More of it protrudes posterior and superior to the ear canal than anterior and inferior. From an evolutionary perspective, this gives an acoustic advantage to any sound source that is in front of or below the subject, which is useful information for finding prey or avoiding being eaten.

The ridges and furrows on the auricle function acoustically as a number of tiny acoustic panels, each one reflecting an incident sound wave with slightly different amplitude and phase features. The combination of the tortuous structure of the pinna and its asymmetric position means that sounds approaching the head will enter the ear canal with different amplitude and phase characteristics if they come from different locations in space. Given this structure, it should not be surprising that humans can tell the difference between a sound emanating from directly in front of the head and a second identical sound of equal level coming from behind the head. In addition, even though you may have learned that the auditory localization ability of humans depends on the relative levels and times of arrivals of sound at each ear, people who are completely deaf in one ear can still localize sounds, albeit not as well as those with binaural hearing. Undoubtedly, the detailed acoustic "signature" of the pinna contributes to this ability.

In addition to providing spectral and phase cues, the pinna also serves as a sound collector. Everyone knows that if you put your hand behind your ear while listening to someone speaking, their voice will sound louder. Try it. Put your hand behind your ear and listen to the background noise wherever you are. Now, before you do anything, think about how you are holding your hand. Is it cupped or held flat? It is probably cupped and held in such a fashion to extend the length and the shape of the pinna. Now, keep your hand behind the pinna, but open it so it is now flat, like you are

reaching to shake hands with someone. You should notice the loudness decreasing somewhat when you flatten your hand.

The increase in loudness occurs because the sounds that bounce off the pinna and your hand reflect down the ear canal and, effectively, add up with the energy in the direct wave. This causes an increase in energy density and the resultant sound pressure at the tympanic membrane, effectively increasing the velocity of the movement of the tympanic membrane. It is well known in acoustics that a horn that is gradually tapered does the best job of collecting the incoming sound wave; when you flattened out your hand, you changed the shape of the "horn" and reduced its efficiency by sending some of the reflected sound away from the ear canal.

Before the advent of electronic hearing aids, ear trumpets were commonly used by people who were hard of hearing. An example of an ear trumpet, cosmetically disguised to look like a headband with a flower, is shown in Figure 3-7. The basic structure is a small exponential horn connected to a tube that fit into the ear canal. The gain function of this ear trumpet, measured in an anechoic chamber on an acoustic manikin, is about 10 dB at 2,000 Hz (not a bad hearing aid for people with mild high-frequency hearing losses). It was attractive, functional, and did not use batteries.

The human ear canal is open at the entrance to the ear and is bounded at its proximal end by the tympanic membrane. Acoustically, the ear canal functions as an open tube resonator. That is, it serves to amplify sounds at some frequencies and not others. You can observe the acoustic characteristics of an open tube resonator by blowing across the top of a partially empty soda bottle. Although the blowing sound you make is relatively wideband, you will hear a sound with a distinct pitch. This is because of the resonance characteristics of the bottle. If you empty the bottle a little and blow again, the pitch will go down. This occurs because you are lengthening the column of air in the bottle and creating a resonant frequency with a longer wavelength (i.e., lower pitch). Specifically, both the soda bottle and the open ear canal follow the

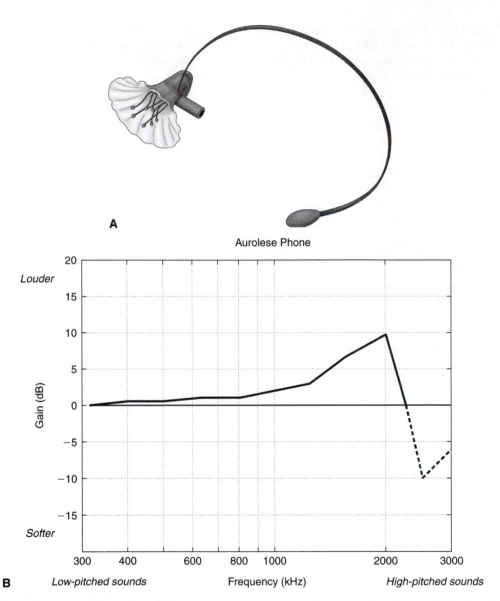

A

Aurolese Phone

B   *Low-pitched sounds*   Frequency (kHz)   *High-pitched sounds*

FIGURE 3-7 (A) Example of an ear trumpet disguised as a headband. Floral Aurolese Phone (1802). The Phone provided an acoustic benefit up to 10 dB over a limited frequency range and was appropriate for a person with a mild hearing loss. (B) Gain function shown below. (B) Chart showing the amplification of external sounds provided by the Aurolese Phone. The gain is the difference in dB measured at the eardrum with and without the Phone, as a function of frequency. (Used by permission from *Deafness in disguise: concealed hearing devices of the 19th and 20th centuries.* From http://beckerexhibits.wustl.edu/did/index.htm, by permission from Becker Medical Library, Washington University School of Medicine. Accessed August 22, 2006.)

so-called **quarter-wavelength rule.** This rule states that the resonant frequency of a simple open tube resonator is that frequency whose wavelength is four times the length of the tube.

$$\text{Resonant frequency (Hz)} = \frac{\text{Speed of sound (feet/sec)}}{4 * \text{length of tube (feet)}}$$

An average human ear canal is about 1 inch. Therefore, resonant frequency is the speed of sound divided by 4 inches (4 times the length of the canal):

$$\text{Resonant frequency (Hz)} = \frac{1143 \text{ feet/sec}}{0.33 \text{ feet}}$$
$$= \sim 3{,}464 \text{ Hz}$$

Therefore, from the length of the ear canal alone, if we measured the SPL at the entrance to the ear canal and just next to the tympanic membrane and varied the frequency of a test signal, we would expect an amplification of approximately 15 to 20 dB in the frequency range around 3 kHz, due solely to the resonance effects. An example of a typical gain function is provided in Figure 7–4.

The overall effects of the transfer function due to the torso, head, pinna, and ear canal have been documented by a number of investigators. Perhaps the most comprehensive and often cited study was completed by E. A. G. Shaw and published in 1974. A summary of his findings, showing the transformation of SPL from the eardrum to the free field as a function of azimuth, is shown in Figure 3-8. The series of graphs depicts the transfer function, in decibels. The figure is broken into measures made in front of the subject, to the side, and behind. Each graph depicts a separate transfer function obtained in the horizontal plane. The degree angle is measured with respect to the front of the listener. Notice that for all measures, the transfer function exhibits a slow increase from about 200 to about 1,400 Hz, with gains of 0 = 10 dB, a range between about 2,000 and 7,000 Hz, where the gain increases to a maximum of just more than 20 dB, and a decline at frequencies greater than 7,000 Hz. The other feature that can be seen in the graph is that

the gain function is broadest (i.e., encompasses the widest frequency range) for sounds that emanate from the front (see Figure 3-8, top).

In summary, the pinna and external ear canal serve to amplify sounds that occur in the field over a range of approximately 2 to 7 kHz, and they do a little better job for sounds emanating from the front of the listener than from the side or behind. The amount of the gain is approximately 20 dB. Next, we consider the effects of the middle ear on sound transmission.

Transfer Function of Middle Ear

The functional characteristics of the middle ear are examined fully in Chapter 7. This chapter limits the discussion to how the middle ear filters the sound as it travels through it. Like any filter, its function can be described by comparing its input with its output and plotting the difference in the frequency and time domains. In the case of the middle ear, the input is the sound pressure in the ear canal, and the output is the movement of the stapes footplate in the round window. Although the measures are difficult to conduct, recent advances in laser interferometry methods allowed measures of the transfer functions in human cadaver ears (i.e., Gan, Wood, & Dormer, 2004; Aibara, Welsh, Puria, & Goode, 2001). In these studies, the displacement of the tympanic membrane is compared with stapes displacement. A summary of the findings is shown in Figure 3-9. The top panel of Figure 3-9 describes the magnitude of the transfer function, expressed in arbitrary dB units; that is, the middle ear acts as a low-pass filter. The cutoff frequency is the resonant frequency of the middle ear, and signals within the passband are passed with equal gain. Above the resonant frequency, the filter response attenuates signals at a rate of about −12 dB per octave.

The phase of the middle ear response is shown in the bottom panel of Figure 3-9. It can be seen that signals within the passband pass, for the most part, without delay, but those above the passband are delayed by increasing amounts with increasing frequency. The slope of the phase function is about −120 degrees per octave. So what does all this mean to the cochlea?

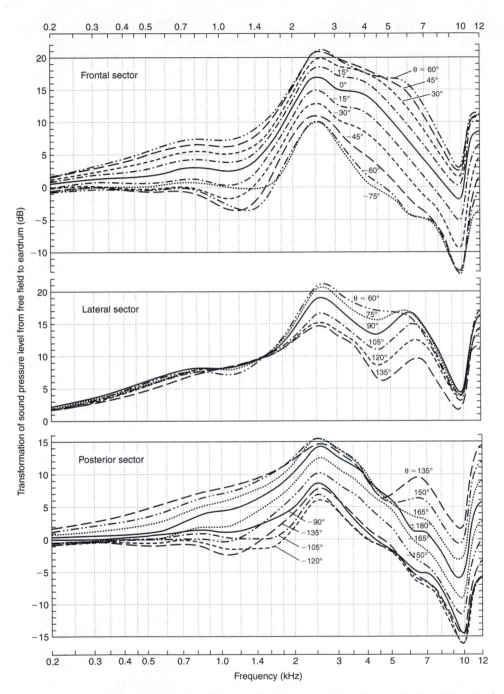

FIGURE 3-8 Free field-to-eardrum transformation for humans as a function of azimuth. For clarity, the functions are separated into frontal, lateral, and posterior sections. (Reprinted with permission from Shaw, E. A. G. (1974). Transformation of sound pressure level from the free field to the eardrum in the horizontal plane. *Journal of the Acoustical Society of America, 56,* 1848–1861. Copyright 1974, American Institute of Physics.)

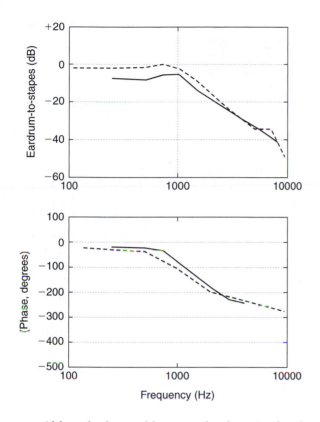

FIGURE 3-9 Middle ear transfer functions for human cadaver ears. (top) Eardrum to stapes gain in decibels. (bottom) Phase shifts at stapes relative to eardrum. (Adapted from Gan, 2004.)

Although the cochlea can also be stimulated through direct vibrations of the skull (i.e., bone conduction), it is far more sensitive to airborne sound vibrations that travel in air through the external and middle ear to the cochlea. As such, under normal listening conditions, the sole source of acoustic energy delivered to the cochlea comes through the vibrations of the stapes footplate in the oval window. Therefore, it should not be surprising that hearing sensitivity depends, in large part, on the filter characteristics of the pinna and external and middle ear.

⚜ SUMMARY ⚜

This chapter has explained that the pinna serves as a power collector and increases the SPL at entrance to the ear. The ear canal has a resonant frequency of about 3 kHz and amplifies incoming sounds between about 2 and 7 kHz by up to 20 dB over the equivalent SPLs in the free field. The middle ear provides a flat gain (see Chapter 7) of about 25 dB for the frequencies below about 1.0 kHz; at higher frequencies, the gain falls off by about 12 dB per octave. Because incoming sound must travel through both the external and middle ears to reach the stapes, the combined frequency domain transfer function is the sum of the effects of each filter independently. Therefore, a "real-world" sound, for example, a white noise, would be transmitted quite well to the stapes at frequencies up to about 7 kHz, with the middle ear providing the amplification at 1 kHz and below and the external ear providing gain above 1 kHz and up to about 7 kHz. At greater than 7 kHz, the relative input to the stapes would continue to fall off. Many scientists believe that the acoustic characteristics of the external and middle ear are major determinants of mammalian hearing sensitivity (e.g., Rosowski, 1991), although recent evidence suggests the cochlea also is a major contributor to hearing bandwidth (Ruggero & Temchin, 2002).

Amplification

It is natural and appropriate to consider the ear as an acoustic instrument. The topics reviewed in this chapter demonstrate that the external and middle ear combine to affect the transduction of incoming sound waves dramatically. These effects include altering the spectrum, amplitude, and phases of signals before they reach the cochlea. In a sense, sound in the environment is "distorted" by the external and middle ears before it gets to the receptors in the inner ear. But in this case, "distortion" is "natural"; it is part of the normal hearing process.

But when an audiologist seeks to treat a patient with hearing loss by fitting a hearing aid, he or she will alter the mechanoacoustic properties of the ear. An earmold placed in the ear canal creates two acoustic effects: It shortens the length of the air column in the canal because it occludes the distal part, and it changes the canal acoustically from an open tube resonator to a closed tube resonator. Occluding the canal with an earmold, therefore, will increase the resonant frequency of the canal by more than twofold. In addition, because the normally open canal is now blocked at the distal end, the patients will often notice an occlusion effect. This effect occurs because bone-conducted sound compresses the air column in the ear canal, and if it is blocked distally, the pressure changes excite the tympanic membrane, particularly at low frequencies. These are just some of the reasons audiologists need to know about filters, spectra, and the processing of the acoustic signal on its way to the cochlea.

KEY TERMS

Aperiodic waveform
Band-pass filter
Band-reject filter
Complex waves
Fast Fourier transform (FFT)
Filter

Fourier transform
Fundamental
High-pass filter
Inverse Fourier transform
Low-pass filter
Octave

Ohm's acoustic law
Periodic waveform
Pink noise
Q of filter
Quarter-wavelength rule
Spectrum

Superposition
Transfer function
Waveform
White noise

STUDY QUESTIONS

1. Why should an audiologist care about spectral processing and filtering?
2. What differentiates "white" noise from "pink" noise?
3. What are the lower and upper cutoff frequencies of a 1/3 octave band of noise centered at 8.0 kHz?
4. Three filters are designed for use in an automobile stereo. All three filters have Q_{3dB} values of 4.0, but different CFs. Do they have the same bandwidth?
5. Assume a complex signal is made up of three sinusoids: 500, 3,000, and 8,000 Hz. Explain how each of these signals would be effected by the acoustic effects of the outer and middle ears.

⌒REFERENCES⌒

Airbara, R., Welsh, J. T., Puria, S., & Goode, R. L. (2001). Human middle-ear sound transfer function and cochlear input impedance. *Hearing Research, 152,* 100–109.

American National Standards Institute (ANSI). (1996). *American National Standard Specification for Audiometers.* ANSI S 3.6-1996. New York: American National Standards Institute, Inc.

Gan, R. Z., Wood, M. W., & Dormer, K. J. (2004). Human middle ear transfer function measured by double laser interferometry system. *Otology and Neurology, 25,* 423–435.

Rosowski, J. J. (1991). The effects of external-and middle-ear filtering on auditory threshold and noise-induced hearing loss. *Journal of the Acoustical Society of America, 90,* 124–135.

Ruggero, M. A., & Temchin, A. N. (2002). The roles of the external, middle, and inner ears in determining the bandwidth of hearing. *Proceedings of the National Academy of Sciences, 99,* 13206–13210.

Shaw, E. A. G. (1974). Transformation of sound pressure level from the free field to the eardrum in the horizontal plane. *Journal of the Acoustical Society of America, 56,* 1848–1861.

⌒SUGGESTED READING⌒

Hartmann, W. M. (1997). *Signals, sounds, and sensations.* New York: AIP Press. Comprehensive mathematical treatment of issues generally related to psycho-acoustics.

Haughton, P. (2002). *Acoustics for audiologists.* New York: Academic Press. A good quantitative source, especially useful for students with electrical engineering backgrounds.

Chapter

4

Essentials of Cell Structure and Function: An Introduction to Cell Biology

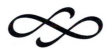

Brian T. Faddis, Ph.D.
Assistant Professor of Otolaryngology
Washington University School of Medicine
St. Louis, Missouri

As students of the science of hearing, you will dwell at some length on both the complexity and rather astonishing capability of the organ of hearing, the ear. You will study tissue specializations such as the organ of Corti and stria vascularis that function together to enable one of the most sensitive information-gathering systems known to humans. At the root of all this complexity is the smallest unit of life, the cell. Cells are not simply the building blocks of tissues. They are individually capable of every type of activity that the whole organism is capable of, including movement, communication, feeding, getting rid of waste products, and any other basic process you can imagine. This chapter explains the anatomy of the cell and some of its basic functions. You will come to appreciate how genetically identical cells can alter their gene expression to create a multitude of different tissues. In fact, more than 200 such tissue specializations exist in the human body. A basic understanding of cellular and subcellular anatomy and physiology will enhance your appreciation of how the ear works and how disease processes affect hearing. You also will have a much easier time understanding new advances in the field of hearing science.

ANATOMY OF THE CELL

The anatomy of the cell can be divided into just a few general components: the membrane system, the structural support system, and organelles specialized for manufacturing needed proteins. In addition, there are specialized cell structures, such as microvilli and stereocilia, which only exist on certain cell types and permit very specialized activities. The following sections deal with each of these cell components in some detail.

MEMBRANE SYSTEM

Individual cells, and the organelles within a cell, are encased by membranes. Although they function as a kind of "skin," membranes are remarkably fluid in nature. This section discusses the different parts of the cell that are most associated with membranes.

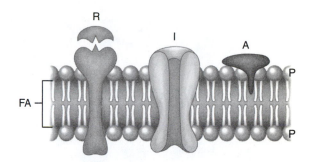

FIGURE 4-1 (See Color Plate) An artist's rendition of the lipid bilayer common to most cell membranes. Each lipid molecule possesses a hydrophilic phosphate head group (P) and hydrophobic fatty acid chains (FA). This structure makes the membrane impermeable to most ions and molecules. Proteins are commonly found embedded in the membrane that serves as a receptor (R), ion channels (I), and anchoring points (A) used to stabilize the cell within the extracellular environment. Proteins such as these allow the cell to control its intracellular environment by making the membrane selectively permeable to desirable ions and molecules.

Plasma Membrane

The cell is bound by a **lipid bilayer** known as the **plasma membrane** (Figure 4-1). Lipid molecules possessing phosphate head groups spontaneously arrange themselves in this bilayer such that the hydrophobic lipid chains constitute the interior of the membrane and the hydrophilic phosphate head groups lie in contact with the aqueous environment both inside and outside the cell. This arrangement prevents most molecules from crossing the membrane. A variety of lipid molecules exist in plasma membranes, and their relative concentrations can affect a number of membrane properties such as permeability, fluidity, and interactions with the extracellular environment. Proteins are another important constituent of the plasma membrane. They can be embedded on the external surface, internal surface, or traverse the membrane completely. They function in a wide variety of roles, including stabilization of the membrane, selective transport of both ions and large molecules, anchoring the membrane to adjacent cells and substrates, cellular motility, and communication. They provide an essential

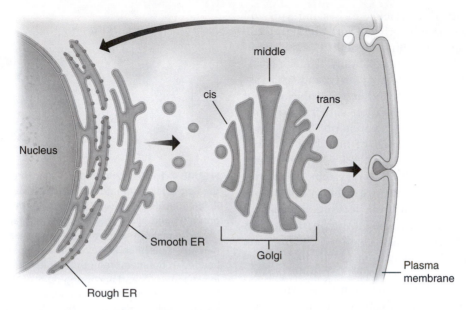

FIGURE 4-2 (See Color Plate) The membrane system of the cell includes the nuclear envelope, rough and smooth endoplasmic reticulum (ER), the Golgi apparatus, and the plasma membrane. These membrane-bound structures are functionally connected and communicate with one another by direct physical connections and through budding vesicles. The unidirectional flow of macromolecules through this system allows the orchestrated modification, folding, and packaging of raw peptides that is required to make them fully functional and delivered to the correct cellular location. Molecules may also be engulfed by the cell membrane and fuse with the ER for proper modification before use by the cell.

link between the extracellular and intracellular worlds, allowing the cell to adjust an immeasurable number of activities according to changes in its environment.

As seen in Figure 4-2, the plasma membrane is functionally, if not physically, continuous with the membrane of the nucleus, **endoplasmic reticulum** (ER), and Golgi complex. These organelles actually pass membrane-bound vacuoles from one compartment to another as manufactured proteins are modified, packaged, and delivered to their appropriate destination, whether that be inside or outside the cell.

Endoplasmic Reticulum

The ER is a system of flattened tubes or sacs that is continuous with the membrane of the nucleus. The plasma membrane of the ER constitutes roughly half of the total membrane in a typical eukaryotic cell and may occupy more than 10% of the cell vol-

ume. The ER plays a central role in the synthesis of proteins and lipids and is also important in the storage of calcium ions in the cell. Calcium activates a number of cellular responses to extracellular signals, so it must be sequestered when not required. Specific calcium-binding proteins and calcium pumps known as Ca^{2+}-ATPases help to sequester calcium from the cytosol. It is the rapid release of calcium from the ER of muscle cells that modulates the contraction of muscle fibrils.

There are two general types of ER: smooth ER and rough ER. These types refer to the absence (smooth) or presence (rough) of **ribosomes** on the surface of the ER membrane. Ribosomes are organelles that translate genetic material into proteins. Their association with the ER allows the ribosome to insert proteins into the lumen of the ER as they are made. In general, proteins that will stay in the ER, be secreted by the cell, or be sent to the lumen of other organelles are the only proteins that will be inserted into the ER. Rough ER is the more abundant type present in most cells. The portion of ER that is smooth is usually minimal. It is from this region of ER that vesicles will bud and transport to the Golgi complex. Some cells specialized for lipoprotein synthesis and lipid metabolism can have abundant smooth ER. The amount of ER can fluctuate considerably in response to the overall activity of the cell. New polypeptides translocated into the lumen of the ER will be folded and assembled into their correct conformation by resident ER proteins. Most will also have sugar molecules attached, a process called *glycosylation*. The ER is also responsible for producing most of the lipids needed to fabricate new plasma membranes.

Golgi Complex

The Golgi complex, or **Golgi apparatus,** is similar to the ER in that it is also a complex series of tubules. However, it possesses a level of order that is not inherent to the ER. It is a primary site of carbohydrate synthesis and serves as a relay station for peptides and proteins made by the ER. It thus serves to supplement the packaging and modification of lipids and proteins already in production. Some of the carbohydrates produced in the Golgi apparatus are attached as oligosaccharide side chains to these lipids and proteins.

The tubules of the Golgi apparatus are arranged as a flattened series of membrane-bound disks often described as a stack of plates. These disks or plates are called *cisternae* (singular, cisterna). A cell may have one large stack of cisternae or many hundred smaller stacks. The Golgi apparatus is often situated close to the nucleus and possesses two distinct sides: a cis side or face and a trans face. The cis face is oriented closer to the nucleus and is typically characterized by the presence of vesicles derived from the ER. The trans face is opposed to the plasma membrane and is also characterized by the presence of vesicles, but these vesicles are derived from the Golgi apparatus itself and are destined, as secretory vesicles, to fuse with the plasma membrane and release their contents to the exterior of the cell. Additional Golgi vesicles transport lipids

and proteins between the various cisternae. This fusion of membrane-bound vesicles is a common occurrence in the cell and is similar to the fusion of two soap bubbles, except that it occurs with astonishing specificity (Vaughan, 2005).

Transport along the membrane system of the cell may then occur as follows. First, a peptide or lipid is manufactured in the ER. As it is transported along the ER, it is modified and folded. Only properly folded proteins and lipids are then shuttled via free vesicles to the cis face of the Golgi. These elements undergo additional modifications as they are transported from cis to medial to trans compartments of the Golgi. In the trans compartment, lipids and proteins are segregated into distinct transport vesicles to be delivered to a specific target site within the cell.

CYTOSKELETON

The supporting system of the cell is the **cytoskeleton.** Although is may appear to be not much more than a supporting scaffold (Figure 4–3), this system does much more than simply dictate the shape of the cell. It is intimately involved in a wide variety of cellular processes such as feeding, motility, intracellular transport, polarization, and cell division. The cytoskeleton is composed of a collection of protein filaments of three different sizes, as well as numerous types of cytoskeleton-associated proteins that serve to link these filaments to one another and to other parts of the cell and to transport organelles along the filaments. The following subsections describe each type of filament in turn and discuss their functional contributions to cellular activity.

Microtubules

The largest cytoskeletal filament in the cell, measuring 25 nm in diameter, is the **microtubule.** It is a hollow tube made from a protein called *tubulin*. The functional building block of the microtubule is actually a heterodimer of two closely related polypeptides called α- and β-*tubulin*. The hollow core structure of the microtubule is composed of

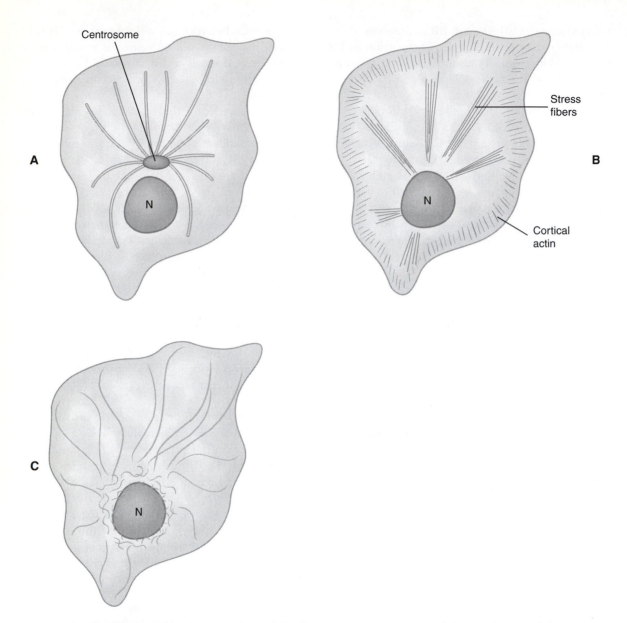

FIGURE 4-3   Simplified graphic representations of the three primary components of the cytoskeleton: (A) microtubules; (B) actin filaments; and (C) intermediate filaments. Microtubules and actin filaments are quite labile and constantly undergoing growth and destruction, a feature that lends itself to cell motility and division. Intermediate filaments are much more stable and play a larger role in cellular stability and resistance to mechanical stress.

13 tubulin molecules arranged as protofilaments around the core. This particular arrangement allows the microtubule to be polarized, consisting of a fast-growing plus end and a slower growing minus end.

The microtubule is the only polarized cytoskeletal element; how this plays a role in its ability to segregate molecules to different parts of the cell is discussed later in this chapter.

Although you may not suspect a major structural component of the cell to be labile, the entire microtubule scaffold within the cell is constantly turning over. A structure called the *centrosome,* typically found near the nucleus of the cell, plays an important part in initiating microtubule formation. If you were to watch a growing microtubule as it radiates out from the centrosome, you would see it grow steadily for a while, then suddenly shrink back, sometimes shrinking only partially before starting to grow again, and sometimes shrinking back completely to ultimately disappear. The minus or slow-growing end of the microtubule is associated with the centrosome. Because it is possible to stabilize a formed microtubule by "capping" the plus end, microtubules can promote a structural polarization of the cell by selectively being capped in one region of the cell (Wittmann & Desai, 2005).

In addition to being structurally polarized, cells can be functionally polarized with the aid of microtubules and specialized motor molecules that associate with them. Two such motor molecules that have been widely studied are kinesin and dynein. Both these molecules consist of two heavy chains and several light chains. The heavy chains bind to the microtubule, whereas the light chains bind to specific cell components. How the heavy chains convert energy from **ATP** hydrolysis into lateral movement along the microtubule is not yet known. The important difference between these two motor molecules is that kinesin only travels outward from the centrosome, toward the plus end of the microtubule, and dynein travels back to the centrosome, or toward the minus end of the microtubule. This difference is important in establishing the polarity of nerve cell processes known as axons and dendrites. Dendrites collect information and transmit it to the neuron cell body, and axons project information away from the cell body.

Additional microtubule-associated proteins (MAPs) do not function as motors, but they can modify the properties of microtubules. Such proteins serve to link microtubules to one another and to other cytoskeletal elements and cell components, perhaps most importantly the plasma membrane. These MAPs help to stabilize microtubules once formed and promote the initiation of new microtubules. Examples of MAPs include such molecules as MAP-1, MAP-2, and tau. Tau and MAP-2 represent a classic example of cellular compartmentalization in nerve cells. Tau is found only in the axonal processes of nerve cells, whereas MAP-2 is found only in the dendritic processes and cell body.

One specialized function of microtubules is that of ciliary motion. The beating movement of cilia or flagella is responsible for moving fluids across the surface of a cell or for propelling a cell through a fluid environment. This beating is caused by the bending of the axoneme, a structure at the center of the cilium or flagellum. This axoneme possesses a special arrangement of nine pairs of microtubules surrounding two individual microtubules. An accessory protein called *ciliary dynein* causes adjacent microtubules to slide against one another, resulting in a bending of a region of the axoneme. A coordinated sliding propagated along the length of the axoneme produces the resultant ciliary or flagellar beating pattern. You will discover later that the kinocilium of the stereociliary bundle found on top of auditory hair cells is a true cilium, possessing the characteristic nine plus two arrangement of microtubules.

Actin Filaments

Actin filaments are the smallest of the cytoskeletal elements, measuring only 8 nm in width. They are composed of actin, one of the most abundant proteins in most types of cells. Like microtubules, actin filaments are polarized with a slower growing minus end and a faster growing plus end. Although actin filaments are thinner, more flexible, and generally shorter than microtubules, the total actin filament length within a cell is much greater than the total microtubule length. Actin filaments also tend to cross-link into aggregates or bundles for increased strength.

Actin is involved in quite a stunning array of cellular activities, from mechanical strength to phagocytosis to motility. Indeed, probably the most well-known function of actin is in the contraction of muscle cells. Three common actin motifs are present in many cells: actin stress fibers, an actin cell cortex, and filopodia. Actin stress fibers consist of rather densely packed actin filaments arranged with alternating orientations of the plus end. These stress fibers are composed of actin filaments and myosin molecules such that they resemble tiny muscle fibers. One end of the stress fiber is anchored to the plasma membrane, where it is closely attached to the underlying substrate or a neighboring cell. The other end is attached to a dense cytoskeletal network near the nucleus. Stress fibers function as anchoring points for the cell, allow for increased mechanical strength of certain tissues, relay extracellular signals to the cytoskeleton, and allow cells to exert tension on the underlying substrate.

Actin formations are particularly important in the cortex of the cell, that region just beneath the plasma membrane. The cortical actin network can consist of a variety of actin formations. In general, actin in the cortical region of the cell is cross-linked by a wide variety of actin-binding proteins and serves to determine the shape and mechanical properties of the cell (Lambrechts, Van Troys, & Ampe, 2004).

A third specialization of actin formations is the finger-like projections known as microvilli and filopodia. These extensions of the plasma membrane are filled with dense arrays of actin filaments all oriented with their plus ends away from the cell body. Actin-binding proteins known as villin and fimbrin are important for cross-linking the actin filaments to provide structural integrity to these finger-like extensions. Microvilli are commonly used to increase the surface area of a cell to maximize its ability to absorb agents from the environment. Filopodia are slender extensions certain cells use for locomotion and to explore the environment (Samaj, Baluska, Voigt, Schlict, Volkmann, & Menzel, 2004).

Actin-binding proteins, the equivalent of MAPs, play an important role in determining the function of a specific actin formation. Table 4-1 lists some of the major classes of actin-binding proteins and the attribute or function they commonly impart to actin filaments.

TABLE 4-1   Some of the Major Classes of Actin-Binding Proteins

Actin-Binding Protein	Function
Tropomyosin	Strengthens individual filaments
Fimbrin, villin, α-actinin	Cross-link or bundle filaments
Gelsolin	Fragments or dissolves filaments
Myosin	Slides filaments and moves vesicles along filaments
Spectrin, ankyrin	Attach filaments to plasma membrane

Intermediate Filaments

Intermediate filaments are so named because their size, 8 to 10 nm in diameter, placed them between the fine actin filaments and thicker myosin filaments in muscle cells where they were first described. They are prominent in cells that are subject to mechanical stress, and they serve to provide a mechanical stability to most cells. A dense network of intermediate filaments called the *nuclear lamina* underlies the nuclear envelope. The intermediate filament cytoskeleton is a uniquely stable skeleton, not subject to the rapid dissolution and regrowth that is characteristic of actin filaments and microtubules. These tough stable filaments are commonly composed of tetramers of fibrous proteins. There are three major classes of intermediate filaments in vertebrate cells: keratins, vimentin, and neurofilaments.

Keratin filaments are primarily found in epithelial cells. They constitute the most diverse family of intermediate filament proteins, with more than 20 varieties found in human epithelia alone. Keratins are tough filaments, indeed; in fact, human hair and fingernails are composed of certain hard varieties of keratins.

Nonepithelial cells are more likely to form intermediate filaments from vimentin and vimentin-like proteins. Unlike actin filaments and microtubules, intermediate filaments have been described in only multicellular animals. Furthermore, not all the cells of a multicellular animal will possess intermediate filaments. The function of intermediate filaments is as varied as the functions of other cytoskeletal elements, although mechanical support appears to be a universal feature. For example, desmin filaments cross-link individual myofibrils in skeletal and cardiac muscle cells. The glial filaments of astrocytes in the nervous system can undergo a dramatic increase when brain tissue is injured, allowing sheets of astrocytes to form an effective scar and seal off the injured area.

Neurofilaments, as their name implies, are found in neurons. They are the most abundant cytoskeletal element in neurons and are found as three different classes, referred to as low-, middle-, and high-molecular-weight classes. All three classes tend to coexist in any given neuron.

THE NUCLEUS

Clearly, the most conspicuous organelle within the cell has to be the nucleus. Often referred to as the brains of the cell, the nucleus contains all the genetic information of the individual in the form of deoxyribonucleic acid (DNA). The nucleus is enclosed by a lipid bilayer known as the nuclear envelope. Two networks of intermediate filaments support this membrane. The nuclear lamina lies just beneath the membrane, and another, less organized network is found at the external surface. Small holes or nuclear pores pierce the membrane to allow access for molecules that will activate transcription of DNA when needed and to allow transcribed messenger ribonucleic acid (mRNA) to exit the nucleus.

Each DNA molecule is packaged in a separate chromosome. Humans possess 24 different pairs of chromosomes; each pair contains one chromosome inherited from the mother and one from the father. Chromosomal DNA is a complex code based on only four simple molecules called nucleotides: adenine, cytosine, guanine, and thymine. Precise three-nucleotide sequences provide a code for each of the 20 amino acids from which all cellular proteins are built. But how are proteins built from this simple code? This sequence starts in the nucleus. You may

have heard that DNA exists as two complementary strands of nucleotides running in opposite directions. The two strands are bound tightly together by hydrogen bonds, which always pair the following bases: adenine with thymine and guanine with cytosine. This DNA double helix can be induced to unravel when the code must be read and a copy made to be used as a blueprint or template for the production of needed proteins. This template is called *mRNA,* and it differs from DNA in two respects: First, the sugar unit incorporated is ribose, rather than deoxyribose; second, the nucleotide base thymine is replaced by one called *uracil.* RNA exists as a single-stranded molecule that is short-lived and is the complement of the DNA strand from which it was transcribed. RNA molecules can also be cleaved and chemically modified before being translated into proteins.

So how does translation occur? This process not only involves mRNA, but another form called *transfer RNA* (tRNA). tRNA molecules are the carriers of the specific amino acids that will be assembled into proteins according to the mRNA code. This activity also requires the presence of another cell organelle called the *ribosome.* You recall that rough ER is so named because its surface is studded with ribosomes. At the ribosome, tRNA molecules carrying specific amino acids are selected that match the code found on the mRNA strand. Start and stop signals are also evident in the mRNA strand that are recognized by the ribosome. Recall that the newly assembled polypeptide or protein can be released into the cytoplasm or inserted into the ER for further modification, packaging, and delivery to specific cellular sites (reviewed in Alberts, Johnson, Lewis, Raff, Roberts, & Walter, 2002, and Stryer, 1999).

Another organelle residing in the nucleus is the **nucleolus.** The nucleolus is a highly organized portion of the nucleus that contains high concentrations of RNA and proteins. Its primary function is the manufacture of ribosomes. The size of the nucleolus is a reflection of its activity and, therefore, differs greatly from cell to cell, depending on the rate of protein synthesis. The nucleolus dissolves when the cell is in the process of division (mitosis), but it is reassembled in each of the daughter cells when this process is completed.

MITOCHONDRIA

It should be quite evident that cells are active manufacturing plants. However, all this activity requires energy, energy that is made by another organelle, the **mitochondria.** The energy currency used by most cells is found in a molecule called *adenosine triphosphate* (ATP). ATP is formed at the inner membrane of the mitochondria as a by-product of a several processes known collectively as *respiration*. For example, the breakdown of 1 molecule of glucose yields 36 molecules of high-energy ATP for use by the cell. Mitochondria are located in the cytoplasm of the cell and can be segregated to distinct regions of high activity, if needed. They can vary tremendously in number, size, and shape between cell types, but are commonly oval or kidney shaped in profile, measuring 0.5 to 1.0 μm in diameter. The relative activity of a cell can be inferred by the abundance of mitochondria or lack thereof. Mitochondria are enclosed in a double membrane. The outer membrane is simple and permeable to many small molecules. The inner membrane is relatively impermeable and is extensively folded, causing the characteristic cristae that are seen in cross sections of these organelles.

ADDITIONAL ORGANELLES

Many additional organelles exist within most cells. These include vacuoles such as lysosomes and peroxisomes specialized for the isolated degradation of cell waste and destruction of hydrogen peroxide, respectively. Other vacuoles are used for routine storage of substances manufactured by the cell. A simplified diagram of a typical animal cell with its various organelles is shown in Figure 4-4. Plant cells contain specialized organelles called *chloroplasts,* which are required for photosynthesis, the means by which plants derive energy from sunlight.

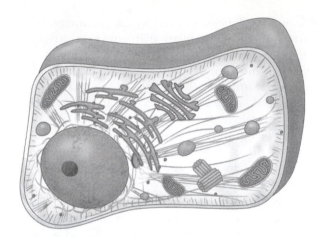

FIGURE 4-4 (See Color Plate) The individual cell requires a diverse and complex array of organelles for both structural and metabolic support at the cellular, tissue, and organismal levels. Through the coordinated efforts of these organelles, the cell can control its internal environment, manufacture needed molecules, become motile, interact with other cells to form tissues, and even alter these processes as changes in the extracellular environment dictate.

CELL DIVISION

Most cells, even when mature, maintain the capacity to replicate or divide. It is not within the scope of this chapter to discuss the intricate details and multiple steps involved in cell division. It is briefly outlined here as an exercise to see how all the parts of the cell we have investigated thus far play exquisitely organized roles in this process (Doxsey, Zimmerman, & Mikule, 2005). Cells will not generally divide unless they receive a signal from another cell or the extracellular environment. This requires some kind of receptor protein on the surface of the target cell. Once the decision is made to divide, the cell must condense its genetic material into compact chromosomes, each pair of which will be split among the daughter cells. During this time, the nuclear envelope also must dissolve. Two mitotic spindles will form and move to opposite ends of the cell. These are composed mainly of microtubules and associated proteins. Each spindle will extend microtubules toward the chromosomal pairs and attach a single microtubule to a single chromosome. After attachment,

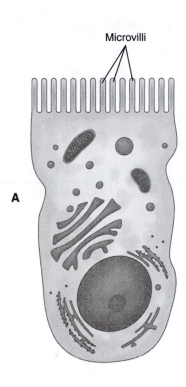

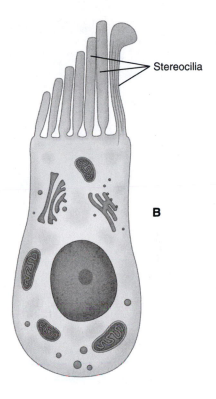

Microvilli on the apical surface
of intestinal epithelial cell

Stereocilia at the tip of
an auditory hair cell

FIGURE 4-5   (See Color Plate) Certain cells possess specializations that impart unique functional attributes to the cell. (A) Finger-like extensions of membrane, called *microvilli,* increase the apical surface area of epithelial cells in the small intestine to enhance the absorption of water and molecules as they pass through the gut. (B) The stereocilia found on top of sensory hair cells in the inner ear activate cellular signaling mechanisms when deflected in the proper direction, allowing for exquisite sensitivity to auditory signals.

the individual chromosomes will be drawn back toward the spindle pole, effectively separating the chromosomes into two equal groups. Once this is accomplished, a nuclear envelope begins to regenerate at each pole and a contractile actin ring forms in the middle of the parent cell. This process is known as *cytokinesis.* The actin ring contracts until the plasma membrane breaks, creating two independent daughter cells. All the cytoplasmic contents, including ER and Golgi apparatus, will have been split roughly equally among the daughter cells. After cytokinesis, the nuclear chromosomes decondense in preparation for continued cellular activity.

SPECIAL ATTRIBUTES AND CELL STRUCTURES

This chapter to this point has discussed cells as a rather generic entity in terms of shape and size. In truth, cells differ dramatically in their shape, from spherical to very oblong to quite random. They also exist in dramatically different sizes, from only a few to several hundred micrometers in diameter. Other specializations are also present that impart unique characteristics to certain cell types (Figure 4-5). For instance, cells that must specialize in absorption typically contain an area of dense microvilli that lie in contact with the absorption environment. These

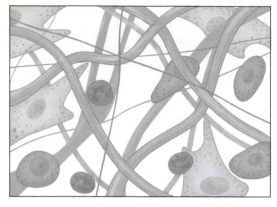

Connective tissue

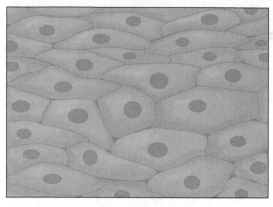

Epithelium

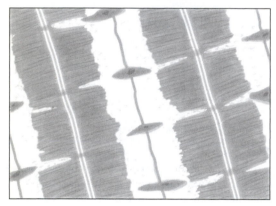

Muscle

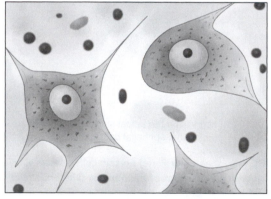

Nervous tissue

FIGURE 4-6 The five classic tissues of the body include blood (not shown), connective tissue, epithelium, muscle tissue, and nervous tissue. These tissues vary considerably in appearance because of differences in organization, cell types, and the amount of extracellular matrix. For example, the loosely organized connective tissue with its abundant extracellular matrix is in sharp contrast with tissues such as epithelium and muscle that are highly organized and contain little extracellular matrix.

microvilli serve to increase the absorptive surface of the cell dramatically without necessitating a large increase in cell size. Some of the most unique cells are those specialized for sensory reception. The stereocilia hair cell bundles atop cochlear hair cells are exquisitely sensitive to movements induced by sound. Similarly, photoreceptors in the retina of the eye can detect a single quantum unit of light. Some cells, such as neurons, have processes that can stretch for several feet to enable the uninterrupted transfer

of messages to the brain. Remember, although all cells possess the same anatomic parts, they possess rather diverse abilities and functional attributes.

CELLS ASSOCIATE TO FORM COMPLEX TISSUES AND ORGANS

With the exception of blood cells and immune cells, most cells form long-term associations with one another that result in recognizable tissues.

Tissues can then associate to form specialized organs. There are more than 200 types of cells in the human body. These associate to form such varied tissues as epithelia, connective tissue, muscle tissue, and nervous tissue. Epithelial tissues, such as skin, form sheets of cells that line the internal and external surfaces of the body. Connective tissues fill the spaces between organs and tissues. These tissues include bone, fat, and an extracellular matrix that is secreted by the cells themselves. We have already discussed how the cytoskeletal elements in muscle cells allow muscles to produce force by contracting. Nervous tissue is specialized for communication. A network of neurons and specialized supporting cells allows the brain to receive information from the environment and to give commands to muscles and other specialized tissues and organs. Figure 4-6 presents several common types of tissues.

⌁SUMMARY∿

Basic cellular anatomy and physiology have been presented as a background for understanding the complex nature of tissues and organs. The functional anatomy of the plasma membrane and organelles such as the nucleus, ER, Golgi apparatus, ribosomes, and mitochondria are discussed. The membranous and cytoskeletal components of cell structure are described as functionally cooperative assemblies designed to meet the various needs of the cell, including signal transduction, production of macromolecules, and proliferation. Cells can form long-term associations with one another to produce various types of tissues such as epithelia, muscle tissue, and connective and nervous tissue.

⌁KEY TERMS∿

Actin filament

ATP

Cytoskeleton

Endoplasmic reticulum

Golgi apparatus

Intermediate filament

Lipid bilayer

Microtubule

Mitochondria

Nucleolus

Nucleus

Plasma membrane

Ribosome

⌁STUDY QUESTIONS∿

1. Draw a diagram of a living cell. Label the important organelles.

2. List four components of the membrane system. Discuss how these components communicate with one another.

3. List the three types of cytoskeletal elements and the important functions of each.

4. Research an organ found in the human body (your choice). Identify several different types of cells and tissues found in that organ. Consider how the different cells or tissues must interact to ensure proper organ function.

⤳REFERENCES⤶

Alberts, B., Johnson, A., Lewis, J., Raff, M., Roberts, K., & Walter, P. (Eds.). (2002). *Molecular biology of the cell* (4th ed.). New York: Garland Publishing.

Doxsey, S., Zimmerman, W., & Mikule, K. (2005). Centrosome control of the cell cycle. *Trends in Cell Biology, 15*(6), 303–311.

Lambrechts, A., Van Troys, M., & Ampe, C. (2004). The actin cytoskeleton in normal and pathological cell motility. *International Journal of Biochemistry & Cell Biology, 36,* 1890–1909.

Samaj, J., Baluska, F., Voigt, B., Schlict, M., Volkmann, D., & Menzel, D. (2004). Endocytosis, actin cytoskeleton, and signaling. *Plant Physiology, 135,* 1150–1161.

Stryer, L. (1999). *Biochemistry* (4th ed.). New York: W. H. Freeman and Company.

Vaughan, K. T. (2005). Microtubule plus ends, motors, and traffic of Golgi membranes. *Biochimica et Biophysica Acta, 1744,* 316–324.

Wittmann, T., & Desai, A. (2005). Microtubule cytoskeleton: A new twist at the end. *Current Biology, 15*(4), R126–R129.

Chapter

5

Introduction to Neurons and Synapses

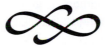

William W. Clark, Ph.D.
Director, Program in Audiology
and Communication Sciences
Washington University School of Medicine
St. Louis, Missouri

Many students who are attracted to the fields of communication sciences—audiology, speech-language pathology, hearing or speech science—do so because of an interest in the communication process. Communication is generally thought of as a process that facilitates interaction between individuals and is accomplished by transmitting a physical stimulus, such as speech, from a sender to a receiver. In a physiologic sense, it refers to the ability of our nervous system to sense and interact with the environment. This is accomplished entirely (as far as we know) through the senses—sight, hearing, taste, smell, and touch.

Communication is also necessary within an organism. This chapter explores one of the most fundamental communication processes known to humans: the exchange of information within and between the individual cells of the nervous system. In virtually every multicellular organism, cells are the building blocks of organs and tissues that perform unique functions or communicate with the external environment. These organs are controlled by other specialized cells that make up the nervous system. Nerve cells, or **neurons,** are the communicators of the internal environment, signaling to each other and to glands and muscles. Neurons also communicate with the other major cell type in nervous systems, called **glial cells.** Through a complicated "wiring" network, nerve cells can sense changes in the internal environment, initiate appropriate "corrective" action, and cause a physiologic change that restores the internal environment within preset limits. This process is called **homeostasis** (derived from Greek, meaning "keep the same"). A good example of a homeostatic mechanism is blood pressure regulation.

When you stand up from a sitting or horizontal position, your blood tends to stay put; that is, its weight stretches the vessels in your legs and lower torso, and it accumulates in your lower extremities and flows downward out of your head (not a good thing!). However, receptors, called *baroreceptors,* are located in the carotid arteries just below the skull. When you stand up, blood flowing out of your head creates a pressure reduction that is sensed by these receptors, and an electrical signal is sent first to centers in the brain, then to cardiac muscle, and finally to smooth muscle around peripheral blood vessels. As a result, heart rate increases, smooth muscle tightens around the blood vessels in the body, particularly in the lower extremities, and the blood is squeezed out of the lower extremities and pumped toward the head, resulting in a restitution of blood flow to the brain. When the carotid baroreceptors are no longer stimulated by low pressure, the reflex is turned off and normal control of blood flow resumes. This reflex is a good example of a **homeostatic mechanism** within an organism, and it is one of thousands of reflexes that are ongoing as animals maintain their internal environment, sense and explore their world, and learn. A key component of all homeostatic mechanisms, in addition to the sensors and muscles, is the "wiring" that connects them, neurons and synapses.

This chapter presents a basic introduction to nerve cells and synapses. It is intended to give a general overview of the structure and function of nerve cells and to provide a foundation for the more comprehensive information about the auditory nervous system provided in Chapters 11, 12, and 14. Because most audiology students have been exposed to the basic concepts of neurophysiology in undergraduate biology courses, this chapter provides only a general review. (For more comprehensive reviews, see the References at the end of this chapter.)

STRUCTURE OF THE NEURON

The structure of the nervous system basically follows its **ontogenetic development.** That is, as we develop from an embryo into a complex individual, our cellular structure and organization become more complex and interconnected. As one moves upward from the spinal cord, increasingly complex neural connections are observed in the brainstem and subcortical structures, as well as the cerebellum; the most complex interactions are located in cortical regions. But first, let us consider the neuron itself.

Neurons are the basic building blocks of the nervous system. Their function is to communicate information. Communication is achieved by transmitting input from one or many sources through

Function   Regions   Structure

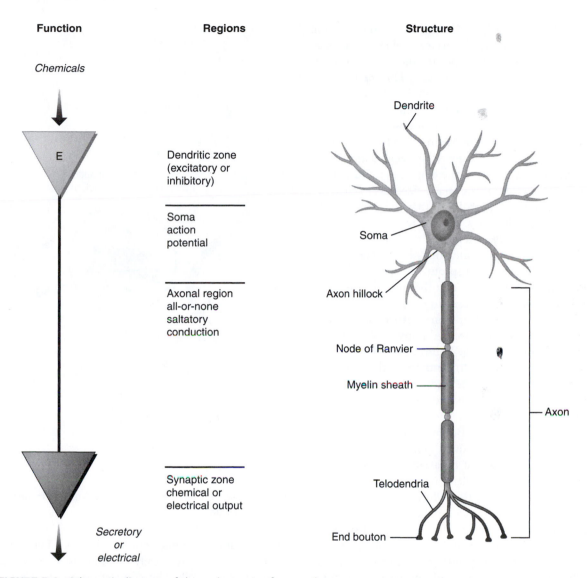

Chemicals

E

Dendritic zone
(excitatory or
inhibitory)

Soma
action
potential

Axonal region
all-or-none
saltatory
conduction

Synaptic zone
chemical or
electrical output

Secretory
or
electrical

Dendrite

Soma

Axon hillock

Node of Ranvier

Myelin sheath

Axon

Telodendria

End bouton

FIGURE 5-1 Schematic diagram of the major parts of a generic neuron.

the neuron to a target, which can be another neuron, organ, gland, muscle fiber, or sensory receptor. Similarly, the input to the neuron can come from another neuron, from a muscle or gland, or from a sensory receptor. Figure 5-1 presents a schematic representation of a generalized neuron. Remember, actual neurons in vertebrates take on many forms, and there are several variants of the described general structure.

The neuron is composed of four general zones: (1) an "input" zone where specific chemical stimuli provide excitatory or inhibitory input, (2) an "action" zone where the input is summed and an electrochemical output is generated, (3) a "transmission" zone that carries the output to its target, and (4) an "output" zone where the neuron secretes chemical or electrical output to another neuron or to a receptor.

Although Figure 5-1 illustrates a single neuron in isolation, it is important to remember that all neurons connect on either end to other neurons or receptors, or to muscles or organs. The *input zone* is called the **dendrite,** and information from the dendrites is transmitted toward the cell body, called the **soma.** Many neurons are composed of complex dendritic extensions, sometimes called **dendritic arborization,** and the dendrites receive input from numerous cells. Input to the dendrites is either electrical or chemical; it is characterized as "excitatory" if it increases the probability that the cell will discharge, and "inhibitory" if it decreases the probability of subsequent cell activity.

The *action zone* includes the cell body, the soma, and the root that sprouts the axon, called the **axon hillock.** It is here that the input to the cell is summed, and the resulting electrical voltage changes create the all-or-none **action potential.**

The *transmission zone* is the axon. It carries the electrical discharge of the neuron from the source to the destination, the **telodendria.** Although axons are relatively short in the auditory system, they can be long (a few feet) in the neurons that control musculature of the legs and feet (and as long as 20 feet in the squid!). Because electrical activity is transmitted relatively slowly along the axon, many neurons are surrounded by a fatty **myelin sheath.** The myelin sheath insulates the axon along most of its length and prevents the diffusion of ions across the cell wall. Interspersed along the myelin sheath are segmented nonmyelinated areas called **nodes of Ranvier.** The nodes speed up electrical conduction along the axon by permitting the electrical current to "jump" from node to node, rather than diffusing along the entire length of the membrane. This type of conduction is called **saltatory conduction,** and it is much faster than conduction created by diffusion of ions along the length of an unmyelinated axon.

The *output zone* is called the *telodendria.* It is composed of long, thin strands of neural tissue that end in **terminal boutons.** These "buttons" are packed with neurotransmitters that can be released when the neuron is activated. Neurons are connected to each other in chainlike fashion, with the output zone of an activating neuron connecting

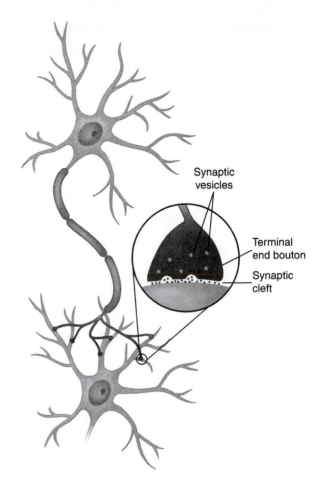

FIGURE 5-2   Terminal end bouton, synaptic cleft, and synaptic vesicles.

closely with the input zone of the next. The connection is not anatomically continuous; a small gap exists between cells. The connection between neurons is called a **synapse.** It includes the terminal bouton, the **synaptic cleft,** and the cell wall of the receptor neuron(s) or tissue. Stimulation of the neuron causes release of neurotransmitters into the synaptic cleft. These neurotransmitters are absorbed by the dendrites or cell body of the adjacent neuron, causing electrochemical changes. The boutons also contain mitochondria that provide the energy source for the release, reuptake, and regeneration of the neurotransmitters. Figure 5-2 presents a schematic of the terminal bouton and synaptic cleft.

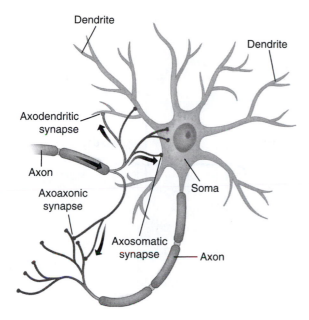

FIGURE 5-3 Axodendritic, axosomatic, and axoaxonic synapses.

Neurons are linked to each other by their synapses. Although the synapse commonly occurs on the dendrite (axodendritic) or the soma (axosomatic) of the target neuron, some axons connect directly to other axons (axoaxonic). Figure 5-3 provides a schematic of these types of connections.

Several types of neurons exist in the central nervous system (CNS). **Unipolar** neurons have a single, bifurcating process that comes off the cell soma. **Multipolar neurons** have more than two processes. Neurons in the auditory system are **bipolar neurons;** that is, they have two processes and resemble the structure shown in the schematic of Figure 5-1.

The majority of the estimated 10 billion neurons in the nervous system are called **interneurons,** which connect one neuron to another (Lorente de No, 1981). Neurons are further classified as afferent or efferent. **Afferent** neurons conduct information toward the brain from the periphery. Sensory input, including audition, is afferent in nature. **Efferent** neurons conduct information away from the brain toward the periphery. Motor neurons are efferent in

nature, and they control movement of a glands or muscles. Chapters 11 and 12 explain that the auditory system is composed of both afferent and efferent fibers. The afferent fibers conduct auditory (sensory) information toward the brain, and the efferent fibers control the sensitivity of the outer hair cells of the cochlea.

FUNCTION OF NEURONS

Neurons represent the primary messenger system within the nervous system. Through their interconnections, they perform an astonishing variety of tasks. In the cochlea, for example, hundreds of outer hair cells may be connected to a single neuron; in contrast, dozens of neurons may terminate on a single inner hair cell. These quite different "wiring diagrams" imply important functional differences between outer and inner hair cells and, as discussed in later chapters, provide the basis for a new understanding of active and nonlinear processing in the ear.

Although neural connections are extremely complicated, the basic function of the neuron is quite simple. Neurons are simple pulse generators that accept input from other neurons or cells, add up that input in the cell body, and trigger a pulse output to other neurons or cells that are connected to the axon. These functions are said to be electrochemical in nature, and a summary of the principal components of neural transduction follows.

Resting Potentials

Like other cells in the body, the neuron has a multi-layer cell wall that separates its internal environment from the extracellular fluids. And, like other cells, the neuron maintains a chemical separation from the extracellular fluids that produces voltage differential across the cell walls. The voltage differential is due to both passive and active processes. When chemicals are dissolved into solutions, they form molecules that carry electrical charge. The value of the charge depends on whether an electron has been added or subtracted from the molecule. For example, potassium (K^+) has one positive charge, and chloride (Cl^-) has one negative charge. The cell wall of a neuron is permeable to ions, and if the sum of the positive and negative charges on each side of the membrane is equal, there will be no net flow of ions across the membrane. However, if the ionic concentrations differ across the cell wall, an **electrochemical gradient** will exist across the cell wall. Consider the example illustrated in Figure 5-4. In Figure 5-4A, a beaker that is divided into two compartments is separated by a **semipermeable membrane.** The membrane is said to be semipermeable, because although many ions can pass through it, they may do so at different rates, and large molecules cannot pass at all. The beaker is filled on both sides with a fluid that contains potassium and chloride in equal concentrations. A voltmeter is connected to electrodes inserted into the fluid on either side of the membrane. The voltmeter displays the potential difference (in volts) across the membrane. Because the concentrations, and the resultant electrical charges, are the same on both sides of the membrane, there will be no "pressure" for the ions to move, and the electrical charge (i.e., the sum of the positive and negative charges on either side of the membrane) will be zero, resulting in a voltage difference across the membrane of 0 V.

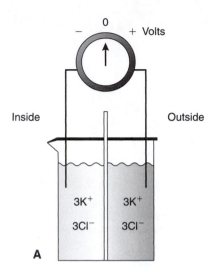

FIGURE 5-4   The effect of an ionic concentration gradient on the potential (voltage) difference across a semipermeable membrane. (A) A beaker contains potassium and chloride ions in the same concentrations across a semipermeable membrane stretched across the center. Because the concentrations of the ions are the same on both sides of the beaker, there is no concentration gradient, and a voltmeter with leads inserted into each side will record a zero charge difference (0 V). (B) The concentration of potassium (K^+) ions is increased by 10-fold on the right side of the beaker. The voltmeter now records a negative voltage, because the number of positive ions on the right side of the beaker now exceeds the positive ions on the left. (C) The concentration gradient and the voltage gradient produced by the action indicated in (B). The greater concentration of potassium on the right side causes a flow of potassium ions across the membrane from high concentration to low. Conversely, the voltage gradient produced by the unequal concentrations moves in the opposite direction, toward electric neutrality.

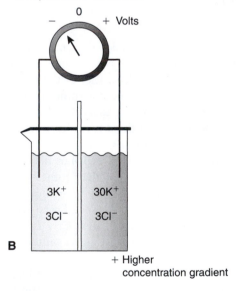

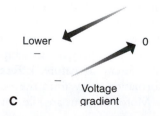

Now, let us pour some potassium into the right half of the beaker, until the concentration of potassium on the right side is 10 times that on the left, as shown in Figure 5-4B. Now, a concentration imbalance exists, and a **concentration gradient** is created that reflects the much greater concentration of positively charged potassium ions on the right side (Figure 5-4C). The imbalance also results in an excess of positively charged ions on the right side of the beaker, creating a voltage difference across the membrane that is recorded as a negative voltage on the meter, because the left side of the beaker contains fewer positive ions than the right side. Immediately after the potassium is poured into the right side, the potassium ions diffuse passively across the barrier, and the rate of diffusion depends on the size of the pores in the membrane, the temperature, and the relative differences in concentration on the two sides. The movement of potassium ions down the concentration gradient also transfers positive ions from the right side of the beaker to the left, reducing the voltage concurrently back toward 0 V. Eventually, the concentrations of all the ions would equalize again across the membrane, and the voltage differential would return to 0 V.

In reality, electrodes inserted into nerve cells record a potential difference of about −50 millivolts (mV) with respect to the outside of the cell. Unless the cell is acted on in some way, this potential is stable and is called a **resting potential.** It is created by an active process that "pumps" ions across the membrane and creates a concentration gradient and voltage difference. The keys to the active process are two proteins, **adenosine triphosphate (ATP)** and **sodium–potassium ATPase (Na-K, ATPase).** Na-K, ATPase is essentially a mechanical motor, pushing potassium (K^+) ions out of the cell and transmitting sodium (Na^+) ions into it. The "fuel" for the motor comes from the breakdown of the ATP protein into two components, ADP and P, which releases energy into the pump. Metabolic energy is then expended within the cell to reconstitute the ADP and P back into an ATP protein, and the process starts again. Figure 5-5 is a schematic of the action of the pump.

The key to the action of the pump is that it is not electrically neutral; for every rotation, three

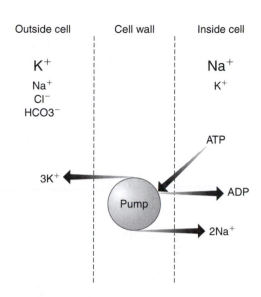

FIGURE 5-5 Role of the active sodium-potassium pump on intracellular and extracellular concentration of potassium and sodium. The pump maintains an ionic concentration difference, and resulting charge and voltage difference across the cell membrane.

potassium ions are discharged from the inside of the cell into the extracellular environment, and only two sodium ions are pumped into the cell. Because sodium and potassium ions each have one positive charge, the result is a charge difference across the cell membrane with more positive ions on the outside than on the inside, creating a voltage difference across the cell wall, with the internal cell environment being negative. It should be remembered that the pump is actually pushing ions against the concentration gradient, thereby increasing the concentration differences across the membrane and increasing the force of the concentration gradient in opposition to the pump process. When these forces just equal the force of the pump, the system is said to be in a state of electrochemical equilibrium. Most nerve cells have equilibrium, or "resting" potentials, of about −50 mV.

An analogy might help to illustrate this concept. Imagine a fancy nightclub that is equally attractive to men and women, and the number of men and women who come to the club are approximately equal. The doors to the club are wide open, and men and women can freely pass in and out. At any time, the mix of men and women would be approximately the same inside and outside the club. But now imagine the club owner hires a big, tough bouncer who is assigned to eject three men from the club for every two he admits. After a while, the distribution of men inside and outside the club changes: more and more of the men end up outside the club, clamoring to get back in, and fewer men are inside. Because the bouncer uses up energy in the process, he has to be fed to restore his strength. Furthermore, as he continues to throw out more men than he admits, his job gets harder, because the men accumulate around the door, pushing to get back in to the club. Eventually, a new steady state is obtained, one in which there are more men outside the club than inside it. More importantly, the force of the men trying to diffuse back into the club is equal to the force of the bouncer pushing them out. This is the state of things inside a normal nerve cell. Because there are more potassium (men) ions outside than inside the cell, and relatively fewer sodium (other men) ions inside, a resting potential of about -50 mV is maintained.

Synaptic Transmission between Nerve Cells

Describing the sequence of events that leads to the activation of a neuron is a little circular. Because all neurons have an input and an output, there is no "starting place" for describing the action. However, given that we now have our idealized neuron sitting at a potential difference between the inside and the outside of the cell of -50 mV, let us consider what happens to the internal electrical potential when the dendrite is stimulated by electrical or chemical input. Although the "normal" mode of neural transmission in the auditory system is exclusively through chemical synapses, all neurons can be activated electrically. In fact, neurons in cardiac tissue communicate normally by electrical transmission. That auditory neurons can be stimulated electrically, as well as neurochemically, allows individuals with profound sensorineural hearing loss to use cochlear implants effectively to stimulate surviving auditory nerve fibers electrically.

For our purposes, it is sufficient to remember that the auditory system can be stimulated electrically, even though the "normal" route of synaptic transmission is chemical. Both modes of stimulation lead to changes in the resting potential of the cell, which affect its excitability. Further complicating our discussion is that a specific dendrite, such as that shown schematically in Figure 5-1, is called *presynaptic* within that cell because it exists along the chain before the synapse. However, remember that the dendrite gets its input "downstream" from other neurons, and its dendrite is "after" the synapse of the preceding cell (see Figures 5-2 and 5-3). Therefore, any voltage change induced in the dendrite that is created by input from the synapse from a previous cell is called *postsynaptic*.

The dendrites contain specific receptor molecules that combine with neurotransmitters coming into contact with the dendrite. The actions within the target neuron fall into two classes: one rather rapid process that affects *ion channels* in the neuron, and another, slower process that creates biochemical changes in the neuron.

For the purposes of this chapter, we are limiting the discussion to the ion-channel effects. Ion channels are formed by the proteins of the plasma membrane, and they provide routes for facilitated diffusion of molecules down their concentration gradient. Ion channels are selective; that is, they are structured to allow only specific ions to pass through the membrane wall. An additional characteristic of many ion channels is that they can be closed or opened by external events. For example, in neurons, a reduction in voltage across the membrane opens sodium ion channels, resulting in an influx of Na^+, which further reduces the voltage inside the cell and serves to propagate the impulse down the axon.

Neurotransmitters binding to the receptor molecule on the dendrite or soma can be excitatory or inhibitory, depending on whether their activity results in a **depolarization** (a reduction in the negative potential) or a **hyperpolarization** (increasing negativity) of the target neuron. The changes in resting membrane potential caused by the transmitter are referred to as **inhibitory postsynaptic potentials (IPSPs)** or **excitatory postsynaptic**

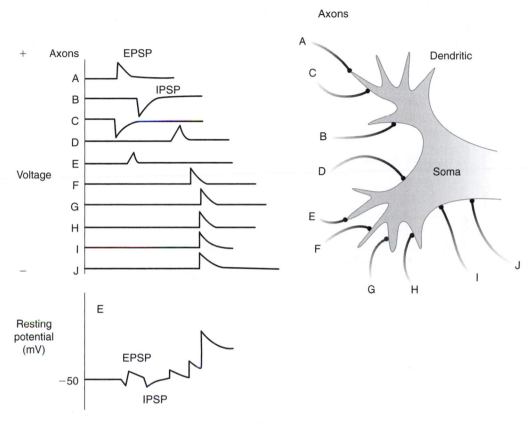

FIGURE 5-6 Illustration of temporal and spatial summation of excitatory (EPSPs) and inhibitory postsynaptic potential (IPSPs). The resting potential inside the cell soma is affected by the excitatory and inhibitory potentials of all the activated neurons that are connected to it. (left) The transient input voltages of the many axons that synapse on the cell. (right) The summed effects on the resting potential measured inside the soma. Note the minipotentials sum both in time (temporally) and over the surface of the dendrite and cell body (spatially).

potentials (EPSPs). These potentials are short-lived, causing an initial abrupt change in receptor potential that decays or "dies out" exponentially. The effects of these mini potentials add up spatially over the region of the dendrite, and they also add up temporally because of the time course of each IPSP or EPSP. An example of spatial and temporal summation and its effect on the resting potential of a cell is given in Figure 5-6.

Initiation of the Action Potential

When the sum of the individual IPSPs and EPSPs creates a critical depolarization near the axon hillock, an action potential is triggered. This action potential is characterized by a rapid and dramatic reversal of membrane potential such that the inside of the cell becomes positive, thought to be due to a rapid influx of Na^+. After the initial "spike" discharge, voltage-activated Na^+ and K^+ channels open sequentially, first creating a hyperpolarization of the cell, and then a gradual recovery to the normal resting potential (see Figure 5-7 for a graphical description). The action potential is then propagated down the axon toward the terminal boutons, with the depolarization opening sodium and potassium channels ahead of the advancing discharge.

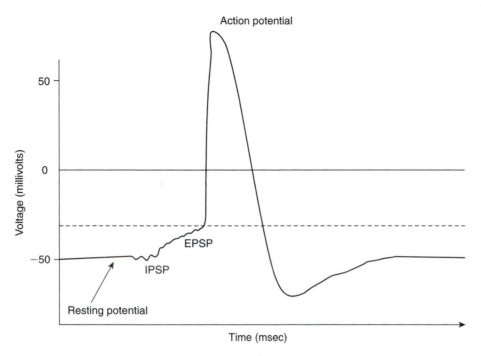

FIGURE 5-7 Voltage change measured in a cell during an action potential. Resting potential: −50 mV. EPSP, excitatory postsynaptic potential; IPSP, inhibitory postsynaptic potential.

Because the action potential is an all-or-nothing phenomenon, it cannot convey information about the strength of its input to the next neuron in the chain. The only information it can transmit is that the sum of the excitatory and inhibitory inputs to the neuron reached a "threshold" depolarization that excited it sufficiently to fire.

Another important factor is that the neuron cannot fire again immediately after generating an action potential. Because the polarization of the neuron is dependent on ion flow, it takes a little while for the active pumps in the neuron to restore its internal ionic environment after an action potential. Immediately after firing, a neuron cannot be reactivated for a period of about 0.5 to 1 millisecond. This period is called the **absolutely refractory period,** during which it cannot fire again, no matter what the stimulus. After the absolutely refractory period, but before the resting potential of the neuron is restored, it is said to be in its **relatively refractory period,** meaning the

neuron can fire, but because it is hyperpolarized, more stimulation is needed. The relatively refractory period extends about 1 millisecond beyond the absolutely refractory period.

From the perspective of the audiologist or hearing scientist, the refractory period of auditory neurons has important consequences. Because the auditory nerve cannot fire at rates greater than about once every millisecond, hearing frequencies that have periods shorter than 1 millisecond (i.e., >1,000 Hz) must require another strategy for coding frequency. Because humans can detect and discriminate signals up to 20,000 Hz, the resolution for coding stimulus frequency is up to 20 times faster than the speed of action potentials from individual auditory nerve fibers. Similarly, designers of cochlear implants must develop alternative stimulus-encoding strategies to allow patients to hear sounds at frequencies that exceed the upper rate limit of individual neurons. These topics are covered in further detail in Chapters 10 and 15.

Propagation of the Action Potential along the Axon

The conduction of a nerve impulse down the axon depends on the passive electrical characteristics of the membrane, its capacitance and its conductance (Best & Taylor, 1966). As current flows from the initial site (the axon hillock), the membrane capacitance is discharged in a spreading pattern, permitting the depolarization of the membrane opening of voltage-gated ion channels ahead of the active region.

The rate of propagation depends on the diameter of the neuron, with larger diameter neurons supporting faster propagation rates. However, even the largest neurons propagate slowly unless a boost is given. The myelination of neurons provides a great "accelerator" for neuron conduction velocity. Nature has solved the "slow speed of conduction" problem in a creative way. Many neurons are wrapped in a myelin sheath that is interrupted periodically along the axon by the nodes of Ranvier. The myelin insulates the membrane, and its high resistance (i.e., low conductance) prevents flow of electricity across the insulated portion of the membrane. In contrast, the nodes of Ranvier are uninsulated and contain the voltage-gated Na^+ channels. This arrangement allows the action potential to "jump" from node to node, greatly increasing conduction velocity. This mode of conduction is called *saltatory conduction.* Most of the neurons in the auditory system are surrounded by myelin sheaths. In fact, the neurons of the auditory nerve are myelinated along most of their length and they lose the sheath only as they pass into the cochlea through small openings in the modiolus, called **habenula perforata.**

Synaptic Zone

The synaptic zone, including the telodendria, the terminal boutons, and the synaptic cleft, is the manufacturing center for the packaging, distribution, and recycling of neurotransmitters. Neurotransmitters are transported in *synaptic vesicles,* which are protein structures that serve as microscopic dump trucks for the loading, transport, and dumping of neurotransmitters. Synaptic vesicles are assembled in the cell soma and transported by an intracellular mechanism to the synaptic zone. Once they reach the synaptic zone, they mature into specialized structures that are coded by their shape for specific neurotransmitters. In the synaptic zone, they open and are loaded with a tiny amount (a "quantum") of a specific neurotransmitter. Loaded synaptic vesicles then coalesce near the thick membrane of the synaptic cleft as individual vesicles, each loaded with a small quantity of neurotransmitter.

When the action potential reaches the synaptic zone, voltage-gated calcium channels activated by the membrane depolarization open and cause an influx of calcium ions into the presynaptic terminals. The influx of calcium ions causes the synaptic vesicles to attach to the presynaptic cell membrane, to open into the synaptic space, and to release their contents into the synaptic cleft. Each packet is called a *quantum,* and the number of vesicles, and therefore quanta, released is determined by the influx of calcium. After the transmitter is released, the membrane of the synaptic vesicle is resorbed into the presynaptic neuron for reuse.

NEUROTRANSMITTERS

Neurotransmitters are defined as chemical substances that are synthesized by neurons, released into synaptic spaces by activation of the neuron, and have specific actions on target cells, muscles, or glands (Brown, 2001, p. 85). Many of the chemical substances identified as neurotransmitters are amino acids. Of these, γ-aminobutyric acid (GABA) is a major inhibitory transmitter found throughout the vertebrate CNS. Another amino acid, glutamate, has been shown to be a major excitatory transmitter. Other neurotransmitters are found among the biogenic amines, including catecholamine, adrenaline, noradrenaline, dopamine, histamine, and serotonin. The other low-molecular-weight transmitters are acetylcholine and ATP.

Several types of neurotransmitters are found within the auditory system, including GABA and glutamate. The known roles of specific transmitters are discussed in Chapters 10, 11, and 12, and how various neurotransmitters affect normal and pathologic auditory processes is an area of active investigation. In the auditory system, glutamate appears to be the major excitatory neurotransmitter for the afferent fibers connected to inner hair cells. Chapter 12 explains that the efferent fibers, which carry information from the brain to the sensory cells of the cochlea, are inhibitory in nature, and most contain GABA. Normal auditory function, therefore, depends on a delicate balance among the supply, utilization, and efferent (inhibitory) and afferent (excitatory) activities in the sensory cells.

⌁SUMMARY⌁

At its core, the basis of all human communication is electrochemical. Organisms must depend on complex neural signaling systems to sense and interact with the environment and other organisms, to maintain control of internal systems, and to react to threats and opportunities. Like any other sense, hearing depends on complex interactions of excitatory and inhibitory stimuli, active metabolic events, and chemical reactions to maintain sensitivity and do its job. The goal of this chapter was to introduce fundamental concepts about the structure and function of neurons to aid in understanding the processes related to hearing that are described more fully in Chapters 11, 12, and 15.

⌁KEY TERMS⌁

Absolutely refractory period
Action potential
Adenosine triphosphate
Afferent
Axon hillock
Concentration gradient
Dendrite
Dendritic arborization
Depolarization

Efferent
Electrochemical gradient
EPSP, IPSP
Glial cells
Habenula perforata
Homeostasis
Homeostatic mechanism
Hyperpolarization
Interneurons
Multipolar neurons

Myelin sheath
Neurons
Neurotransmitter
Nodes of Ranvier
Ontogenetic development
Relatively refractory period
Resting potential
Saltatory conduction
Semipermeable membrane

Sodium–potassium ATPase
Soma
Synapse
Synaptic cleft
Telodendria
Terminal boutons
Unipolar, bipolar neurons

⌁STUDY QUESTIONS⌁

1. How does a nerve cell maintain its resting potential?

2. What is the biological advantage of myelination of nerve fibers, and how does it work?

3. What are the four functional zones of neurons, and how do they differ from each other?

4. What would happen to the membrane potential of a neuron if the active pump was poisoned?

5. Describe the process by which synaptic vesicles are created and released into the synaptic cleft.

⌁REFERENCES⌁

Best, C. H., & Taylor, N. B. (1966). *The physiological basis of medical practice.* Baltimore: Williams & Wilkins.

Brown, A.G. (2001). *Nerve cells and nervous systems: An introduction to neuroscience* (2nd ed.). London: Springer-Verlag.

Lorente de No, R. (1981). *The primary acoustic nuclei.* New York: Raven Press.

Seikel, J. A., King, D., & Drumwright, D. (2005). *Anatomy and physiology for speech, language, and hearing* (4th ed.). Clifton Park, NY: Thomson Delmar Learning.

Part
II

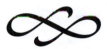

Anatomy and Physiology

Chapter

6

Development of the Ear

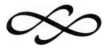

Dwayne D. Simmons, Ph.D.
Associate Professor of Otolaryngology
Washington University School of Medicine
St. Louis, Missouri

The development of the ear is one of the more remarkable examples of engineering in the vertebrate body. The ear is a composite structure with a complex embryonic origin. It is organized into three anatomic parts that differ from each other in structure and embryonic origin. The inner ear consists of organs for hearing and balance and is embedded in a petrous temporal bone. The middle ear consists of a tympanic space with three auditory ossicles and an auditory tube. The external ear consists of the **auricle** (pinna), the external acoustic (auditory) meatus, and the tympanic membrane (eardrum). The external and middle parts of the ear regulate the transfer of sound waves from the environment to the inner ear.

Although a lot of information has been obtained from studies of the human embryo (e.g., Bredberg, 1967, 1968; Tanaka, Sakai & Terayama, 1979), by far the majority of what we know comes from studies of rodent embryos and postnatal pups. Most of what is known about the genes involved in the formation of the inner ear comes from studies of ear defects found in various gene deletion (null) mutations in mouse models. The inner, middle, and external ears begin to develop a little after 3 weeks' **gestation** and are complete before the end of the third **trimester.** In the embryo, the inner ear is the first to develop and originates as epidermal placodes (thickenings or discs) that appear on either side of the head at the level of the future hindbrain. The **otic placode** then develops into an **otocyst,** or otic vesicle, a structure that has highly differentiated, sharply defined tissue borders. The otocyst gives rise to the hearing (cochlea) and vestibular (saccule, utrical, and semicircular canals) organs. While the inner ear is differentiating, the external and middle ears develop from structures of the first and second **pharyngeal arches** and from the intervening pharyngeal cleft (groove) and pouch. Toward the beginning of the third trimester (roughly 28–29 weeks), much of the development has occurred and the fetus is capable of responding to sounds. Figure 6-1 illustrates the development of the inner, middle, and external ears. In the fetus, the ear starts to function as the auditory system matures, and by birth, it is fully capable of analyzing sounds in the environment. Immediately after birth, hearing capability continues to mature through early childhood. These postnatal improvements include absolute thresholds, frequency discrimination, and binaural hearing.

MORPHOGENESIS OF THE EAR

Embryogenesis of the Inner Ear

The formation of the inner ear is extremely complex. To form highly specialized organs of hearing and balance, specific afferent and efferent innervation patterns, and exquisite tuning of sensory structures, the inner ear requires the progress and interaction of multiple cellular events and numerous tissues. During the first and second trimesters of pregnancy, rudimentary gene networks play fundamental roles in the initial patterning of the inner ear. The **morphogenesis** of inner ear organs requires cellular specification, followed by fate determination, and it is dependent on multiple signaling cues from surrounding mesodermal and endodermal tissues. During inner ear formation, activation of specific genes is required to guide the subsequent commitment and fate determination of auditory and vestibular cells. Furthermore, this process must be orchestrated with neural growth and synapse formation to achieve normal hearing and balance function.

Signals are released from the developing hindbrain (rhombencephalon), the area that will become the cerebellum and medulla oblongata, and stimulate the exterior lining of the embryo to form a thickened concentration of embryonic cells on each side. A number of genes are expressed either in or adjacent to the ectodermal area that will become the inner ear (Figure 6-2). Candidate genes for inner ear induction include members of the fibroblast growth factor *(Fgf)* family and a number of transcription factors, including members of the *Pax* gene family. These genes are believed to have some role in inducing the ectodermal tissues toward placode formation, and ultimately inner ear formation. Ear induction begins with a state of placode competence, followed by the specification of the otic field, and then a progressive acquisition of identity and commitment to the otic fate until an irreversible state of

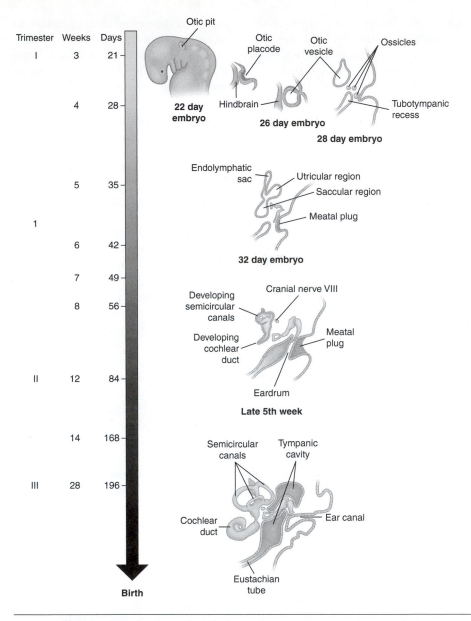

The external ear develops from six auricular hillocks located on the facing margins of the first and second pharyngeal arches.

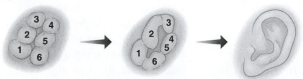

FIGURE 6-1 Developmental timeline of the inner, middle, and outer ears. (Adapted from W. J. Larsen, 1997, and D. D. Simmons, 2003.)

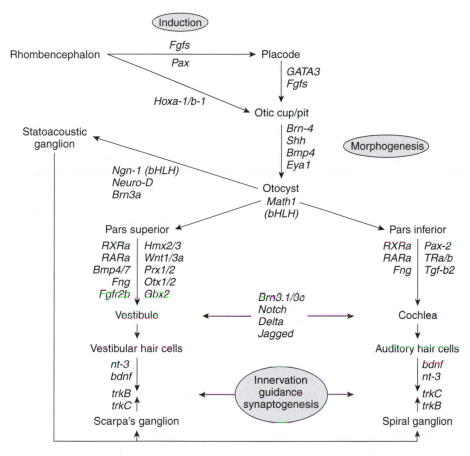

FIGURE 6-2 Flow chart of tissues and some of the known genes that are involved in the development of the inner ear. (Adapted from Frenz et al., 2001.)

determination is reached (Larsen, 1997; Steel & Bock, 1985, Noramly & Grainger, 2002; Simmons, 2003). A common early phase of ear development results in placode induction and otocyst formation. Each of these two developmental pathways appears to follow a largely similar trajectory, using molecular variations on a common set of genes such as basic helix loop helix *(bHLH)* genes *(Math1, Ngn1, NeuroD)*, POU transcription factors *(Brn3* family), and neurotrophins and their receptors (brain-derived neurotrophic factor/neurotrophin-3 [BDNF/NT3], tyrosine receptor kinase B [trkB]/trkC).

Thickenings of the surface **ectoderm** or placodes are found in the 22-day-old embryo (roughly 2 mm in length). During the fourth week, otic placodes rapidly fold inward and form hollow vesi-

cles called *otocysts.* Over the next 7 to 14 days, each vesicle gives rise to a membranous labyrinth from which all inner ear sensory organs and the endolymphatic duct form. During the sixth to eighth gestational week, the saccule forms a tubular outpocketing at its lower pole that penetrates the surrounding **mesenchymal** tissue. This outgrowth, the cochlear duct, begins to coil until it has completed two-and-one-half turns and begins to resemble the shell shape called the *cochlea.* Its connection with the remaining portion of the saccule is then confined to a narrow pathway, the ductus reunions.

Morphogenesis transforms the otocyst into the three-dimensional shape of the inner ear, a labyrinth of ducts and recesses. The morphogenesis of the ear is accomplished in a series of interdependent steps that include patterning, growing, and sculpting. The morphogenesis of the otocyst is governed by a set of patterning genes that includes zinc finger proteins such as GATA3, members of the bone morphogenic proteins (BMP), FGF, homeodomain transcription factors *(Hox),* and *Pax* transcription factors (see Figure 6-2). Periotic mesenchymal tissues surrounding the cochlear duct are further stimulated to form the protective bony labyrinth and membranes that separate different areas of the inner ear. This process begins in the 10th gestational week in which the cartilaginous shell of the cochlear duct undergoes vacuolization (cavitation), and two perilymphatic spaces, the scala vestibuli and scala tympani, are formed. The cochlear duct is then separated from the scala vestibuli by the vestibular (Reissner's) membrane and from the scala tympani by the basilar membrane. The lateral wall of the cochlear duct remains attached to the surrounding cartilage by the spiral ligament, whereas its medial portion is connected to and partly supported by a long cartilaginous process, the modiolus, the future axis of the bony cochlea (see Figure 6-1).

Before focusing on sensory hair cells and synapses, we summarize the general trends of cochlear maturation. The coiled cochlea follows a general gradient of development from base to apex—a gradient applicable either to gross morphologic development or to the maturation of subcellular components, mechanism, or both. The most apical part of the cochlea retains some underdeveloped features into adulthood. This appears true both from a morphologic point of view and from a general physiologic perspective. Studies in rodents demonstrate that at the onset of auditory function, when most cochlear structures are still underdeveloped, the physiologic responses of the cochlea have high thresholds and poor tuning (Walsh, McGee & Javel, 1986; Walsh & McGee, 1990). However, some active properties can be detected quite early in basal regions of the cochlea, and they mature quickly. Apical regions of the cochlea develop much slower, and the most apical parts retain primarily passive behavior, rather than the active cochlear mechanics associated with basal regions.

The growth of the otocyst is paralleled by the sculpting of the canals and the formation of neurons that innervate specific sensory epithelia.

GATA enhancer binding protein *(GATA3),* transcription coactivators such as *Eya1,* and Fgf proteins are essential for the growth and overall development of the ear past the otocyst. These genes are expressed in the ear and promote their effect by interacting with other genes expressed in the ear and may change their expression in null mutants. Genes that result primarily in a cochlear or ventral otocyst defect affect ventral patterning either through a diffusion gradient, such as for sonic hedgehog *(Shh),* or by being differentially expressed, such as with *Pax2.* Mutations in these genes form only a short cochlear duct. The vestibular system forms at least the vertical canals in such mutations. Genes that cause primarily a vestibular phenotype when mutated exert their effect from their expression in the brain. Genes that fall into this category are *Wnt1/3a* and possibly *Gbx2.* Other genes expressed in the ear such as *Hmx2/3* cause almost as much defect as *Wnt1/3a* double-null animals. The phenotype of such mutants is an elongated sack that may be composed of the endolymphatic duct and parts of the cochlea. Other genes exert their effects via expressions in the otocyst. Despite different expression patterns, *Fgf10* null mutations have a phenotype somewhat similar to *Gbx2* null mutations, but they also have lost the horizontal canal. The *Otx1* transcription factor null mice lack only a horizontal canal and show a confluence of utricle and saccule. An Fgf receptor *(Fgfr2b)* null mouse develops a sacklike ear somewhat similar to the homeodomain *Hmx2/3* and *Wnt (1/3a)* factor null mice. Figure 6-2 summarizes some of the known genes that guide inner ear formation.

Development of Sensory Hair Cells

Superimposed on the development of the inner ear are also patterning processes that ultimately result in the generation of hair cells and sensory neurons. In general, hair cell and sensory neuron formation each depend on a single proneuronal gene, the mammalian atonal homologue gene *(Math1)* and neurogenin 1 *(ngn-1),* respectively. Null mutation studies show that in addition to *Math1,* POU domain transcription factor *Brn3.1/3c,* as well as other transcription factors such as *Notch, Delta,* and *Jagged* are essential for hair cell development. Intracellular receptors for retinoic acid (Rxr and Rar) and thyroid hormone (TRα and TRβ) are also implicated in controlling cochlear **differentiation,** and especially hair cell number. Initially, epithelial cells of the cochlear duct are alike. With further development, however, epithelial cells of the cochlear duct separate into an inner and an outer ridge. The inner ridge forms the future spiral limbus and associated structures. The outer ridge forms the future sensory epithelium (organ of Corti), where it differentiates into one row of inner and at least three rows of outer hair cells. An acellular, gelatinous substance, the tectorial membrane, attaches to the spiral limbus and eventually extends to the outer hair cells where their stereocilia tips insert. The sensory hair cells, support cells, and the tectorial membrane together will constitute the organ of Corti (Figure 6-3).

Both scanning and transmission electron microscopy indicate the presence of an undifferentiated sensory epithelium with a field of microvilli and kinocilia at the luminal surface. Nerve fibers are already invading this epithelium at a precise location (great epithelial ridge). A few days after invading fibers are seen, hair cells can be distinguished from neighboring support cells. Initially, both types of cochlear hair cells are similar in shape: cylindrical but with a slightly swollen base. Quickly, inner hair cells distinguish themselves by increasing in size and obtaining their characteristic pear-shape. The shape of outer hair cells remains immature longer, until the supporting structures and spaces mature. In general, outer hair cell maturation occurs later than for inner hair cells, and it coincides with changes in the functional properties of cochlea, such as increasing sensitivity gain and frequency selectivity.

The general pattern of differentiation of stereocilia bundles has been described in the mammalian cochlea as a four-stage process. The earliest stages of stereociliary differentiation are similar in both types of cochlear and vestibular hair cells. In the earliest stage, future stereocilia are not significantly morphologically different from surrounding microvilli but are arranged in round and densely packed clusters. In the cochlea, stereociliary differentiation begins with inner hair cells. From the primitive round tuff, a "V-shaped" bundle of stereocilia develops, with the tip

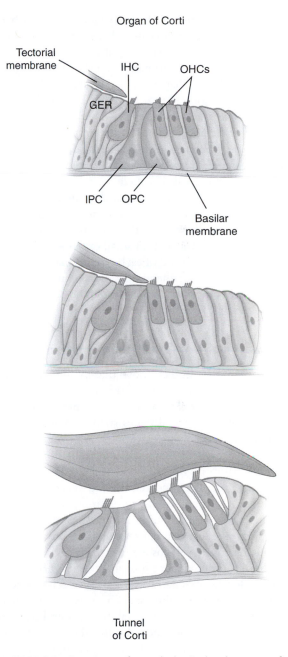

FIGURE 6-3 Sequence of morphologic development of the organ of Corti. IHC, Inner hair cell; OHC, outer hair cell; IPC, inner pillar cell; OPC, outer pillar cell.

of the "V" centered on the kinocilium. On inner hair cells, the V-shaped bundle quickly becomes almost linear. Microvilli and extra stereocilia disappear, and the remaining stereocilia arrange themselves into three or four parallel rows that are graded in length. The tallest stereocilia are located near the kinocilium in the most external row. Before the onset of function, the kinocilium regresses and disappears, first on outer hair cells and then on inner hair cells. The final length of the tallest stereocilia appears to be correlated with the final length of the hair cell itself.

While cells of the cochlear duct are differentiating, the utricular portion of the otic vesicle differentiates sequentially to form the anterior, posterior, and lateral semicircular ducts. A small expansion, the ampulla, forms at one end of each semicircular duct. The hair cell sensory epithelium in the ampullae and the utricle are responsible for detecting the accelerations and orientation of the head.

Development of Hair Cell Innervation

Null mutation studies show that *Ngn-1,* a *bHLH* gene, is essential for the formation of all sensory neurons in the ear. Sensory neuron precursors also express other essential genes such as *NeuroD.* Hair cell innervation involves expression of members of the nerve growth factor family of neurotrophins, namely, BDNF and NT-3, within the sensory epithelium and their corresponding receptors (*trkB* and *trkC*) within the sensory neurons. Sensory neurons develop precise initial projections of their axons into the central nervous system and of their dendrites to the various end organs of the inner ear. Although the neurotrophins most likely play a role, the molecular mechanisms for these precise projection patterns are unknown. The organ of Corti is innervated by the peripheral fibers (dendrites) of the spiral ganglion tucked into the coil of the cochlea. The spiral ganglion, the central fibers of which form the cochlear branch of the vestibulocochlear nerve, innervates the sensory epithelium before the first signs of hair cell differentiation can be observed (about 9–10 weeks' gestation in human fetuses). Scarpa's ganglion, the central fibers of which form the vestibular branch of the vestibulo-

cochlear nerve, innervates vestibular hair cells just before hair cell differentiation as in the cochlear duct. Impulses received by the inner ear sensory organs are transmitted to the brainstem by ganglion neurons whose central axons compose cranial nerve VIII, and they terminate in the brainstem.

Adult cochlear hair cells are innervated by two types of spiral ganglion nerve fibers that send information to the cochlear nuclei. Type I spiral ganglion fibers are contacted directly by the inner hair cells, whereas type II spiral ganglion fibers are contacted by outer hair cells. Two different kinds of efferent nerve fibers from the superior olive in the brainstem also innervate the cochlea: lateral efferents contact the afferent fibers immediately below the inner hair cells, whereas medial efferents make direct (axosomatic) contact with outer hair cells. The development of afferent and efferent innervation is illustrated in Figure 6-4. Afferent nerve fibers invade the cochlear epithelium quite early, even before morphologic differentiation of hair cells can be observed. A characteristic of radial afferents early in development is the dramatic sprouting of nerve fiber endings below inner hair cells. During normal development, this primitive branching is followed by a pruning mechanism that results in the adult unbranched configuration. Mature afferent synapses can be seen in a 12-week-old fetal cochlea, first at inner hair cells and then a few days later at outer hair cells. At this stage, stereocilia are just beginning to grow, and the onset of cochlear function is still 6 to 8 weeks ahead.

Efferent and afferent nerve fibers apparently invade the fetal cochlea about the same time, which is well before the first signs of hair cell differentiation. However, efferent fibers lag somewhat behind afferent fibers in contacting hair cells. Also, the first arriving efferent fibers enter the developing organ of Corti and stay at the inner hair cell level before they go on to invade the outer hair cell region. That efferents destined for (axosomatic) contact with outer hair cells may wait below inner hair cells has been hypothesized to play an important role in the maturation of cochlear function.

By the 14th gestational week, inner hair cell innervation patterns are nearly adult-like. Afferent

Immature cochlear innervation

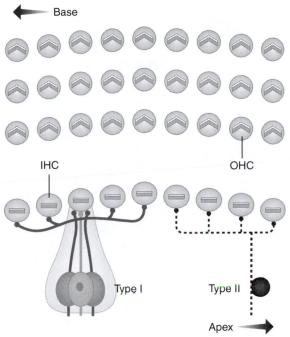

Mature cochlear innervation

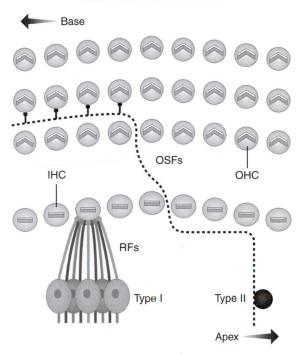

FIGURE 6-4 Development of organ of Corti innervation in the embryonic cochlea. The peripheral fibers from spiral ganglion neurons form radial fibers (RFs) and outer spiral fibers (OSFs) that innervate developing hair cells. *(Left)* RFs in contact with inner hair cells (IHCs) represented by their stereociliary hair bundles. The earliest innervation patterns show single RFs having multiple contacts with IHCs, which is different from the mature pattern where a single RF contacts a single IHC. *(Right)* OSFs in contact with outer hair cells (OHCs). Initially, immature OSFs contact IHCs, then mature OSFs contact the OHCs. (Adapted from Simmons et al., 1991.)

dendrosomatic connections are made with sensory cells, and efferent axodendritic synapses are made among the neuropil underlying inner hair cells. Only afferents are identified in the outer cell region as late as gestational week 16. By week 22, efferent axosomatic synapses are present among outer hair cells, but they are underdeveloped. Surface features such as stereociliary patterns are adult-like at this age. Table 6-1 summarizes the development of sensory and neural structures in the fetal cochlea.

TABLE 6-1 **Timing of the Development of Sensory and Neural Structures in the Human Cochlea**

Event	Period
Afferent fibers in cochlear epithelium	9th gestational week
Distinguishable inner and outer hair cells	10–11th gestational week
Appearance of stereocilia on inner and outer hair cells	11–12th gestational week
First synapse-like contacts between fibers and hair cells	12th gestational week
First efferent endings below inner hair cells	14th gestational week
Opening of tunnel of Corti, formation of Neul's spaces	18–20th gestational week
Mature appearance of stereociliary bundles	20–22nd gestational week
Formation of efferent axosomatic synapses with outer hair cells	20–30th gestational week
Morphologically mature outer hair cells	30th gestational week

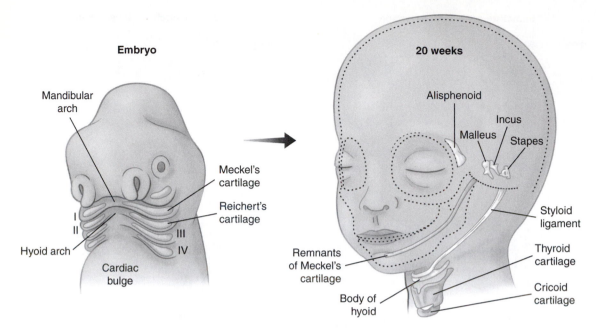

FIGURE 6-5 The middle ear ossicles (malleus, incus, and stapes) and external ear pinna or auricle form from tissues of the first (I) and second (II) pharyngeal arches. The first pharyngeal arch is also associated with bony structures of the mandible. The second pharyngeal arch causes structures associated with the larynx such as the hyoid.

EMBRYOGENESIS OF EXTERNAL AND MIDDLE EARS

As the inner ear differentiates, the middle ear also forms (see Figure 6-1). The **endoderm** of the first pharyngeal pouch will line the middle ear (tympanic) cavity and auditory (Eustachian) tube. The middle ear derives from the first pharyngeal pouch and extends as a tubotympanic recess. During gestational week 5, the distal part of the recess widens and gives rise to a primitive tympanic cavity, and the mesoderm between the two canals forms the tympanic membrane. The stalk of the recess remains narrow and forms the Eustachian tube, through which the tympanic cavity communicates with the nasopharynx. The middle-ear ossicles develop from the cartilage of the first and second pharyngeal arches (Figure 6-5). The malleus and incus are derived from cartilage of the first pharyngeal arch, and the stapes is derived from cartilage of the second arch. The tympanic cavity enlarges to incorporate the ossicles and coats the ossicles with epithelium. Although the ossicles appear during the first half of

fetal life, they remain embedded in mesenchyme until the eighth month, when the surrounding tissue dissolves. The endodermal epithelial lining of the primitive tympanic cavity then extends along the wall of the newly developing space. The tympanic cavity is now at least twice as large as before. When the ossicles are entirely free of surrounding mesenchyme, the endodermal epithelium connects them in a mesentery-like fashion to the wall of the cavity. The supporting ligaments of the ossicles develop later within these mesenteries.

The external ear pinna or auricle also forms from tissues of the first and second pharyngeal arches. During the sixth gestational week, six tissue swellings termed auricular **hillocks** become apparent. Three hillocks develop on the first arch and three on second arch. The pinna originates on the embryonic neck below the lower jaw; then as the mandible develops, the external ear moves relatively higher with a more vertical orientation. By gestational week 9, each of the auricular hillocks has formed a distinctive portion of the definitive external ear. For example, hillock 1 forms the tragus and hillock 6 forms the antitragus, as well as part of the helix. The lobule of the ear is not derived from the hillocks.

The outer (external) auditory meatus develops from the dorsal portion of the first pharyngeal cleft. The outer meatus develops around week 5, where it extends inward toward the pharynx. Toward the end of trimester 1, epithelial cells at the bottom of the meatus proliferate, forming a solid epithelial plate, the meatal plug until week 18. In the seventh month (trimester 3), this plug dissolves, and the epithelial lining of the floor of the meatus participates in forming the tympanic membrane (eardrum). Occasionally, the meatal plug persists until birth, resulting in congenital deafness.

The eardrum is made up of three embryonic tissues: the ectodermal epithelial lining at the bottom of the auditory meatus, the endodermal epithelial lining of the tympanic cavity, and an intermediate layer of connective tissue that forms the fibrous stratum. The major part of the eardrum is firmly attached to the handle of the malleus, and the remaining portion forms the separation between the external auditory meatus and the tympanic cavity.

DEVELOPMENT OF HEARING FUNCTION AND BEHAVIOR

Prenatal Hearing

The functional development of the cochlea occurs during trimesters 2 and 3. It is likely that by the middle of prenatal life and definitely by 26 through 29 gestational weeks, the fetus can hear and respond to sounds. Myelination of the auditory pathway commences after the onset of hearing. Moreover, during trimester 3, the fetus is capable of discriminating between different frequencies and between speech stimuli. Fetal hearing, which occurs in a fluid environment, is via bone conduction. The quantity and type of sound that typically reaches the fetus and its effect is unknown. Most likely, the mother produces nearly all of the sound reaching the fetus, including speech, because her body reduces sound from the environment and produces noises that mask others.

Despite the limitations of hearing *in utero*, fetuses hear maternal speech and remember something of what is heard after they are born. New-

borns prefer to listen to speech in their native language, indicating that some type of auditory learning has taken place *in utero*. A newborn infant will recognize his or her mother's but not father's voice immediately after birth. Also, if a mother reads a rhythmic story to her fetus in the last weeks of pregnancy, her newborn will recognize the story even if another female reads it.

Currently, little evidence exists that prenatal auditory stimulation enhances development. As reported by Werner (2003), studies claiming to show that fetuses exposed to certain types of sound stimulation *in utero* are more intelligent or better adjusted have not been substantiated by subsequent research. Likewise, no data have been reported that show children who are deaf or hard of hearing are at a disadvantage because they did not receive *in utero* stimulation. Thus, studies claiming to show that infants and children are more intelligent or better adjusted if they are exposed to certain types of music (i.e., "the Mozart effect") have not been substantiated by subsequent research. Perhaps the best conclusion we can draw from studies of fetal experience with sound and speech is that it actually serves to fine-tune the basic circuitry of the auditory system and makes infants more responsive to speech after birth. You might say that it gets them into a language-learning mode.

Postnatal Hearing

The general maturation of postnatal hearing is summarized in Table 6-2. Absolute thresholds and frequency discrimination mature first at high and then at low frequencies. Absolute threshold measures are available from the newborn period through childhood and adolescence and into adulthood. A few days after birth, neonates tend to have evoked auditory-brainstem thresholds that are 30 to 70 dB higher than those of adults. The audibility curves are more or less flat at this age. Thresholds improve progressively during infancy. During the first 6 postnatal months, the improvement is greater at high than at low frequencies. By 6 months, thresholds for frequencies greater than approximately 4 kHz are actually closer to those of adults than are thresholds at lower frequencies. The "high-frequency-first" pattern of development continues through the

TABLE 6-2 Summary of Development of Three Major Auditory Behaviors

Hearing Behavior	Onset	Mature
Intensity processing (thresholds, discrimination, loudness)	26–29 weeks	By 6 years of age
Frequency processing (resolution, discrimination, representation)	Third trimester	By 1 year of age
Localization and binaural processing (masking-level differences, localization)	Birth	By 5 years of age

remainder of childhood: Mature thresholds are observed at progressively lower frequencies as a child grows, until about 10 years of age, when thresholds are mature across the frequency range. The pattern of threshold development before 6 months is most likely a direct reflection of middle ear and central neural auditory development. Nonsensory processes such as attention or motivation also make a contribution to early threshold development.

Adults can discriminate about a 1-dB change in the intensity of a pure tone whether the tone is barely audible or at a high intensity. The ability to discriminate small changes in a stimulus is usually referred to as the difference limen or jnd. During the postnatal period from infancy (6 months old) through middle childhood (4 years old), there is a definite improvement in intensity discrimination from about 6 dB to about 3 dB. There is general agreement that the intensity difference limen (dL, the smallest change that can be detected) approaches adult values around 6 years of age.

Both frequency resolution and discrimination depend on the width of the so-called auditory filter, the psychophysical concept depicting the frequency analysis performed within the cochlea. Auditory filter width and critical bandwidth mature early but last at high frequencies. By most physiologic measures of frequency resolution, such as otoacoustic emissions and auditory brainstem responses, auditory filter widths appear to mature by 6 months of age. However, elevated masked thresholds are commonly measured up until roughly 10 years of age. If the auditory filter widths are relatively constant, but masked thresholds are elevated above adult levels, then it suggests an inefficient filter or signal-to-noise ratio required for detection. This immaturity may be because infants and children have greater difficulty distinguishing signal from noise or are monitoring the wrong filter or

multiple filters. Three-month-old infants are rather poor at frequency discrimination, particularly in high-frequency ranges. However adult-like frequency discrimination occurs rather quickly, and by 6 months, infants have frequency difference limens at 4,000 Hz around 2%.

Localization and binaural hearing cues in adults depend on interaural intensity and interaural time differences, as well as the minimum audible angle, or threshold for detection of a change in sound source location. Newborn infants are capable of making at least crude localizations of a sound source. Within a few days of birth, infants make slow long-latency head turns (left or right) toward a sound source. This response depends on the duration and repetition rate of the sound stimulus. Interestingly, the response appears to disappear around 2 months, then reappear with a quicker and shorter latency. The accuracy with which infants turn to face a sound source increases progressively until about 18 months of age. Interaural cue discriminations improve throughout the postnatal period and into childhood. The minimum audible angle progressively decreases from 2 months until sometime between 18 months and 5 years of age.

COMMON DEFECTS ASSOCIATED WITH DEVELOPMENT

Each year in the United States, about 24,000 newborn infants have some form of significant hearing impairment. Most types of congenital deafness are usually associated with deaf-mutism and are caused by genetic factors. In many cases, the genes involved in congenital deafness have been identified. Recessive inheritance is the most common cause of congenital deafness. Congenital deafness may be caused by abnormal development of the membranous and bony labyrinths or by the abnormal formation of the middle ear ossicles and eardrum. In extreme cases, the tympanic cavity and external meatus are absent. Congenital deafness may also be caused by environmental factors that interfere with normal development of the internal and middle ears. For example, a rubella viral infection during the seventh or eighth week of development can cause severe damage to the organ of Corti and result in sensorineural deafness. It has also been suggested that poliomyelitis, erythroblastosis fetalis, diabetes, hypothyroidism, and toxoplasmosis can cause congenital deafness.

External ear defects are common and may serve as an indicator of a specific pattern of congenital anomalies (Figure 6-6). The external ears

Normally developed newborn outer ear

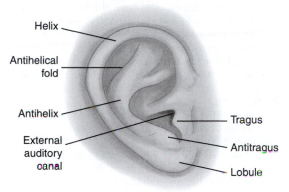

- Helix
- Antihelical fold
- Antihelix
- External auditory canal
- Tragus
- Antitragus
- Lobule

Abnormal size, shape, and rotation of newborn outer ear

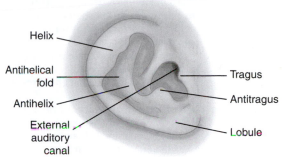

- Helix
- Antihelical fold
- Antihelix
- External auditory canal
- Tragus
- Antitragus
- Lobule

Adult outer ear with ear tags

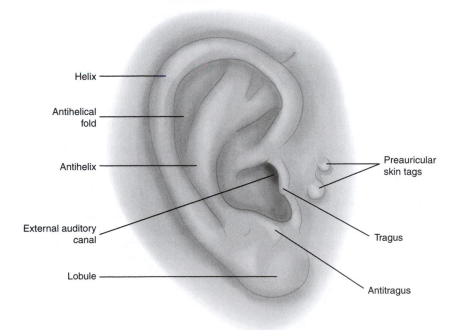

- Helix
- Antihelical fold
- Antihelix
- External auditory canal
- Lobule
- Preauricular skin tags
- Tragus
- Antitragus

FIGURE 6-6   Common external ear defects.

How Is Hearing Loss Inherited?

Current estimates suggest that half of all childhood deafness is due to hereditary factors. People have 23 pairs of chromosomes, including a pair of sex chromosomes. Each pair consists of one chromosome inherited from the mother and one chromosome inherited from the father. The sex chromosomes determine the sex of a person. Girls inherit two X chromosomes (one from each parent), and boys inherit one X chromosome (maternal) and one Y chromosome (paternal). Chromosomes are made up of genes that contain the instructions necessary for the characteristics or traits that make up each person. Except for the XY chromosome pair, every person thus has two copies (alleles) of every gene because there are two pairs of chromosomes. In total, each person has about 30,000 genes that are grouped into 23 pairs of chromosomes.

Genes are made of specific sequences of deoxyribonucleic acid **(DNA).** Four kinds of chemical bases (adenine [A], thymidine [T], guanine [G], and cytosine [C]) comprise DNA. Little variation exists in the DNA sequences of genes across individuals. However, when there are differences in gene sequences, these are usually the result of some type of alteration (referred to as a *mutation*) in the DNA. A simple substitution of one chemical base (e.g., an A to a C) can be enough to alter the function of the DNA sequence that makes a gene. Although mutations may occur that do not interfere with the health of an individual, mutations that disrupt the function of a gene can have serious consequences not only for the individual but also for his or her offspring.

Much of what is known about genetic inheritance patterns originated with the work of Gregor Mendel using garden-variety peas. In Mendelian genetics, gene mutations can be autosomal dominant or recessive. If only one altered gene allele is needed for an individual to be affected, the mutation is considered dominant. Thus, even if a person inherits one normal copy of the gene from a parent, the mutated gene will be stronger than the normal gene and cause the expression of the altered trait or characteristic. A mutation can also be recessive. In such a case, the altered gene is weaker than the normal gene and will only cause the altered trait or characteristic when the individual inherits two identical altered gene copies. If a person inherits one altered gene allele and one normal gene allele, that individual is not affected. Such a person, however, can pass on the mutated gene allele to his or her children. Such a parent will be a carrier, but with no obvious altered gene function.

An additional form of gene inheritance involves the X and Y sex chromosomes. Recessive mutations on the X chromosome do not have corresponding alleles on the Y chromosome. This type of inheritance pattern is called **sex-linked inheritance.** A male child receiving the recessive gene on the X chromosome from his mother would almost invariably express the altered trait. For the recessive gene to be expressed in a female child, the daughter would have to receive a copy of the mutated gene from the X chromosome of both parents.

In genetics, non-Mendelian inheritance is the passing on of a trait in a form other than through chromosomal inheritance. Forms of non-Mendelian inheritance include the inheritance of mitochondrial diseases, some of which are associated with hearing loss. Mitochondria are small cellular structures that provide energy for cells and that have their own unique set of genes. If a mutation is in one of the mitochondrial genes, the mutation can be passed to offspring through the mitochondria. Mitochondrial inheritance behaves differently from autosomal and sex-linked inheritance. Mitochondria typically contain from 5 to 10 gene copies, all inherited from the mother. When mitochondria divide, the copies of DNA present are divided randomly between the two new mitochondria, then those new mitochondria make more copies. As a result, if only a few of the DNA copies inherited from the mother are altered, mitochondrial division may cause most of the defective copies to end up in just one of the new mitochondria. Mitochondrial disease begins to become apparent once the number of affected mitochondria reaches a certain level. An example of this form of inheritance is the A1555G mutation, which makes people more likely to lose their hearing if they are treated with certain antibiotics. In addition, specific (point) mutations in mitochondrial DNA have been found to be associated with diabetes mellitus and deafness. The most common mutation leads to an A-to-G transition.

Waardenburg's Syndrome

Waardenburg's syndrome (WS) is a genetic disorder that has the following main characteristics: (1) a wide bridge of the nose; (2) pigmentary disturbances such as two different colored eyes (generally one is brown and the other bright blue, although occasionally patches of brown and blue are mixed in the same eye), white forelock (lock of hair growing from the front part of the head), white eyelashes and premature graying of the hair; and (3) some degree of cochlear deafness. In addition to these primary features, there may also be cleft lip and/or cleft palate and enlargement of the colon. However, these features are less common than the primary features.

Type I of the disorder is characterized by displacement of the fold of the eyelid, whereas type II does not include this feature. However, the frequency of deafness is greater in type II. Other than hearing loss, most people with WS do not have any particular medical problems. The facial features and pigmentary changes merely help in making the diagnosis and cannot be considered abnormal.

Because WS is inherited in dominant fashion, researchers typically see families with several generations who have inherited one or more of the features. Many of these people are unaware that they have the gene because the accompanying symptoms can be so mild. The chance of "carriers" passing on the gene to their children is 50%, regardless of the features they possess. Of course, someone in a WS family who does not have the gene cannot pass it on.

WS may be much more common in our population than previously believed. As many as 2 to 3 of every 100 children in schools for the deaf may have WS. Because the majority of those with the gene have little or no hearing loss, experts believe that for every child they see with WS and severe hearing loss, there are four to five family members who have relatively normal hearing but also have the gene.

The discovery of the human gene that causes WS, *pax3*, came about after scientists speculated that "splotch mice," which have splotchy coloring in their coats, might have the same gene that causes WS in humans. They located the gene that causes the irregular coloring in mice, then found the same gene in humans. With a mouse model to draw from, scientists are learning much about how *pax3* causes WS.

---

are often abnormal in shape and low-set in infants with chromosomal syndromes, such as trisomy 18, and in infants affected by maternal ingestion of certain drugs (e.g., trimethadione). Auricular appendages (skin tags) are also common and result from the development of accessory auricular hillocks. Microtia (small auricle) results from suppressed development of the auricular hillocks. This anomaly often serves as an indicator of associated anomalies, such as atresia (obstruction) of the ear canal and middle ear anomalies. All of the frequently occurring chromosomal syndromes and most of the less common ones have ear anomalies as one of their characteristics. The reported incidence of significant sensorineural hearing loss in young children varies from 1:1,000 to 1:2,000 depending on the population studied. Approximately 20% of patients with congenital sensorineural hearing loss have radiographic anomalies of the inner ear. Congenital ear malformation results from a defect in the de-velopment of the membranous labyrinth, the osseous labyrinth, or both.

Absent obvious ear, head, or neck deformities, congenital hearing loss can present as an invisible disability at birth. Complete labyrinthine **dysplasia** is rare, and it was first described early in the twentieth century. It has been associated with several syndromes. Labyrinthine dysplasias are characterized by a collapse of the cochlear duct and saccule. It is probably the most common form of inner ear pathology in patients with congenital deafness. Another type of labyrinthine dysplasia is characterized by malformation of the cochlear basal turn and is related to familial high-frequency sensorineural hearing loss.

Complete labyrinthine aplasia, known as Michel's deformity, represents one of the most severe forms of inner ear defect. It is bilateral complete bony and membranous aplasia of the inner ear. It is extremely rare. The otic placode differentiates into structures of the inner ear during the third week of gestation. Cochlear aplasia results from the

Ear and Kidney Developmental Linkage

A number of genetic and nongenetic disorders affect both ears and kidneys (Figure 6-7). However, the types of problems may be different, and the reasons that both ears and kidneys are involved may be due to different processes in development. The kidney problems can include malformed or missing kidneys or problems at a microscopic level; the ear problems may include malformation of the external ear or the ossicles (small bones) of the middle ear, or microscopic changes in the cochlea. These point to several areas of similarity between the ears and kidneys. These are similarities in structure, function, or in the timing of prenatal development, that is, the period of development of the fetus during pregnancy.

When seen through the microscope, the kidney and the cochlea of the inner ear have similar membranes, which are held together with a substance called *collagen*. These membranes are similar in function and in structure (the way they are put together). In both cases, these membranes help to maintain the

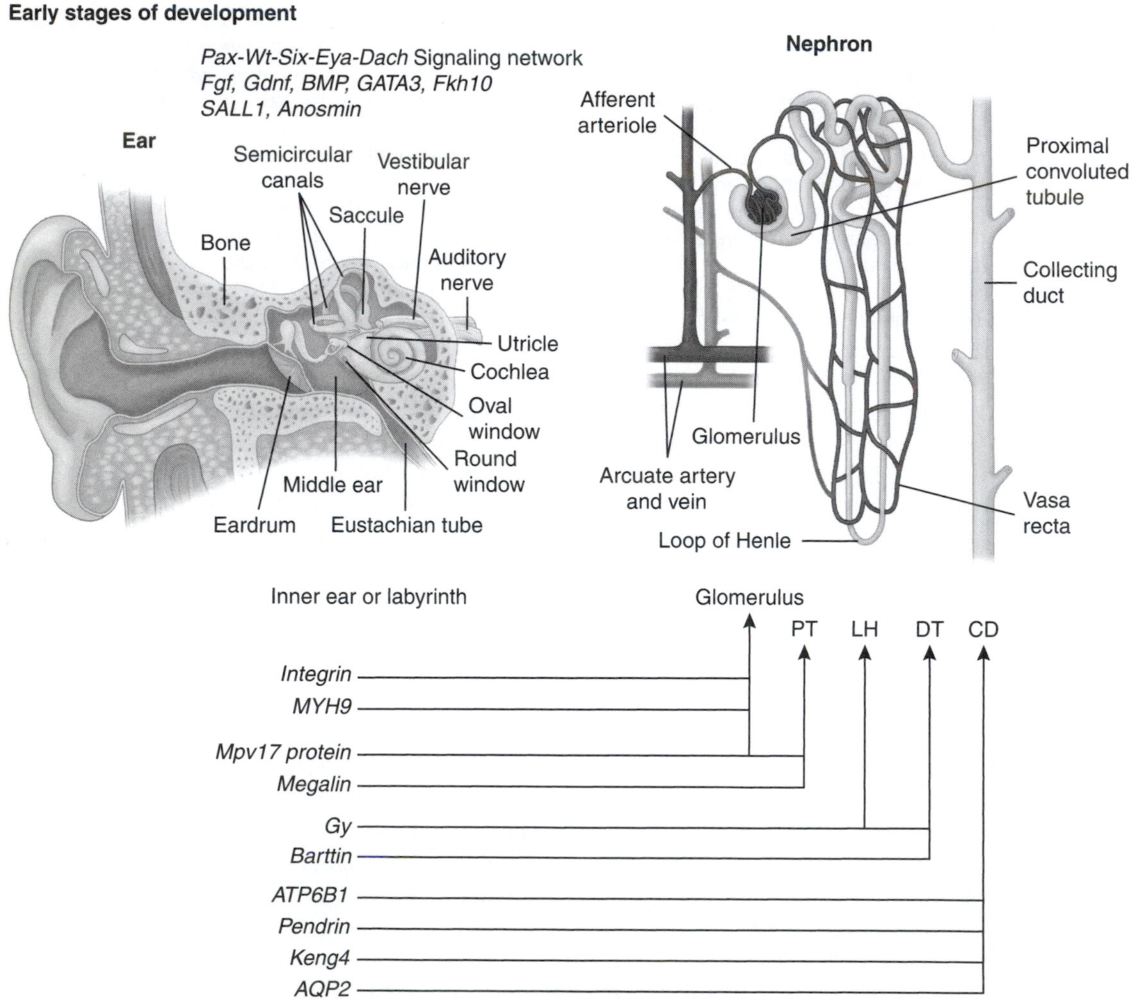

Early stages of development

FIGURE 6-7 (See Color Plate) Ear and kidney genetic linkages. CD, Collecting duct; DT, distal tubule; LH, loop of Henle; PT, proximal tubule. (Adapted from Izzedine et al., 2004.)

chemical balance of the fluids of the kidney and inner ear. Because of similar molecular structure, they can be damaged by the same drugs, such as overdose of diuretics.

In the developing fetus, both the ear and kidney develop around the fifth to eighth week of pregnancy. Thus, a genetic problem in coordinating development at that time, or a nongenetic problem, such as an infection, might affect the development of both areas at the same time. Several examples can be given to show how different problems can influence both the ears and the kidneys in different ways. The branchio-oto-renal syndrome (BOR) involves the external and middle ear structures together with the kidneys. Some people have also been found to have a duplication of the ureters, which are the tubes leading from the kidney to the bladder. Because this has been found to be more common in some families than in others, it has been suggested that it might be a separate syndrome and has been named both BOU syndrome, for branchio-oto-ureteral, and BOUU, to remind one of the duplication. These conditions are quite variable, and a person with the gene may have only one of the minor characteristics, or they may have serious hearing and kidney problems. In both of these syndromes, the ear and kidney problems appear to be primarily problems of prenatal development. One researcher, Dr. Michael Melnick, has suggested the reason ears and kidneys are both affected is because they develop at the same time. For example, something specific may affect cell division at that particular point in prenatal development.

Other syndromes affect the ear and the kidney more at the biochemical level. Alport's syndrome is a genetic condition characterized by the progressive loss of kidney function and hearing. Alport's syndrome can also affect the eyes. The presence of blood in the urine (hematuria) is almost always found in this condition. In 1927, Dr. Cecil A. Alport first identified it in a British family. Presumably, the cause of these functional problems involves the molecular similarities between the cochlea and the kidney. Alport's syndrome is caused by mutations in *COL4A3, COL4A4,* and *COL4A5,* which are all collagen biosynthesis genes. Mutations in any of these genes prevent the proper production or assembly of the type IV collagen network, which is an important structural component of basement membranes in the kidney, ear, and eye. Basement membranes are thin, sheetlike structures that separate and support cells in many tissues. When mutations prevent the

formation of type IV collagen fibers, the basement membranes of the kidneys are not able to filter waste products from the blood and create urine normally, allowing blood and protein into the urine. The abnormalities of type IV collagen in kidney basement membranes cause gradual scarring of the kidneys, eventually leading to kidney failure in many people with the disease. Interestingly, correction of the kidney problems by transplantation sometimes halts the progression of the hearing loss, which suggests that additional factors in the blood, such as the toxicity that goes along with kidney failure, may further damage the hearing. Thus, in these syndromes, there is not a problem with formation of the kidney or cochlea, but rather in their continued function.

Examples of other syndromes with hearing loss and renal problems include:

- *Charcot–Marie–Tooth disease and deafness:* Charcot–Marie–Tooth disease is an autosomal dominant condition. It is a progressive nerve disease that causes gradual decrease of muscle function in the legs. The hearing loss is sensorineural and usually is noted in adolescence and gets progressively worse. Some people also have nephritis, or kidney disease, with this condition.

- *Epstein's syndrome (macrothrombocytopathia, nephritis, and deafness):* Epstein's syndrome is an autosomal dominant syndrome that is similar to Alport's syndrome, except that it also includes a defect of the platelets, the cells of the blood that aid in clotting. Another similar condition, called *Fechtner syndrome,* has abnormalities of the white blood cells as well.

- *Muckle–Wells syndrome (urticaria, deafness, and amyloidosis):* Muckle–Wells syndrome is an autosomal dominant condition with recurrent fever, skin rash (urticaria), joint pain, progressive sensorineural hearing loss, and amyloidosis of the kidneys, which is an accumulation of a protein in the kidney, which gradually blocks its function. The hearing loss usually begins in childhood, whereas the other problems may not be seen until adolescence.

- *Renal tubular acidosis and hearing loss:* Renal tubular acidosis is an autosomal recessive condition that involves sensorineural hearing loss and formation of kidney stones. It appears to have two types. In one type, the hearing loss is profound and present at birth, and the kidney problems, which occur

Continues

Ear and Kidney Developmental Linkage–*Continued*	
early in infancy, can be severe if not treated. In the other type, the kidney stones and hearing loss do not appear until adolescence. The kidney problems are milder, and the hearing loss is progressive. • *Townes–Brock syndrome:* Townes–Brock syndrome is autosomal dominant condition that can be quite variable within families. The characteristics include lack of an opening for the anus, which must be repaired at birth, abnormal bones of the hands or feet, kidney problems (usually small, poorly formed kidneys), "lop"-shaped (droopy) ears, and mild sensorineural hearing loss. • *Otorenal-Genital syndrome:* Otorenal-genital syndrome is a rare recessive condition that involves abnormal middle ear ossicles, incomplete formation	of the kidneys, and abnormalities of the reproductive organs. Genetic research into syndromes with both renal and auditory problems will be valuable in explaining how the damage is done to these two systems and hopefully will provide means of therapy, particularly for life-threatening renal disease. SOURCE: Harvard Medical School Center for Hereditary Deafness (http://hearing.harvard.edu/index.htm), Boys Town National Research Hospital (www.boystownhospital.org), and the National Institute on Deafness and Other Communication Disorders (NIDCD; http://www.nidcd.nih.gov, accessed February 1, 2007).

arrested development of the cochlea during the fifth week. The cochlea fails to form and appears as a single cavity. The vestibule and semicircular canals may be normal or malformed. Incomplete partition deformity, also well known as Mondini's deformity, represents a small cochlea with incomplete or no scalae. The cochlea is usually flat and has one-and-a-half turns instead of the normal two-and-a-half turns. Arrest of maturation at the gestational seventh week may result in Mondini's deformity. Patients with a wide internal auditory canal may be predisposed to cerebrospinal fluid leaks, resulting in recurrent meningitis (Brookhouser, 1996).

A thorough clinical, audiologic, and radiologic evaluation should be made of all patients suspected of having these deformities. Clinical history should include possible exposure to teratogen during pregnancy, family history of hearing impairment, progression and/or fluctuation of the hearing loss, and associated vestibular symptoms. A routine audiologic evaluation is required. Workups can be helpful in determining possible causative factors. Workups include TORCH (toxoplasmosis, other infections, rubella, cytomegalovirus, and herpes simplex) titers, FTA-ABS (fluorescent treponemal antibody absorption), urinalysis, and thyroid function tests. High-resolution

computed tomography provides excellent visualization of the bony labyrinth of the inner ear.

ENVIRONMENTAL INFLUENCES

Human fetuses pass through a period of extreme auditory immaturity late in the second and early in the third trimester of gestation. From a clinical point of view, the incidence of hearing loss among premature infants is much greater than that observed in the normal population, and it is becoming increasingly clear that critical developmental periods exist during which the mammalian auditory system is particularly vulnerable to environmental agents and are remarkably plastic. In this context, the long-term consequences of environmental noise and ototoxins on the development of function in the premature infant population are of great concern. Because morbidity and mortality rates for premature infants are decreasing, and because human auditory development continues into the third trimester of gestation and beyond, premature infants subjected to potentially ototoxic and acoustically traumatic environments of intensive care nurseries, as well as those drugs exposed *in utero*, may be prone to develop long-term pathologic sequelae.

ᘯ SUMMARY ᘰ

The ear is a composite structure with a complex embryonic origin. Although a great deal of information has been obtained from studies of the human embryo, by far the majority of what is known comes from studies of rodent embryos and postnatal pups. Most of what is known about the genes involved in the formation of the inner ear comes from studies of ear defects found in various gene deletion (null) mutations in mouse models. The inner, middle, and external ears begin to develop a little after 3 weeks' gestation and are complete before the end of the third trimester. In the embryo, the inner ear is the first to develop and originates as epidermal placodes (thickenings or discs) that appear on either side of the head. Inner ear development is dependent on multiple signaling cues from surrounding tissues. While the inner ear is developing, the external and middle ears also develop from structures of the first and second pharyngeal arches and from the intervening pharyngeal cleft (groove) and pouch. The result is that the middle ear consists of a tympanic space with three auditory ossicles and an auditory tube. Separately, the external ear consists of the auricle (pinna), the external acoustic (auditory) meatus, and the tympanic membrane (eardrum). Toward the beginning of the third trimester (roughly 28–29 weeks), much of the development has occurred and the fetus is capable of responding to sounds. In the fetus, the ear starts to function as the auditory system matures, and by birth, it is fully capable of analyzing sounds in the environment. Immediately after birth, hearing capability continues to mature through early childhood. Congenital deafness may be caused by abnormal development of the membranous and bony labyrinths or by the abnormal formation of the middle ear ossicles and eardrum.

ᘯ KEY TERMS ᘰ

Auricle	Endoderm	Morphogenesis	Pharyngeal arches
Differentiation	Gestation	Otic placode	Sex-linked inheritance
Dysplasia	Hillock	Otocyst	Trimester
Ectoderm	Mesenchymal		

ᘯ STUDY QUESTIONS ᘰ

1. How does the inner ear form during embryogenesis?

2. Describe the formation of hair cells and hair cell innervation.

3. Give the primary events and structures during the formation of the middle and external ears.

4. When is the fetus capable of responding to sounds?

5. What are the typical causes of congenital deafness?

⌁REFERENCES⌁

Boys Town National Research Register for Hereditary Hearing Loss: http://www.boystownhospital.org

Bredberg, G. (1967). The human cochlea during development and ageing. *Journal of Laryngology and Otology, 81,* 739–758.

Bredberg, G. (1968). Cellular pattern and nerve supply of the human organ of Corti. *Acta Otolaryngologica Supplementum, 236,* 1+.

Brookhouser, P.E. (1996). Sensorineural hearing loss in children. *Pediatric Clinics of North America 43,* 1195–1216.

Frenz, D., McPhee, J., & Van De Water, T. (2001). Structural and functional development of the ear. In J.F. Jahn & J. Santos-Sachi (Eds.), *Physiology of the Ear,* 2nd ed. (pp. 191-214). San Diego: Singular.

Harvard Medical School Center for Hereditary Deafness: http://hearing.harvard.edu/index.htm

Izzedine, H., Tankere, F., Launay-Vacher, V., & Deray, G. (2004). Ear and kidney syndromes: molecular versus clinical approach. *Kidney International, 65,* 369-385.

Larsen, W. J. (1997). *Human embryology* (2nd ed.). New York: Churchill Livingston.

National Institute on Deafness and Other Communication Disorders (NIDCD): http://www.nidcd.nih.gov

Noramly, S., & Grainger, R. M. (2002). Determination of the embryonic inner ear. *Journal of Neurobiology, 53,* 100–128.

Simmons, D. D., Manson-Gieseke, L., Hendrix, T. W., Morris, K., & Williams, S. J. (1991). Postnatal maturation of spiral ganglion neurons: a horseradish peroxidase study. *Hearing Research, 55,* 81-91.

Simmons, D. D. (2003). The ear in utero: An engineering masterpiece. *Hearing Health Magazine, 19,* 10–14.

Steel, K. P., & Bock, G. R. (1985). Genetic factors affecting hearing development. *Acta Otolaryngologica Supplementum, 421,* 48–56.

Tanaka, K., Sakai, N., & Terayama, Y. (1979). Organ of Corti in the human fetus: Scanning and transmission electron microscope studies. *Annals of Otology, Rhinology, and Laryngology, 88,* 749–758.

Walsh, E. J., & McGee, J. (1990). Development of auditory coding in the central nervous system: Implications for in utero hearing. *Seminars in Perinatology, 14,* 281–293.

Walsh, E. J., McGee, J., & Javel, E. (1986). Development of auditory-evoked potentials in the cat. I. Onset of response and development of sensitivity. *Journal of the Acoustical Society of America, 79,* 712–724.

Werner, L. (2003). Prenatal auditory stimulation: Truth, fiction or moot point. *Hearing Health Magazine, 19,* 2.

⌁SUGGESTED READING⌁

Hereditary Hearing Loss Home Page: http://webhost .ua.ac.be/hhh

Minoli, I., & Moro, G. (1985). Constraints of intensive care units and follow-up studies in prematures. *Acta Otolaryngologica Supplementum, 421,* 62–67.

Chapter

7

Structural and Functional Anatomy of the Outer and Middle Ear

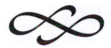

Brian T. Faddis, Ph.D.
Assistant Professor of Otolaryngology
Washington University School of Medicine
St. Louis, Missouri

In this chapter, we start to explore the structural complexity of the more peripheral portions of the organ of hearing, the outer and middle ear. The anatomic relations of these discrete regions of the auditory system are shown in Figure 7-1. The outer and middle ear regions have developed to actually enhance the collection and the relevance of audi-tory signals before they even reach that part of the ear where the sensory receptors are located. No other sensory system, except perhaps the eye, has adapted such an intricate mechanism to ensure that proper perceptual information is extracted from a stimulus. This chapter proceeds with descriptions of the structural components or gross anatomy of both

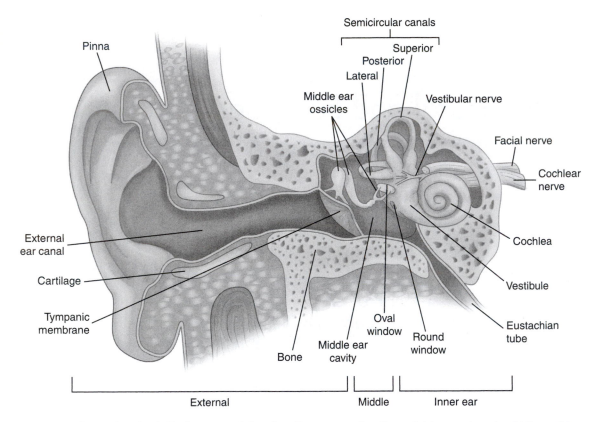

FIGURE 7-1 (See Color Plate) The human peripheral auditory system has three divisions: external, middle, and inner ears. The external ear consists of the pinna (or auricle) and the external ear canal (or external auditory meatus). The tympanic membrane (or eardrum) closes off the medial end of the external ear canal. The middle ear is an air-filled cavity that contains the three middle-ear ossicles: malleus (M), incus (I), and stapes (S). The middle-ear cavity is con-nected to the nasopharynx by the Eustachian tube. The inner ear (or membranous labyrinth), which is housed within the petrous portion of the temporal bone, includes the cochlea, vestibule (containing the saccule and utricle), and three semicircular canals (lateral, posterior, and superior). The cochlea contains the end organ for hearing. Its sensory cells are innervated by the cochlear branch of the 8th cranial nerve. The vestibule and three semicircular canals contain the end organs for balance and motion detection, respectively. Sensory cells in these end organs are innervated by the vestibular branch of the 8th cranial nerve. There are two openings from the middle to the inner ear: the oval window into which is fitted the footplate of the stapes, and the round window, covered by the round window membrane.

the outer and middle ear regions and discusses the functional relevance of this anatomy to the perception of auditory signals, particularly as they relate to human oral communication.

OUTER EAR

The outer or **external ear** consists of the **auricle** (or pinna) and the external auditory canal. The auricles provide one of the most prominent features of the human visage and are the subject of a great deal of superstition and folklore. Why is it that leprechauns and Santa's elves have pointy ears? And why do people ask if your ears were burning when they were talking about you? Aside from the nose, the ears are probably the most characteristic feature of the human head, helping to lend a uniqueness that makes our appearance truly our own. However, study of the outer ear and its capabilities will certainly convince you that the auricles were designed for more than outward appearance or to simply support the frames of eyeglasses.

Auricle

The auricle or pinna protrudes from the middle of each side of the human head, a rather unique location compared with most species. In humans, the auricles are roughly equivalent in size and shape. They are a somewhat rigid structure, acquiring their shape from the underlying elastic cartilage to which the skin of the ear is closely applied. The shape of the ear follows closely that of the cartilage frame primarily because of the lack of a fatty layer that is present in most other parts of the body. Thus, although ears always look fit and trim, they are also the first part of the body to suffer when exposed to cold temperatures. For this reason, they are also the area most subject to frostbite and one of the most obvious sites when blood flow increases because of embarrassment or nervousness.

Although ears can and do present vast differences in appearance, they are composed of a consistent array of structures that have all been named. These structures help to demarcate distinct regions

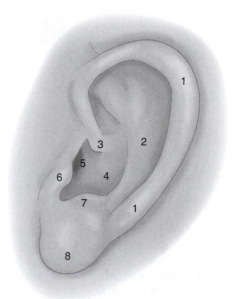

FIGURE 7-2   Anatomic landmarks of the outer ear include the following structures: (1) helix, (2) antihelix, (3) crus of the helix, (4) concha, (5) external auditory meatus, (6) tragus, (7) antitragus, and (8) lobule. The opening to the external auditory meatus is barely visible at this angle. Only the lobule is not supported by a cartilaginous substructure.

of the auricle that offer their own functional consequences to incoming auditory signals. The anatomic structures of the auricle are labeled in Figure 7-2. The outermost ridge, called the **helix,** runs in C-shaped fashion from the most anterior-superior aspect of the auricle down to the inferior aspect, ending at the lobule or **earlobe.** Just inside the helix runs a second ridge called the **antihelix.** The crus of the helix is a third ridge that runs roughly horizontal from an anterior position just above the **external auditory meatus** or ear canal back to the antihelix. These three ridges provide the majority of the structural integrity of the auricle. Without these ridges, especially the characteristic C shape of the helix and antihelix, the auricle would move quite freely because of head movements or changes in the wind. (Imagine how difficult it would be to

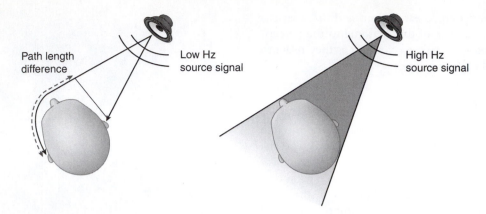

FIGURE 7-3 Effects of the head and external ear on localization of sounds in space. (left) Diagram showing how low-frequency sound waves wrap around the structures of the head to enable the brain to localize sound in space using temporal differences in the arrival of the signal at each ear. (right) Diagram showing how the head and outer ear can baffle or reduce the amplitude of high-frequency sounds, allowing the brain to localize these signals using differences in intensity of the signal at each ear.

hear continuously if this were the case.) The prominent protrusion or tubercle at the anterior edge of the external auditory meatus is known as the **tragus.** An opposing tubercle located at the inferior end of the antihelix ridge is called the **antitragus.** The tragus and antitragus help to define a conical portion of the auricle known as the **concha,** which leads directly into the ear canal. The earlobe is the only part of the auricle that is not supported by a cartilaginous substructure.

Functional Significance of the Auricle

The auricle does much more than just look pretty. The conical shape of the auricle actually enhances the collection of sound waves. The shape and location of the auricles can also help to localize sounds in space if they are of the right frequency. Low-frequency sounds are long wavelengths that easily wrap around the auricle and are therefore not shadowed or reduced in intensity as they enter the ear canal. Sounds of low frequency can therefore be located in space by comparing the time of arrival of a signal at each ear. That is, the sound appears to be

located on the side of the earlier arrival (Figure 7-3). High-frequency sound, however, represents a shorter wavelength that is subject to shadowing by the head and auricle, and thus is reduced in intensity at the offside ear. Localization of these frequencies is accomplished using intensity cues; the sound appears to be located at the side of greater intensity (see Figure 7-3) (Möller, 2000; Goode, 1988; Tonndorf, 1988).

The physical properties of the external ear can also modify the sound wave as acoustic vibrations are transferred to the eardrum, or **tympanic membrane.** This is due to a property called **resonance.** *Random House College Dictionary* describes *resonance* as "the state of a system in which an abnormally large vibration is produced in response to an external stimulus," occurring when the frequency of the stimulus (the sound wave) matches the natural vibration frequency of the system (the auricle and ear canal). In humans, the external ear resonates with sound-wave stimulation, particularly in the frequency range of 2 to 7 kHz, a range, probably not coincidentally, that is characteristic of human speech. Thus, the human outer ear can not

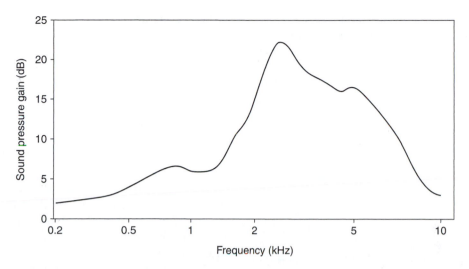

FIGURE 7-4   Histogram of an external ear transfer function showing the gain in sound pressure caused by resonance of external ear structures. In this example, most of the gain, seen between 2 and 7 kHz, is primarily due to contributions from the concha and external auditory meatus. This transfer function shows that sound levels may increase more than 20 dB in hearing level while being transmitted from the auricle to the tympanic membrane, and that the gain is frequency dependent.

only change the phase characteristics of a sound stimulus, it can actually amplify these wavelengths, increasing the sound pressure at the tympanic membrane. The combination of phase and amplitude changes that results from the effects of intervening structures is known as a **transfer function.** Transfer functions can describe effects of the head and torso on interaural time difference, as well as resonance-mediated increases in amplitude of a signal (Figure 7-4) (Tonndorf, 1988; Yost, 2000).

EXTERNAL AUDITORY MEATUS

The concha of the auricle feeds directly into the remaining portion of the external ear, the ear canal or external auditory meatus. In adult humans, the ear canal is approximately 2.5 cm long and 0.7 cm in diameter. The outer one-third to one-half of the canal has a flexible cartilaginous frame, much like the rest of the external ear. The remaining inner portion is attached to the temporal bone of the skull. The canal is slightly elliptical in shape. The path of the ear canal

is slightly twisted or S-shaped. The outer cartilaginous portion runs superior/posterior, and the inner bony portion runs inferior/anterior. This lazy S shape can be straightened for otoscopic examination of the tympanic membrane by pulling the auricle gently in a posterior/superior direction (see Figure 7-1) (Gray, 1996).

Functional Significance of the External Auditory Meatus

In addition to its resonance capabilities, the ear canal protects the tympanic membrane and middle ear by both anatomic and physiologic means. Anatomically, the length and diameter of the canal impede foreign objects that might enter and damage the delicate tympanic membrane. The S-shaped course of the canal also aids protection in this respect. The physical properties of the ear canal also help to ensure that the middle and inner ear will not be influenced by external temperature changes. Given the pronounced effect that temperature would have on the viscosity of inner ear fluids, imagine how differently our hearing sensitivity might change as we moved from one environment to the next if this were not the case.

Physiologic protection is afforded by a variety of different mechanisms. First, hairs located in the outer third of the canal, which all point outward, provide an effective barrier to both animate (bugs) and inanimate objects (small beads and beans). Second, sebaceous and ceruminous glands, also located in the cartilaginous portion, secrete wax that has antibacterial and antifungal properties. Last, the external or epidermal layer of the tympanic membrane and that of the ear canal actually migrates outward, a characteristic quite unique to this part of the body. The mechanism of this shedding is unknown. Migration occurs at a rate of 0.5 to 1.0 mm/day and functions to keep the tympanic membrane and ear canal free of shed skin cells, called *keratinocytes,* and dried cerumen, as well as any other small debris (Johnson, Hawke, & Jahn, 1988). In other parts of the body, this shedding process is achieved by daily friction or rubbing against the skin, obviously not an option deep in the ear canal. Impaired migration of epidermis may contribute to the devastating middle ear disorder cholesteatoma (cholesteatoma is discussed in Chapter 17). In addition to clearing debris, epithelial migration also encourages the rapid and spontaneous healing of tympanic membrane perforations.

MIDDLE EAR

The external ear ends at the tympanic membrane, a delicate boundary between the external and middle portions of the ear. The middle ear couples sound energy from the external auditory meatus to the inner ear, or cochlea, and in doing so, helps to match the relatively low impedance of the air in the ear canal to the high impedance of the fluids in the cochlea. We discuss why this is important later in this chapter, but first, the following subsections examine the anatomic structures of the middle ear.

Temporal Bone

The central portion of the external auditory meatus, the middle ear cavity, and the structures that comprise the inner ear are all situated within the petrous portion of the temporal bone. The human temporal bone is formed from four separate bones: the squamous, petrous, tympanic, and mastoid bones (Figure 7-5). Only the squamous, petrous, and tympanic portions are present at birth. These bones grow and fuse through childhood as the fourth part, or mastoid portion, develops. The squamous portion is a flat, sheetlike bone on the lateral superior surface of the temporal bone. It forms the roof of the bony external auditory canal. The zygomatic process extends from the inferior edge of the squamous temporal bone. The tympanic portion is a horseshoe-shaped structure that forms the floor and the anterior and posterior walls of the bony external auditory canal. The mastoid portion is a bulky bone with a large prominence that can be felt just behind the ear. This prominence provides the attachment site for several of the strap muscles of the neck. These portions of the temporal bone provide for muscle attachments and bony support of the external ear. Three muscles—the anterior, superior, and posterior auricularis muscles—attach the auricle to the temporal bone (Gray, 1996). In most humans, these are almost useless because we readily turn our heads to assist with localization of sound in space. Many animals, however, must limit movement to avoid detection by predators, and therefore need and have much greater control over movements of their pinnae.

The final portion of the temporal bone is the petrous portion. It is the petrous portion that actually houses the middle and inner ear (Figure 7-6). The base of this pyramid-shaped bone is attached to the medial surface of the other temporal bones, and the apex projects inward toward the brain. An opening on the posterior surface of the petrous temporal bone, the **internal auditory meatus** (see Figure 7-5, right), allows passage of the auditory and vestibular nerves from the inner ear to the brain and nerve processes from the brain to the inner ear as well.

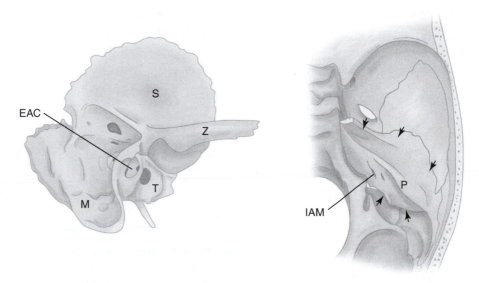

FIGURE 7-5   The right human temporal bone shown in lateral view (left) and superior view (right). The squamous bone (S), tympanic bone (T), and mastoid bone (M) can be seen in the lateral view. Other structures include the zygomatic arch (Z) and the external auditory meatus (EAC). The outer layer of the mastoid bone has been drilled away in this sample to show the mastoid air cells. The petrous portion (P, *arrowheads*) of the temporal bone must be viewed from the interior of the skull, where it forms the floor of the middle cranial fossa (bottom). The internal auditory meatus (IAM) transmits the auditory nerve.

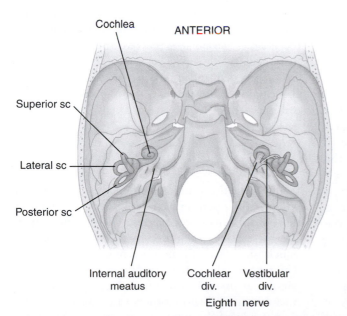

FIGURE 7-6   The base of the human skull showing the orientation of the membranous labyrinth in the temporal bone. Visible structures include the cochlea; the superior, lateral, and posterior semicircular canals (sc); and the internal auditory meatus through which the 8th cranial nerve (i.e., vestibulocochlear) enters the temporal bone. Shown at the left is a stained horizontal section through the middle of the temporal bone.

Tympanic Membrane

The eardrum, or tympanic membrane, is a delicate film or sheet of tissue that stretches across the border between the external and middle ears. It is approximately 9.0 mm in diameter in adult humans and is oriented such that the inferior edge is anchored more medially than the superior edge, creating a 55-degree angle with the floor of the ear canal (Gray, 1996). It is also concave in shape, an attribute that lends some flexibility to the membrane and, in doing so, adds to the functional significance of the middle ear, as we shall discuss. The membrane in humans is roughly five to eight cell layers thick, though this varies widely among animal species. The tympanic membrane transmits vibrational energy to the bones of the middle ear via its attachment to the manubrium of the **malleus.**

The tympanic membrane has been divided extensively into distinct anatomic regions based on both location and physical properties (Figure 7-7). It is commonly divided into quadrants, named for their anterior/posterior and superior/inferior locations. Most of the perimeter of the tympanic membrane is a thickened fibrocartilaginous ring, the annulus, fixed to the tympanic portion of the temporal bone. The superior edge of the membrane is not similarly fixed, but it is connected by two folds, the anterior and posterior malleolar folds, to the lateral process of the malleus. The small triangular-shaped region of membrane above these folds is more lax than the rest of the membrane and is called the *pars flaccida.* The majority of the membrane, which is tauter like the skin of a drum, is known as *pars tensa* and is much better adapted for the transmission of sound-induced vibrations into the middle ear. The membrane is concave because of its attachment to the manubrium of the malleus, which draws it inward. The most recessed portion of this concavity is known as the *umbo.*

The thickness of the tympanic membrane is composed of three layers. The outermost lateral or cutaneous layer is continuous with the epithelial lining of the ear canal. It is this layer that migrates to aid in clearing of debris and spontaneous healing of tympanic membrane perforations. The intermediate or fibrous layer is actually composed of two types of fibers: a radiate layer of laterally directed fibers that

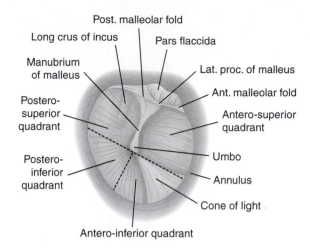

FIGURE 7-7   Lateral view of the tympanic membrane as if through a speculum or otoscope. The tympanic membrane can be divided into quadrants. The anterior and posterior malleolar folds define the region known as pars flaccida. The manubrium of the malleus can be seen at its attachment to the medial side of the membrane, where it creates the most concave region known as the umbo. The long arm of the incus can often be seen on the other side of the posterior superior quadrant of pars tensa.

extend from the manubrium outward and a circular layer of fibers that are more prominent at the periphery of the membrane. The innermost layer, known as the *medial* or *mucous layer,* is derived from the lining of the middle ear cavity. The tympanic membrane is well innervated, and thus quite sensitive to pressure. Branches of cranial nerves V and X innervate the lateral aspect of the membrane, and cranial nerve IX innervates the medial surface (Gray, 1996).

Ossicles

Connecting the tympanic membrane to the oval window, the opening to the inner ear, is a chain of three small bones or **ossicles.** Despite their small size, these bones are joined by true articular joints, which allow significant movement of the chain. The first ossicle or malleus possesses a head, neck, handle or manubrium, and short process. The manubrium and short process are attached to the medial side of the tympanic membrane. The head of the malleus articulates with the body of the second ossicle, the **incus.** The incus has two processes or crura, one short and one long. The short process extends back to the posterior bony wall of the middle ear and acts as the fulcrum or pivot point for incus rotation. The long process articulates with the head of the third ossicle, the **stapes.** Attached to the head of the stapes are two crura that connect to the footplate. The footplate of the stapes is sealed to the entry of the inner ear or oval window by means of an annular ligament. The relation of the three ossicles and their associations with the tympanic membrane and oval window are shown in Figures 7-7 and 7-8.

The ossicles are suspended in the middle ear cavity by several ligaments, the most important of which are the posterior ligament of the incus and the anterior ligament of the malleus. Tension along the ossicular chain is dependent on movement of the flexible tympanic membrane as sound waves impinge on it, but it can also be modulated by the actions of two small muscles that help to anchor the ossicles to the bony walls of the middle ear. The **tensor tympani** muscle arises from a bony canal on the anterior wall of the middle ear, just above the opening of the **Eustachian tube.** It is attached to the neck of the malleus and, when contracted, serves to increase tension on the tympanic membrane by pulling the manubrium of the malleus inward. The tensor tympani is innervated by a branch of the fifth cranial nerve (the trigeminal nerve). The **stapedius** muscle arises from the posterior wall and inserts into the neck of the stapes. It is the smallest skeletal muscle in the human body. Contraction of the stapedius muscle pulls the stapes rearward, orthogonal to its plane of piston-like movement, to fix the footplate in the oval window. The stapedius is innervated by a branch of the seventh cranial nerve (the facial nerve). Contractions of these middle ear muscles may play important roles in protection of the hearing apparatus, speech discrimination, and pressure equilibration (see later).

Acoustic Middle Ear Reflex

In humans, the **acoustic middle ear reflex** represents a contraction of the stapedius muscle in response to sound. In many animal species, con-

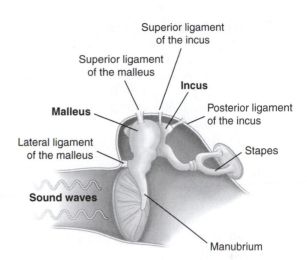

FIGURE 7-8 The functional/structural arrangement of the ossicular chain in the middle ear. Pictured is the malleus with its long process or manubrium embedded in the medial surface of the tympanic membrane. The head of the malleus is attached to the body of the incus whose short process extends to the posterior wall and acts as the fulcrum for ossicular movement. The long process of the incus is fixed to the head of the stapes. Two crura of the stapes connect the head to the footplate, which is sealed onto the round window membrane by the annular ligament. The ossicular chain is suspended in the cavity by way of several ligaments, including the superior and lateral ligaments of the malleus and the posterior and superior ligaments of the incus.

tractions of both the stapedius and tensor tympani muscles are used by this reflex. The threshold of the acoustic reflex is about 85 dB in normal-hearing adults. The strength of the stapedius contraction increases with increasing amplitude of the sound stimulus, and the latency of the response decreases from about 100 milliseconds at threshold to approximately 25 milliseconds for a high-intensity stimulus. Even when a stimulus is presented to only one ear, the reflex is present in both ears, but it is stronger in the ear that received the stimulus. The acoustic middle ear reflex is most commonly studied by examining changes in the acoustic impedance of the ear using noninvasive tympanometry, which is available in most clinical settings.

The neural pathways responsible for the acoustic middle ear reflex start with the first synapse in the ventral cochlear nucleus. From there, two main pathways of the stapedius reflex exist. One direct pathway travels from the ventral cochlear nucleus to the ipsilateral facial motor nucleus without additional synapses. Facial nerve fibers then communicate directly with the stapedius muscle through a small branch off the facial nerve called the *stapedius nerve.* The other and less direct pathway travels through the trapezoid body, synapsing in the lateral and medial superior olivary complexes before ascending to both ipsilateral and contralateral facial motor nuclei (Moller, 2000).

The acoustic middle ear reflex may serve two useful purposes. First, contraction of the stapedius muscle stiffens the ossicular chain, which may prevent noise damage to middle and inner ear structures, particularly to sudden loud noises. Second, stiffening of the ossicular chain preferentially reduces transmission of low-frequency sounds, and may therefore enhance the perception of high frequencies that can be masked by low frequencies. This has been shown to be important for the discrimination of loud speech because it has been observed that patients with paralyzed stapedius muscles have reduced speech discrimination scores at speech levels greater than 90 dB. However, we typically do not encounter speech at levels of 90 dB, so the functional significance of this remains in question. Because both middle ear muscles may be contracted by the initiation of speech production, this reflex may serve to mask the bodily sounds of speech mechanics so we do not have to listen to the sounds of our own breathing and tongue and jaw movements as we speak.

Eustachian Tube

If the middle ear were a closed chamber, it would suffer from pressure alterations caused by changes in temperature and altitude. The Eustachian tube (sometimes referred to as the auditory tube) is a small channel, approximately 36 mm in length, that connects the middle ear to the lateral wall of the nasopharynx. The first 12 mm is bony and begins in the anterior wall of the middle ear cavity. The Eustachian tube allows air to pass from the nasopharynx to the middle ear to equalize pressure on either side of the tympanic membrane. Middle ear pressure must equal the external atmospheric pressure to maintain the full movement of the tympanic membrane. Although the tube is normally closed, it commonly opens briefly during swallowing by the action of the salpingopharyngeus and dilator tubae muscles of the palate, which are innervated by cranial nerve XI, the spinal accessory nerve. It is possible to force the Eustachian tube open by trying to blow air against the resistance of a closed mouth and nose (the Valsalva maneuver). Experienced scuba divers can hold their Eustachian tube open or open it briefly at will by swallowing. The inexperienced diver that is unable to equilibrate pressure in the middle ear will experience the painful consequences after descending only a few feet underwater. Unfortunately, at this point, the pressure increase only makes it more difficult to open the Eustachian tube.

Summary of the Middle Ear Cavity

It might be useful at this point to take an overall look at those structures both within and adjacent to the middle ear cavity because they may also be affected by diseases of the middle ear. If you were to stand in the external auditory canal, peering through the transparent tympanic membrane with the ossicles removed, you would see something similar to Figure 7-9. On the anterior wall of the chamber, to your right, is the opening to the Eustachian tube. On the medial wall straight ahead is a bump called the *promontory* that indicates the location of the underlying basal turn of the cochlea. Overlying the promontory can be seen the tympanic nerve plexus, a branch of cranial nerve IX. Just above and posterior to the promontory is the oval window that leads to the vestibule of the inner ear and is normally covered by the stapes footplate. Slightly posterior to the promontory is the round window opening to scala tympani of the cochlea. Also seen in the posterior superior corner

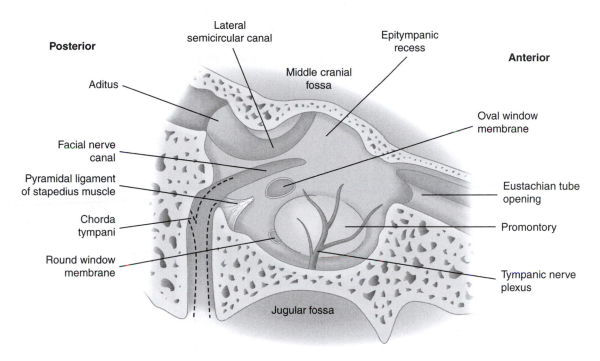

FIGURE 7-9 Lateral view of the right middle ear cavity as if peering through the tympanic membrane. The ossicles have been removed to permit observation of other structures. Adjacent anatomic structures are labeled and their relations with the middle ear cavity are outlined in the text.

of the medial wall is a prominence that indicates the underlying horizontal (or lateral) semicircular canal. This is the only part of the vestibular system that is exposed for visual inspection using noninvasive means. Along the superior anterior aspect of the medial wall is the canal that transmits the tensor tympani muscle that will attach to the manubrium of the malleus. On the posterior wall, we find a recess called the *aditus* that extends into the mastoid bone and a prominence called the *pyramid* to which the stapedius muscle is attached. Running vertically up the outer posterior wall is the chorda tympani, a branch of the facial nerve that carries taste sensation from the anterior two thirds of the tongue. The base or floor of the middle ear is composed mostly of the bony canal that surrounds the internal jugular vein. The roof is a layer of bone that separates the middle ear from the middle cranial fossa of the skull base. The epitym-

panic recess that extends upward into the roof allows the head of the malleus and body and short process of the incus to sit above the superior edge of the tympanic membrane (O'Rahilly, 1983).

Functional Significance of the Middle Ear

The middle ear is responsible for an important aspect of the transmission of sound waves, that of impedance matching. **Impedance** can be described as an obstruction or hindrance to movement. Why is impedance important for the transmission of energy from airborne sound waves to the fluids of the cochlea? Well, consider what happens when light rays hit the surface of water. The light is reflected. In fact, almost all of the light is reflected. The same thing would happen in the ear if airborne sound waves were to impinge directly on the oval window of the fluid-filled cochlea. It is estimated that more than 99.9% of the sound energy would be reflected off the oval window membrane, creating an inefficient vehicle for sound reception because of this impedance mismatch (Pickles, 1988). So, how does the middle ear accomplish impedance matching? The structures of the middle ear actually use several different mechanisms to increase the force applied to the oval window through the stapes footplate, effectively matching the impedance of the air in the ear canal to that of the cochlear fluids. These mechanisms are summarized in Figure 7-10 and also discussed further later; Relkin (1988) also analyzes these mechanisms in detail.

First and most important, the area of the tympanic membrane is much greater than that of the stapes footplate or oval window. The functional area of the tympanic membrane in this respect is that which is stiffly connected to the manubrium, which measures approximately 55 mm^2. The area covered by the stapes footplate is only about 3.2 mm^2. Since pressure is equal to force per unit area ($p = F/A$), the increase in force on the oval window is equivalent to the ratio of the size differences, or 55 mm^2/3.2 mm^2, which equals 17. Thus, the decrease in size between the tympanic membrane and the stapes footplate contributes a 17-fold increase in force to help overcome the impedance mismatch.

A second mechanism takes into account the flexibility and conical shape of the tympanic membrane. As this membrane moves in and out, it buckles, allowing the arm of the malleus to move less than the membrane. This results in an increase in force but a decrease in velocity, again increasing the pressure on the oval window accordingly. This mechanism contributes approximately a twofold increase in pressure to the oval window.

The third contribution to impedance matching comes from the lever action of the ossicles. Because the arm of the incus that articulates with the head of the stapes is shorter than the manubrium of the malleus, the resultant action on the stapes is again one of increased force and decreased velocity. This mechanism contributes a 1.3-fold increase in force on the oval window. Studies in the cat have shown that the contributions of these three mechanisms are sufficient to meet the increased

impedance of the cochlear fluids, with the tympanic membrane/oval window ratio contributing more than 85% of the needed change in force. The gain achieved by the human middle ear is frequency dependent, but measures roughly 30 dB in the midfrequency range.

Additional functional attributes of middle ear structures would include the protection afforded by acoustic reflex contraction of the stapedius muscle in response to loud noise and the directing of applied forces to the oval window exclusively. Another opening to the cochlea, the round window, is covered by a thin round window membrane that allows pressures transmitted into the cochlea to be dissipated from the opposite side of the basilar membrane. This allows for a unidirectional flow of pressure into and out of the cochlea. If during sound wave transmission pressure were applied equally to both the oval and round window membranes, there would be no resultant movement within the cochlea because the cochlear fluids are incompressible.

BLOOD FLOW AND INNERVATION TO THE OUTER AND THE MIDDLE EAR

Blood flow to the auricle is supplied by the posterior auricular artery, a branch of the external carotid, the anterior auricular branch of the superficial temporal artery, and a branch from the occipital artery (Figure 7-11). Arteries that supply the external auditory meatus include branches from the posterior auricular, maxillary, and temporal arteries (Gray, 1996). Sensory nerves that supply the auricle include the greater auricular nerve, from the cervical plexus; the auricular branch of the vagus nerve; the auriculotemporal branch of the mandibular nerve (trigeminal origin); and the lesser occipital nerve from the cervical plexus (Peuker & Filler, 2002). Nerves that supply the external auditory meatus include the auriculotemporal branch of the mandibular nerve and the auricular branch of the vagus (Gray, 1996).

Blood flow to the middle ear is provided by six different arteries: the tympanic branch of the maxillary artery (tympanic membrane), the stylomastoid branch of the posterior auricular artery

Mechanism	Ratio of force increase	Relative force increase
Area	$A_{TM} : A_{OW}$	$17\times$
Velocity	$V_{TM} : V_{Malleus}$	$2\times$
Lever action	$L_{Man} : L_{Incus}$	$1.3\times$

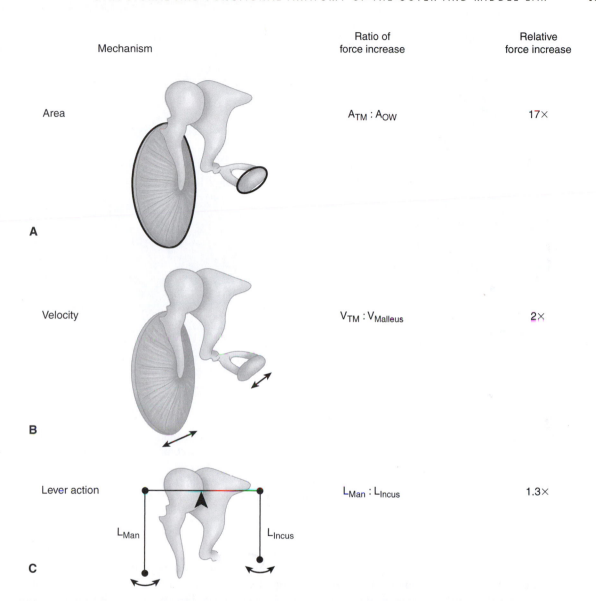

A

B

C

FIGURE 7-10 The three mechanisms used to increase the force on the oval window (OW), relative to that on the tympanic membrane (TM). (A) Because pressure = force/area, the force applied to the oval window becomes a function of the ratio of the areas of the two structures, which is approximately 55 mm²/3.2 mm², or an increase of 17 times the pressure at the TM. (B) The flexible nature of the TM allows it to be displaced more than the manubrium, which means the velocity of TM movement is increased relative to the manubrium. Because the product of velocity and pressure must remain equal, and the velocity of the manubrium is less than the TM, the pressure (force) on the manubrium must be greater than that on the TM. (C) The lever action of the malleus/incus chain results in a larger force and decreased velocity on the stapes compared with the TM because the manubrium (L_{man}) is longer than the long process of the incus (L_{incus}).

Blood supply

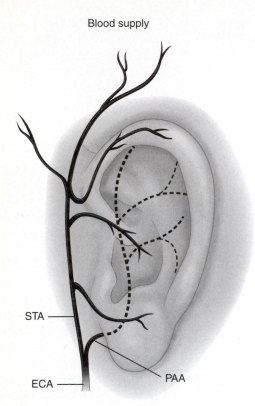

Nerve supply

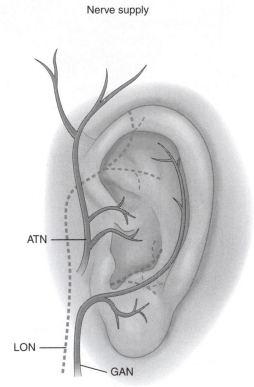

FIGURE 7-11   Blood supply and innervation of the outer ear. Diagrams of the major blood supply (left) and innervation (right) of the human auricle. Blood supply to the auricle is accomplished via two branches of the external carotid artery (ECA), the superficial temporal artery (STA) and the posterior auricular artery (PAA). Innervation of the auricle is by great auricular nerve (GAN), auriculotemporal nerve (ATN), and the lesser occipital nerve (LON). Vessels and nerves that project to the posterior portions of the auricle are denoted by broken *(dotted)* profiles.

(posterior wall and mastoid), the petrosal branch of the middle meningeal artery, a branch of the ascending pharyngeal, the tympanic branch of the internal carotid, and a branch from the artery of the pterygoid canal. Several nerves innervate the middle ear and contribute to the tympanic plexus, a meshwork of nerves that lies over the surface of the promontory. These nerves include the tympanic branch of the glossopharyngeal nerve and the superior and inferior caroticotympanic nerves from the sympathetic carotid plexus. From the tympanic plexus, nerves are distributed to the mucosal lining of the middle ear cavity, the round and oval window membranes, and the Eustachian tube. Interestingly, pathology to the other areas supplied by these same nerves can cause "referred pain" sensations to the middle ear, a common cause of otalgia or ear pain (Gray, 1996).

↭ SUMMARY ↝

This chapter explores the anatomy and functional significance of the external and the middle ear. The external ear consists of the auricle and external auditory meatus, which promote and enhance the airborne transmission of sound waves through a process called *resonance*. The middle ear structures are designed to enhance the pressure of the airborne wave so it will match the greater impedance of the cochlear fluids. The tympanic membrane, together with the three ossicles, the malleus, incus, and stapes, provide a moving chain of structures that successfully performs this impedance matching task. Two small middle ear muscles, the stapedius and tensor tympani, when contracted, are capable of stiffening the ossicular chain to both protect the inner ear from sudden loud noises and to enhance the perception of high-frequency sounds.

↭ KEY TERMS ↝

Acoustic middle ear
  reflex
Antihelix
Antitragus
Auricle
Concha
Earlobe

Eustachian tube
External auditory
  meatus
External ear
Helix
Impedance
Incus

Internal auditory
  meatus
Malleus
Ossicles
Resonance
Stapedius
Stapes

Tensor tympani
Tragus
Transfer function
Tympanic membrane

↭ STUDY QUESTIONS ↝

1. Discuss how the external ear can aid in auditory perception. Does this differ for low- and high-frequency sounds? Explain why.

2. Define resonance. Tell what frequencies are enhanced by the specific resonance capabilities of the outer ear. Why are these frequencies important for human hearing?

3. What is the acoustic middle ear reflex? What is the likely functional significance of such a reflex?

4. How does the middle ear prevent airborne sound waves from being reflected as they hit the tympanic membrane?

5. Discuss the three different mechanisms the middle ear uses to match the impedance of air in the external ear canal to the fluids of the inner ear. Which of these mechanisms is the most important? What would be the result if impedance was not matched?

↭ REFERENCES ↝

Goode, R. L. (1988). Auditory physiology of the external ear. In Fahn, A. F., & Santos-Sacchi, J. (Eds.), *Physiology of the ear* (pp. 147–159). New York: Raven Press, New York.

Gray, H. (1996). In Williams, P. L. (Ed.), *Gray's anatomy* (pp. 1068–1097). New York: Elsevier Press.

Johnson, A., Hawke, M., & Jahn, A. F. (1988). The nonauditory physiology of the external ear canal. In Fahn, A. F., & Santos-Sacchi, J. (Eds.), *Physiology of the ear* (pp. 41–58). New York: Raven Press.

Möller, A. R. (2000). *Hearing: Its physiology and pathophysiology* (pp. 5–67). San Diego: Academic Press.

O'Rahilly, R. (1983). *Basic human anatomy* (pp. 391–399). Philadelphia: WB Saunders.

Peuker, E. T., & Filler, T. J. (2002). The nerve supply of the human auricle. *Clinical Anatomy, 15,* 35–37.

Pickles, J. O. (1988). The outer and middle ears. *An Introduction to the Physiology of Hearing* (3rd ed.). San Diego: Academic Press.

Relkin, E. (1988). Introduction to the analysis of middle ear function. In Fahn, A. F., & Santos-Sacchi, J. (Eds.), *Physiology of the ear* (pp. 103–123). New York: Raven Press.

Tonndorf, J. (1988). The external ear. In Fahn, A. F., & Santos-Sacchi, J. (Eds.), *Physiology of the ear* (pp. 29–39). New York: Raven Press.

Yost, W. A. (2000). *Fundamentals of hearing: An introduction* (p. 65–78). San Diego: Academic Press.

Chapter

8

Cochlear Anatomy

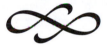

Barbara A. Bohne, Ph.D.
Professor of Otolaryngology
Washington University School of Medicine
St. Louis, Missouri

Gary W. Harding, M.S.E.
Associate Professor of Otolaryngology
Washington University School of Medicine
St. Louis, Missouri

Although the middle ear is important for enhancing one's sensitivity to airborne sound, you can hear loud sounds even if part of the middle ear is missing or blocked (see Chapter 17). In contrast, the **cochlea** (i.e., hearing portion of the inner ear) is absolutely essential for hearing. It contains the sensory cells (i.e., inner [IHC] and outer **hair cells** [OHC]) responsible for converting mechanical waves into electrical activity that is transmitted to the brain and perceived as sound. Sensory cells can be destroyed by excessive exposure to noise (see Chapter 18), certain drugs (see Chapter 19), infections in the inner ear, or aging (see Chapter 21). Permanent loss of sensory cells is manifested functionally as a sensorineural hearing loss. This chapter describes the basic structure of the cochlea, the complicated hearing organ (i.e., **organ of Corti**), the specialized sensory cells and their innervation, and the fluids and fluid spaces in the cochlea.

GROSS STRUCTURE OF THE INNER EAR

The temporal bone is one of the major bones of the skull. It forms part of the floor and lateral side of the skull (Figure 8-1). Both the middle and inner ears are completely contained within the petrous (i.e., rock hard) portion of the temporal bone (see Figure 8-1, black dashed line).[1]

The temporal bone must be removed from the skull and dissected open, or decalcified, embedded in a support medium, then cut into thin slices (i.e., sections) using a precision sectioning machine called a *microtome* to view middle- and inner-ear structures. The sections are stained to show various

---

[1]Within the inner ear, there are eponyms for a number cell types and structures based on the descriptions of early anatomists, including Boettcher, Claudius, Corti, Deiters, Hensen, Huschke, Nuel, Reissner, and Rosenthal. An excellent history of the discoveries pertaining to the inner ear and the changes in nomenclature over time can be found in articles by Hawkins (2004a, b) and Schacht and Hawkins (2004).

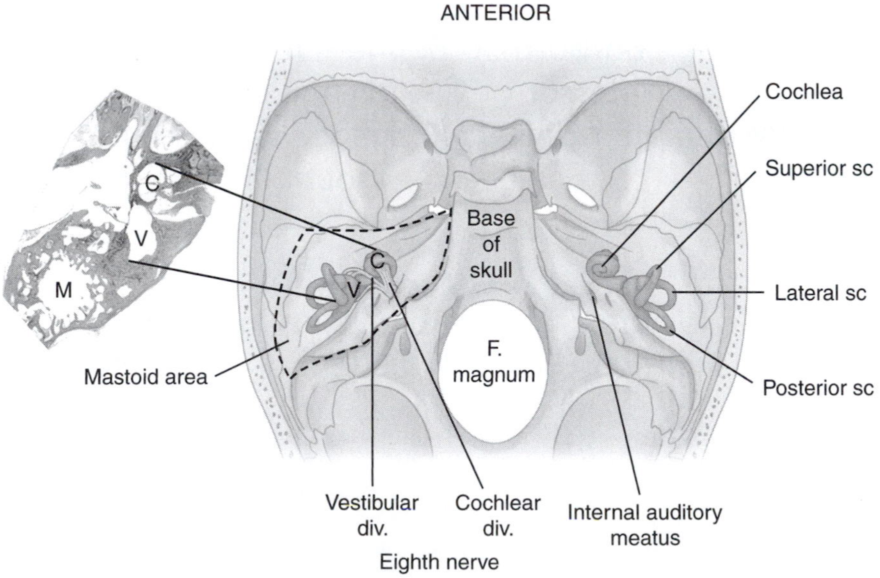

FIGURE 8-1 View of the base of the human skull with silhouettes of the left and right inner ears superimposed on the petrous portion of the temporal bone (outlined by *black dashed line*). C, cochlea; F. magnum, hole (foramen) in basal part of skull through which the spinal cord joins the brainstem; M, mastoid air cells; sc, semicircular canal; V, vestibule. The anatomical relations of key structures are indicated on the horizontal section through the left temporal bone.

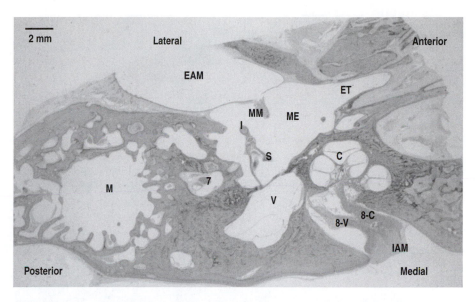

FIGURE 8-2 Horizontal section (20-μm thick) through the middle of the human temporal bone (same section as in Figure 8-1). C, cochlea; EAM, external auditory meatus; ET, Eustachian tube; I, incus; IAM, internal auditory meatus; M, mastoid; ME, middle-ear cavity; MM, manubrium of malleus; S, stapes; V, vestibule; 7, facial nerve; 8-C, cochlear division of vestibulocochlear nerve; 8-V, vestibular division of vestibulocochlear nerve.

tissues and cells, mounted on glass slides, and examined by light microscopy. An overview of the relations among the external, middle, and inner ears can be obtained by examining a horizontal section through the middle of the temporal bone. Figure 8-2 shows a section through a normal human temporal bone at the level of the external auditory meatus (EAM) and **internal auditory meatus** (IAM). The three-dimensional appearance of the middle-ear cavity is comparable with a rectangular box. The top is formed by the tegmen tympani, a thin plate of bone that separates the middle-ear cavity from the brain in the middle cranial fossa. The bottom is formed by the bone of the hypotympanum, separating the middle-ear cavity from the jugular bulb. The four walls are formed, respectively, by the tympanic membrane laterally, the cochlea (C) and vestibule (V) medially, the mastoid air cells (M) posteriorly and the Eustachian tube (ET) anteriorly. The most posterior portion of the mastoid appears as a bump behind the auricle. In the

middle-ear cavity (ME), portions of the ossicles (i.e., manubrium of the malleus [MM] attached to the tympanic membrane, long process of the incus [I] and stapes [S]) are visible. The vertical descent of the seventh cranial nerve (i.e., **facial nerve** [7]) through the temporal bone is visible in the posterior wall of the middle-ear cavity. Both the cochlear division (8-C) and vestibular division (8-V) of the eighth cranial nerve (i.e., **vestibulocochlear nerve**) are seen in the IAM.

The cochlea (Latin meaning "snail shell") consists of a spiral canal that, in humans, makes two and a half turns around a spongy central core termed the **modiolus.** Dividing the cochlea in half shows the centrally placed modiolus (M) and five radial sections through the cochlear turns and fluid spaces (i.e., **scala vestibuli** [SV], **scala tympani** [ST], **scala media** [Figure 8-3, box]). The bodies of the **spiral ganglion cells** (i.e., primary auditory neurons) are found in **Rosenthal's canal** (rc), a spiral canal located at the periphery of the modiolus (M).

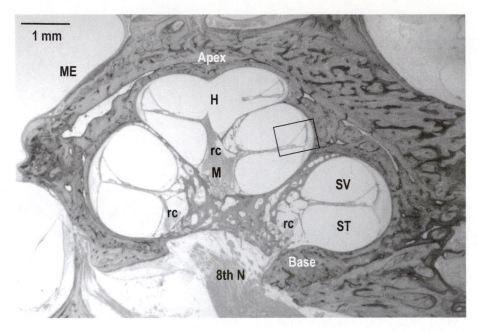

FIGURE 8-3   High-power photomicrograph of a midmodiolar section through the human cochlea. *Box* denotes the boundaries of one turn of the membranous cochlea that is shown at a higher power in Figure 8-4. 8th N, cochlear division of vestibulocochlear nerve; H, helicotrema; M, modiolus; ME, middle-ear cavity; rc, Rosenthal's canal; ST, scala tympani; SV, scala vestibuli.

The central processes (i.e., axons) of the ganglion cells form the cochlear division of the vestibulo-cochlear nerve (8th N) that exits the temporal bone at the base of the cochlea.

FLUID SPACES IN THE COCHLEA

Scala vestibuli and scala tympani are both filled with **perilymph,** a fluid that has a low concentration of potassium ions and a high concentration of sodium ions. This fluid is similar in ionic composition to cerebrospinal fluid (CSF). At the base of the cochlea, the oval and round windows provide openings from the middle ear into the vestibule and scala tympani, respectively. The stapes footplate is tightly held in the oval window by the annular ligament. The round window is closed by the relatively thin, semipermeable round-window membrane. Near the base of scala tympani, the

cochlear aqueduct connects scala tympani to the CSF space in the cranium. Scalae vestibuli and tympani are in communication with one another at the cochlear apex via the **helicotrema** (H) (see Figure 8-3).

Scala media is a triangular-shaped space that is located between scala vestibuli and scala tympani. Its boundaries are **Reissner's membrane,** the **basilar membrane,** and the **stria vascularis** (Figure 8-4). The boundaries of the **cochlear duct** or **endolymphatic space** are the epithelial covering on the superior surface of the basilar membrane, the superior surface of the **spiral limbus,** the inferior layer of Reissner's membrane, and the inner surface of the stria vascularis. The endolymphatic space is filled with **endolymph,** a fluid that has a low concentration of sodium ions and a high concentration of potassium ions, making it similar in ionic concentration to intracellular fluid.

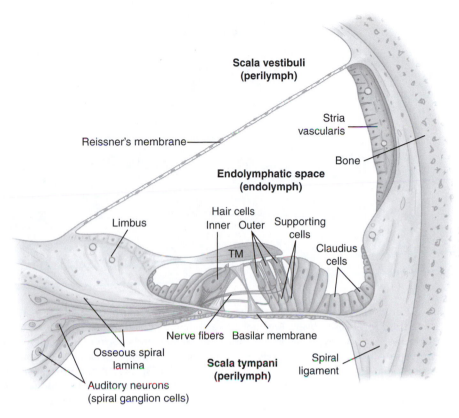

FIGURE 8-4   (See Color Plate) Schematic view of a portion of the membranous cochlea. C, Claudius cell; TM, tectorial membrane. (Adapted from Davis and Associates, 1953, by B.A. Bohne, 2004.)

COCHLEAR DUCT

The cochlear duct spirals around the modiolus from the base to the apex of the cochlea. A radial view of one turn of the cochlear duct is shown diagrammatically in Figure 8-4. All cells that form the endolymphatic boundary are derived from the embryonic cell layer called the *neuroectoderm* and are joined at their apical ends by tight junctions (i.e., **zonulae occludens**). Tight junctions prevent the passage of ions between the different fluid compartments in the cochlea.

The superior boundary of the endolymphatic space is formed by Reissner's membrane. This membrane is composed of two layers of squamous (i.e., flattened) cells. The cells in the inferior layer are joined by tight junctions. The lateral boundary of the endolymphatic space is formed by the stria vascularis. The cells on the surface of the stria vascularis facing the modiolus are joined by tight junctions. The inferior boundary of the endolymphatic space is formed by the superior surface of the organ of Corti, Claudius cells, inner sulcus cells, and the epithelial cells on the superior surface of the limbus. Boettcher cells (not shown in Figure 8-4) are found laterally on the basilar membrane in the basal turn. Their apical surfaces are entirely covered by

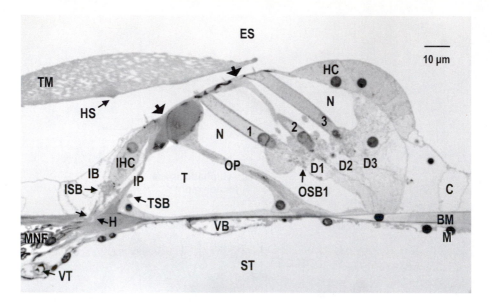

FIGURE 8-5   Radial section of the organ of Corti from the second turn of a control chinchilla. 1, 2, 3, outer hair cells in the first, second, and third rows, respectively; BM, basilar membrane; C, Claudius cell; D1, D2, D3, Deiters' cell in first, second, and third rows, respectively; ES, endolymphatic space; H, habenula perforata (between *arrows*); HC, Hensen's cell; HS, Hensen's stripe; IB, inner border cell; IHC, inner hair cell; IP, inner pillar cell; ISB, inner spiral bundle of nerve fibers; M, mesothelial cell; MNF, myelinated nerve fibers; N, Nuel's space; OP, outer pillar cell; OSB1, first outer spiral bundle of nerve fibers; ST, scala tympani; T, tunnel; TM, tectorial membrane; TSB, tunnel spiral bundle of nerve fibers; VB, vessel of the basilar membrane; VT, vessel of the tympanic lip of the osseous spiral lamina.

Claudius cells. The exact function of the Boettcher cells is unknown, but it may involve ion or fluid transport, or both.

The limbus is attached to the superior lip of the **osseous spiral lamina** (i.e., double layer of thin bone projecting from the modiolus). The limbus consists of a network of fibrocytes, capillaries, and numerous filaments. The epithelial cells on the superior surface of the limbus are called *interdental cells*. These cells are separated from one another by the teeth of Huschke, short projections of the connective tissue of the limbus. The medial edge of the **tectorial membrane** (TM) is attached to the interdental cells of the limbus. These latter cells are thought to be responsible for maintaining the structure of the TM. The TM is a gelatinous matrix, with embedded fibrils, that is about 96% water. It overlies the superior surface of the organ of Corti. In the living ear, the lateral edge of the TM is at-

tached to the apical surfaces of **Hensen's cells** (HC) (Figure 8-5).

The peripheral processes of spiral ganglion cells and efferent fibers enter or leave the organ of Corti by passing between the two lips of the osseous spiral lamina. Innervation of the organ of Corti is discussed in a later section.

ORGAN OF CORTI

The organ of Corti (see Figure 8-4) is a lacy network of sensory and supporting cells with interposed fluid spaces. The sensory cells, called IHCs and OHCs, occupy the superior half of the organ of Corti. Hair cells were named for the small "hairlike" projections (i.e., **stereocilia**) from their apical surfaces. In the organ of Corti, the supporting cells extend from its superior to its inferior surface.

Because fixation of human temporal bones is generally not optimal and because all mammalian organs of Corti have substantially the same appearance, detailed structure of the organ of Corti can best be seen in sections of animal cochleas. Figure 8-5 is a photomicrograph of a radial section through the organ of Corti from a normal chinchilla. The thin, flexible basilar membrane (BM) is covered on its superior surface by the organ of Corti, inner sulcus cells medially, and Claudius cells (C) laterally, whereas mesothelial cells (M) and blood vessels (i.e., vessel of the basilar membrane [VB]; vessel of the tympanic lip of the osseous spiral lamina [VT]) are found on its inferior surface. The basilar membrane itself is composed of extracellular matrix material in which heavy, radially oriented fibrils are embedded. Scala tympani (ST) is inferior to the basilar membrane.

Extending from the cochlear base to apex, the organ of Corti contains two types of sensory cells: a single row of IHCs and three rows of OHCs. Supporting cells are found medial to and in between adjacent IHCs (i.e., inner border [IB]; inner phalangeal [p]; Figure 8-6), inferior and lateral to the OHCs (i.e., Deiters' cells [D1, D2, D3]; HC], and at the margins of the **tunnel** (T) (i.e., inner pillar cell [IP]; outer pillar cell [OP]). The **pillar** and **Deiters' cells** contain parallel, intracellular bundles of microtubules that extend from the bases of the cells on the basilar membrane up to their heads or phalangeal processes, respectively, at the superior surface of the organ of Corti. The inner and outer pillar cells have a triangular relation in the radial direction. The inner pillars are offset such that the thin head plate that projects from each inner pillar head generally overlaps part of two outer pillar heads. In the apical-basal (i.e., spiral) direction, the outer pillar feet are slightly apical to their heads and Deiters' cell processes angle basally across three to four OHCs before reaching the superior surface of the organ of Corti and forming phalangeal processes. These supporting cell relations provide stiff, yet lightweight, connections between the basilar membrane and endolymphatic surface of the organ of Corti.

A view of the endolymphatic surface of the organ of Corti in the first turn of a chinchilla cochlea is shown in Figure 8-6. The apical surface of each hair cell is separated from neighboring hair cells by phalangeal processes from different supporting cells. Adjacent IHCs are separated by phalangeal processes (p) from inner phalangeal cells. OHCs in the first row (see Figure 8-6, region 1) are separated by phalangeal processes from the outer pillar head (pop). OHCs in the second row (see Figure 8-6, region 2) are separated by phalangeal processes (D1) from the first row of Deiters' cells. OHCs in the third row (see Figure 8-6, region 3) are separated by phalangeal processes (D2) from the second row of Deiters' cells. Phalangeal processes (D3) from the third row of Deiters' cells are lateral to the third row of OHCs. Figure 8-6 shows that third-row OHCs are on a straight line directly lateral to the first-row OHCs. In contrast, second-row OHCs are offset in a spiral direction by half the diameter of an OHC.

The tunnel (T) and the **spaces of Nuel** (N) are fluid-filled spaces within the organ of Corti. The latter spaces surround the body of each OHC. All fluid spaces in the organ of Corti communicate with one another. The superior surface of the organ of Corti is termed the **reticular lamina** (see Figure 8-5, heavy arrows). It is composed of the head plates of the inner pillar cells and the apices of the hair cells alternating with phalangeal processes from the inner phalangeal cells, Deiters' cells, and outer pillar cells (see Figure 8-6). Tight junctions exist between all cells that form the reticular lamina. Therefore, the tunnel and Nuel's spaces are not in communication with the endolymphatic space (ES). A number of studies have shown that the fluid in the organ of Corti is perilymph or is similar to perilymph in its ionic composition.

The peripheral processes (myelinated nerve fibers [MNF]) of the spiral ganglion cells are myelinated until they enter the organ of Corti through a series of small holes in the basilar membrane called **habenulae perforata** (H; see Figure 8-5, small opposing arrows) that are located inferior to the IHCs. Within the organ of Corti, the nerve fibers form nonmyelinated bundles inferior to the

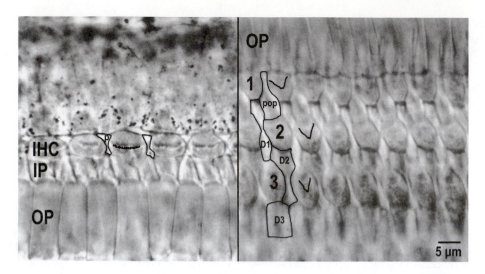

FIGURE 8-6   Horizontal view of the reticular lamina of the organ of Corti as seen from the direction of Reissner's membrane. 1, 2, 3, outer hair cell in first, second, and third rows, respectively; D1, D2, D3, phalangeal process from Deiters' cell in first, second, and third rows, respectively; IHC, inner hair cell; IP, inner pillar head; OP, outer pillar head; p, phalangeal process from inner phalangeal cell; pop, phalangeal process from outer pillar head. Arrangement of stereocilia on the hair cells is drawn in black.

IHC (i.e., inner spiral bundle [ISB]), within the tunnel space (i.e., tunnel spiral bundle [TSB]), and inferior to each row of OHCs (i.e., outer spiral bundles [e.g., OSB1]) (see Figure 8-5).

In most histologic preparations, the TM is shrunken and displaced from its *in vivo* location because of dehydration. Even with preparation artifacts, several features of the TM are visible, including its tapering lateral edge and **Hensen's stripe** (HS), which appears as a small, dark protrusion from its inferior surface (see Figure 8-5).

INNER AND OUTER HAIR CELLS

The intracellular organelles and surface specializations on IHCs and OHCs can best be appreciated in transmission electron micrographs (Figure 8-7). The IHC (I) has a flask-shaped body, a centrally located nucleus with organelles, such as mitochondria and lysosomes, scattered in the cytoplasm. Just inferior to the apical surface of the cell is an electron-dense structure called the *cuticular plate* (cp). The specializations on the apical surface [i.e., stereocilia (st)] of the

cell that project into the endolymphatic space (ES) are similar to elongated, parallel microvilli. Rootlets project into the cuticular plate from each stereocilium. On the IHCs, three to four rows of stereocilia are arranged in nearly a straight line, which is oriented in an apical-basal direction (see Figure 8-6). The stereocilia are graded in length with the shortest on the medial side and the tallest on the lateral side of the cell. *In vivo*, the tallest stereocilia are in contact with the lateral side of HS. Tight junctions (see Figure 8-6, arrows) are found between the inner pillar (IP) and the apex of the IHC, as well as the inner border cell (IB) and the IHC. Cross-sectioned nerve fibers (nf) are visible where the nerve fibers synapse on the hair cell base. The tunnel space (T) is visible lateral to the inner pillar body (see Figure 8-7A).

The OHC (O1) is long and cylindrical with its nucleus located near the base of the cell. The base of each OHC and its nerve endings (E) sit in the cup region (D) of a Deiters' cell. Intracellular organelles (i.e., mitochondria, lysosomes, and microbodies) are clustered in the region inferior to the cuticular plate (cp). A group of mitochondria inferior

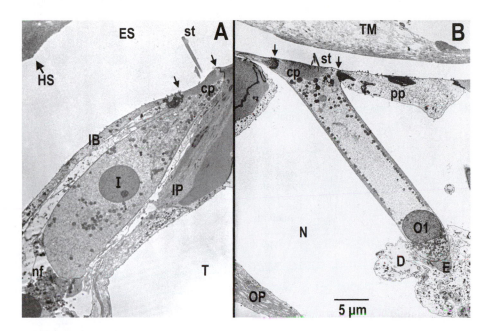

FIGURE 8-7 Transmission electron micrographs of (A) third-turn inner hair cell and (B) first-turn outer hair cell from a control chinchilla. cp, cuticular plate; D, cup region of Deiters' cell; E, nerve ending; ES, endolymphatic space; HS, Hensen's stripe; I, inner hair cell; IB, inner border cell; IP, inner pillar cell; N, Nuel's space; nf, nerve fibers; O1, first row outer hair cell; OP, outer pillar body; pp, phalangeal process from supporting cell; st, stereocilia; T, tunnel; TM, tectorial membrane.

to the nucleus fills the region where the nerve endings (E) synapse. A single row of mitochondria is found adjacent to the lateral plasma membrane of the cell. On the OHCs, three to five rows of stereocilia (st) are arranged in a "W-" or "V-shaped" pattern on the cell surface with the points facing laterally (see Figure 8-6). The stereocilia on the OHCs are also graded in length from the medial to the lateral side of the cell. *In vivo,* the tips of the tallest (i.e., lateralmost) stereocilia are embedded in the TM. Tight junctions (see Figure 8-7, arrows) are found between the hair cell apex and the phalangeal process (pp) of the adjacent supporting cells. Nuel's space (N) surrounds the OHC body (see Figure 8-7B).

HAIR CELL INNERVATION

The hair cells in the organ of Corti have both **afferent** and **efferent** innervation (Figure 8-8). The bipolar spiral ganglion cells, the bodies of which are located in Rosenthal's canal, provide afferent innervation to the hair cells. The central (i.e., axonal) processes of these cells traverse the modiolus, exit the temporal bone via the IAM, and synapse in the cochlear nuclei of the brainstem. Their peripheral processes traverse the osseous spiral lamina, pass through the holes in basilar membrane (i.e., habenulae perforata; see Figure 8-5), and enter the organ of Corti to synapse on the hair cells.

Type I spiral ganglion cells have large bodies and large, round nuclei. In some species other than humans, the bodies of type I ganglion cells and their peripheral processes (as far as the habenulae perforata) are myelinated. Depending on species, type I cells comprise 85% to 95% of the spiral ganglion cell population and exclusively innervate IHCs. The peripheral process of each type I ganglion cell exits a habenula perforata, runs directly to the nearest IHC, and forms a small bouton ending on the base or basolateral side of the hair cell. These fibers are called

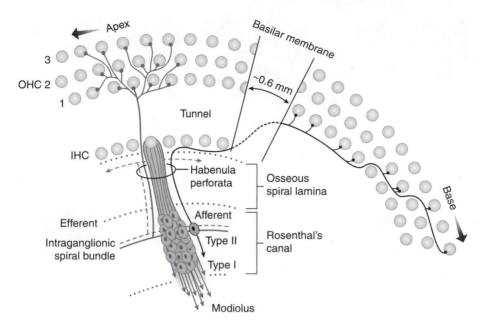

FIGURE 8-8   Summary of hair cell innervation in the organ of Corti. IHC, inner hair cells; OHC 1, 2, 3, outer hair cells in first, second, and third rows, respectively. (Adapted from Spoendlin, 1984, by B.A. Bohne, 2004.)

radial afferents, and depending on species and cochlear location, each IHC synapses with about 10 to 20 of these fibers. Within the IHC adjacent to afferent nerve endings, it is common to find synaptic bodies surrounded by synaptic vesicles.

Type II spiral ganglion cells have small bodies and lobular, eccentrically located nuclei, and they are thinly myelinated or not myelinated at all. Type II cells comprise 5% to 15% of the spiral ganglion cell population and exclusively innervate OHCs. These cells are located laterally in Rosenthal's canal near the origin of the osseous spiral lamina. Their peripheral processes exit the habenulae perforata, travel a short distance in the inner spiral bundle, pass between adjacent inner pillar feet, and then cross near the floor of the tunnel as basilar fibers. The fibers enter one of the outer spiral bundles, turn in a basal direction, and travel as much as 0.6 mm before forming bouton nerve endings on a variable number of OHC bases (e.g., 6–60) in one or more rows. Each OHC synapses with multiple (but an

unknown number) afferent fibers. Within the OHC adjacent to the afferent nerve endings, synaptic bodies are found in some species (e.g., human, guinea pig, and chinchilla), but not others (e.g., cat).

The neurons that provide efferent innervation to the hair cells are located in the brainstem (see Chapter 14). These neurons are found in both the ipsilateral and contralateral superior olivary complexes. The efferent fibers exit the brainstem with the vestibular division of the vestibulocochlear (8th) nerve, then cross (via Oort's anastomosis) to the cochlear division within the IAM. In all mammals, the number of efferent fibers innervating the cochlea is considerably smaller than the number of afferent fibers, although the exact number has been reported for only one species. In the cat, about 500 efferent fibers (crossed [i.e., contralateral] and uncrossed [i.e., ipsilateral]) enter each IAM. The efferent fibers then enter the intraganglionic spiral bundle that runs at the periphery of Rosenthal's canal. From their point of entry, these fibers run both apically and basally. Many of the fibers in the intraganglionic spiral bundle are non-myelinated. At various points, individual or small groups of fibers turn laterally to enter the osseous spiral lamina. These fibers pass through the habenulae perforata together with the afferent fibers and enter the organ of Corti. Efferent fibers to the IHCs turn and enter the inner spiral or tunnel spiral bundle, traveling for a variable distance before synapsing on the radial afferent fibers that, in turn, are synapsing on the IHC bases. Efferent fibers to the OHCs are myelinated before crossing the habenulae perforata. Once in the organ of Corti, these fibers may spiral in the inner spiral bundle for a short distance, pass to the tunnel spiral bundle, and then cross the tunnel as upper tunnel crossing fibers in most species. Lateral to the tunnel, the fibers immediately divide into multiple branches that run both apically and basally in the outer spiral bundles. On the bases of the OHCs, the efferent fibers form large endings that contain many synaptic vesicles and large mitochondria. A flattened cisterna of smooth endoplasmic reticulum (i.e., subsynaptic cisterna) is adjacent to each efferent nerve ending on OHCs.

SPIRAL LIGAMENT AND STRIA VASCULARIS

The **spiral ligament** (SpL) is positioned lateral to the cochlear duct, between the cochlear bone and the lateral side of the stria vascularis (see Figure 8-4). It contains fibrocytes, extracellular matrix material, and blood vessels (Figure 8-9). Perilymph fills its intercellular spaces. The spiral ligament thus provides a second route of communication between scalae tympani and vestibuli, in addition to the helicotrema. Reissner's membrane is attached to the spiral ligament near its superior end where the superior end of the stria vascularis is located. The basilar membrane inserts into the spiral ligament near its inferior end.

The stria vascularis (i.e., vascular stripe) consists of three cell layers (i.e., marginal [M], intermediate [I], and basal [B]) and an intraepithelial network of capillaries (C) (see Figure 8-9). The marginal (M) cells are known as chromophils because they stain

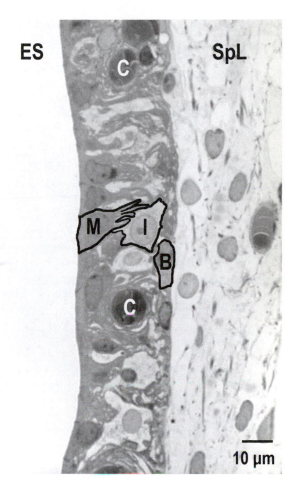

FIGURE 8-9   Radial section of stria vascularis and spiral ligament (SpL). B, basal cell of the stria vascularis; C, capillary; ES, endolymphatic space; I, intermediate cell of the stria vascularis; M, marginal cell of the stria vascularis.

darkly. They abut the endolymphatic space (ES) and are joined by tight junctions at their luminal margins. Their basolateral surfaces are deeply infolded and the folds contain numerous mitochondria. The marginal cells are thought to secrete potassium that is found in a high concentration in endolymph.

Intermediate (I) cells are known as chromophobes because they stain lightly. These cells are melanocytes because in all pigmented mammals they contain a variable number of melanin granules.

TABLE 8-1   Cochlear Parameters in Selected Species

Cochlear Parameter	Human	Chinchilla	Mouse
Organ of Corti (OC) length	Mean (male): 37.11 mm[a] Mean (female): 31.9 mm[a] Range: 28–40 mm[c]	Mean (male and female): 18.4 mm[b] Range: 16–21.6 mm[b]	Mean (male and female): 6.06 mm[b] Range: 5.66–6.43 mm[b]
Frequency range of hearing	20–20,000 Hz[d]	90–22,800 Hz[e]	1,000–100,000 Hz[e]
Total inner hair cells	Mean: 3,480[f] Range: 3,035–4,390[f]	Mean: 1,800[b] Range: 1,600–2,030[b]	Mean: 705[b] Range: 684–746[b]
Inner hair cell density	Mean: 109/mm OC[f] Range: 93–125[f]	Mean: 100/mm OC[b] Range: 96–103[b]	116/mm OC[b] Range: 109–123[b]
Total outer hair cells	Mean: 13,345[f] Range: 11,220–16,040[f]	Mean: 7,150[b] Range: 6,300–8,280[b]	Mean: 2,398[b] Range: 2,331–2,483[b]
Outer hair cell density	Mean: 415/mm OC[f] Range: 387–459[f]	Mean: 405/mm OC[b] Range: 391–416[b]	Mean: 395/mm OC[b] Range: 371–419[b]
Total spiral ganglion cells	Mean: 30,500[g]–33,600[h] (cell bodies in Rosenthal's canal)	Mean: 23,550[i] (myelinated fibers in cochlear nerve)	Mean: 12,600[j] (myelinated fibers in cochlear nerve)

aSato, Sando, & Takahashi, 1991.
bBohne and Harding, 2004, unpublished data.
cWright, Davis, Bredberg, Ulehlova, & Spencer, 1987.
dDallos, 1986.
eFay, 1988.
fBredberg, 1968.
gRasmussen, 1940.
hHinojosa, Seligsohn, & Lerner, 1985.
iBoord & Rasmussen, 1958.
jEhret, 1979.

These cells are thought to generate the positive potential (i.e., +80 to +100 mV) in the endolymphatic space.

The basal (B) cells are flat and overlapping and form a continuous layer that separates the interior of the stria vascularis from the spiral ligament. These cells are joined to one another by tight junctions. They form a sleeve around each capillary entering and leaving the stria vascularis. Because of the tight junctions between adjacent marginal cells and between overlapping basal cells, the interior of the stria vascularis is separated from perilymph in the spiral ligament and endolymph in the endolymphatic space.

BLOOD SUPPLY OF THE INNER EAR

The arterial blood supply to the inner ear comes from the labyrinthine artery that enters the temporal bone through the IAM along with the seventh and eighth cranial nerves. This artery is a branch of the anterior inferior cerebellar artery that, in turn, is a branch of the basilar artery. Within the modiolus, the artery divides into arterioles that supply capillary beds in Rosenthal's canal, the spiral ligament, stria vascularis, limbus, and osseous spiral lamina. To supply capillaries in the stria vascularis and spiral ligament, the arterioles radiate over scala vestibuli before entering the superior portion of the spiral ligament.

The only capillaries near the organ of Corti are the vessel of the tympanic lip of the osseous spiral lamina and the vessel of the basilar membrane (see Figure 8–5). These latter vessels form discontinuous arcades inferior to the basilar membrane. The capillary beds in the spiral ligament and stria vascularis join collecting venules that run radially within the bone around scala tympani. These venules ultimately join the labyrinthine vein in the modiolus that, in turn, exits the temporal bone via the IAM. The labyrinthine vein drains into the transverse or inferior petrosal sinus.

VARIATIONS IN COCHLEAR PARAMETERS

Both within and across species, considerable variability exists in cochlear parameters such as the length of the organ of Corti/basilar membrane complex, the total number of sensory and spiral ganglion cells, and the density of hair cells per millimeter of the organ of Corti. Some of these variations have functional consequences for hearing, such as the range of audible frequencies and the difference limen for frequency. Table 8-1 shows some of these parameters for the human, chinchilla, and mouse. The latter two animals are often used to study normal and abnormal hearing.

CLINICAL RELEVANCE

At birth, the normal human organ of Corti contains approximately 3,400 IHCs and 13,000 OHCs. These numbers are considerably less than the 110 million rods and 5.5 million cones in the retina. A variety of external agents result in the death of cochlear hair cells, including excessive exposure to noise (i.e., military, industrial or recreational), systemic treatment with certain drugs (e.g., aminoglycoside antibiotics, anticancer agents), and physical trauma to the temporal bone. Hair cells are also lost with advancing age. Because there are relatively few sensory elements in the cochlea, small losses of these cells can result in a permanent sensorineural hearing loss. The high-frequency portion (i.e., base) of the cochlea is more vulnerable to damage from drugs, noise, and aging than the low-frequency portion (i.e., apex). This accounts for the progressive loss of high-frequency hearing that is found in many older humans.

✌ SUMMARY ∻

The inner ear consists of the *cochlea,* which contains the sensory organ responsible for hearing, and the *vestibule,* which contains the sensory organs for balance and equilibrium. This chapter describes the morphological structure of the cochlea, including the *organ of Corti,* the end organ for hearing, which contains sensory cells (i.e., *inner and outer hair cells*), supporting cells, and *spiral ganglion cells* (i.e., primary auditory neurons); the *basilar membrane,* which is set in motion by movement of the tympanic membrane and ossicular chain; and fluid spaces (i.e., *scalae vestibuli, media,* and *tympani*). The inner and outer hair cells are responsible for transducing the mechanical waves of the basilar membrane into electrical impulses that are transmitted by the spiral ganglion cells to the brain for the perception of sound.

✌ KEY TERMS ∻

Afferent nerve
Basilar membrane
Cochlea
Cochlear duct
Deiters' cell
Efferent nerve
Endolymph
Endolymphatic space
Facial nerve
Habenula perforata

Hair cell
Helicotrema
Hensen's cell
Hensen's stripe
Internal auditory
    meatus
Spiral limbus
Modiolus
Organ of Corti
Osseous spiral lamina

Perilymph
Pillar cell
Reissner's membrane
Reticular lamina
Rosenthal's canal
Scala media
Scala tympani
Scala vestibuli
Spaces of Nuel

Spiral ganglion cells
Spiral ligament
Stereocilium
Stria vascularis
Tectorial membrane
Tunnel
Vestibulocochlear
    nerve
Zonula occludens

⤳ STUDY QUESTIONS ⤲

1. Describe the gross structure of the inner ear and how it relates to the middle ear.

2. Describe the three fluid compartments and their boundaries and the two fluids of the cochlea.

3. Describe the cochlear duct and its boundaries. What is special about its boundaries?

4. Name the cells of the organ of Corti. Describe their relation to one another, as well as to the basilar membrane and TM.

5. Describe the afferent innervation of IHCs and OHCs. How does it differ?

⤳ REFERENCES ⤲

Boord, R. L., & Rasmussen, G. L. (1958). Analysis of the myelinated fibers of the acoustic nerve of the chinchilla. *Anatomical Record, 130,* 395.

Bredberg, G. (1968). Cellular pattern and nerve supply of the human organ of Corti. *Acta Otolaryngologica Supplementum, 236,* 1–135.

Dallos, P. (1986). *The search for the mechanisms of hearing.* Leesburg, VA: The World & I, Washington Times Corporation.

Davis, H., Benson, R.W., Covell, W.P., Fernandez, C., Goldstein, R., Katsuki, Y., Legouix, J.P., McAuliffe, D.R., & Tasaki, I. (1953). Acoustic trauma in the guinea pig. *Journal of the Acoustical Society of America, 25,* 1180–1189.

Ehret, G. (1979). Quantitative analysis of nerve fibre densities in the cochlea of the house mouse *(Mus musculus). Journal of Comparative Neurology, 183,* 73–88.

Fay, R. R. (1988). *Hearing in vertebrates: A psychophysics databook.* Winnetka, IL: Hill-Fay Associates.

Hawkins, J. E. (2004a). Sketches of otohistory. Part 1. Otoprehistory: How it all began. *Audiology and Neuro-otology, 9,* 66–71.

Hawkins, J. E. (2004b). Sketches of otohistory. Part 3. Alfonso Corti. *Audiology and Neuro-otology, 9,* 259–264.

Hinojosa, R., Seligsohn, R., & Lerner, S. A. (1985). Ganglion cell counts in the cochleae of patients with normal audiograms. *Acta Otolaryngologica, 99,* 8–13.

Rasmussen, A. T. (1940). Studies of the VIIIth cranial nerve of man. *Laryngoscope, 50,* 67–83.

Sato, H., Sando, I., & Takahashi, H. (1991). Sexual dimorphism and development of the human cochlea. Computer 3-D measurement. *Acta Otolaryngologica, 111,* 1037–1040.

Schacht, J., & Hawkins, J. E. (2004). Sketches of otohistory. Part 4. A cell by any other name: Cochlear eponyms. *Audiology and Neuro-otology, 9,* 317–327.

Spoendlin, H. (1984). Primary neurons and synapses. In I. Friedmann & J. Ballantyne (Eds.), *Ultrastructural atlas of the inner ear* (pp. 133–164). London: Butterworths.

Wright, A., Davis, G., Bredberg, G., Ulehlova, L., & Spencer, H. (1987). Hair cell distributions in the normal human cochlea. *Acta Otolaryngologica Suppletum, 444,* 1–48.

⤳ SUGGESTED READING ⤲

Durrant, J. D., & Lovrinic, J. H. (1995). Structure of the mammalian cochlea. *Bases of hearing science* (pp. 115–137). Baltimore: Williams & Wilkins.

Schuknecht, H. (1993). *Pathology of the ear.* Malvern, PA: Lea and Febiger.

Slepecky, N. B. (1996). Structure of the mammalian cochlea. In P. Dallos, A. N. Popper, & R. R. Fay (Eds.), *The cochlea* (pp. 44–129). New York: Springer.

Chapter

9

Macromechanics: Basilar Membrane Responses

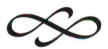

William W. Clark, Ph.D.
Director, Program in Audiology
and Communication Sciences
Washington University School of Medicine
St. Louis, Missouri

The travel of an acoustic signal as it passes through the outer and middle ear has been described in previous chapters. Along the route, an acoustic signal is changed quite dramatically in amplitude, bandwidth, and phase. This chapter considers how the airborne sound pressure disturbance is delivered to the basilar membrane (BM) and ultimately to the sensory receptors, the outer and inner hair cells. We begin rather passively with a description of the classic view of mechanical tuning of the BM, and then we "liven up" our discussion by considering relatively recent discoveries about how the BM/organ of Corti sharpens tuning with active processes. Because the active and passive processes coexist, familiarity with both is necessary to understand the basis of normal hearing function, as well as the effects of disease or defect of heredity or external agent on function. Although an understanding of the spherical nature of Earth does not require

knowledge about the theories that it was flat, coexistence of passive and active processes in the cochlea requires understanding of both processes.

PASSIVE MECHANICS

Because the cochlea is such a complex, three-dimensional structure, it is easier to visualize how it works by unrolling it from the modiolus and considering it as a long, graduated, straight tube (Figure 9-1).

As detailed in Chapter 8, the cochlea includes three chambers, separated by membranes and bony projections. For purposes of this discussion, the cochlea can be thought of as a graduated or tapering tube, divided into two fluid-filled compartments by a bony shelf with a slit in it and a hole at the end. Stretched across the slit is the BM, a "rubbery" membrane of graduated width and thickness.

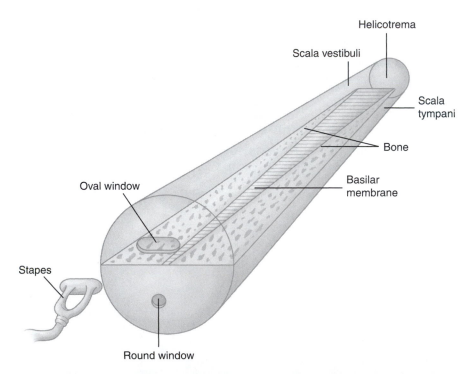

FIGURE 9-1 Model of the cochlear duct. Note that the cross-sectional area of the duct decreases from the base to the apex, but the width of the basilar membrane increases as the membrane extends apically.

Note in Figure 9-1 that the taper of the BM is arranged exactly opposite to the taper of the cochlea: it is thin and stiff near the stapes and gets wider, thicker, and looser near the apex. It may be helpful to think about the membrane as a piano, with the low notes (and longer, more massive strings) near the apex and the high notes (with shorter, stiffer strings) near the base. The model has two "windows," one on each side of the BM. Both windows are covered by a thin membrane, and the stapes is attached into the upper, or oval, window. The stapes is attached by a ligament at its posterior aspect, and it "rocks" into and out of the oval window as it is moved by acoustic stimulation. Physical models such as this were constructed by physiologist George von Békésy in the 1940s and 1950s, and they helped him to develop the classic theory about cochlear excitation, for which he was awarded the Nobel Prize in Physiology or Medicine in 1961.

Excitation of the Model

The normal input to this model is the rocking movement of the stapes. Because the model of the cochlear duct has hard walls and is completely filled with incompressible fluid, the only way the stapes can move inward is if there is a "pressure relief" valve that allows the fluid somewhere to go. That is the function of the round window membrane—for each movement inward of the stapes, there is an equal and opposite movement outward of the round window membrane. The fluid is thus displaced in a to-and-fro manner as the stapes is displaced.

What if the model did not have a stapes? In that case, we would have two identical membranes placed closely together. Now consider the approach of a sound wave at a frequency where the human ear is exquisitely sensitive: 1,000 Hz. Recall from Chapter 2 that the wavelength of a 1,000-Hz sinusoid in air is about 1 foot; that is, the distance between a pressure peak and a pressure minimum would be about 6 inches. Because a life-size model of the cochlea is small compared with the wavelength of the signal, the sound wave would "push" or "pull" on both windows simultaneously, even if the wave approached at an angle, resulting in

no fluid displacement, even for extremely high-pressure changes (Figure 9-2A).

The only way to get a pressure *difference* across the membranes would be to arrange the model so that a positive pressure occurred at the oval window at the same time as a negative pressure at the round window. For a signal of 1,000 Hz, the windows would have to be 6 inches apart—not a very good solution for humans with heads of only 8 inches in diameter! Fortunately, nature and physics have a better solution. Displacement of the cochlear fluids and movement of the BM can occur by selectively delivering the signal to only one window and by protecting the other window from the airborne sound as shown schematically in Figure 9-2B. As we have already learned, the middle ear handles the job quite nicely, which is why it is appropriate to consider the round window membrane a pressure relief valve.

Fluid Dynamics and Stimulation of the Basilar Membrane

Look at the model in Figure 9-1 again. If the BM were rigid and incapable of movement, pressing inward on the stapes would push fluid down the scala vestibuli, through the helicotrema, and back up the scala tympani to the round window. Although there would be fluid displacement, there would be no movement of the BM. If, however, the BM were flexible with a uniform "flex" along its longitudinal dimension, then amount and location of the displacement of the BM with stapes vibration would depend on the pressure difference above and below the partition along its length. Pressure differences along the membrane could occur if the wavelength of the transmitted sound were short enough to produce "local" maxima and minima along its length. In fact, this might be a good way to send input of differing frequencies to different locations along the membrane: for high-frequency sounds, the wavelength is short, and therefore maximum stimulation would be toward the base of the cochlea; for low-frequency sounds with longer wavelengths, the maximum would be displaced toward the apex. Sounds good, doesn't it? All that we need to do to "prove" this theory is to calculate the wavelengths

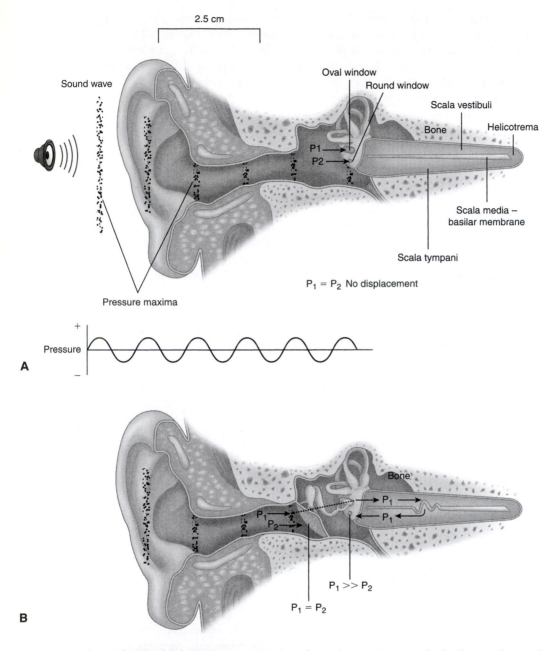

FIGURE 9-2 (See Color Plate) Schematic representation of sound transmission to the basilar membrane. (A) Without a middle ear, the positive pressures (P_1 and P_2) in a sound wave will strike both the oval window and the round window nearly simultaneously. Because the cochlear fluids are nearly incompressible, pressing inward on each window will cause no net movement of fluid and no displacement of the basilar membrane. (B) The middle ear transmits and amplifies the pressure gradient (P_1) to the stapes and oval window, and protects the round window from airborne sound (that is, P_2 is much smaller than P_1). In this case, the inward "push" of the stapes causes a displacement of fluid toward the round window membrane, which serves as a pressure relief valve. The net result is a displacement of the basilar membrane.

for audible sounds and determine whether they fit reasonably along the membrane. The length of the cochlea in humans is about 3.2 cm. Chapter 2 explains that the wavelength of a sound is equal to the speed divided by the frequency. In water, sound travels at about 161,000 cm/sec. Therefore, the wavelength for a 1-kHz sinusoid in water is 1.6 meters (m); for a 20,000-Hz sound (the upper limit of human hearing), the wavelength is 8 cm, more than twice the length of the cochlear duct. As a practical issue, the pressure increase created by stapes movement inward is instantaneously distributed almost uniformly along the length of the BM, even for the highest frequency audible sounds. The way to think about this is to consider that the duct is pushed everywhere nearly at once by stapes movement; it is not pushed at one end and pulled at the other as the pressure wave front travels through the cochlea.

So why does the BM not just move up and down as a single unit as the stapes moves in and out? The answer lies in structure of the BM, which gradually shifts from a thin, stiff membrane at the base to a thick, elastic membrane near the apex. The nineteenth-century physicist Helmholtz argued that such a structure would "resonate" at different places depending on the frequency of the incoming sound (Helmholtz, 1863). Tuned like the strings of a harp or a piano, Helmholtz argued that the high frequencies would stimulate the base of the cochlea and the low frequencies the apex. Complex sounds, composed of multiple frequencies, would create local maxima representing the components that made up the sounds and, of course, stimulate differentially the population of sensory cells distributed along the BM. According to Helmholtz, the BM was made up of a series of stretched strings of continuously varying length and mass loosely coupled together. Hearing occurs by sympathetic vibration; that is, a complex signal containing many components would cause vibrations of all the strings tuned to each component simultaneously. The principle can be easily demonstrated with a piano. Sit in front of the piano and press the foot pedal to take the dampers off. Now sing a clear note of a particular pitch loudly and stop abruptly. You will hear the piano continue

to "sing" back a sound of the same pitch briefly. This is because the complex signal you created with your vocal chords caused "sympathetic" vibration in individual strings of the piano tuned to the frequencies of your vocalization. The principle of sympathetic vibration forms the foundation of the so-called resonance or place theory of hearing.

Helmholtz's ideas received considerable support from George von Békésy, as mentioned earlier. von Békésy, a telephone engineer by training, sought to observe directly the action of sound on the BM in the cochlea. He worked first on physical models of the cochlea, and he was the first to report the existence of traveling waves (see von Békésy, 1960, for a review of his early work). Two observations made by von Békésy were most noteworthy. First, because the pressure increase created by inward movement of the stapes is distributed uniformly across the length of the cochlear duct, if BM motion is controlled by the graduated stiffness and mass of the organ of Corti, then the excitation pattern should not depend on where the stapes is located within the cochlear duct. von Békésy built models with the stapes located near the apex and confirmed that BM motion always proceeded from base to apex, no matter where the stapes was located. von Békésy also observed that the pressure increase created a traveling wave that always traveled from the base of the cochlea, where the cochlear duct is large and the BM narrow and stiff toward the apex, where the cross-sectional area of the cochlear duct is small, but the BM is wide and massive. He also observed that the wave decreased in velocity as it traveled from base to apex, from about 15,000 cm/sec at the base to about 1,000 cm/sec at the apex. Note that even at its fastest, the wave travels much more slowly than the pressure wave in fluid (161,000 cm/sec).

It may be useful to think about a not-quite-correct analogy. If you tie a long rope to a door handle, stretch it slightly, and then shake the free end of the rope up and down, you will create a "traveling wave" in the rope. Note that the wave always starts near the "base" (your hands) and travels toward the fixed end at the door handle. If you shake the rope gently, the wave disturbance

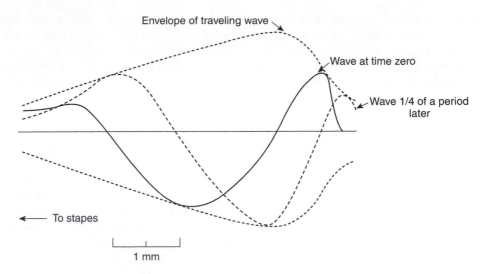

FIGURE 9-3 Detail showing the displacements of the cochlear partition at two points in time for a single sinusoidal signal. A continuous "movie" of this graph would show a wave traveling from left to right, reaching the maximum displacements identified at the *dotted lines* above and below the membrane. (Adapted from Békésy, G., von (1960). *Experiments in hearing.* New York: McGraw-Hill Book Company, by permission.)

will travel down the rope and dissipate before it reaches the end, and no obvious reflections will occur from the fixed end of the rope. This is what happens in the cochlea: the energy dissipates before reaching the helicotrema.

Basilar Membrane Vibration with Sinusoidal Stimulation

Now let us consider how the BM/organ of Corti complex responds to continuous sinusoidal stimulation. Figure 9-3 presents a "freeze-frame" depiction of BM motion taken at two points in time. The solid line depicts the movement of the membrane at time = 0, and the heavily dotted line shows the amplitude of the membrane movement a quarter wavelength later. It can be seen that the displacement of the membrane "travels" from the base toward the apex. As noted earlier, it will also be slowing down as it travels. As the wave makes its way down the cochlear duct, its displacement gradually increases to a maximum and then "dies out"

apically. The outside dotted line in Figure 9-3 represents the "envelope" of the wave, outlining the limits of excitation as a function of place. Because the stiffness and mass of the membrane are graduated from base to apex, stimulation at different frequencies results in maxima at different places. Lowering the stimulus frequency shifts the maximum displacement toward the apex, and increasing the stimulus frequency shifts the maximum toward the base. Changing the intensity of the stimulus does not change the rate of travel or the point of maximum stimulation but does increase the amplitude of motion (within limits).

Another characteristic of the tuning of the BM is apparent in Figure 9-3. By varying the frequency of the stimulus sinusoid and observing the "place" of maximum stimulation, it is possible to map precise coordinates relating frequency to place of stimulation. This so-called tonotopic map actually confirmed the place theory of hearing, which was originally proposed by Helmholtz. The "sharpness" of the mechanical tuning, therefore, is represented by the rate at which the maximum amplitude falls off at places adjacent to the point of maximum stimulation; that is, the slopes of the traveling wave envelope define the filter characteristics of the BM/organ of Corti complex.

To validate the findings from physical models, von Békésy also studied the BM vibration patterns in cadaver ears. He used stroboscopic illumination and studied the response of the BM to high-level acoustic stimulation. For the preparation, cochleas were immersed in water and the round window membrane was driven by vibrations of a rubber membrane. Because his technique required him to drill open the cochlea, he could only observe in the apical half of the cochlea; observing the basal half would have required destroying the apex and would have changed the mechanical system. von Békésy's measurements for pure tone stimuli between 25 and 1,600 Hz are shown in Figure 9-4.

Once again, we can see evidence of **tonotopic organization** and broad tuning. To determine more precisely the degree of sharpness, or selectivity of the BM/organ of Corti, von Békésy made measurements at discrete locations along the cochlear partition and determined the relative amplitude of the response as he varied the stimulus frequency with constant amplitude at the stapes (von Békésy's results are shown in Figure 9-5).

The amplitudes of each curve are expressed as the normalized amplitude to the maximum value, 1.0. The chief characteristic of these curves is the broad tuning they exhibit. Remember from our study of decibels and filters in Chapters 2 and 3 that a reduction in amplitude of 50% is 3 dB, then the half-power or 3-dB bandwidth for all stimuli is quite large. At 400 Hz, for example, the bandwidth extends from 200 Hz on the low side to around 500 Hz on the high side. Given this poor frequency resolving power, it was difficult for von Békésy and others to explain the relatively sharp tuning observed in auditory nerve fibers (see Chapter 11) and in the psychoacoustic response of the normal listener. By the 1960s it was known that the inner ear was capable of much sharper frequency resolving power than that displayed in von Békésy's observa-

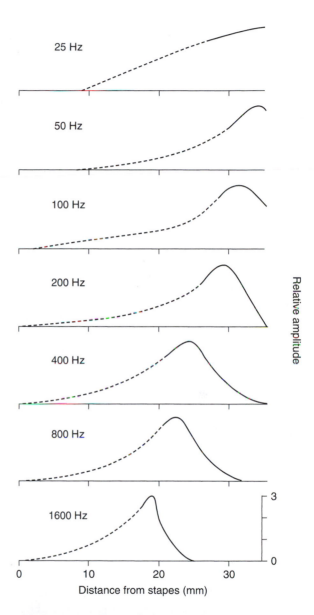

FIGURE 9-4 Patterns of vibration of a cadaver specimen for various frequencies. *Dashed lines* indicate the measures are inexact, because it was necessary to destroy the more apical portion of the cochlear partition to observe the amplitudes of movement toward the stapes. (From Békésy, G., von (1960). *Experiments in hearing.* New York: McGraw-Hill Book Company, by permission.)

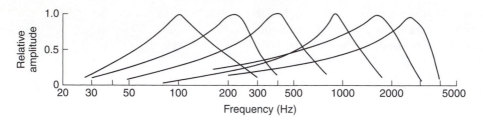

FIGURE 9-5 Resonance curves for the cochlear partition of mammals measured at several locations. Note the relatively poor frequency selectivity of the response, as reflected by the wide band width over which the response was within 3 dB (0.5) of the maximum. (From Békésy, G., von (1960). *Experiments in hearing.* New York: McGraw-Hill Book Company, by permission.)

tions. As a matter of fact, the so-called critical bandwidth for hearing, calculated from measures of masking of pure tones by bands of noise and by studies of loudness summation, displays bandwidths nearly 10 times as sharp as those observed in von Békésy's cadavers. Of even more importance was the observation that the tuning characteristics of primary auditory neurons were much sharper than the excitation patterns that von Békésy described (see Chapter 11). The disconnect between mechanical tuning, discrimination ability, and neural tuning led scientists on a two-decade mission to identify how the auditory system managed to "sharpen" up the mechanical response of the cochlea before transmitting frequency-specific information up the auditory nerve. Students of audiology in the 1960s and 1970s had to learn about "second filters," "lateral inhibition," and other hypothesized mechanisms that were proposed to explain the tuning observed in the nerve fiber. Regarding the conclusion that the ear was a linear device, these students also were taught that if one extrapolated the displacement measurements made by von Békésy downward to threshold values (about 10-dB sound pressure level [SPL] at 1 kHz), then that would mean the ear could detect BM movement on the order of 1 millionth (1/1,000,000) of the diameter of a hydrogen atom (about 1 millionth the thickness of the membrane covering the surface of one stereocilium!). Furthermore, it could pick those displacements out of the continuous bombardment by the relatively "giant" red blood cells as

they coursed through the inner ear, which, of course, is preposterous.

The Nonlinear Nature of Basilar Membrane Responses

The so-called place theory of hearing, proposed by Helmholtz and developed and refined by von Békésy, assumed the basilar membrane response to acoustic input was linear and passive. Both assumptions turned out to be wrong. Nearly everyone assumed that von Békésy's observations represented the behavior of the living cochlea working at normal stimulation levels. However, von Békésy made it clear that his studies had to be made at extremely high levels, around 120-dB SPL, so he could see the motion of the BM, and they were made on dead ears. Their applicability to the "normal" situation would hold only if the ear were a passive and linear system. And now scientists know that the living mammalian ear, receiving acoustic input at "normal" sound levels (e.g., within about 50 dB above threshold) is neither passive nor linear. Advances in our understanding about cochlear mechanical tuning came from a number of disciplines within audiology, including psychoacoustics, neurophysiology, applied mathematics, and otopathology. As scientists developed more sensitive methods and tools to study the behavior of the living ear with stimuli near threshold, clues began to accumulate suggesting that the students' disbelief about linearity of BM response were well founded.

Some clues came from psychoacoustics. It had long been known that complex sounds presented at high levels could result in the perception of extra tones that were not present in the stimulus. Known as "combination," "distortion," or "Tartini" tones, these phenomena referred to that if a listener heard two closely spaced tones, f1 and f2, at fairly high stimulus levels, above about 80-dB SPL, he or she could perceive extra signals at multiple combinations of the two tones, the most predominant one being the so-called cubic distortion tone at $2f1-f2$ (Plomp, 1965). These tones were clearly audible even though they were not present in the stimulus, and clearly showed that the ear was nonlinear at high stimulus levels. It was thought that the combination tones were created by nonlinear mechanical motion of the BM at high stimulus levels. In 1967, Julius Goldstein, an electrical engineer at the Massachusetts Institute of Technology, developed a clever way to measure the presence of "combination" or "distortion" tones (Goldstein, 1967). He presented two stimuli simultaneously in one ear of sufficient strength to create a distortion product. For example, two tones presented simultaneously to one ear at frequencies of 2,400 and 2,800 would create an audible distortion product at 2,000 Hz ($2 \times 2,400$ Hz $= 4,800$ Hz $- 2,800$ Hz $= 2,000$ Hz). Goldstein demonstrated the perception by presenting a second tone to the other ear, at a frequency that was slightly mistuned to the $2f1 - f2$ signal, for example, 2,003 Hz. The combination tone in the ipsilateral ear and the second tone in the contralateral ear combined to produce the perception of "beats" at the difference frequency (3 Hz). The surprising finding from Goldstein's study was that combination tones could be perceived at low stimulus levels, near threshold in some cases, for normal listeners. If Goldstein was correct, then it must be concluded that the hearing mechanism reflected in the sensation of tonal signals is nonlinear even at threshold. This was such an astonishing finding that many people did not believe him.

However, between 1967 and the mid-1980s, scientists in a variety of disciplines began to accumulate evidence that the ear was not a passive mechanical device. The presence of otoacoustic emissions from normal ears (reviewed in Chapter 13) and the physiologic representation of two-tone distortion as recorded in the whole-nerve action potential (see Chapter 11) both indicated that the inner ear is nonlinear at low stimulus levels. Another puzzling observation was that if the ear was damaged, either by mechanical insult, application of drugs, or hypoxia, it became more linear; that is, these "extra" responses disappeared. In the ultimate damage case—the death of the subject—the response of the BM/organ of Corti complex was entirely linear.

BASILAR MEMBRANE VIBRATIONS IN LIVING SUBJECTS: NONLINEAR AND ACTIVE PROCESSES

It should be clear at this point that understanding how the BM vibrates at threshold requires direct observation at low stimulus levels in living preparations. Using newly developed computer and measurement technology, Johnstone and Boyle (1967) in Australia and later Rhode (1971) at the University of Wisconsin reported measurements of BM movements in living animals. Using the **Mössbauer technique,** which involved placing a small radioactive probe on the underside of the BM and recording the emission of gamma rays with a sensitive detector, they were able to measure the velocity of the malleus and the BM made in living mammals at moderate stimulus levels. A summary of Rhode's findings, reported in 1971, is shown in Figure 9-6.

Figure 9-6 shows the ratio of the amplitude of the BM displacement to the displacement of the malleus as a function of frequency at a particular spot on the squirrel monkey cochlea. The "place" of the measurement had a characteristic frequency of approximately 7 kHz. The results differed remarkably from those that von Békésy reported in cadaver ears. First, the tuning of the membrane was much sharper in the living ear. The slopes of the **tuning curve** reached about 24 dB per octave just below the so-called characteristic frequency, and nearly 100 dB per octave on the high-frequency side of

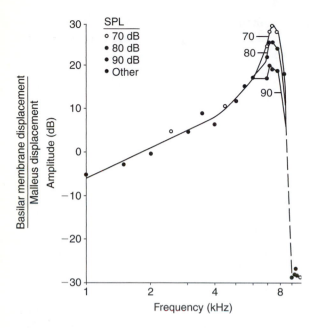

FIGURE 9-6 Plot showing the ratio of amplitude of displacement for the basilar membrane and the stapes as a function of frequency. Measurements were made in the squirrel monkey cochlea at a place corresponding to a characteristic frequency of 7 kHz. Stimuli were presented at 70, 80, and 90 dB SPL. (From Rhode, W. S. (1971). Observations of the vibration of the basilar membrane in squirrel monkeys using the Mossbauer technique. *Journal of the Acoustical Society of America, 49,* 1218–1231, by permission. Copyright 1971 American Institute of Physics.)

the peak. The second, and in some ways even more remarkable, observation was that the sharpness of tuning *increased* as the stimulus level decreased. That is, as the stimulus level was reduced from 90 to 70 dB SPL, the selectivity of the **BM response** increased. Another way of saying this is to conclude that the damping of the BM is reduced at low stimulus levels compared with high stimulus levels. In fact, to explain the sharp tuning, it was necessary to propose that the membrane somehow could exhibit **negative damping.** Negative damping means that not only is the BM a sharply tuned resonator, but it also requires that energy be added to the system to explain the tuning. Conceptually, the term *negative damping* can be understood by thinking about a car

traveling down a road at 60 miles/hour. If you press on the accelerator, you will speed up; if you step on the brake, you will slow down. Acceleration, in this analogy, could be called *negative braking,* and it means that additional energy is pumped into the system from another source, in this case, the motor of the car. In the case of the BM, negative damping really means "amplification." We now know that the outer hair cells are the motors that "amplify" the BM response to weak signals (our current understanding of this process is detailed in Chapter 10).

Although the reports by Johnstone and Boyle (1967) and Rhode (1971) were monumental, they still did not explain completely the sharp tuning observed in the auditory nerve fiber response. But remember that the techniques they used were still invasive. Although the radioactive source used in the Mössbauer technique was tiny, it still loaded the BM by its mass and required a hole to be drilled into the scala tympani. More recent studies of BM movement have been conducted using sensitive **laser velocimetry** techniques, and some of the results that Ruggero and his colleagues (Ruggero, Narayan, Temchin, & Recio, 2000) reported are redrawn in Figures 9-7 and 9-8. These measures were made at the 3.5-mm site along the BM of a chinchilla. The 3.5-mm place on the chinchilla cochlea corresponds to a frequency of about 9 kHz.

Figure 9-7A shows measurements of BM velocity as a function of input SPL. At high stimulus levels (100 dB SPL), the BM response is quite broadly tuned, as von Békésy reported. As the stimulus level is decreased in 10-dB steps, however, the BM response shows differing characteristics. For stimuli with frequencies distant from the point of measurement, less than 8 kHz and greater than 12 kHz, the response of the BM is nearly linear. That is, for each 10-dB decrement in stimulus intensity, there is a corresponding decrease in BM response. At frequencies near the recording point, however, the response falls far less than 10 dB per 10-dB decrement, and the frequency of maximum response shifts upward. This is more easily seen in Figure 9-7B, which depicts the "gain" or amplification of the sharply tuned portion of the BM response with the response normalized to stimulus

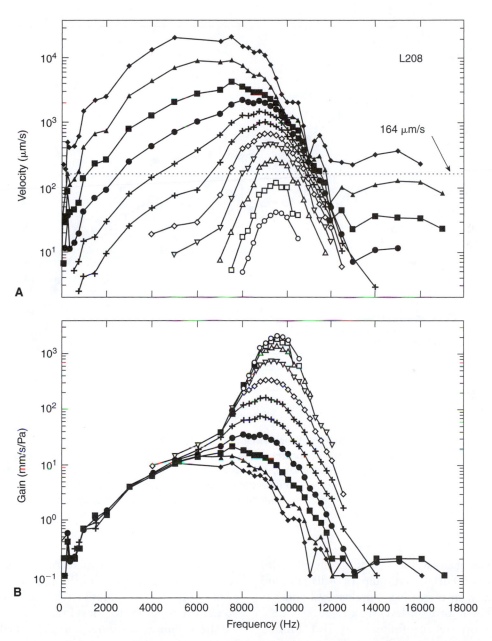

FIGURE 9-7 Magnitudes of the basilar membrane response to pure tone stimuli measured at one location in the chinchilla cochlea. (A) Stapes velocity. (B) Gain normalized to stimulus pressure. The parameter is the level of stimulation (0–100 dB sound pressure level). Note the nonlinear and linear portions of the velocity function (A) and the gain provided by the so-called cochlear amplifier (B). (From Ruggero, M., Narayan, S. S., Temchin, A. N., & Recio, A. (2000). Mechanical bases of frequency tuning and neural excitation at the base of the cochlea: Comparison of basilar-membrane vibrations and auditory-nerve-fiber response in chinchilla. *Proceedings of the National Academy of Sciences, 97,* 11744–11750, by permission. Copyright 2000 National Academy of Sciences, USA.)

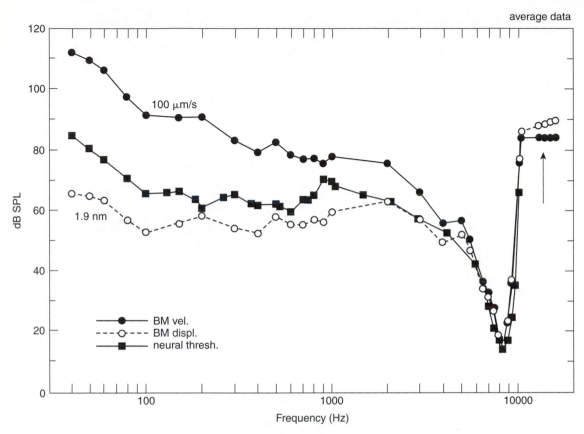

FIGURE 9-8 Comparison of frequency tuning of the basilar membrane (BM) and auditory nerve fibers at a specific site in the chinchilla cochlea. Note the similarity of the curves, particularly at the center frequency. SPL, sound pressure level. (From Ruggero, M., Narayan, S. S., Temchin, A. N., & Recio, A. (2000). Mechanical bases of frequency tuning and neural excitation at the base of the cochlea: Comparison of basilar-membrane vibrations and auditory-nerve-fiber response in chinchilla. *Proceedings of the National Academy of Sciences, 97,* 11744–11750, by permission. Copyright 2000 National Academy of Sciences, USA.)

pressure. The gain at the center frequency (CF) place is about 50 dB for a stimulus of 0-dB SPL, and it decreases with increasing stimulus level and becomes minimal for high-level signals.

The more recent findings of BM tuning, therefore, show us that the "motor" in the cochlea provides about a 50-dB "boost" to the input signal from the stapes that is most observable at very low stimulus levels (Ruggero, 2000). It also indicates that the "boost" is nonlinear and, in fact, is called a **saturating nonlinearity,** meaning that

the gain decreases with increasing stimulus level. This makes physical and biological sense: We really only "need" to amplify the low-level signals to get the input up to a level that can be detected by the receptor, the inner hair cell. Furthermore, if the two components, the "active" one and the "passive" one, are adding to each other at high levels (i.e., greater than about 70 dB SPL), the "passive" component will "swamp" the active one. This appears to be what is happening in the cochlea.

☙ SUMMARY ❧

We know that the BM vibration has two important components that contribute to its mechanical response to acoustic stimuli. One is a passive component that generates a broadly tuned response to signals of high level. The other is an active component, acting in parallel with the passive component, which provides amplification of low-level inputs and sharpens the frequency response of the BM significantly. The active component comes from the hair cell complex, is dependent on metabolic energy for its operation, and although it is present at all stimulus levels, it provides gain only for levels less than about 50-dB SPL.

The final question to be resolved about BM tuning before we move on to a discussion of the micromechanical processes of the BM is whether the tuning as demonstrated in BM response matches that seen in the response of the primary auditory nerve fiber. If they match, then we know that the tuning is controlled by BM response characteristics, and we can cease looking for the second filter.

Figure 9-8 shows just such a comparison. These data come from studies of BM tuning and frequency threshold curves of many chinchillas with normal hearing. It does not require much imagination to see that the two measures fall nearly on top of each other, particularly at frequencies near the CF of the auditory nerve fiber. It is clearly evident that the sharpness of the frequency response of the auditory nerve is already contained in the BM response; there is no need to invoke explanations of additional filtering to explain the tuning characteristics of the auditory nerve fiber. Therefore, in the next chapter, our attention is directed toward the BM complex, which includes the organ of Corti and the hair cell complex, to learn how the ear accomplishes such a remarkable feat.

☙ KEY TERMS ❧

BM (basilar membrane) response
Frequency tuning curve

Laser velocimetry
Mössbauer technique

Negative damping
Saturating nonlinearity

Tonotopic organization

☙ STUDY QUESTIONS ❧

1. What mechanical features of the BM/organ of Corti complex allow it to respond maximally in different places to signals of different frequencies?

2. What is the difference between a nonlinear process in transduction and an active process? How does each contribute to frequency tuning on the BM?

3. What observation from the field of psychoacoustics led to the hypothesis that the ear was nonlinear at low sound pressure levels?

4. What paradoxical finding has been reported in numerous studies of normal and disordered hearing?

5. What does the term "negative damping" mean in terms of basilar membrane responses to sounds?

⌁REFERENCES⌁

Békésy, G., von (1960). *Experiments in hearing*. New York: McGraw-Hill Book Company.

Goldstein, J. L. (1967). Auditory nonlinearity. *Journal of the Acoustical Society of America, 41,* 676–689.

Helmholtz, H., von (1863). *Die Lehr von Tonemfundungen.*

Johnstone, B. M., & Boyle, A. J. F. (1967). Basilar membrane vibration examined with the Mossbauer technique. *Science, 158,* 390–391.

Plomp, R. (1965). Detectability threshold for combination tones. *Journal of the Acoustical Society of America, 37,* 1110–1123.

Rhode, W. S. (1971). Observations of the vibration of the basilar membrane in squirrel monkeys using the Mossbauer technique. *Journal of the Acoustical Society of America, 49,* 1218–1231.

Ruggero, M., Narayan, S. S., Temchin, A. N., & Recio, A. (2000). Mechanical bases of frequency tuning and neural excitation at the base of the cochlea: Comparison of basilar-membrane vibrations and auditory-nerve-fiber response in chinchilla. *Proceedings of the National Academy of Sciences, 97,* 11744–11750.

⌁SUGGESTED READING⌁

Durrant, J. D., & Lovrinic, J. H. (1995). *Bases of hearing science*. Baltimore: Williams & Wilkins.

Moller, A. R. (1982). *Auditory physiology*. New York: Academic Press.

Pickles, J. O. (1982). *Introduction to the physiology of hearing*. New York: Academic Press.

Wever, E. G. (1949). *Theory of hearing*. New York: John Wiley & Sons.

Wever, E. G., & Lawrence, M. (1954). *Physiological acoustics*. Princeton, NJ: Princeton University Press.

Chapter

10

Micromechanics: Transduction and Hair Cell Function

Kevin K. Ohlemiller, Ph.D.
Associate Professor of Otolaryngology
Washington University School of Medicine
St. Louis, Missouri

This chapter continues to develop the coding of sounds in the cochlea as a cascade of events. The frequency tuning of the healthy basilar membrane is sufficiently sharp to account for normal perceptual ability to distinguish between sound frequencies. It may therefore be anticipated that all cochlear hair cells need to do is retain this sharpness of tuning in transmitting excitation to afferent neurons. In the case of **inner hair cells** (IHCs), this is essentially true, although these cells also distort and filter incoming signals in ways that significantly influence afferent neuronal responses and perception. This chapter also explains that the transfer of information from the basilar membrane to the organ of Corti is bidirectional, so that **outer hair cells** (OHCs) participate in a **feedback loop** that influences the response properties of the basilar membrane and, in turn, IHCs. IHCs and OHCs thus play different roles, typically described as a *coding* role for IHCs and an *amplification* role for OHCs. Both respond electrically to sound, as a result of sheering motion of their **stereociliary bundle.** Yet, only OHCs respond mechanically to modify the movement of the basilar membrane. This chapter therefore differentiates between two parallel processes: a feed-forward loop (basilar membrane→hair cells) and a feedback loop (OHCs→basilar membrane). In examining this step in the cascade of information flow, we have moved from the realm of **macromechanics** (large-scale movements such as the traveling wave itself) to **micromechanics** (movement of individual cells or their components).

Historical Highlights	
1851–1863	A. Corti first observes cochlear hair cells (Corti, 1851). V. Hensen first describes stereocilia and proposes a role in hair cell excitation (Hensen, 1863).
1930	E. Weaver and C. Bray first record the cochlear microphonic in cats, noting that the amplified potential, when put through a loudspeaker, reproduced words spoken into the animal's ear (hence the name microphonic). They believed they were recording from neurons.
1958–1969	Ultrastructural studies led by H. Engstrom (1958; Engstrom, Ades, & Hawkins, 1962) and R. Kimura (1966) and innervation studies by H. Spoendlin (1966, 1969) point to different functional roles for inner (IHCs) and outer hair cells (OHCs).
1954–1968	Studies led by I. Tasaki (Tasaki, Davis, & Eldredge, 1954) and H. Davis (1958, 1965, 1968) identify the reticular lamina as the locus of origin of the cochlear microphonic and OHCs as its primary generator. Davis first proposes that is it produced by sound modulation of a resistance.
1974–1980	Investigations led by P. Dallos point to an amplification role for OHCs. These studies used kanamycin to eliminate OHCs, so that the physiologic effects of their absence could be observed.
1978	I. Russell and P. Sellick obtain the first intracellular recordings from IHCs.
1980–1985	Y. Tanaka and colleagues obtain first recordings from OHCs (Tanaka, Anasuma, & Yanagisawa, 1980). P. Dallos and colleagues provide first high-quality recordings from OHCs, demonstrating significant functional differences between IHCs and OHCs (Dallos, Santos-Sacchi, & Flock, 1982; Dallos, 1985).
1977–1982	A. J. Hudspeth and colleagues characterize gating of ion currents by movement of the stereocilia bundle in frog hair cells and lay the foundation for the reverse process as the basis of the cochlear amplifier.
1983–1985	OHC motility is first directly observed in studies led by W. Brownell.
2001–2002	Studies by P. Dallos, D. Oliver, and B. Fakler identify prestin as the motor protein underlying OHC somatic motility.
2005	A. J. Hudspeth and D. Chan demonstrate force generation by the cochlear hair cell stereocilia bundle in gerbils.

THE FEED-FORWARD CASCADE

The process by which basilar membrane motion (a mechanical event) is converted to hair cell excitation (an electrical event) is termed **transduction.** This name refers to the conversion of one type of energy into another, and it is in keeping with terminology whereby all energy-converting devices (e.g., microphones, speakers) are transducers. So that the "goal" of basilar membrane motion is to immediately identify the structure that appears most closely linked to the energy conversion from mechanical to electrical as the hair cell stereociliary bundle. Recall that the motion of the basilar membrane at any one location is principally perpendicular to the membrane itself. On first analysis, this would only seem to compress hair bundles into the tectorial membrane and might suggest that stereocilia are activated somewhat like the valves on a trumpet. Instead, the prevailing picture relies on the fact that the basilar membrane and tectorial membrane both move in response to sound, but do not rotate around the same axis (Figure 10-1). The basilar membrane and organ of Corti are attached at their margins to nonmoving structures (the osseous spiral lamina and spiral ligament) (see Chapter 8). The tectorial membrane is attached to the reticular lamina at its lateral margin, but medially is fixed to another nonmoving structure, the spiral limbus. The difference in points of attachment of the basilar membrane and tectorial membrane creates relative motion between the tectorial membrane and reticular lamina as the basilar membrane moves (see Figure 10-1). This results in shearing force that displaces the stereocilia back and forth as the basilar membrane and organ of Corti move up and down, translating the direction of mechanical excitation by 90 degrees. Normal stereocilia appear quite stiff; thus, this motion involves pivoting of each stereocilium around its point of insertion into the hair cell cuticular plate, with little bending. Note that shearing forces will arise regardless of whether the tips of stereocilia are attached to the tectorial membrane. Indeed, most evidence indicates that the stereocilia of OHCs are attached to the tectorial membrane, whereas those of IHCs are not (Slepecky, 1996). Shearing forces applied to IHC bundles appear mediated by the viscous drag of fluids around the bundle. Direct contact between OHC stereocilia and tectorial membrane is probably required for force generation in the feedback loop.

Stereocilia Motion and Ion Channel Activation

How does motion of the stereociliary bundle cause ionic currents and electrical excitation of hair cells? The stringent requirements of hearing appear to have precluded biochemical mechanisms involving many intermediates, whereby A activates B, which activates C, and so on. Each step in such a cascade would impose a delay, including time required for each signaling intermediate molecule to reach its target, then bind to the target, then unbind. Because mammals can collectively hear at frequencies exceeding 100 kHz (consider bats and aquatic mammals), the transducer must be able to operate at comparable speeds. That is, the transducer must be able to turn currents on and off, cycle by cycle, within a few microseconds. To solve this problem, evolution seems to have favored a direct gating mechanism in which the motion of the hair bundle causes ion channels to be transiently pulled open. Several types of evidence support this notion, including recordings of mechanically activated currents at the top of the hair bundle by James Hudspeth and colleagues (Hudspeth & Jacobs, 1979) and the characterization of filaments connecting the tips of adjacent rows of stereocilia that probably mediate channel opening (Pickles, Comis, & Osborne, 1984). Lateral motion of the hair bundle is thought to cause differential displacement of adjacent rows of stereocilia and to directly pull ion channels open (Figure 10-2). Positively charged ions then flow into stereocilia from the endolymphatic space and into the cell body, depolarizing (exciting) the hair cell. The actual number of such channels may be small—perhaps only one per stereocilium, according to Hudspeth's work (Hudspeth, 1982). Importantly, even in the absence of sound, these channels open and close randomly at a low rate. Therefore, even at rest, some fraction of channels are

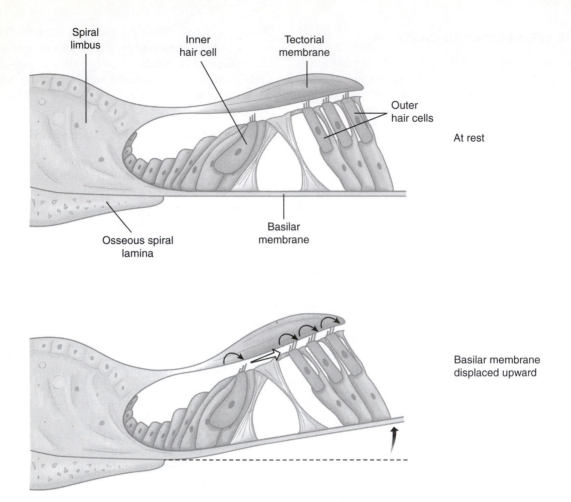

Spiral limbus

Inner hair cell

Tectorial membrane

Outer hair cells

At rest

Osseous spiral lamina

Basilar membrane

Basilar membrane displaced upward

FIGURE 10-1 Schematic representation of organ of Corti showing how different points of attachment for the basilar membrane and tectorial membrane can cause shearing movements of the hair cell stereocilia *(unfilled arrow)* when the basilar membrane is displaced vertically. Stereocilia of outer hair cells are moved by virtue of direct connection to the tectorial membrane. Inner hair cell stereocilia are moved by viscous drag of surrounding fluids.

always open and positive current is flowing through the hair cell, leaving it less negatively charged than it would otherwise be. This is a critical feature, considering that the basilar membrane can move either up or down from its resting position. For the hair cell to generate an electrical response that follows the motion of the basilar membrane, it must be able to modulate its membrane potential in either the positive or negative direction.

Electrochemical Gradients and Ion flow

Ion channels are not "pumps," but simply doorways. Their activation will not lead to positive ion flow into hair cells unless external forces are operating to drive those currents. Recall from Chapter 5 that ion flow obeys two types of gradients: voltage gradients and concentration gradients (collectively known as electrochemical gradients). Voltage gradients arise from the mutual repulsion of like-charged particles

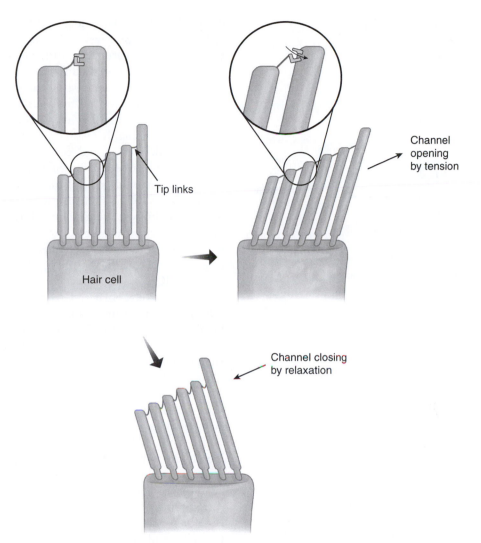

FIGURE 10-2 Schematic representation of attachments between stereocilia (tip links) and how these might be affected by movements of the hair bundle in opposite directions. Movement toward the tallest row places tension on links and opens ion channels. Movement toward the shortest row relaxes links and allows channels to close. At rest, a small population of channels will be open at any given time due to random opening and closing.

(ions). Positively charged ions will move away from each other, into regions that have a more negative net charge, that is, down a voltage gradient. In addition, all particles, whether charged or uncharged, will distribute themselves homogenously in a medium by flowing down their concentration gradient. Both of these gradients are required to understand positive current flow through hair cells.

Cochlear scala media is a uniquely composed extracellular compartment (Figure 10–3). Endolymph, which fills this space (and the entire membranous labyrinth), has a high potassium (K^+) concentration typically characteristic of the *inside* of cells (roughly 150 millimolar [mM]) (Wangeman & Schacht, 1996). Endolymph also has a low sodium (Na^+) concentration (about 1 mM). Perilymph,

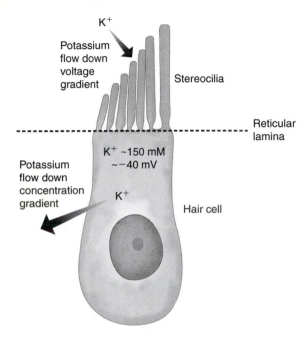

Scala media (endolymph)
High potassium (~150 mM)
High positive charge (~+80 mV)

K^+
Potassium flow down voltage gradient

Stereocilia

Reticular lamina

K^+ ~150 mM
~−40 mV

Potassium flow down concentration gradient

K^+

Hair cell

Scala tympani (perilymph)
Low potassium (~5 mM)
Low positive charge (~0 mV)

FIGURE 10-3 Schematic representation of chemical and electrical gradients that give rise to ionic currents through hair cells. Scala media contains high potassium levels and is highly positively charged. Hair cells also contain high potassium, but are negatively charged. Potassium ions flow into hair cells by flowing down the resulting electrical gradient. Fluid around the base of the cell is positively charged (compared with inside the cell), but low in potassium. Potassium flows down concentration gradient, out of the cell.

which fills scala tympani and scala vestibuli (recall that these connect), is low in K^+ (about 5 mM) and high in Na^+ (about 150 mM), as is typical of most extracellular fluids, and overall is similar in composition to cerebrospinal fluid surrounding the brain. If one were to place the positive lead of a voltmeter inside scala media and the negative lead into

the perilymphatic space, it would be observed that scala media is positively charged. This positive **endocochlear potential** (EP), normally around +80 to 90 mV, is directly linked to active pumping of K^+ ions into scala media by the stria vascularis. Sodium ions are removed from scala media in this process. Note that the flow of K^+ from endolymph to perilymph is highly favored in this arrangement, because both voltage and concentration gradients are aligned to drive K^+ out of scala media. That is exactly what would occur if the cells that make up the boundary of scala media were not joined by special seals known as **tight junctions.** Instead, the lowest resistance path for K^+ to escape scala media is through hair cells via the stereocilia transduction channels. Like scala media, the inside of the hair cell is high in K^+. Unlike scala media, however, the hair cell is negatively polarized (roughly −40 mV for IHCs). This is because hair cells, like neurons, are highly permeable to K^+ along their basolateral membranes and are "pulled" toward the equilibrium potential for K^+ (typically about −70 mV) (see Chapter 5). The following scheme thus emerges: Potassium ions flow down a voltage gradient from scala media into hair cells, even though there is no concentration gradient between them (see Figure 10-3). The voltage gradient driving this flow is loosely the sum of the hair cell resting potential and the EP. Potassium ions then flow down their concentration gradient from the hair cell body into the surrounding perilymphatic space, even though the latter step is counter to the voltage gradient across the cell membrane.

Hair cells may be considered to balance their membrane potential based on the relative resistances of the mechanically gated channels on the stereocilia and the K^+ channels that line the basolateral membrane of the cells. When no sound is present, the resistance of the mechanically gated channels is dominant. The cell then hyperpolarizes toward the equilibrium potential for K^+ and sits in a low state of excitation. When sound is present, the resistance of the mechanically gated channels is reduced as more of these channels open. The basolateral membrane resistance then dominates, and the cell depolarizes toward the EP. The reason that K^+

is the major current carrier in hair cells is that K^+ is the dominant positive ion in endolymph. The mechanically activated channels on the stereocilia are themselves not very selective for specific ions.

Having arrived in the spaces around the hair cells, K^+ is "recycled" back to stria vascularis so that the loop can be repeated, efficiently using potassium that is already available. There exists a web of connections between supporting cells of the organ of Corti and different types of fibrocytes in the spiral ligament for just this purpose (Slepecky, 1996). These include special channels called **gap junctions,** which join cells directly and promote ion flow from cell to cell. It is fundamentally the movement and distribution of K^+ around the scala media → scala tympani → scala media loop that makes possible the proper function of hair cells. That distribution is primarily established by the ion-pumping action of the stria vascularis. This process requires energy in that adenosine triphosphate (ATP, the "currency" of cellular energy) is necessary. Other steps in the K^+ cycle (diffusion through the organ of Corti and spiral ligament en route to the stria) are passive. In this arrangement, the most energy-expensive functions are conducted away from the organ of Corti. From an evolutionary perspective, reducing the energy load on hair cells may have obviated the need for elaborate vascularization of the organ of Corti. Placing blood vessels within the organ would likely increase the intrinsic background noise, and thereby decrease hearing sensitivity. A design whereby hair cells gate ion flow, rather than pump ions, may also help protect them from injury related to the metabolic demands of noise exposure.

Receptor Potentials

We now have the necessary concepts to construct a **receptor potential,** the electrical response of a hair cell to an acoustic stimulus (Figure 10-4). In this and the next few sections, most of the discussion is directed toward IHCs and bears on how sounds are coded. Nevertheless, IHCs and OHCs are similar in their electrical responses and how these arise.

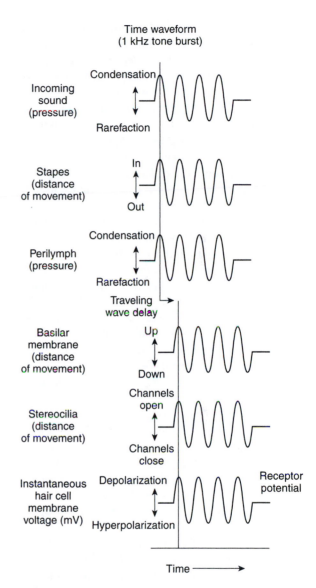

FIGURE 10-4 Schematic showing representation of a simple tonal stimulus at various points in the cochlear cascade of events up through the hair cell receptor potential. For a low-level stimulus, the waveform is essentially preserved, with the introduction of a delay for the traveling wave. At each point the stimulus is represented either as the movement of a structure, as compression/rarefaction in a medium (air, cochlear fluids), or as a change in electrical potential.

Let us assume that a 1 Hz tone burst is input to the ear at some moderate intensity, and we want to compare the time waveform depicting the response of the basilar membrane and an IHC at the 1 kHz location. Before the stimulus is turned on, the basilar membrane is in its resting position, and therefore so is the cell's hair bundle. This means that most, but not all, of the mechanically gated channels are closed. Because the stimulus contains only a single frequency, and we are examining the place of maximal response, we can expect the waveform of the stimulus itself to be preserved at every stage. Thus, the up-and-down displacements of the basilar membrane reflect rarefactions and condensations in the tone-burst waveform transmitted through the ossicles to the perilymph. Transmission through the perilymph is essentially instantaneous, but there will be an interposed delay for the traveling wave to reach the 1 kHz location (see Chapter 9). For each cycle, as the basilar membrane moves up, the stereocilia bundle is displaced away from the modiolus, and the hair cell will depolarize from its resting membrane potential. As the basilar membrane moves down, the bundle is displaced toward the modiolus, and the hair cell hyperpolarizes beyond its initial membrane potential. In this cycle-by-cycle manner, the analog waveform of the tone will be represented in the receptor potential. In the terminology used by engineers, the rapid hair cell voltage changes that define the receptor potential are termed *AC*, for "alternating current." Among engineers, AC generally refers to any rapidly varying signal, or part thereof. The term was extended to hair cell responses in the first classic studies of hair cell function (Russell & Sellick, 1978; Dallos et al., 1982; Dallos, 1985). In our simple scenario, the AC component of the hair cell response is a sinusoid that recapitulates the original stimulus.

Unfortunately, we would quickly exhaust the conditions under which such a simple scenario might apply, finding that they are limited to low-stimulus intensities and stimulus frequencies less than a few kilohertz.

Effect of Stimulus Intensity Because a "high-fidelity" representation of the acoustic world would appear desirable, it may be surprising that the sys-

tem has apparently evolved to sacrifice some amount of fidelity as part of a trade-off. What features of hair cells impart reduced fidelity and why? The first is level-dependent nonlinearity of the transducer (Hudspeth & Corey, 1977). This is best understood by examining the relation between the displacement of the stereociliary bundle and the resulting deviation of the hair cell membrane potential from the resting potential. For small movements in either direction, the relation falls on a straight line, and thus adheres to the formal definition of linearity (Figure 10-5A). For a low-level sinusoidal input, the simple case from the preceding section applies: The time-varying movement of the hair bundle will also be sinusoidal, as will the pattern of change in the membrane potential of the cell. However, for larger bundle displacements in either direction, the relation begins to flatten out, or "saturate." At the point of saturation and beyond, increased bundle displacements will yield progressively smaller incremental responses. If the input pattern is a sinusoid, the response acquires a "squared-off" appearance (see Figure 10-5B). The term usually applied to the level-dependent saturation of the transducer response—and thus the hair cell response—is "compression." The transducer incorporates a **compressive nonlinearity.**

Note further that the point of saturation is reached much more quickly in the hyperpolarizing direction than in the depolarizing direction. This reflects that most mechanically gated channels are closed at rest, and more channels are available to be opened than closed. Hence, the second key feature of the transducer nonlinearity is **asymmetry.** The consequence is that truncation (squaring off) of the sinusoid input is more pronounced on the bottom of the waveform than on the top. This means the hair cell will show net depolarization during the stimulus. Still, it is notable that no matter now large the bundle deflection, the hair cell **membrane voltage** never becomes positive. From a typical resting potential near -40 mV, the maximal positive excursions of the membrane potential might reach, say, -25 mV for an intense stimulus, but this still leaves the hair cell negatively charged. In this regard, hair cells differ in their manner of excitation from

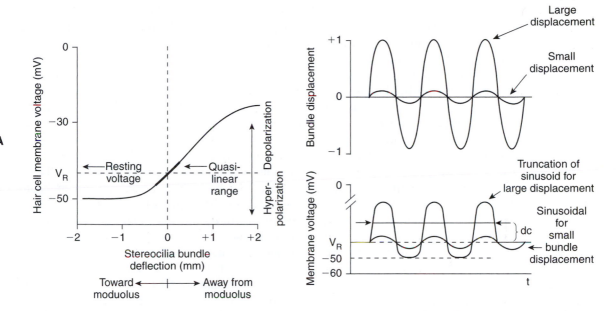

FIGURE 10-5 (A) Schematic representation of the compressive nonlinear conversion of stereociliary displacement into changes in the hair cell membrane potential. Small sinusoidal variation in bundle position leads to sinusoidal variation in membrane potential. (B) shows how hair cell membrane potential changes with time as the stereociliary bundle is displaced back and forth in a sinusoidal pattern. Large sinusoidal bundle displacements lead to truncated and asymmetric variations membrane potential. Thus, the stimulus waveform shows nonlinear distortion and is no longer faithfully represented.

neurons, which briefly become positively charged during an action potential (see Chapter 5). In viewing Figure 10-5A, keep in mind that the seemingly small overall range of movement of the stereociliary bundle (±2 μm in Figure 10-5A) covers the entire intensity range of hearing, which exceeds 10^6-fold variation in sound pressure. Low sound levels would yield barely measurable movements of the bundle along the x-axis.

In truncating and altering the symmetry of the input waveform, the transducer imposes **distortion.** The signal-distorting properties of the transducer impact not only IHC responses, but also OHC responses, and the feedback provided by the latter on the basilar membrane (discussed later). Transducer nonlinearities are thus far-reaching, impacting the response of the basilar membrane, neurons, and perception itself. In engineering, as well as in hearing science, distortion has specific

meaning. Recall from Chapter 3 that not all changes in the shape of a waveform constitute distortion. Filtering a complex tone (sinusoids of different frequencies added together), for example, may change the waveform, but this is not distortion. The key difference is that filtering *reduces* the frequency content of a signal, whereas distortion actually *adds* frequencies that were not present originally. Because tonotopy and frequency analysis are foundational to cochlear function, and ultimately perception (see Chapters 9 and 15), the implication is that the transducer subverts an accurate representation of the acoustic environment. In essence, in most settings, we perceive components of sounds that do not exist. What do we gain? It is clear that the great advantage of compression is **dynamic range.** As we said, the range of sound pressures we must detect and act on in the environment exceeds 6 orders of magnitude, or more than 120 dB. Over that range, we can detect changes in intensity on the order of 1 dB, or about 10%. One reason we retain the ability to distinguish small changes in intensity at high sound levels is that our hair cells do not "run out" of dynamic range. Their responses continue to grow at high levels, albeit nonlinearly. Thus, to gain dynamic range, we tolerate error in the encoding of the stimulus spectrum. Accuracy with regard to the stimulus spectrum is arguably more important at lower sound levels, when our cochleas function more linearly. Near threshold, where we may require optimal discernment of the spectrum, the transducer—and thus the cochlea—is nearly linear.

As a result of transducer asymmetry, the hair cell is depolarized from its resting state for large bundle displacements. If we were to present the same stimulus many times, each time using a different starting phase, and then average all the values in the receptor potential at times t_1, t_2, t_3, and so forth, we would observe this depolarization, because the AC component will average out. Low-pass filtering of the receptor potential would yield a similar result. In the vernacular of engineers, slow shifts are termed *direct-coupled* (DC) shifts. Again, in keeping with the engineering perspective of the pioneering investigators into hair cell function (Russell & Sellick, 1978; Dallos et al., 1982; Dallos, 1985), the slow offset component of the hair cell receptor potential has been termed the **DC potential.** If one were conversely to measure the peak-to-peak magnitude of the receptor potential, or high-pass filter the waveform, one would isolate the complementary **AC potential.**

If the compressive character of the transducer has advantages for perception, what about the asymmetry that causes the DC potential? Although this issue is considered more in-depth in Chapter 11, we can state that the major goal of hair cell response, whether AC or DC, is to influence the rate and timing with which each hair cell (principally each IHC) releases excitatory neurotransmitter into the synaptic junction it forms with approximately 20 to 30 afferent neurons. The more depolarized the hair cell is, the more neurotransmitter that is released, and the more rapidly the neurons will exhibit action potentials (or "spikes") (see Chapter 5).

Thus, the amplitude of the receptor potential DC component largely determines the **spike rate** of auditory neurons.

The transducer is not the only contributor of nonlinearities to hair cell responses. Ion channels in the basolateral membrane of the cells also play a role. More significantly, OHCs modify the mechanical drive to IHCs such that the latter actually receive a compressed version of the sound stimulus at their input. Nevertheless, changes in hair cell responses as a function of stimulus intensity essentially (Figure 10-6) follow from the relation laid out in Figure 10-5. Figure 10-5 predicts that the **intensity-response curve** will have two segments: a quasi-linear segment at lower sound intensities, and a saturating segment at high intensities. Note here that we have switched from consideration of the cycle-by-cycle instantaneous relation between the stimulus and hair cell response to the overall magnitude of each. Hair cell intensity response curves (also called input-output curves) thus share the major features of analogous curves for the basilar membrane. This applies to both AC and DC components of the response. The AC potential can be estimated either from the peak-to-peak value of the response envelope or the calculated root-mean-square (RMS) value. As stated earlier, low-pass filtering, or averaging the response to many stimuli presented in random phase, will isolate the DC component. Compared with the AC component, the **intensity curve** for the DC component of the receptor potential is usually shifted to the right on the x-axis. This is expected, because it reflects asymmetric truncation of peaks at higher sound levels. Note from Figure 10-6A that, although the rate of increase of the response amplitude with increasing stimulus level slows at high intensities, both the AC and DC response do continue to grow—the principal advantage of compression.

As an exercise, we can even work backward from the original response waveforms, shown in Figure 10-6A, to recreate the compressive character of the cycle-by-cycle response of the hair cell. For the peak rarefactions and compressions in the sound wave (expressed in Pascals) at each intensity applied, we can plot the corresponding positive and negative peaks of

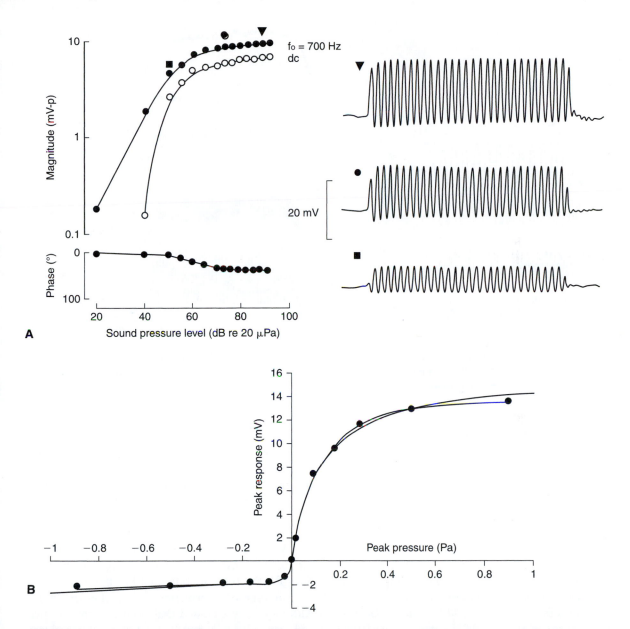

FIGURE 10-6 (A) Intensity response curves for the AC and DC receptor potential of an inner hair cell, together with the phase of response for the AC component. Raw response waveforms are shown at right for the indicated intensities. (B) Peak sound stimulus condensation and rarefaction for several stimulus levels versus maximum positive and negative excursions of the hair cell membrane potential. This indirect method largely recapitulates the transducer relation of Figure 10-5. (From Dallos, P., & Cheatham, M. A. (1992). Cochlear hair cell function. *Sensory transduction* (pp. 372–393). New York: Rockefeller University Press, by permission.)

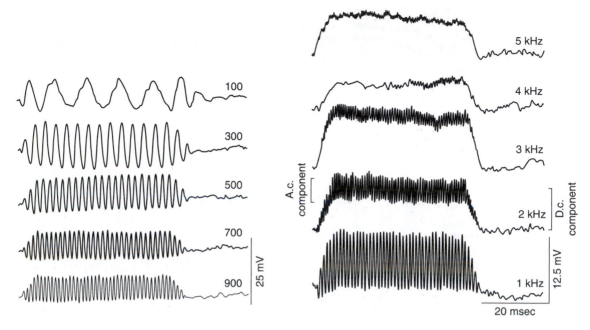

FIGURE 10-7   Raw response traces from an inner hair cell in the guinea pig cochlear base show changes in the response with increasing stimulus frequency. As the frequency increases, the AC component becomes less prominent. (Adapted from Palmer & Russell, 1986.)

the hair cell waveform (in millivolts), as the investigator has done in Figure 10-6B. The resulting plot strongly resembles Figure 10-5A, precisely because it largely reflects the characteristics of the transducer.

Low-Pass Filtering of the AC Response Component   Under most real-world conditions, both AC and DC components would be observed in the receptor potential. The AC component, however, is subject to a limitation that the DC component is not. Recall that the AC component can be removed by low-pass filtering. In fact, *all hair cells are low-pass filters* because of the parallel resistance-capacitance circuit formed by their cell membrane. For stimuli at frequencies above roughly 4 to 5 kHz, the AC component contributes progressively less to the receptor potential. Hair cells tuned to higher frequencies, when presented with a high-frequency tone, generate receptor potentials containing primarily or solely the DC component. Figure 10-7 shows original hair cell responses illustrating

this point. Each trace in Figure 10-7 is a single recorded receptor potential elicited by a tone at the accompanying stimulus frequency. This basal hair cell responds well to loud tones at all frequencies presented, yet note the progressive loss of the rapid AC component as the stimulus frequency increases. At 4 to 5 kHz, only the DC component remains.

As we will revisit in Chapter 11, the removal of the AC response by low-pass filtering has implications for the type of code used by afferent neurons and the type of information that reaches the brain. Although it was argued that both the compressive and asymmetric character of the hair cell transducer have benefits, any benefit conveyed by the loss of the AC response component of hair cells at high stimulus frequencies currently is unclear. Perhaps low-pass filtering by cell membranes simply presented mechanosensory organs with a difficult problem that there has been no pressing need to "solve" (from an evolutionary perspective) because of the availability of other coding options.

Effect of Stimulus Frequency

If we include both AC and DC responses, hair cells are principally band-pass filters, just as is the basilar membrane at any location. The frequency tuning (or passband) of any filter may be determined in

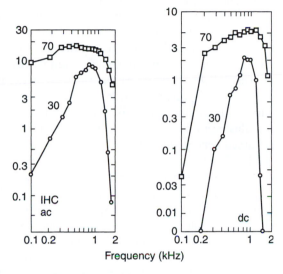

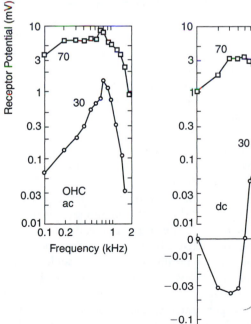

two different ways, depending on the question being asked. First, one may sweep across frequencies at a fixed stimulus level and derive an **iso-level curve.** This can be done for basilar membrane velocity or displacement, as depicted in Chapter 9 (see Figure 9-7). For hair cells, it could be done while measuring the magnitude of either the DC or AC component of the receptor potential. These yield generally similar results, although the AC potential may be undetectable in basally located hair cells. For a low-to-moderate level stimulus and a healthy cochlea, there will be a clear **best frequency** (BF) that elicits the maximal response (Figure 10-8). What would happen if we repeat the process using a much higher level stimulus? If the cell (or any filter we might be examining) is linear and the response axis uses a log scale, any curve obtained will have the same shape but will be shifted vertically. A 20 dB increase in the stimulus level would simply shift the curve upward 10-fold (i.e., 20 dB) on the y-axis. The same degree of frequency tuning would be apparent, independent of the stimulus level used. This is decidedly *not* what we would find for hair cells. As shown in Figure 10-8, iso-level curves obtained at high stimulus levels typically show low-pass filter characteristics, with no clear BF. The change in the shape of the curve is caused by another complexity of the compressive nonlinearity of the hair cell response: It is stimulus frequency dependent. The growth of the response is compressive near the BF, but nearly linear below the BF. Thus, the curve flattens out at high stimulus levels, because most of the growth in the response occurs below the BF.

FIGURE 10-8 Iso-level curves for inner (IHC; top) and outer hair cell (OHC; bottom). Both AC and DC response show clear frequency tuning at lower stimulus levels. At high levels, tuning broadens, so that band-pass filter characteristic becomes low-pass. Curves for OHCs are superficially similar, although the DC component of the receptor potential may be negative below the best frequency. (From Dallos, P., & Cheatham, M. A. (1992). Cochlear hair cell function. *Sensory transduction* (pp. 372–393). New York: Rockefeller University Press, by permission.)

How can stimulus level dependence in the shape of hair cell iso-level curves arise? This chapter has attributed most of the compressive nonlinearity of hair cell responses to the stereociliary transducer, which functions similarly in IHCs and OHCs. No aspect of transducer operation was suggested to be frequency dependent. To explain how the same transducer can cause near-linear growth of the response below the BF *and* compressive growth near the BF, we must return to distinctions between IHC and OHC function. Chapter 9 described how an **active process** was needed to account for the sharp tuning and sensitivity of the basilar membrane, and we have said that OHCs generate mechanical feedback that enhances the movement of the membrane, and thereby the responses of IHCs. Amplification of basilar membrane motion by OHCs reflects not only the nonlinearity of their transducer, but also other nonlinearities that are part of the feedback mechanism.

OHCs incorporate not one transducer, but two. The first is the "forward" transducer in the hair bundle, which converts motion into an electrical signal. A second transducer exclusive to OHCs converts their electrical response back into motion that is fed back into the basilar membrane. The identity of the "reverse" transducer remains controversial (and is considered later), but its role is widely accepted. Moreover, this transducer is both asymmetric and compressive. When considering the nature of the feedback provided to the basilar membrane by OHCs, we are confronted by two nonlinear transduction steps that act in series to alter the motion of the basilar membrane, which, in turn, alters the input to the OHCs. Despite much research, it has proved difficult to untangle this knot of cause and effect. Conceptual models may instead refer to the "basilar membrane-OHC-tectorial membrane complex" (e.g., Cheatham & Dallos, 2000). The implication is that compression observed in IHC responses near the BF reflects both the influence of the IHC transducer *and* additional compressive contributions from the OHC-based amplifier. When the IHC is stimulated well below its BF, the amplifier is "turned off" and the response is less compressed. The different roles of IHCs versus OHCs, and the different influences on their responses, are demonstrated in part by iso-level curves for their DC response. Note in Figure 10-8 that the DC response in OHCs can actually be negative below the BF. Net hyperpolarization of OHCs below their BF may be essential to how their amplification role is disengaged below the BF.

The second way that tuning of a filter can be determined is typically reserved for nonlinear systems and has been heavily used in the study of the cochlea. Chapter 9 introduced **frequency tuning curves** in the context of basilar membrane responses. For a given location (or hair cell), these curves address the question, "How loud must the stimulus be to obtain a response?" When this is determined over a wide range of frequencies for a hair cell in a healthy cochlea, a narrow range of frequencies will be found where the threshold for a criterion response is minimal. This is again the BF (also called the *characteristic frequency,* although the latter term is most often applied to cochlear neurons) and would be found to be the peak frequency of an iso-level curve obtained from the same hair cell. In a linear system, these two curves would have exactly the same shape, only inverted. (Thus, little value exists in constructing both types of curves in a linear system.) However, in healthy, nonlinear hair cells, these two curves will yield different information.

Frequency tuning curves are also referred to as **iso-response curves,** because by definition, they connect all frequency-intensity pairs that yield the same level of response. What will be called a *response* necessarily involves a subjective decision. We cannot know what magnitude of response in a hair cell corresponds to the perception of a sound. Moreover, we often are limited by the level of background noise in the electrophysiologic recording setup. The chosen criterion response, therefore, ends up being somewhat arbitrary. In practice, the criterion chosen is typically as near as possible to the recording noise level, the goal being to obtain a threshold near the BF that can be compared with behavioral/perceptual thresholds across laboratories or species. Because the nonlinearities considered in this chapter increase with stimulus level, tuning curves will be most similar to iso-level curves obtained at lower stimulus levels. In the healthy cochlea, curves such as those shown in Figure 10-9 generally emerge. Figures 10-9A and B show tuning curves obtained from the same IHC for the DC and AC components of the receptor potential, respectively. The cell's BF is approximately 17 kHz.

Two features of these curves are typical for high-BF hair cells. Approaching the BF from lower frequencies, the threshold declines steeply, reaches a minimum at the BF, then abruptly rises. This is the **tip** region of the curve. Below the BF is a region termed the **tail**, a flat segment extending to the

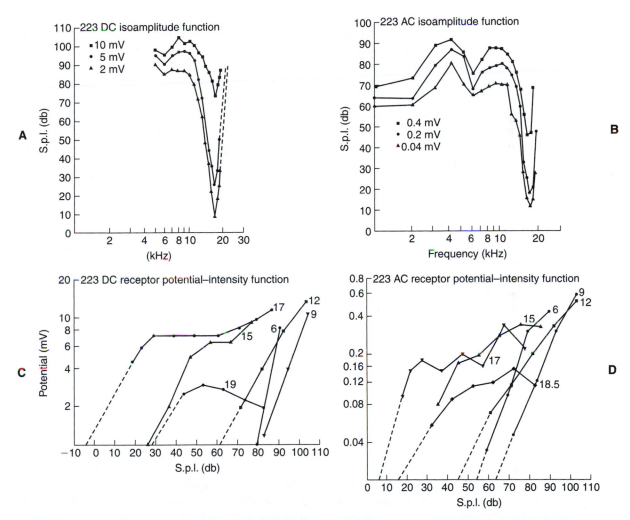

FIGURE 10-9 (A, B) Frequency tuning curves for a single basal inner hair cell. The best frequency of this cell is about 17 kHz. Curves for DC (A) and AC (B) components include effects of increasing the response criterion, as indicated. Tuning of DC and AC components are similar. The magnitude of the AC component was compensated for the calculated affects of low-pass filtering by the hair cell membrane. (C, D) Intensity response curves for the DC (C) and AC (D) response components. Curves obtained near the best frequency (BF) are shifted to the left (more sensitive) and show pronounced compression. Curves obtained below the BF are linear. (From Russell, I. J., & Sellick, P. M. (1978). Intracellular studies of hair cells in the mammalian cochlea. *Journal of Physiology, 284*, 261–289, by permission from Blackwell Publishing.)

lowest frequencies tested (more prominent for the AC tuning curve in this example). Within each panel, the investigators in this classic demonstration (Russell & Sellick, 1978) also show the effect of increasing the response criterion, so that the cell is required to generate a larger response. As the criterion is made more stringent, louder stimuli are needed to elicit a response, and the curve shifts upward, as expected. However, the shape is not retained. The tip-length is shortened, so that the tip/tail ratio decreases. This blunting of tuning at higher stimulus levels is analogous to that shown in Figure 10-8 for iso-level curves and arises from the same mechanisms. How compressive nonlinearities cause these changes in the shape of tuning curves can be elucidated by examining vertical "slices" at different stimulus frequencies in Figures 10-9A and B. Each slice yields an intensity-response curve, several of which have been constructed in the Figures 10-9C and D (a few more points have been added). To interpret these, let us begin with Figure 10-9C (DC response) by considering the curve obtained with a 17 kHz (BF) stimulus. Because the hair cell is tuned to this frequency, this curve is shifted to the left, meaning that a low-level stimulus elicited a response. Over the course of about 30 dB, this curve saturates (flattens out), so that large changes in stimulus amplitude are needed to obtain an increase in the response. This is exactly why the tip of the tuning curve shifts dramatically upward as the response criterion is increased. Now, for a stimulus above the BF (19 kHz), note that even an intense stimulus yields a poor response (Figure 10-9C). The tuning curve accordingly rises steeply at this frequency. Finally, for intensity curves obtained at frequencies below the BF, note that intense stimuli are needed to obtain a response. Once threshold is reached, however, the response increases quickly over a narrow intensity range. The intensity curves obtained at frequencies below the BF rise in a straight line, that is, without compression. This is why increases in response criterion lead to parallel shifts in the tail region of the tuning curve. Although the points illustrated here were in reference to the DC response, the same general observations can be made for the AC response.

We have now come full circle on the concept of compression, beginning with intensity-response curves, proceeding to iso-level and frequency tuning curves, and re-creating intensity curves by cutting slices through the tuning curves. The goal—and it is an important one—is to achieve familiarity and a level of comfort with how the prominent theme of compression echoes through hair cell (and neural) responses, no matter how we examine them. In the demonstration in Figure 10-9, you may have noticed a seeming contradiction. How were AC responses recorded in a hair cell tuned to 17 kHz? This feat relied on an engineering method for estimating how large the AC component would be in the absence of hair cell low-pass filtering and "compensating" responses accordingly. This allowed inferences regarding how the growth and tuning of the AC component would compare with that of the DC component, regardless of whether the AC component would really have been large enough to be biologically significant.

Frequency tuning curves obtained in healthy cochleas will always show a well-defined tip and (for mid and high BFs) a much less sensitive tail. For any cochlear location, hair cell and basilar membrane tuning curves share these key features and will show similar tuning curves overall. This is expected, of course, because the hair cell tuning is based on the tuning of the basilar membrane. The prominent tails of high BF tuning curves may seem a surprising feature, inconsistent with a conception of the cochlea as a bank of "labeled line" filters. True "labeling" would mean that each filter responds only for stimuli near the BF. Yet, both tip and tail responses of the basilar membrane, hair cells, and ultimately neurons play a role in stimulus coding. The existence of tuning curve tails follows directly from the character of the traveling wave. Recall that the traveling wave begins in the cochlear base, proceeds apically to a point of maximum excitation, and then extinguishes rapidly. Thus, a given stimulus, if presented at sufficiently high levels, will excite not only its own preferred location, but also all points basal to it. Restated, any location will respond to its own BF, as well as to lower frequencies. That is exactly what tuning curve tips and tails show.

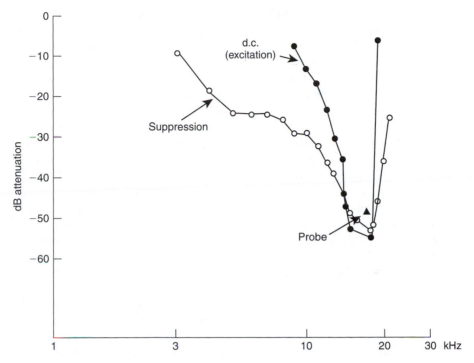

FIGURE 10-10 Excitation and suppression tuning curves for the DC response component of a single inner hair cell from the cochlear base. The suppression area was derived by presenting a probe tone at the best frequency at the level indicated and measuring the level of a simultaneous second tone needed to reduce the DC response magnitude at many frequencies. (From Sellick, P. M., & Russell, I. J. (1979). Two-tone suppression in cochlear hair cells. *Hearing Research, 1,* 227–236, by permission.)

Two-Tone Suppression

Yet another manifestation of nonlinearity in hair cell responses is what happens when a second, non-BF tone is added to a "probe" tone presented near the BF. If the system were linear, then the response to the two tones would be the sum of responses to each of the tones in isolation. Let us consider two cases, one in which the second tone falls within the frequency tuning curve (i.e., is excitatory on its own), and one in which the second tone falls outside the tuning curve (and thus has no effect by itself). In the first instance, the temporal response of the stereociliary transducer will be impacted by interactions between the two stimuli. At any moment, these may augment or cancel each other, as might any two sinusoids added together. When the "net"

stimulus waveform is put through the compressive transducer nonlinearity, the response to both tones together may be either enhanced, or **suppressed,** relative to the response to the probe alone. If we are recording from an IHC, the overall effect of a second tone will affect the IHC directly *and* any amplification by OHCs, because the transducers of both cell types will come into play. In summary, the effect of a second tone that falls within the tuning curve on either the AC or DC response is difficult to predict.

Now let us consider the case where the second tone lies outside the tuning curve and appears to produce no DC response. Surprisingly, the DC response to the probe may be reduced. Figure 10-10 shows an example of this. Flanking the boundaries of the excitatory response area is a large **suppression area.**

The key to how this arises may lie in the AC response of this high-BF hair cell's transducer (Cheatham & Dallos, 1992). Below the DC tuning curve, we may consider there to exist a "virtual" AC curve, like those revealed by compensation methods in Figure 10-9. Whereas the cell generates little AC response to any stimulus near the BF, neither the motion of the hair bundle nor the resulting transduction currents are subject to low-pass filtering. Hair bundle motion related to the suppressor tone thus may effectively *bias* the position of the transducer, so that the currents elicited by the probe are reduced. This would apply to both IHCs and OHCs, so that amplification is reduced. This type of suppression is not limited to hair cells with high BFs: Throughout the cochlea, stimuli that fall within the region between the DC and real (low BF) or "virtual" AC tuning curves (high BFs) could produce such a bias. Figure 10-10 shows that the suppression area disappears near the BF. Near the BF, the distinction between probe and suppressor essentially disappears. Finally, note that the term *suppression* is preferred over inhibition in this context, because within neuroscience, "inhibition" is restricted to synaptic mechanisms. Suppression is purely mechanical and requires that the probe and suppressor be presented simultaneously.

FEEDBACK LOOP

A host of observations led to early proposals that IHCs and OHCs serve different functions. Foremost, they look quite different, including the arrangement of their stereociliary bundles, and they possess a different complement of organelles. Their placement in the organ of Corti also suggests different roles: OHCs occupy the middle region of the basilar membrane, where displacements are largest, whereas IHCs rest at least partly over the stationary osseous spiral lamina. As mentioned earlier, the stereocilia of the OHCs make direct contact with the tectorial membrane, whereas those of the IHCs are not generally believed to do so. Substantial differences in innervation also suggested different functions (Spoendlin, 1966, 1969). IHCs receive roughly 95% of all afferent contacts (radial afferents), each of

which makes contact with only one or a few hair cells. OHCs receive the remaining 5%. Moreover, the spiral afferent neurons may contact dozens of OHCs while meandering over half a cochlear turn. This arrangement would not be predicted to yield sharp frequency tuning in these neurons, and it suggests a role for these other than coding.

Even before direct observations on OHC physiology, functional evidence also pointed to a modulatory role for OHCs. Efferent neurons make direct contact with the bodies of OHCs, but principally with the afferent dendrites contacting IHCs (see Chapter 12). Most efferents that contact the OHCs reach the cochlea by crossing the midline of the head in a manner that has allowed the effect of selectively activating these to be explored. Electrically shocking these fibers in experiments with animals was observed to decrease the sensitivity and sharpness of frequency tuning of both IHCs and their afferent neurons (e.g., Brown, Nuttall, & Masta, 1983). Activating the efferents also reduces the amplitude of otoacoustic emissions recordable from the ear canal (Siegel & Kim, 1982). Finally, selective application of ototoxic drugs such as kanamycin can yield regions of the cochlea that have seemingly normal IHCs, but a complete absence of OHCs. In such preparations, the sharpness of frequency tuning and sensitivity of IHCs and radial afferent neurons are reduced (Dallos & Wang, 1974; Dallos & Harris, 1978). These findings and others have provided strong evidence that OHCs affect the mechanical environment of the IHCs.

Direct physiologic recordings from OHCs have been much more difficult to obtain than those from IHCs; thus, our understanding of IHC function matured much more rapidly. In hindsight, we know that this difficulty arose not merely from the narrow shape and location of OHCs, but from the dual character of their responses to sound. As data from OHC recordings began to accumulate, some puzzling differences in receptor potentials of these two cell types were noted. For example, we saw that, for low-level stimuli below the BF, OHCs generate hyperpolarizing DC potentials (see Figure 10-8). We now know that the explanation of this lies in the fact that OHCs interact mechanically with their environment and effectively modify their own input. Even though this was suspected, electrical recordings from OHCs did not provide definitive clues to the primary contribution of OHCs to hearing.

Mechanical Responses of Outer Hair Cells

The critical piece of the puzzle regarding the contribution of OHCs to hearing required isolating intact cells, placing them in a chamber of artificial perilymph, delivering depolarizing current pulses, and *watching*. OHCs were found to shorten when depolarized and to lengthen from their resting state when hyperpolarized (Brownell, 1983; Brownell, Bader, Bertrand, & deRibaupierre, 1985). As confirmed in many subsequent studies, the overall change in length can be on the order of 5% to 10%. This **somatic motility** is directly linked to the membrane potential, and thus follows the receptor potential during a stimulus. It may lie at the heart of the **cochlear amplifier,** by providing cycle-by-cycle enhancement of the motion of the basilar membrane. The essential membrane element underlying fast motility is a voltage-sensing protein, recently identified and named prestin (Oliver et al., 2001; Dallos & Fakler, 2002). Prestin exhibits either a short or long conformation, depending on the voltage across it, so that length changes across the entire hair cell arise through the collective action of thousands of prestin molecules. Although prestin can change its shape sufficiently rapidly to drive the cochlear amplifier throughout the entire range of hearing, an apparent limitation of somatic motility as the basis for the cochlear amplifier is the need for an adequate AC receptor potential in OHCs, to provide cycle-by-cycle drive. As emphasized, the AC component in hair responses is filtered out by the hair cell membrane for frequencies above a few kilohertz. Thus, frequency limitations of the electrical response of the hair cell, rather than limitations of the motile mechanism itself, could limit the role played by OHC motility.

Another candidate process for the cochlear amplifier is suggested by characteristics of the mechanically gated transduction channels on stereocilia (Hudspeth, 1997). These may operate in reverse. As the channels open and close, they may alter the stiffness of the hair bundle, because they are directly tied to bundle displacement. As a result, the potential exists for the hair bundle to actively push on the tectorial membrane as channels close. Active force generation by the hair bundle has been demonstrated in amphibians and may well apply to the mammalian cochlea (Chan & Hudspeth, 2005). It does not appear subject to the frequency limitations that could pose a problem for somatic motility. Nevertheless, it appears unlikely that prestin, an apparently highly specialized motor protein that clearly imparts motile properties, has no purpose. Both somatic motility and active hair bundle mechanics are likely to be operating in OHCs, and both may ultimately be necessary to account for the contribution of OHCs to hearing. Both mechanisms have the feature of not having to provide their own filtering. Instead, they need only amplify the output of another filter, the basilar membrane.

Additional contributing factors to nonlinear mechanics have recently found support and merit at least brief mention. Pillar cells, which form a stiff tripod-like structure, and thus lend rigidity to the organ of Corti, may vary their stiffness in response to local molecular signals. Efferent terminals have been demonstrated on Deiters' and Hensen's cells, raising the possibility that these may alter their stiffness or length (Okamura, Shibahara-Maruyama, Sugai, & Adams, 2002). In fact, mechanical responses of Deiters' cells to chemical signals have been demonstrated (Bobbin, 2001). Future versions of this text may need to incorporate surprising contributions of supporting cells whose roles have been assumed to be passive.

GROSS REFLECTIONS OF HAIR CELL ELECTRICAL RESPONSES

Cells undergoing polarization changes, such as hair cells responding to sound, act like antennas. If they lie in a highly organized epithelium, like the organ of Corti or retina, then the responses of hundreds or thousands of cells add together and can be detected from a distance. Thus, an electrode placed inside the cochlea, within the middle ear, or on the tympanic membrane can record the reflections of hair cell

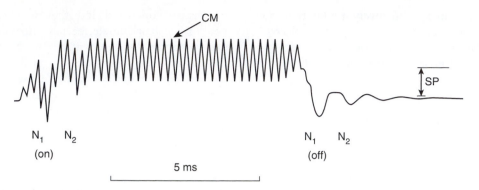

FIGURE 10-11 Cochlear electrical response to tone burst as recorded at the round window. Without random-phase averaging or filtering, the response contains elements of neuronal response (N_1, N_2) and analogs of the hair cell AC (cochlear microphonic [CM]) and DC responses (summating potential [SP]).

receptor potentials, summed across many hair cells. Electrical potentials recorded at a distance from the cells that generate them are referred to as **gross potentials.** Gross potentials take many forms and are a common basic science and clinical tool. Properly interpreted, they provide basic physiologic information and permit inferences about health versus pathology. They are easier to obtain than single-cell recordings and require less invasive procedures; therefore, they can be repeated within a subject. Typically, monitoring gross potentials requires a recording configuration known as **differential recording,** whereby signals detected by two electrodes are compared. One of these is placed as close as possible to the epithelium to be monitored (the "active" electrode), and the other is placed some distance away, where the activity of the epithelium should be weak or unrecordable (reference electrode). In differential recording, the signal detected by the reference electrodes at any time is subtracted from that detected by the active electrode, and this difference is multiplied. Assuming that any activity picked up by the reference electrode is noise, and unrelated to the epithelium of interest, differential recording detects and amplifies only those potentials that reflect the response of the epithelium. Whether the polarity of the signal is positive or negative at a given moment depends on

whether the active electrode is closest to a region where current is flowing into cells (referred to as a "current sink") or out of cells (a "current source"). Generally, a current sink seen by the active electrode will yield a negative deflection, and a source will produce a positive deflection.

In the presence of a stimulus, an electrode placed near the round window will record a complex waveform that includes contributions from both afferent neurons and hair cells (Figure 10-11). The neuronal component, known as the **compound action potential** (CAP), derives from synchrony of afferent responses at the beginning of a stimulus (see Chapter 11 for a more detailed discussion). When the CAP is removed by filtering, the remaining signal is seen to resemble the canonical hair cell receptor potential. In fact, we can isolate and define two gross electrical potentials that principally reflect the AC and DC components of individual hair cell receptor potentials. These are the **cochlear microphonic** (CM) and the **summating potential** (SP), respectively.

Cochlear Microphonic

Hair cells that are close together will depolarize and hyperpolarize at nearly the same time, because they will be activated by the same basilar membrane displacements. The further apart the cells are, the more likely it is that they will be activated by regions of the basilar membrane that act asynchronously. In the first instance, the activity of the closely spaced hair cells will add together, generating a larger and more readily detectable extracellular response. In the second instance, the activities of more widely separated hair cells will be out of phase and will partly cancel each other, rendering their responses less detectable. These phase considerations specifically apply to the rapidly changing component of the receptor potential, that is, the AC potential. The CM is thought to reflect the AC responses of many hair cells (see Figure 10-11). For simple recording configurations, such as placing the active electrode at the round window or on the tympanic membrane, the cells monitored by the microphonic are mainly OHCs in the basal half of the cochlea. OHCs are favored over IHCs by shear number, because they are more than four times as numerous. Why the base should be favored over the apex requires consideration of the traveling wave. The traveling wave moves from base to apex, slowing down and decreasing in wavelength as it progresses. This means that for any stimulus frequency, the rate of phase variation per unit length of basilar membrane increases apically. Complete mutual cancellation will occur for hair cells located at, and just beyond, the peak of the traveling wave, where response phase changes most rapidly with distance. In the cochlear base, a large segment of hair cells will respond nearly in phase to frequencies that are well below the range of frequencies served by the base. Accordingly, an electrode at the round window or within the basal turn will preferentially detect basal OHCs responding well below their BF. An iso-response curve for the CM recorded in this manner will show little frequency tuning (Figure 10-12), because as the stimulus approaches the BF, phase cancellation at the peak of the traveling wave reduces the response. Other recording configurations, such as placing differential electrodes into scala vestibuli and scala tympani at the same basal–apical location, permit inferences about smaller populations of hair cells, and recording the CM in this manner typically demonstrates a degree of fre-

quency tuning. Sharp tuning of the CM that resembles the tuning of individual hair cells can only be demonstrated using masking stimuli (see later).

Technically, it is not the hair cell body that generates the CM, but rather transduction currents through the stereocilia and hair cell cuticular plate. This is because gross potentials will tend to reflect current flow across large resistances. This becomes an important distinction when it is recalled that the hair cell body acts like a low-pass filter that removes the AC component of the receptor potential at high frequencies. Because the CM reflects transducer currents, rather than whole-cell voltage changes, the CM is recordable at high frequencies where little or no AC potential would be detected in individual hair cells.

Summating Potential

Much of what has been said about the CM can be extended to the summating potential (SP). This slow potential appears to arise largely as a reflection of individual OHC DC responses, although IHCs may contribute more to the SP than to the CM (Dallos, Schoeny, & Cheatham, 1972). Recall that OHC DC potentials may be either positive or negative. Moreover, the polarity of the SP depends on whether the recording electrode is above or below the reticular lamina. These complexities can make the interpretation of the SP somewhat difficult. Generation of the SP requires intact nonlinear properties of the transducer and OHC active mechanics. When these are compromised, the SP is readily affected, whereas the CM is relatively insensitive to moderate pathology. The major clinical use of the SP, although not extensive, has been in the diagnosis of Ménière's disease and endolymphatic hydrops (e.g., Ruth, Lambert, & Ferraro, 1988). It is instructive to consider why the SP may serve in this capacity. Both of these conditions are thought to reflect a fluid imbalance in the inner ear. This imbalance may, in some cases, distend the membranous labyrinth and may bias the position of the basilar membrane (i.e., alter its resting position). With our understanding of transduction and transducer function, we can see how this may alter the DC com-

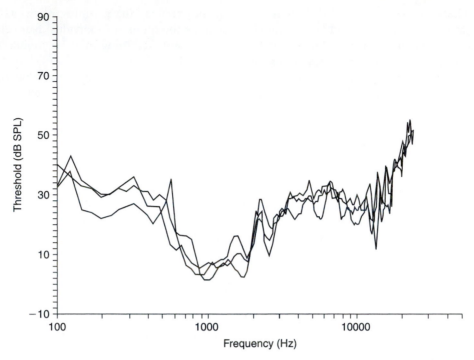

FIGURE 10-12   Iso-response curve for the cochlear microphonic recorded from scala tympani of the cochlear basal turn in gerbil. Curves from three experiments have been normalized. Using a computer, the sound level was varied at each test frequency to identify the level yielding a 3-μV peak-to-peak response. The location of the recording electrode was approximately the 18 kHz location. (From Ohlemiller, K. K, & Siegel, J. H. (1992). The effects of moderate cooling on gross cochlear potentials in the gerbil: Basal and apical differences. *Hearing Research, 63,* 79–89, by permission.)

ponent of hair cell receptor potentials, thereby affecting the SP. Surprisingly, the nature of the effect is often an increase in SP amplitude.

Unlike the CM, the SP is not subject to phase cancellation. Therefore, some degree of frequency tuning can be observed when a single cochlear electrode or differential electrode pair is used for recording. Figure 10-13A shows the result of recording the SP from scala tympani of the basal cochlear turn in the guinea pig. Beginning with the positive SP (SP$^+$), the different curves represent iso-response curves obtained using different response criteria. More stringent criteria shift the curve vertically and are associated with broadened tuning. These curves, as well as the effects of criterion change, are exactly analogous to the hair cell fre-

quency tuning curves of Figure 10-9. This is expected, because they both reflect hair cell tuning near the recording electrode. For stimulus frequencies well below the BF, the polarity of the SP reverses (SP$^-$) and shows tuning that resembles the tails of the curves in Figure 10-9. The reversal presumably reflects both the dominance of OHCs in SP generation and the fact that the DC response component in OHCs can be negative below the BF (see Figure 10-8).

Note that tuning of the SP does not appear as sharp as for single hair cells. This is because the recording electrode picks up signals from many hair cells over some distance. The gap between the sharpness of tuning of single hair cells versus the SP can be narrowed by the addition of a **masker** to a

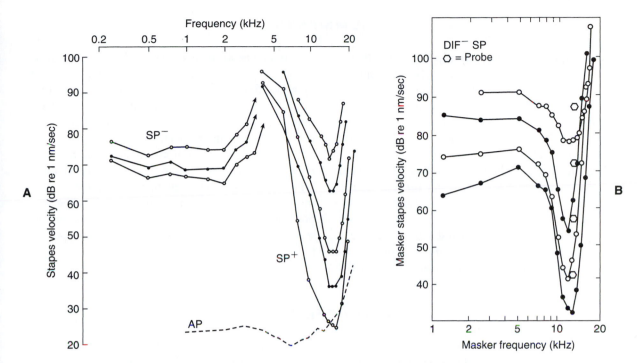

FIGURE 10-13 (A) Frequency tuning curves for the summating potential (SP) recorded in scala tympani of the cochlear base in guinea pig. Nested series of curves shows the effect of increasing the response criterion. Near the best frequency, the SP is positive (SP+) and shows fairly sharp tuning. Well below the BF, the SP is negative (SP−). *Dashed curve* shows the threshold for the compound action potential (AP), which represents the neural response. Stapes velocity (*y*-axis) is scaled in divisions equivalent to sound level in decibels. (B) Frequency tuning curves for the SP recorded in the cochlear basal turn by differential electrodes (hence DIF−) using a masking paradigm. Probe tones were fixed at the frequencies and levels shown *(hexagons),* and a second simultaneous masker tone was varied in frequency and level to find the minimum level that masked the response to the probe. (From Cheatham, M. A., & Dallos, P. (1984). Summating potential (SP) tuning curves. *Hearing Research, 16,* 189–200, by permission from Elsevier.)

near-threshold BF stimulus. Figure 10-13B shows such a procedure applied to the SP recorded using differential electrodes. Each curve represents the minimum presentation level needed for a masking tone (presented at various frequencies) to reduce the SP response elicited by a BF probe at a particular level (see Figure 10-13B, hexagons). At the lowest probe level, we again reproduce an archetypal frequency tuning curve, with tip and tail. Again, in analogy with Figures 10-9 and 10-13A, increasing the probe level (which mimics an increase in response criterion) shifts the curves vertically and leads to broadened tuning. The similarity between the lowest curves in Figure 10-13B and the tuning

curves shown earlier is actually somewhat misleading, in that they do not reflect precisely the same processes. The curves in Figure 10-13B arise partly through suppression (as in Figure 10-10) and by excitation. If the masker excites hair cells near the recording site to an extent similar to the probe, the probe will add no detectable additional response. Competing excitation by the masker shapes the curves principally at the BF (recall that there was no suppression at the tip of the curve in Figure 10-10) and well below BF. The term *masker* applies to any stimulus that interferes with either a physiologic response or a behavioral response and whose basis in suppression may not be clear.

∙∼ SUMMARY ∼∙

Optimal application of currently dominant therapies such as hearing aids and cochlear implants depends on recognizing the contributions to perception of decreased sensitivity, reduced sharpness of tuning, and loss of compression. These qualities reside in the micromechanics of the basilar membrane-OHC-tectorial membrane complex and in the mix of OHC versus IHC and neural pathology. How the normal characteristics of the cochlea arise is important for understanding, treating, and explaining its dysfunction. It also imposes the limits that determine which diagnostic methods are useful and practical. For example, clinicians do not record from individual hair cells of their clients

(too impractical), or even routinely use gross measures such as the CM or SP (too ambiguous), yet they do frequently record otoacoustic emissions (see Chapter 13), because the latter are both accessible and sufficiently interpretable within the context of cochlear micromechanics.

Finally, the success of eventual treatments (e.g., new prostheses, regeneration, stem-cell therapy) will depend on how well they reproduce normal micromechanics. Clinicians should seek to be in a position to evaluate for themselves, based on the research literature, the relative advantages and potential dangers of particular approaches.

∙∼ KEY TERMS ∼∙

AC/DC potential
Active process
Asymmetric
     nonlinearity
Best frequency
Cochlear amplifier
Cochlear microphonic
Compound action
     potential
Compressive
     nonlinearity

Depolarization
Differential recording
Distortion
Dynamic range
Endocochlear potential
Feedback loop
Frequency tuning
     curve
Gap junction
Gross potential

Inner hair cells
Intensity curve
Iso-level curve
Iso-response curve
Macromechanics
Masker
Membrane voltage
Micromechanics
Outer hair cells
Receptor potential

Somatic motility
Spike rate
Stereociliary bundle
Summating potential
Suppression
Suppression area
Tectorial membrane
Tight junctions
Transduction
Tuning curve tip/tail

∙∼ STUDY QUESTIONS ∼∙

1. Explain how basilar membrane motion in one direction can cause stereocilia motion in an orthogonal direction.

2. How does the nonlinearity of the stereocilia transducer channels give rise to the DC component of the receptor potential?

3. Explain why potassium currents flow through hair cells.

4. Describe the two types of mechanical feedback by OHCs that could form the basis of the cochlear amplifier.

5. Compare the frequency tuning and input-output relations of the IHC AC and DC potentials with similar measures for the basilar membrane.

⚹REFERENCES〜

Bobbin, R. P. (2001). ATP-induced movement of the stalks of isolated cochlear Deiters' cells. *Neuroreport, 12,* 2923–2926.

Brown, M. C., Nuttall, A. L., & Masta, R. I. (1983). Intracellular recordings from cochlear inner hair cells: Effects of stimulation of the crossed olivo-cochlear efferents. *Science, 222,* 69–72.

Brownell, W. E. (1983). Observations on a motile response in isolated outer hair cells. In W. R. Webster & L. M. Aitkin (Eds.), *Mechanisms of hearing* (pp. 5–10). Clayton, Australia: Monash University Press.

Brownell, W. E., Bader, C. R., Bertrand, D., & deRibaupierre, Y. (1985). Evoked mechanical responses in of isolated cochlear outer hair cells. *Science, 227,* 194–196.

Chan, D. K., & Hudspeth, A. J. (2005). Ca2+ current driven nonlinear mechanical amplification by the mammalian cochlea in vitro. *Nature Neuroscience, 8,* 149–155.

Cheatham, M. A., & Dallos, P. (1984). Summating potential (SP) tuning curves. *Hearing Research, 16,* 189–200.

Cheatham, M. A., & Dallos, P. (1992). Two-tone suppression in inner hair cell response: Correlates of rate suppression in the auditory nerve. *Hearing Research, 60,* 1–12.

Cheatham, M. A., & Dallos, P. (2000). The dynamic range of inner hair cell and organ of Corti responses. *Journal of the Acoustical Society of America, 107,* 1508–1520.

Corti, A. (1851). Recherches sur l'organ de l'ouie des mammiferes. *Zeitschrift fur Wissenschaft Zoologie, 3,* 109–169.

Dallos, P. (1985). Response characteristics of mammalian cochlear hair cells. *Journal of Neuroscience, 5,* 1591–1608.

Dallos, P., & Cheatham, M. A. (1992). Cochlear hair cell function. *Sensory transduction* (pp. 372–393). New York: Rockefeller University Press.

Dallos, P., & Fakler, B. (2002). Prestin, a new type of motor protein. *Nature Reviews Molecular and Cellular Biology, 3,* 104–111.

Dallos, P., & Harris, D. (1978). Properties of auditory nerve responses in absence of outer hair cells. *Journal of Neurophysiology, 41,* 365–383.

Dallos, P., Santos-Sacchi, J., & Flock, A. (1982). Intracellular recordings from cochlear outer hair cells. *Science, 218,* 582–584.

Dallos, P., Schoeny, Z. G., & Cheatham, M. A. (1972). Cochlear summating potentials: Descriptive aspects. *Acta Otolaryngolica Supplementum, 302,* 1–46.

Dallos, P., & Wang, C. Y. (1974). Bioelectric correlates of kanamycin intoxication. *Audiology, 12,* 227–289.

Davis, H. (1958). Transmission and transduction in the cochlea. *Laryngoscope, 68,* 359–382.

Davis, H. (1965). A model for transducer action in the cochlea. *Cold Spring Harbor Symposium in Quantitative Biology, 30,* 181–189.

Davis, H. (1968). Mechanisms of the inner ear. *Annals of Otology, Rhinology, and Laryngology, 77,* 644–655.

Engstrom, H. (1958). Structure and innervation of the inner ear sensory epithelia. *International Review of Cytology, 7,* 535–585.

Engstrom, H., Ades, H. W., & Hawkins, J. E. (1962). Structure and function of the sensory hairs of the inner hair cell. *Journal of the Acoustical Society of America, 34,* 1356–1363.

Hensen, V. (1863). Zur morphologie der schnecke des menschen und der Saugetiere. *Zeitschrift fur Wissenschaft Zoologie, 13,* 481–512.

Hudspeth, A. J., & Corey, D. P. (1977). Sensitivity, polarity, and conductance change in response to controlled mechanical stimuli. *Proceedings of the National Academy of Sciences, 74,* 2407–2411.

Hudspeth, A. J. (1997). Mechanical amplification of stimuli by hair cells. *Current Opinion in Neurobiology, 7,* 480–486.

Hudspeth, A. J. (1982). Extracellular current flow and the site of transduction by vertebrate hair cells. *Journal of Neuroscience, 2,* 1–10.

Hudspeth, A. J., & Jacobs, R. (1979). Stereocilia mediate transduction in vertebrate hair cells. *Proceedings of the National Academy of Sciences, 76,* 1506–1509.

Kimura, R. S. (1966). Frequency tuning of the basilar membrane and auditory nerve fibers in the same cochlea. *Acta Otolaryngologica, 61,* 55–72.

Ohlemiller, K. K, & Siegel, J. H. (1992). The effects of moderate cooling on gross cochlear potentials in the gerbil: Basal and apical differences. *Hearing Research, 63,* 79–89.

Okamura, H. O., Shibahara-Maruyama, I., Sugai, N., & Adams, J. C. (2002). Innervation of supporting cells in the guinea pig cochlea detected in bloc-surface preparations. *Neuroreport, 13,* 1585–1588.

Oliver, D., He, D. Z., Klocker, N., Ludwig, J., Schulte, U., Waldegger, S., Ruppersberg, J. P., Dallos, P., & Fakler, B. (2001). Intracellular anion as the voltage sensor of prestin, the outer hair cell motor protein. *Science, 292,* 2340–2343.

Palmer, A. R., & Russell, I. J. (1986). Phase-locking in the cochlear nerve of the guinea-pig and its relation to the receptor potential of inner hair-cells. *Hearing Research, 24,* 1–15.

Pickles, J. O., Comis, S. D., & Osborne, M. P. (1984). Cross-links between stereocilia in the guinea pig organ of Corti, and their possible relation to sensory transduction. *Hearing Research, 15,* 103–112.

Russell, I. J., & Sellick, P. M. (1978). Intracellular studies of hair cells in the mammalian cochlea. *Journal of Physiology, 284,* 261–289.

Ruth, R. A., Lambert, P. R., & Ferraro, J. A. (1988). Electrocochleography: Methods and clinical applications. *American Journal of Otology, 9,* 1–11.

Seikel, J. A., King, D. W., & Drumwright, D. G. (2005). *Anatomy & physiology for speech, language, and hearing* (3rd ed.). Clifton Park, NY: Thomson Delmar Learning.

Sellick, P. M., & Russell, I. J. (1979). Two-tone suppression in cochlear hair cells. *Hearing Research, 1,* 227–236.

Siegel, J. H., & Kim, D. O. (1982). Efferent neural control of cochlear mechanics? Olivocochlear bundle stimulation affects cochlear biomechanical nonlinearity. *Hearing Research, 6,* 171–182.

Slepecky, N. B. (1996). Structure of the mammalian cochlea. In P. Dallos, A. N. Popper, & R. R. Fay, (Eds.), *The cochlea* (pp. 44–129). New York: Springer.

Spoendlin, H. (1966). *The organization of the cochlear receptor.* Basel, Switzerland: Karger.

Spoendlin, H. (1969). Innervation patterns in the organ of Corti of the cat. *Acta Otolaryngologica, 67,* 239–254.

Tanaka, Y., Anasuma, A., & Yanagisawa, K. (1980). Potentials of outer hair cells and their membrane properties in cationic environments. *Hearing Research, 2,* 431–438.

Tasaki, I., Davis, H., & Eldredge, D. H. (1954). Exploration of cochlear potentials in guinea pig with a microelectrode. *Journal of the Acoustical Society of America, 26,* 765–773.

Wangeman, P., & Schacht, J. (1996) Homeostatic mechanisms in the cochlea. In P. Dallos, A. N. Popper, & R. R. Fay (Eds.), *The cochlea* (pp. 130–185). New York: Springer.

Wever, E. G., & Bray, C. W. (1930). Action currents in the auditory nerve in response to acoustical stimulation. *Proceedings of the National Academy of Sciences, 16,* 344–350.

ᨒSUGGESTED READINGᨒ

Dallos, P. (1988). Cochlear neurobiology: Some key experiments and concepts of the past two decades. In G. M. Edelman, W. E. Gall, & W. M. Cowan (Eds.), *Auditory function* (pp. 153–188). New York: Wiley and Sons.

Dallos, P. (1992). The active cochlea. *Journal of Neuroscience, 12,* 4575–4585.

Dallos, P. (2002). Outer hair cell: The key to mammalian hearing. In C. I. Berlin, L. J. Hood, & A. Ricci (Eds.), *Hair cell micromechanics and otoacoustic emissions* (pp. 1–24). New York: Singular Press.

Moller, A. R. (2000). *Hearing: Its physiology and pathophysiology.* New York: Academic Press.

Pickles, J. O. (1988). *Introduction to the physiology of hearing.* New York: Academic Press.

Santos-Sacchi, J. (2003). New tunes from Corti's organ: The outer hair cell boogie rules. *Current Opinion in Neurobiology, 13,* 459–468.

Santos-Sacchi, J. (2001). Cochlear physiology. In A. E. Jahn & J. Santos-Sacchi (Eds.), *Physiology of the ear* (pp. 357–391). New York: Singular Press.

Chapter

11

Cochlear Afferent Neuronal Function

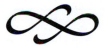

Kevin K. Ohlemiller, Ph.D.
Associate Professor of Otolaryngology
Washington University School of Medicine
St. Louis, Missouri

Our progression through the chain of cochlear events triggered by sound now brings us to the afferent neurons whose responses are driven by hair cells. We have considered in detail how hair cells code stimulus frequency and intensity and have seen that this coding involves trade-offs. To a large extent, hair cells are "labeled line" band-pass filters that signal the presence of a particular frequency band in an acoustic stimulus. Yet, they respond to other frequencies, particularly below their best frequency (BF), in the tails of their **frequency tuning curves.** Hair cells can signal a wide range of sound intensities by incrementing their response magnitude, but this involves compression that distorts the stimulus. Finally, we have noted that unavoidable low-pass filtering by the hair cell membrane causes the cycle-by-cycle information in the stimulus to be lost at higher frequencies. Afferent neurons can transmit only stimulus information that is passed on by hair cells; they cannot reintroduce information discarded by hair cells. Thus, the response characteristics and limitations of the neurons are largely set by the hair cells. Yet we will see that the afferents also "re-encode" the stimulus in a way that virtually replaces the original stimulus waveform. Moreover, the synaptic junction (or simply synapse), by which hair cells communicate with neurons, introduces a new *asymmetric compressive nonlinearity* and new **dynamic range** limitations. These have implications for coding and perception. Nevertheless, the sharp frequency tuning established by the outer hair cell (OHC)-tectorial membrane-basilar membrane complex (see Chapter 10) is passed on to the afferents, so that a best frequency or **characteristic**

Historical Highlights

1937	R. Lorente de Nó publishes authoritative work on cochlear afferent innervation, using the Golgi staining method. Distinct populations of neurons innervating inner and outer hair cells are first noted.
1954	I. Tasaki obtains first recordings from single auditory nerve fibers in guinea pigs. These appeared poorly tuned (an artifact of the methods). Because von Békésy's basilar membrane data also suggested poor tuning, sharp frequency tuning (as demonstrated perceptually) was posited to arise centrally through lateral inhibition.
1965	N. Kiang and colleagues publish definitive description of the responses of normal auditory neurons in frequency, level, and time in cats. Basic features of frequency tuning, intensity curves, rate adaptation, spontaneous activity, phase-locking, and two-tone suppression are reported in the first extensive application of computers in hearing research. It becomes clear that afferent neurons are sharply frequency tuned, in contrast with much of the basilar membrane data of the time. This leads to much debate about what type of sharpening mechanism lies between the basilar membrane and afferent neurons.
1966–1978	Studies by R. Klinke and W. Oertel (1966), as well as R. Bobbin and M. Thompson (1978), indicate that glutamate or an analog is the primary afferent neurotransmitter in the cochlea.
1967–1981	H. Spoendlin (1967, 1974, 1981) extends the anatomic characterization of cochlear neurons, separating radial and spiral afferents by their receptor cell targets, number of cells contacted, and their relative numbers. The role of radial afferents as the primary "coders" is recognized.
1971–1982	Accumulating basilar membrane and afferent neuronal tuning data make it clear that these are similar, and that any "second filter" responsible for normally sharp frequency tuning lies prior to basilar membrane mechanics. Particularly significant in this debate were basilar membrane studies by W. Rhode (1971) and P. Sellick and colleagues (1982).
1978–1982	Studies by M. C. Liberman (1978, 1980, 1982a,b) in cats greatly refine understanding of physiologic and anatomic correlates of afferent characteristic frequency and spontaneous firing rate. Variation in threshold by afferents innervating the same hair cell gains acceptance as a normal phenomenon and probable mechanism for extending dynamic range. The first complete cochlear frequency map is constructed, based on neuronal tracing.

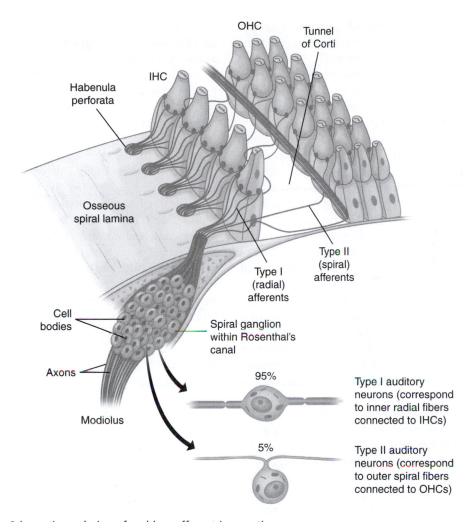

FIGURE 11-1 Schematic rendering of cochlear afferent innervation.

frequency (CF) can be identified for any healthy neuron. Similarities in the shape of intensity, iso-level, and frequency tuning curves of the basilar membrane, inner hair cells (IHCs), and radial afferents are a prominent theme in this chapter.

ANATOMY OF COCHLEAR AFFERENT INNERVATION

There are two major types of afferents, **radial** (or **type I**) and **spiral** (or **type II**), with an overall total of about 40,000 to 50,000 neurons per cochlea

(Spoendlin, 1967, 1974, 1981) (Figure 11-1). Each neuron of either type has its cell body (or **soma**) within **Rosenthal's canal** (see Chapter 8). Each soma projects a single dendrite laterally through the **osseous spiral lamina;** the dendrite then emerges into the organ of Corti through one of many channels in the bone, termed **habenulae perforata.** A second process, the **axon,** extends from the soma into the **modiolus,** en route to the brain. Collectively, all cochlear neuronal cell bodies are referred to as the **spiral ganglion,** reflecting that they spiral around the modiolar "core" of the cochlea and are part of the **peripheral nervous system.** (A ganglion is any cluster of neurons located outside the **central nervous system.**)

Radial afferent neurons, which are the focus of this chapter, are postsynaptic to IHCs and comprise about 90% to 95% of all afferents (Spoendlin, 1967, 1974, 1981). Any single IHC is contacted by about 20 afferent dendrites. In most species examined, radial afferents are myelinated central to the habenulae. Surprisingly, one prominent exception may be humans, wherein myelination of radial afferents appears variable (Ota & Kimura, 1980). Because myelin importantly serves as an insulator that reduces the conduction time for action potentials, such variability among radial afferents is puzzling.

Spiral afferents are postsynaptic to OHCs and comprise the remaining 5% to 10% of afferents. Despite many attempts, no sound-driven response has yet been identified in these neurons. Based on their numbers and innervation pattern, these probably provide information for feedback control of cochlear micromechanics through cochlear efferent neurons.

In terms of neuronal "wiring," the cochlea appears fairly simple, especially compared with, for example, the retina, where there are many more types of neurons and connections. In the retina, neurons serving slightly different locations in visual space are connected so that they inhibit each other. This serves the purpose of sharpening visual acuity (or spatial resolution), which is analogous to frequency tuning in the cochlea. In the cochlea, each radial afferent extends directly radially (hence the name) and contacts only one or a few closely spaced IHCs (Liberman, 1980), and mutual inhibitory connections are not found. The sharpness of tuning of any radial afferent will instead reflect (1) the sharpness of tuning of the basilar membrane at the point of innervation, and (2) the basal-apical range of hair cells contacted. It thus makes sense that each afferent innervates a spatially restricted set of hair cells: If they contacted widely distributed IHCs, they would not be sharply tuned.

Digital Coding by Neurons

At the afferent synapse, the way sound is encoded switches from "analog" to "digital." Chapter 10 examined the representation of the temporal waveform of a sound stimulus at successive points in the cochlear cascade. Changes in the stimulus waveform as reflected in the IHC receptor potential include filtering, compression, and the addition of a DC component. Nevertheless, throughout the cascade up through the hair cell response, sound remains encoded as a time-varying waveform that largely recapitulates the stimulus. This is essentially the definition of **analog coding.** At the IHC/afferent synapse, any similarity between input and output waveforms is sacrificed and converted into the information "medium" of the brain, the action potential (or "spike"; see Chapter 5) (Figure 11-2). The instantaneous compressions and rarefactions characterizing the original sound are replaced by instantaneous variation in **spike probability,** the likelihood that a spike will occur at any moment in time. When a stimulus is present, the average spike probability is increased, so that the **spike rate** in spikes per second also increases. Spike rate and probability are, of course, expected to be correlated. Note that there is no information whatsoever in either the magnitude or overall shape of an action potential. A spike simply occurs, or does not occur, at a particular moment in time—in close analogy to the value of a binary digit in a computer. Thus, spike coding is, in a sense, **digital coding.**

Subdividing Radial Afferents by Spontaneous Firing Rate

Radial afferents are not homogeneous. They vary by **spontaneous firing rate,** the rate of action potentials that occur in the absence of sound (Kiang, Watanabe, Thomas, & Clark, 1965). In all mammalian species examined, the distribution of spontaneous firing rates (SRs) across all afferents shows two major modes (Figure 11-3), with the overall range of SRs extending from 0 to more than 100 spikes/sec. Modes generally appear near 0.0 to 2.0 ("low-SR neurons") and 60 to 70 spikes/sec ("high-SR neurons"). Variation in SR is thought to primarily reflect variation in release from the hair cell of **glutamate,** by consensus the major neurotransmitter at the hair cell/afferent synapse. This release occurs in **quanta,** or "packets" of neurotransmitter that fill small membrane-bound vesicles.

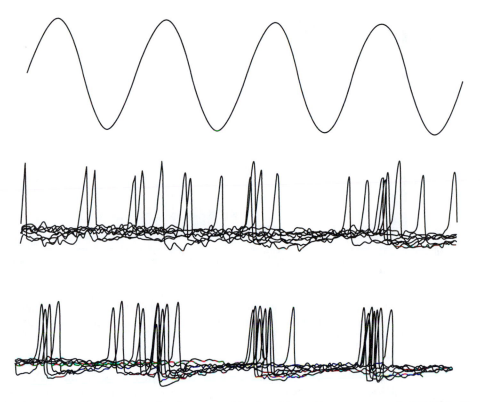

FIGURE 11-2 Superimposed raw traces of action potentials of cochlear afferent neurons. Individual spikes do not at all resemble the sinusoidal stimulus, but rather indicate its presence by their rate of occurrences and their timing. Spikes in the lower trace are phase-locked to the sinusoid. (From Javel, E., McGee, J. A., Horst, J. W., & Farley, G. R. (1988). Temporal mechanisms in auditory stimulus coding. In G. M. Edelman, W. E. Gall, & W. M. Cowan (Eds.), *Auditory function: Neurobiological bases of hearing* (pp. 515–558). New York: Wiley & Sons. Reprinted by permission.)

These fuse with the hair cell membrane and release their contents into the synaptic space.

Recall from Chapter 10 that IHCs are somewhat depolarized in the absence of sound. Although hair cells are not neurons (and do not exhibit action potentials), like neurons they release neurotransmitter at a rate correlated with membrane depolarization. The existence of spontaneous activity in radial afferents, therefore, is not surprising. But the depolarization does not explain variation in SR across neurons contacting the *same* IHC. This puzzle was solved, in part, by M. C. Liberman (1980), who showed in cats that neurons with different SRs tend to innervate different regions of the cell and differ in thickness (Figure 11-4). Pillar versus modiolar

regions of the hair cell membrane may form synapses with intrinsically different rates of neurotransmitter release and contact neurons with different spike initiation thresholds.

What purpose does spontaneous activity, and its variation across neurons, serve? From Chapter 10 we know that the depolarization of IHCs at rest allows them to both depolarize and hyperpolarize around their resting state, and in doing so, to follow the waveform of a sound stimulus. We can think of the hair cell receptor potential as modulating spike probability, so that instantaneous spike probability increases and decreases in a manner that follows the receptor potential. Neurons can code information in this manner only if they are spontaneously active,

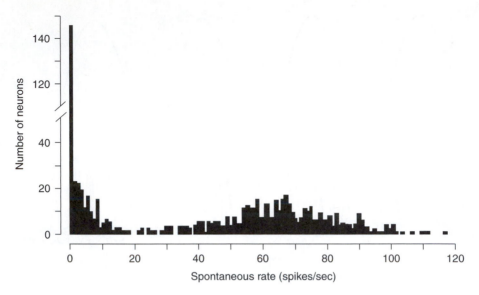

FIGURE 11-3   Distribution of spontaneous firing rates in the auditory nerve of the cat. (From Liberman, M. C. (1978). Auditory nerve responses from cats raised in a low noise chamber. *Journal of the Acoustical Society of America, 63,* 442–455, by permission. Copyright 1978, Acoustical Society of America.)

and thus able to both up- and down-regulate spike probability. It follows that low-SR neurons do not have this ability, because they cannot reduce their firing rate when the hair cell hyperpolarizes. These neurons may serve a special function. Studies in several species have shown that neuronal response thresholds to sound vary inversely with SR, so that low-SR neurons have the highest thresholds (Figure 11-5). The spread of thresholds by SR is considerable. Completely normal neurons with an SR less than 2.0 spike/sec can exhibit thresholds that are increased more than 50 dB relative to their high-SR counterparts. The following sections consider how this may be important for extending the dynamic range of the cochlea.

Converting the Receptor Potential into Spike Rate and Probability

Figure 11-6 depicts a highly idealized relation between the instantaneous IHC membrane potential during a stimulus and the probability of an action potential for hypothetical low- and high-SR neu-

rons innervating the same hair cell. Based on many indirect observations, this relation takes the form of an asymmetric compressive nonlinearity, somewhat similar to that described for the hair cell stereociliary transducer in Chapter 10. Note that the x-axis in Figure 11-6 is essentially the y-axis of Figure 10-5, so that these stages can be conceived as cascaded. For large depolarizations, spike probability approaches 1.0, or 100% probability that a spike will occur. Large hyperpolarizations, however, are *not* associated with negative y-values, because probability cannot be less than zero. If the incoming sound is a low-intensity tone burst that falls within the tuning curve for the hair cell's AC response, the receptor potential will resemble the stimulus. If the hair cell membrane potential remains within the linear range for the high-SR neuron in Figure 11-6, the *time variation in spike probability* for this neuron will also resemble the stimulus. The waveform for spike probability for the low-SR neuron will be quite different, however. It will markedly increase only when the hair cell reaches some threshold amount of depolarization. It will also extend only in one direction and may have narrower peaks than the receptor potential. For both neurons in Figure 11-6, spike probability will be greatest at the positive peaks in the receptor potential, that is, at a particular stimulus phase. This is known as **phase-locking** (Kiang et al., 1965). (The word *locking* unfortunately implies more precision than is found, but it is catchy and easier to say than *phase-correlation*.) Note that the actual phase of the neuronal response relative to the original stimulus will be influenced by interposed delays, including the traveling wave delay, and the brief delay that occurs between the release of neurotransmitter from the hair cell and the initiation of a spike. The former may be several milliseconds, and the latter about 0.5 milliseconds.

Still considering Figure 11-6, what if the tone burst were made louder, so that the hair cell operates outside the quasi-linear range of the high-SR fiber? Even if the hair cell receptor potential remained perfectly sinusoidal, the temporal character of spike probability would become both asymmetric and compressed. As discussed in Chapter 10, the receptor potential itself will, in fact, be distorted and will include a DC component. The effect of the DC component on spike probability is therefore exaggerated by virtue of being cascaded with a similar synaptic nonlinearity. Through this combination of effects, *average* spike probability greatly increases during a suprathreshold stimulus, which is equivalent to saying that the spike rate increases. Through phase-locking and increased spike rate, the stimulus alters both instantaneous spike probability and average spike rate. The brain uses both types of information.

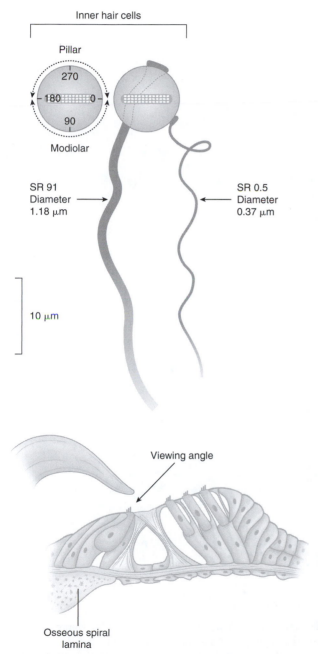

FIGURE 11-4 Schematic showing difference in appearance and location of dendritic endings for representative low and high spontaneous firing rates (SR) neurons in the cat. Low-SR neurons terminate on the modiolar side of the inner hair cell; high-SR neurons terminate on the pillar side and have a larger diameter. (Adapted from Liberman, 1982.)

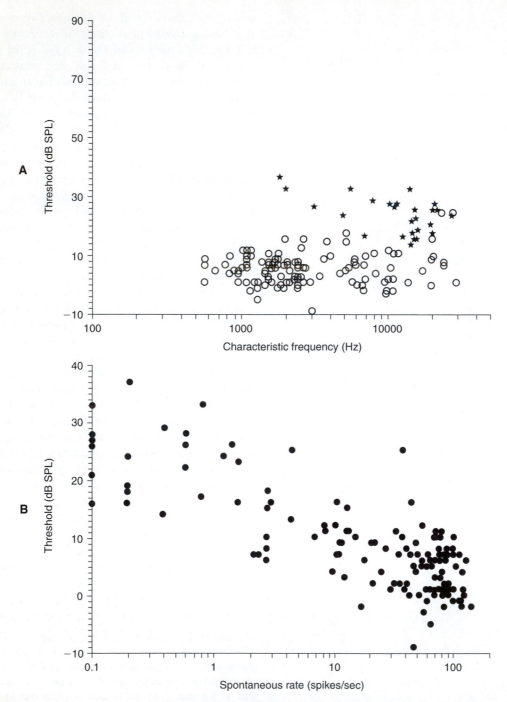

FIGURE 11-5   (A) Neuronal response thresholds at the characteristic frequency versus CF in the gerbil. Neurons have been divided into by spontaneous rate: >2.0 spikes/sec *(unfilled circles);* ≤2.0 spikes/sec *(stars).* (B) CF threshold versus SR. Thresholds increase with decreasing SR. (From Ohlemiller, K. K., Echteler, S. M., & Siegel, J. H. (1991). Factors that influence rate-versus-intensity relations in single cochlear nerve fibers of the gerbil. *Journal of the Acoustical Society of America, 90,* 274–287, by permission. Copyright 1991, American Institute of Physics.)

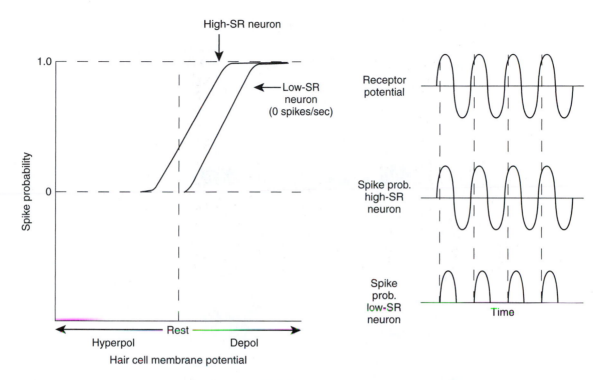

FIGURE 11-6 Schematic representation of the instantaneous relation between spike probability and hair cell membrane potential for a low- and high-spontaneous firing rate (SR) neuron (compare with Figure 10-5). For both neurons, the relation is compressive because spike probability (prob.) saturates near 1.0 for large depolarizations. The relation is asymmetrical because spike probability increases more than it decreases for large changes in the membrane potential. For the high-SR neuron, there is a range over which the relation is quasi-linear, and there is spontaneous activity (reflected by nonzero spike probability) at the resting membrane potential. For the low-SR neuron (in this case, 0.0 spikes/sec), spike probability at the resting membrane potential is near zero. Because the low-SR neuron cannot decrease spike probability when the hair cell hyperpolarizes (cannot have probability less than zero), the time pattern of spike probability during the sinewave stimulus recapitulates only depolarizing excursions of the membrane potential. The fact that the relation is shifted to the right for the low-SR neuron also means that it will have a higher response threshold.

Counting Spikes

Scientists studying the way auditory neurons encode sound have typically done so by recording the activity of one neuron at a time. This involves inserting a needle-like electrode (typically less than 1.0 μm in diameter at the tip) into the spiral ganglion or cochlear nerve and detecting action potentials from individual neurons in the presence of highly controlled, calibrated sounds. The response of any one neuron will not be exactly the same every time the same sound is presented. The goal, therefore, is to present the same sound many times and identify tendencies. This is achieved by con-

structing a response histogram. This process requires a computer to both trigger a stimulus and record all spike times, so that the times of all spikes relative to the beginning of the stimulus **(spike latencies)** can be recorded over many presentations. Depending on the requirements of the experiment, the computer lumps spike latencies into "bins" (typically about 1.0 millisecond in duration). Each time the stimulus is presented, the computer notes the times of all spikes relative to stimulus onset, determines into which bin each spike falls, and increments the total count by one in that bin. Over many stimulus presentations, a **poststimulus time histogram**

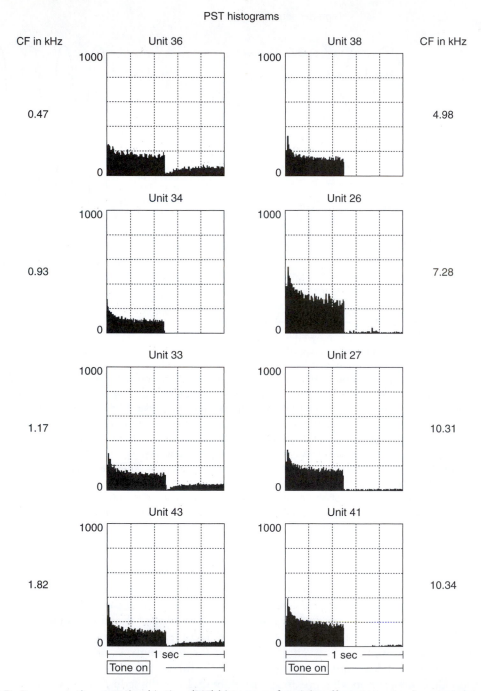

FIGURE 11-7 Representative poststimulus time (PST) histograms for eight afferent neurons in response to character-istic frequency (CF) tones in the cat. CFs are indicated. Note difference in onset versus steady-state firing rate, and delayed recovery of spontaneous activity after the stimulus. (From Kiang, N.-Y. S., Watanabe, T., Thomas, E. C., & Clark, L. F. (1965). *Discharge patterns of single fibers ini the cat's auditory nerve.* Cambridge, MA: MIT Press, by permission. Copyright 1965 The MIT Press.)

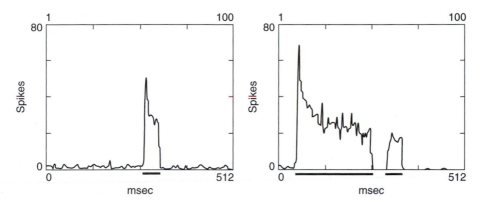

FIGURE 11-8 Effect of a preceding stimulus on the response to a brief probe tone burst. Depending on level and interstimulus delay, the preceding (adapting) stimulus reduces or eliminates the response to the probe. Tone bursts were presented at the times indicated below the graphs. (From Smith, R. L. (1977). Short-term adaptation in single auditory nerve fibers: Some post-stimulatory effects. *Journal of Neurophysiology, 40,* 1098–1112, by permission. Copyright 1977 The American Physiological Society.)

(PSTH) emerges, similar to those shown in Figure 11-7. The histogram reveals that spike rate increases during the time a suprathreshold tone is on, as deduced by the simple fact that there are more spikes per bin while the stimulus is turned on than in the interval afterward. The number of spikes in any bin can be converted into the spike rate by dividing the number of spikes in the bin by the number of presentations and the bin width.

Although not visible in Figure 11-7, a delay will occur between the beginning of the tone burst and the increase in firing rate. The modal time for the first spike after stimulus onset is known as *first spike latency.* This primarily reflects traveling wave and synaptic delays, but may also include delays in the sound system and nerve conduction time. Some surprises also appear in the histograms. First, the increase in spike rate is greatest at the onset of the stimulus, falls rapidly to some roughly constant value, and then slowly declines further. This reduction in spike rate over the course of the stimulus is called **rate adaptation,** and it is believed to reflect a reduction in the amount of neurotransmitter immediately available for release by the hair cell (see Geisler, 1998). Another surprise is that immediately after the tone burst, the rate of firing falls to near zero, then gradually recovers to the spontaneous rate. This recovery is also believed to reflect neuro-

transmitter availability. Although the purpose served by these adaptation and recovery effects is not known with certainty, it is likely that auditory neurons evolved to optimally detect *changes* in the acoustic environment, rather than constancy. Hence, neurons appear to emphasize the onset of a new stimulus in the environment by greatly increasing their firing rate and to emphasize the end of the sound by steeply reducing their firing rate below the spontaneous rate.

The period after the tone response during which spontaneous spikes are reduced is also associated with another significant property. During that period, which may exceed 200 milliseconds, the **rate response** to a second tone will be reduced (Smith, 1977) (Figure 11-8). Therefore, the response of a neuron to a given stimulus may be influenced by its response to a previous stimulus, especially if the first stimulus elicits a large response. This **forward masking** has a counterpart at the perceptual level, such that a given sound may reduce the detectability of a later sound.

Constructing histograms helps us to characterize spike rate increases that would presumably serve to tell the brain a stimulus is present. To facilitate our study of spike rates and patterns, we "cheat" by presenting the same sound many times. Yet, in the real world, sounds that may be critical for survival are usually not conveniently repeated. The brain has solved this problem by redundancy. Many neurons are "polled" to yield a rapid best guess as to the nature of the stimulus. Thus, the brain derives a kind of PSTH from the activity of many neurons from a single real-world stimulus presentation.

The use of bins to count spikes in the laboratory is merely a convention that may capture aspects of the neural coding process. The size of the bin will greatly impact the result. For any feature of the response we wish to detect, there will be an optimal bin width. If bin width were infinitely short, no two spikes would ever be found to have *exactly* the same latency. The histogram would be virtually flat, because no bin would contain more than one spike. At the other extreme, if the bin width were 100 milliseconds, we would be unable to detect rate adaptation or any fine details of the PSTH.

The neurons in Figure 11-7 were presented with moderately loud tone bursts at their characteristic frequency, while keeping stimulus phase constant. For the low-CF neurons (see Figure 11-7, left column), we would expect phase-locking to occur; yet, it is not visible in the PSTHs. This is because the bin width is several milliseconds—much longer than the stimulus period. To observe phase-locking, we must apply a bin width that is much shorter than the stimulus period. Moreover, a different counting strategy is generally used. Figure 11-9 shows examples of both **period histograms** and **interval histograms** obtained for four neurons using stimulus frequencies of 0.5, 1.0, 2.0, and 4.0 kHz. (However, for the moment, ignore the graph.) First, let us consider the period histogram obtained using a stimulus frequency of 0.5 kHz (see Figure 11-9, top left). The total time on the *x*-axis is 2.0 milliseconds, or one stimulus period. Because the histogram contains many bins, the bin width is clearly much shorter than the period. The "zero" time reference used by the computer to compute latencies is also no longer the stimulus onset. It is now a specific phase of the stimulus. The computer has assigned spike times as if the stimulus were "folded over" at multiples of the stimulus period (period histograms are also called *folded histograms*). If the spikes are phase-locked to the stimulus, we predict they would fall within a single mode over a narrow range of

times (phases), within the half of the stimulus period for which the hair cell was depolarized, and that is what is observed.

Continuing with Figure 11-9, consider now the interval histogram obtained using the 0.5-kHz stimulus. Here, yet another counting strategy has been applied, whereby the computer sets the timer to zero every time a spike occurs, and then measures the time to the next spike. With this approach, the distribution of intervals between spikes can be observed. If the spikes are phase-locked, we might predict the interval will tend toward the stimulus period, so that all intervals should distribute around 2.0 milliseconds. However, that is decidedly *not* what we find. Instead, the intervals form several modes at multiples of the stimulus period. Phase-locking does not imply that a neuron fires every stimulus cycle. The neuron may wait several cycles to fire again.

Proceeding clockwise in Figure 11-9, the same analysis is repeated at progressively higher stimulus frequencies (in different neurons, but that is immaterial). Because the time axis of the period histogram has been fixed at 2.0 milliseconds, the period histograms cover multiple stimulus periods. At 1.0 and 2.0 kHz, spike times again fall into modes spaced once per stimulus period, and the interval histograms again show peaks at multiples of the stimulus period. At 4.0 kHz, however (see Figure 11-9, bottom right), the degree of organization of spike times greatly decreases. If we quantify the strength or prominence of phase-locking (now refer to the graph in Figure 11-9), we find a progressive decrease up to roughly 5 kHz, where phase-locking essentially disappears. This decline with stimulus frequency fits well with the low-pass character of the hair cell AC receptor potential (see Chapter 10), which is necessary for phase-locking. It may also partially reflect "jitter" in the precision of spike timing.

It is worth pointing out what seems *not* to determine the upper frequency limit of phase-locking. Recall from Chapter 5 that an action potential has a fixed duration and is followed by a **refractory period,** during which time another spike cannot occur. A single spike may thus "occupy" a neuron for a few milliseconds. If phase-locking depended on the neuron spiking at every period of the stimulus, phase-locking would be

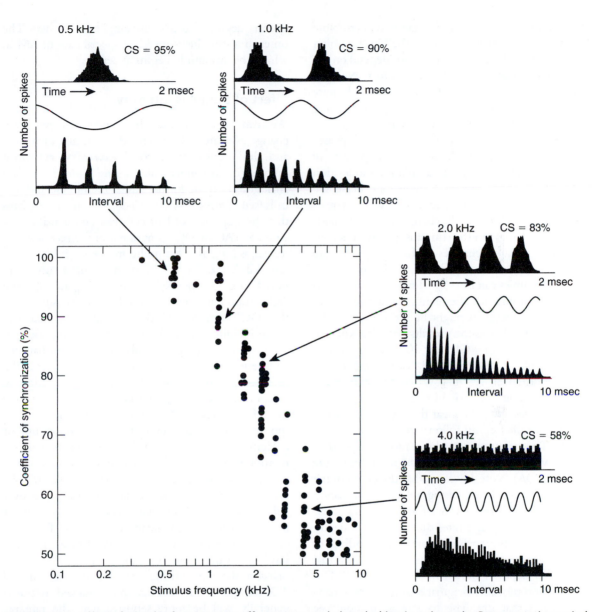

FIGURE 11-9 Effect of stimulus frequency on afferent neuronal phase-locking in guinea pig. Representative period and interval histograms are shown for different neurons at 0.5, 1.0, 2.0, and 4.0 kHz. Modes corresponding to the stimulus period can be seen, but their prevalence declines with increasing frequency. Overall, maximal strength of phase-locking declines above ~1.0 kHz and essentially disappears by 5.0 kHz (bottom left). CS, Coefficient of synchronization.

much more frequency-limited than it appears. Note also that, at least for loud stimuli, the low-pass filter characteristic of Figure 11-9 does not depend on the characteristic frequency of the neuron. Neurons with CFs greater than 5 kHz can phase-lock quite well to tones in the tails of their frequency tuning curves, although not to their own CF.

The principles that underlie neuronal phase-locking are also applicable to dynamic aspects of stimuli, that is, frequency and amplitude modulation (FM and AM, respectively). Simple tone bursts are limited to the laboratory and clinic, whereas real-world stimuli are constantly changing. For any neuron, sudden changes in the stimulus spectrum near its CF will elicit rapid changes in firing rate that are time-locked to these modulations. Responses to stimulus dynamics can be studied systematically by sinusoidally varying the frequency or amplitude of a carrier frequency that might be set to the CF of a neuron. Figure 11-10 shows results obtained when an afferent neuron with a CF near 20 kHz is presented with a stimulus having a 20 kHz carrier, but amplitude modulated at 100 Hz. When the response is examined using period histograms set to the *period of the modulator,* it is clear that the instantaneous firing rate of the neuron follows the period of modulation. The strength of this "modulator-phase-locking" varies with the depth of the modulation (see Figure 11-10A). Note, however, that the depth of the peaks and valleys in the histogram is actually larger than the modulation depth of the stimulus itself. Thus, the neuron exaggerates the modulation depth, thus enhancing the apparent **temporal coding** of AM. The degree of this exaggeration versus the actual modulation depth is shown in Figure 11-10B. This phenomenon probably originates in the same synaptic processes that give rise to rate adaptation (see Figures 11-7 and 11-8). The IHC afferent synapse

appears designed to magnify amplitude changes. The onset of a stimulus is merely a special case of AM in which the amplitude begins at zero.

Effect of Stimulus Intensity

We can now consider how neuronal responses change as stimulus levels are systematically increased, and thus construct neuronal **intensity response curves** (often simply called *intensity curves*) that are analogous to those for the basilar membrane and hair cells (see Figures 10-6 and 10-9). Chapter 10 explains that the responses of hair cells can be quantified for either the AC or DC component of the receptor potential, as long as the stimulus frequency is less than a few kilohertz. In IHCs, both components were noted to give generally similar results, although the AC component is expected to be more sensitive than the DC component. Because afferent neuronal phase-locking and spike rate responses are based on these, we can anticipate similarities between hair cell and neural intensity curves. Let us consider how the receptor potential will influence the generation of spikes as the level of a subthreshold tone burst near the CF is increased. Near threshold, the hair cell response consists primarily of the AC component. For a high-SR neuron, sinusoidal variation in hair cell membrane voltage will translate into similar variation in spike probability (see Figure 11-6). Near threshold, the decrease in spike probability that occurs over half the stimulus period will be balanced by a similar increase in probability during the other half. This, of course, is essentially the definition of phase-locking, but it holds the implication that there is explicitly *no change* in the overall firing rate. Thus, like the hair cell AC response, the neuronal phase-locked response generally will be more sensitive than the rate response (Figure 11-11).

FIGURE 11-10 Amplitude-modulation-following response of an afferent neuron in cat. A tone at the characteristic frequency (CF; 20 kHz) was modulated at 100 Hz, using different modulation depths. (A) Period histograms (at the modulator period) obtained using modulation depths of 0.22 and 0.11 (left column). Modulation of the neuronal response exceeds that of the stimulus waveform (right column). (B) Comparison of modulation of the neuronal response (*circles,* as determined from period histograms as in A) with that of the stimulus waveform at various modulation depths. (From Joris, P. X., & Yin, T. C. T. (1992). Responses to amplitude-modulated tones in the auditory nerve of the cat. *Journal of the Acoustical Society of America, 91,* 215–232, by permission. Copyright 1992 Acoustical Society of America.)

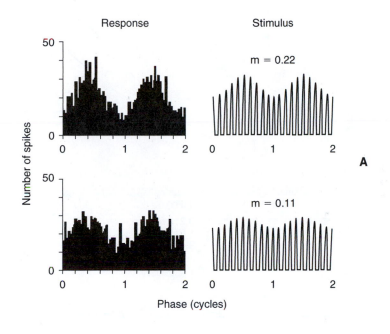

Response   Stimulus

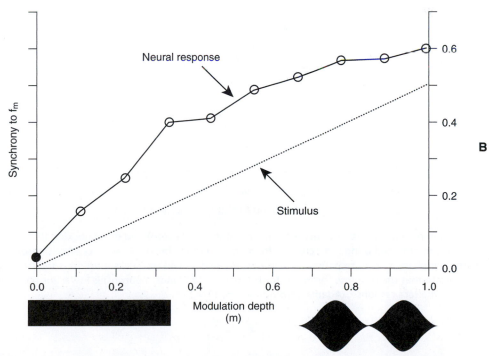

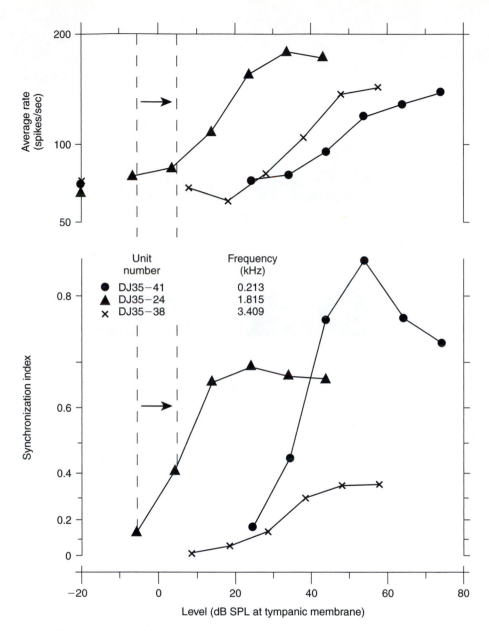

FIGURE 11-11 Comparison of intensity curves for neuronal spike rate (top) and phase-locking (bottom) for three auditory neurons in cat, obtained using characteristic frequency (CF) tone bursts. Phase-locked responses appear more sensitive. Note poor phase-locking response of neuron stimulated at 3.4 kHz. SPL, sound pressure level. Arrows and dashed lines indicate that the response threshold for this neuron (and most neurons) is lower for the phase-locking response than for the rate response. (Adapted from Johnson, 1974.)

As the stimulus level increases further, changes in both the rate and timing of spikes will be observed. By computing both spike rate and the proportion of spikes that are phase-locked at each level, we obtain curves that relate either spike rate or the strength of phase-locking to stimulus level. For any neuron, both quantities will begin to increase at their own distinct thresholds, increase over some range of intensities, and then saturate at high intensities (see Figure 11-11). Average neuronal firing rates usually saturate between 200 and 400 spikes/sec. The degree of phase-locking can be expressed in different ways. The synchronization index, used in Figure 11-11, varies between 0.0 and 1.0, the latter signifying "perfect" phase-locking, whereby all spikes have exactly the same phase. Below threshold, both types of curves reflect only randomly timed spontaneous spikes. Comparison of Figures 11-11, 10-6, and 10-9 shows that the intensity response characteristics of neurons and hair cells are generally similar. However, using either rate or phase-locking measures, neurons show a narrower dynamic range than hair cells, meaning that they increase from threshold to saturation over a more restricted range of sound levels. The dynamic range disparity between hair cells and neurons is thought to reflect the compressive nonlinearity posed by the synapse (see depiction in Figure 11-6). The hair cell transducer itself is also compressive, of course; yet, when these are cascaded, the dominant effect will be due to the more restricted (or "harder" saturating) stage.

Coding of Stimulus Intensity

The limiting influence of the afferent synapse is important when considering what portion of intensity curves conveys the most information. At high stimulus levels, where the neuron's response is saturated, there is no way for it to differentiate between one high level and another. Only over the rising portion of these curves can individual neurons presumably inform the brain about small changes in stimulus level. Curves such as those of Figure 11-11, therefore, present a problem that has been the subject of much speculation and modeling. The psychophysical abilities of humans and animals permit the detection of

stimulus-level changes of only about 1 dB over nearly the entire sensation range (>120 dB) (Moore, 1989). Yet, the effective range of most afferent fibers to steady-state tones is only about 20 to 30 dB. Many candidate explanations as to how the auditory system fills this "dynamic range gap" exist; thus, controversy has mostly involved exactly how these are combined (Viemeister, 1988). Note first that likely strategies do *not* require spread to higher CFs as a significant contributor. To see why this might be proposed, consider that a sufficiently loud tone at nearly any frequency below the CF can activate a given neuron, as long as it falls within the tail of the frequency tuning curve of the neuron (see Figure 11-15). It thus seems reasonable that the key to our intensity discrimination abilities is the engagement of neurons tuned to higher frequencies as a stimulus becomes louder. This does, in fact, occur, and it is the basis of loudness recruitment perceived by hearing-impaired listeners (see Moore, 1989), but it is not the basis of normal intensity discrimination abilities.

So what are likely candidate mechanisms that can account for narrow intensity discrimination? First, many neurons serve hearing at any given frequency (about 20 per IHC). We have seen that these vary widely in threshold, in a manner that is inversely correlated with SR (see Figure 11-5). Moreover, a surprising additional feature linked to both SR and threshold is the shape of the intensity curve itself. Low-SR neurons often combine high thresholds with rate-level curves that do not show "flat" saturation. Instead, these curves continue to increase in a manner that has been termed **sloping saturation** (Sachs & Abbas, 1974) (Figure 11-12). The key to this property is thought to be how the saturating nonlinearity of the hair cell transducer (see Figure 10-5) is cascaded with that of the synapse (see Figure 11-6). Low-SR neurons require comparatively large hair cell depolarizations to increase their firing rate. This means that large movements of the stereociliary bundle are required. But the hair cell response grows more slowly for large bundle displacements, because of the nonlinearity of the transducer. As a result, the slope of the intensity curve of the low-SR neuron will be lower than that of a typical high-SR, low-threshold neuron. A shallow slope means a wider dynamic range.

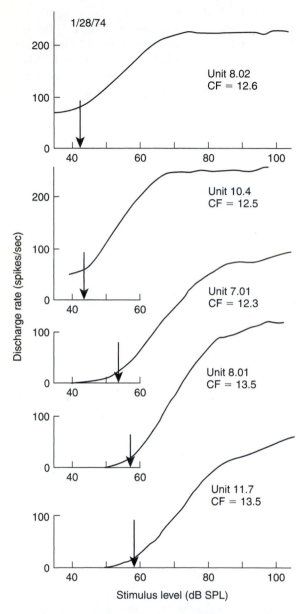

FIGURE 11-12 Rate-intensity curves for auditory neurons in cat, obtained using characteristic frequency (CF) tone bursts. Curves for low-SR neurons exhibit increased thresholds and "sloping saturation." SPL, sound pressure level. (From Sachs, M. B., & Abbas, P. J. (1974). Rate versus level functions for auditory-nerve fibers in cats. *Journal of the Acoustical Society of America, 56,* 1835–1847, by permission. Copyright 1974 Acoustical Society of America.)

The key to yet another way that afferent neurons may extend their dynamic range again lies in the shape of PSTHs (see Figure 11-7). As pointed out earlier, the onset spike rate is greater than the steady-state rate that continues throughout the tone burst. The onset response also has a wider dynamic range than the steady-state response (Smith, 1985) (Figure 11-13), even approaching that of hair cells. Because natural stimuli are dynamic, this may be a significant factor. However, forward masking by background noise may particularly reduce onset responses (see Figure 11-8) and limit the usefulness of this feature.

Effect of Stimulus Frequency

Chapter 10 explored the frequency tuning of hair cells using iso-level and frequency tuning curves. Completely analogous curves can be generated for radial afferent neurons. Just as for hair cells, these can be obtained for the AC (phase-locking) or DC (firing-rate) response. Figure 11-14A shows a family of iso-level curves obtained at several intensities for one neuron. At the lowest stimulus level, the range of frequencies over which the firing rate exceeds the SR (0.0 spikes/sec in this case) is limited to frequencies near 9 kHz, the apparent characteristic frequency. As frequency sweeps are run at higher levels, the curves broaden, mostly toward lower frequencies. This is reminiscent of iso-level curves for IHCs (see Figure 10-8) and the basilar membrane (see Figure 9-7). If we compared iso-level curves from many neurons, we would typically observe pronounced "flattening" of the curves at high stimulus levels, more so than for hair cells. This flattening of iso-level curves for most neurons again derives from saturation of the synapse and has implications for population coding of stimulus spectral shape (see later).

Figure 11-14B shows the frequency tuning curve for the same neuron. Recall that this is obtained by defining an arbitrary response criterion and determining at each of many test frequencies the stimulus intensity required to elicit a response. Typically, a small fixed increase in the number of spikes above the spontaneous rate is chosen. For the

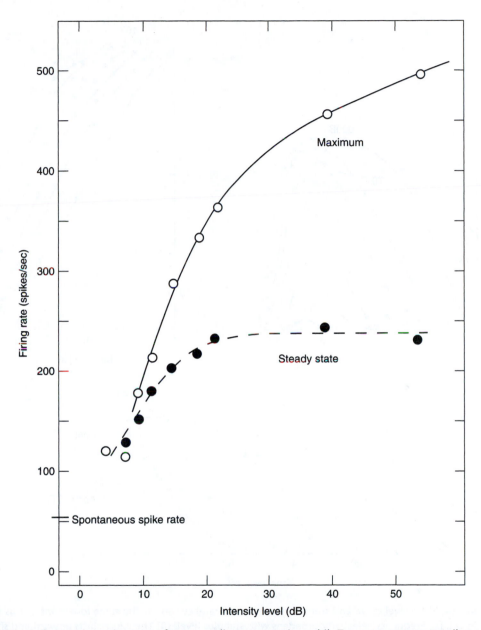

FIGURE 11-13 Spike rate-intensity curves for one auditory neuron in gerbil. *Top curve* represents spikes counted only during the first 5.0 milliseconds of the response (onset response). Bottom curve represents steady-state spike rate. The onset response has a wider dynamic range. (Adapted from Smith, 1985.)

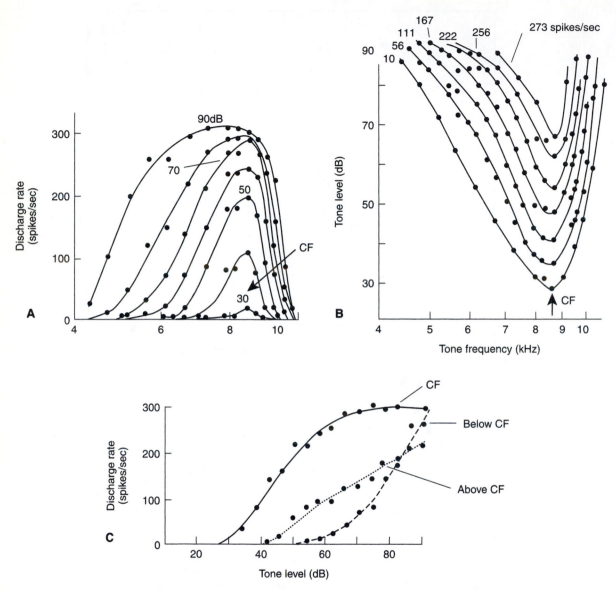

FIGURE 11-14 (A, B) Iso-level curve and frequency tuning (iso-rate) curves for the same low-spontaneous firing rate (SR) neuron in cat. (A) Frequency selectivity broadens with stimulus level. (B) The curve shifts upward and shows progressive reduction in tip length with increasing response criterion. (C) Rate-intensity curves at frequencies at characteristic frequency (CF), and above and below CF. These can be thought of as vertical "slices" through the tuning curves in B. For frequencies below the CF, the threshold is much higher, but the response is more linear (less compressed) at high sound levels. For frequencies above the CF, intensity curves become progressively shallower, yielding the steep cutoff slopes of tuning curves above CF. (Adapted from Evans, 1978.)

neuron shown, the investigators performed an explicit test of the effect of increasing the response criterion, yielding a set of nested curves. All of these have minima at the CF indicated by the iso-level curve in Figure 11-14A. The lowest criterion response, associated with the lowest tuning curve for this low-SR neuron, was 10 spikes/sec. As the criterion was raised, the curve shifted upward and the tip length decreased (tail frequencies were not included in the plot). The changes in the curve that accompany more stringent criteria are similar to those depicted for hair cells in Chapter 10 (see Figure 10-9).

The general features of both iso-level and frequency tuning curves (steep high-frequency cutoff, low-frequency tail response) can be predicted from differences in intensity curves obtained near, and away from, the CF (see Figure 11-14C). Above the CF, the slope becomes progressively shallower, so that large increases in intensity yield little additional response. At some frequency above the CF the intensity curve can be thought of as becoming completely flat; that is, it is impossible to drive the neuron. Near the CF, thresholds are low, but growth of the response is compressive. Below the CF, thresholds are high, but growth is linear, which is why the iso-level curve may become skewed to lower frequencies at high intensities. The relation between intensity curve shape and the changes found for iso-level and frequency tuning curves with increasing level/criterion recapitulates that for hair cells (see similar discussion in Chapter 10) and for the basilar membrane. This is anticipated because the origin of these lies in active basilar membrane mechanics.

Better appreciation of the tip–tail conformation of afferent frequency tuning curves and the orderly variation in their shape with CF can be gained from Figure 11-15. Note that a distinct tail is apparent only for mid- and high-CF neurons. Because rate-intensity curves are monotonic with level (meaning that they increase with intensity, not decrease), we can conceive of the frequency tuning curve as representing the lower boundary of all frequency-intensity pairs that activate the neuron. Within this curve, the neuron may indicate the frequency and intensity of a stimulus by its firing rate. The tuning curve obtained using any criterion, by definition, joins all frequency-intensity pairs eliciting the same response.

For neurons with CFs less than about 5 kHz, one could obtain generally similar phase-locking curves, using strength-of-phase-locking criteria. These typically have lower thresholds than rate-based curves (Figure 11-16), in keeping with the principles outlined for the hair cell AC receptor potential and its reflection in phase-locking. Finally, it is worth emphasizing that the frequency tuning of the basilar membrane, hair cells, and afferent neurons are all similar. IHCs and their afferents appear to be passive recipients of the frequency tuning properties of the basilar membrane.

Correlates of Characteristic Frequency

As discussed earlier, tuning curve shape varies with CF. This section considers some other correlates of CF.

Point of Innervation   Although it had been established from von Békésy's experiments that the cochlea contains a frequency map, most experimental preparations used for basilar membrane or hair cell recording involve only restricted cochlea locations and have not been useful for constructing detailed maps. In the course of recordings from single auditory nerve fibers in cats, M. C. Liberman (1982a,b) filled the neurons with dyes that allowed them to be traced to their point of origin. Figure 11-17 shows a log-linear relation between CF and cochlear termination point. This means that the cochlea allocates space such that relative frequency changes are represented by the same absolute distances. Roughly as many hair cells and neurons are devoted to frequencies covering, for example, the 1- to 2-kHz octave as the 10- to 20-kHz octave.

Latency of Response   The basilar membrane traveling wave proceeds from base to apex, so that the apex responds up to several milliseconds later than the base. Because frequencies are mapped in an orderly way along the partition, we would expect that neurons tuned to low frequencies would respond later

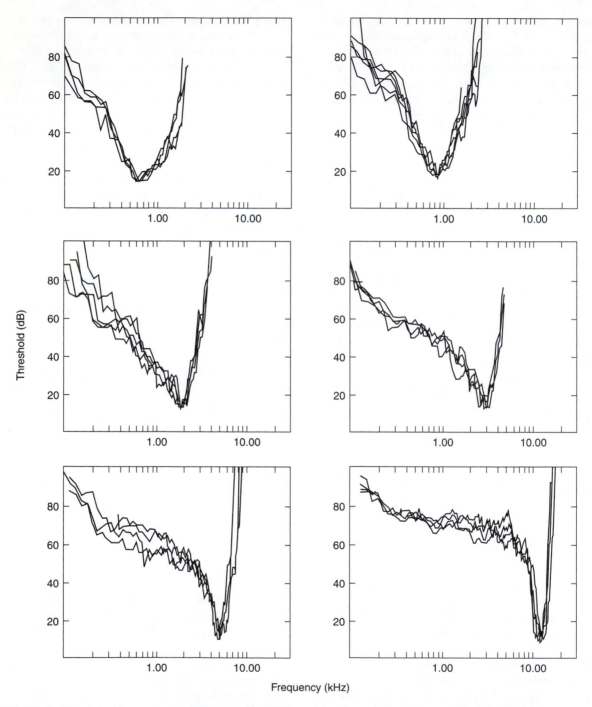

FIGURE 11-15   Typical frequency tuning curves of auditory neurons in gerbils with progressively higher characteristic frequencies (CFs). For each frequency range, tuning curves of several neurons have been superimposed. (Adapted from Ohlemiller, K. K., & Echteler, S. M. (1990). Functional correlates of characteristic frequency in single cochlear nerve fibers of the Mongolian gerbil. *Journal of Comparative Physiology, 167,* 329–338, by permission.)

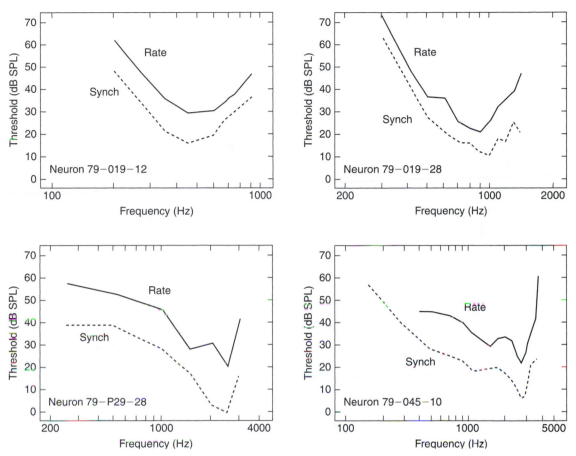

FIGURE 11-16 Comparison of rate and phase-locking frequency tuning curves for four afferent neurons in the cat. For each neuron, an arbitrary increase in firing rate above the spontaneous firing rate (SR) or degree of phase-locking was set, and the sound level required to reach criterion was determined at many frequencies. Rate and phase-locking curves are similar in shape, but offset vertically, the latter being more sensitive. SPL, sound pressure level. (From Javel, E., McGee, J. A., Horst, J. W., & Farley, G. R. (1988). Temporal mechanisms in auditory stimulus coding. In G. M. Edelman, W. E. Gall, & W. M. Cowan (Eds.), *Auditory function: Neurobiological bases of hearing* (pp. 515–558). New York: Wiley & Sons, by permission.)

than those tuned to higher frequencies, and that is, indeed, the case. A plot of first-spike latencies to clicks or CF tones yields a relation like that shown for cats in Figure 11-18. Note that the range of latencies rapidly increases for CFs less than about 800 Hz. This is because the traveling wave slows as it moves apically. By contrast, the basal turn moves nearly synchronously, as indicated by the fact that latencies change little for CFs between about 4 and 20 kHz. The variation in latency with CF poses a challenge for coding schemes based on temporal synchrony, because differ-

ent locations responding to the same temporal feature of the stimulus would do so at slightly different times. If higher auditory centers derive temporal information by monitoring many frequency regions, there must be some way of compensating for these delays. How temporal information is used, and how and whether such compensation occurs, is unclear.

Sharpness of Tuning Figure 11-15 suggests that the tips of afferent tuning curves become narrower with increasing characteristic frequency. This is true,

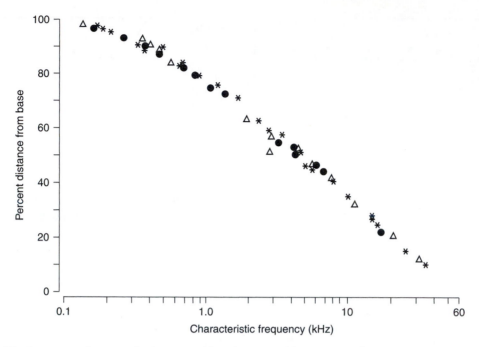

FIGURE 11-17 Frequency-place map in the cat cochlea, determined by recording from individual afferent neurons and then filling them with a dye, so that their place of origin could be determined. Each symbol type identifies data from a single animal. The map is near log-linear, so that equal proportional frequency differences are represented by similar distances along the partition. (From Liberman, M. C. (1982b). The cochlear frequency map of the cat: Labeling auditory-nerve fibers of known characteristic frequency. *Journal of the Acoustical Society of America, 72*, 1441–1449, by permission. Copyright 1982 American Institute of Physics.)

in *relative* terms, as plotted on a log-frequency axis. In *absolute* terms, high-CF curves are much broader: Neurons with CFs less than ~2 kHz have tips whose width is on the order of a few hundred Hertz, whereas neurons with CFs greater than ~5 kHz show tips extending 1 kHz or more. However, in engineering and in auditory physiology, it is customary to compare filter widths on a log axis, so that relative changes are emphasized. As discussed later, this practice is in keeping with our perceptual abilities. Tuning curve width is often quantified using a metric that is analogous to one used by engineers to characterize any band-pass filter: the Q-factor (quality factor). Physiologists use the Q_{10} (or Q_{10dB}), which expresses the ratio of the CF to the absolute bandwidth of the frequency tuning curve 10 dB above CF threshold (Kiang et al., 1965). Figure 11-19 shows that Q_{10} increases with

CF, confirming visual impressions of the curves in Figure 11-15. If we measure the Q-factor at a different point on the tuning curve, the Q_{40} (CF divided by bandwidth 40 dB above threshold), the shape of the relation changes, because this measure is highly sensitive to the emergence of tuning curve tails at mid-CFs.

What is the relevance of neural Q_{10}'s, and their increase with CF, to perception? Two types of comparisons may be made: one having to do with **frequency discrimination,** and the other with **frequency resolution** (see Moore, 1989). To assist our discussion, it is instructive to convert Q_{10}'s to tuning curve tip bandwidth as a percentage of CF. Doing this, we would find that "percent bandwidths" progressively narrow with CF, from about 30% of center frequency at low CFs, down to about 10% at high CFs (see Figure 11-15; Evans, Pratt,

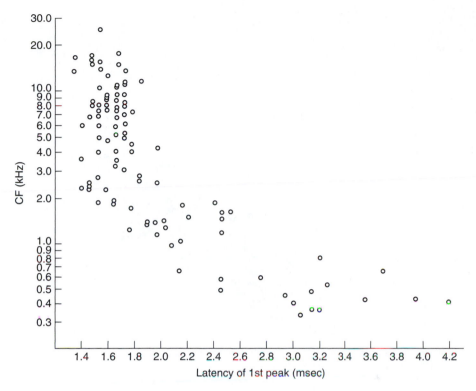

FIGURE 11-18   Latency of response versus characteristic frequency (CF) in the cat. Each data point represents the first spike latency of one neuron, as determined from the poststimulus histogram to a click stimulus. Latency increases with decreasing CF because of traveling wave delays. (From Kiang, N.-Y. S., Watanabe, T., Thomas, E. C., & Clark, L. F. (1965). *Discharge patterns of single fibers in the cat's auditory nerve.* Cambridge, MA: MIT Press, by permission. Copyright 1965 The MIT Press.)

& Cooper, 1989). Q_{10}'s give an exaggerated impression of the sharpening of tuning with increasing CF, in that percent bandwidths change only by a factor of ~3, whereas Q_{10}'s change by a factor of ~6 to 7 (see Figure 11-19). As discussed later, percent bandwidths are more readily comparable with psychoacoustic measures.

Frequency discrimination ability is examined by varying the frequency of a "reference" tonal stimulus and measuring how small a change in frequency can be detected. Detection thresholds less than 1% are typically obtained for frequencies below about 4 kHz (see Moore, 1989). However, detection thresholds increase to more than 5% of the reference frequency at higher frequencies. These values vary in a manner *opposite* to the trend in tun-

ing curve shape. At low frequencies, discrimination thresholds are too small to be explained by tuning curve width (<1% vs ~30%). Yet, the two measures are fairly close at high frequencies, if we consider that the task of detecting a change in frequency in one direction essentially probes half of the width of the tip, or about 5% at high CFs. The discrepancy between tuning curve width and discrimination thresholds at low frequencies has led to the suggestion that phase coding partly underlies our abilities at low frequencies. Frequency discrimination, therefore, may closely reflect tuning curve characteristics only at higher frequencies.

A more general way of considering cochlear neurons as filters pertains to frequency resolution, or how close in frequency two stimuli can be and both still be

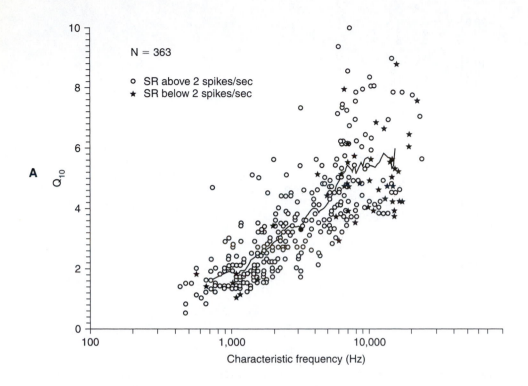

A

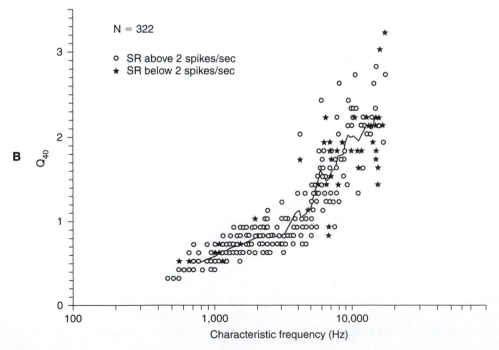

B

distinguished. Psychoacousticians have long recognized the existence of largely independent perceptual frequency channels, known as **critical bands** (Zwicker, Flottorp, & Stevens, 1957). Stimuli engaging different critical bands are readily detectable and show little interaction. Critical bands have been suggested to correspond to roughly constant lengths along the basilar membrane (~0.9 mm in humans). Expressed as a percentage of center frequency, they vary in width from about 30% to 40% at low frequencies to about 20% at high frequencies, although this can depend strongly on how they are measured (see Moore, 1989). This is reasonably close to percent bandwidths for neurons. Discrepancies can be explained by considering that: (1) experimentally determined neural tuning curves merely *reflect* real frequency tuning, and (2) typical procedures for estimating critical bands lead to suppression, so that **suppression areas** become included in the estimate (see later). In summary, frequency tuning in the periphery largely establishes the widths of filters in the central auditory system, and ultimately at the perceptual level.

Two-Tone Rate and Synchrony Suppression

In Chapter 10 we considered the effect of presenting a second tone to an IHC responding to a tone burst near the BF. As the second tone is varied in frequency and level, suppression areas can be identified around the margins of the tuning curve for the DC component of the receptor potential. Because the neuronal firing rate response is driven principally by the hair cell DC response, the same is true for rate-response tuning curves of afferent neurons (Figure 11-20). As for hair cells, only responses to stimuli near the CF can be inhibited. Responses to stimuli within the tuning curve, but well away from the CF, can only be enhanced.

The general similarity between two-tone suppression and surround inhibition in the visual system led to proposals that it may serve in enhancing spectral peaks in complex stimuli such as speech. Little support for appreciable contrast enhancement by suppression has been found. Most evidence instead indicates that tuning of both the hair cell DC response (Cheatham & Dallos, 1992) and neural rate response (see later) are blunted by suppression, so that spectral contrast is reduced.

A related phenomenon known as **synchrony suppression** (Javel, McGee, Horst, & Farley, 1988) may, however, play a beneficial role in perception of complex stimuli. A neuron showing phase-locking to a tone near CF can phase-lock to a second tone at the same time (assuming the second tone lies within the tuning curve). A period histogram at the period of the lower frequency would show modes corresponding to each stimulus period. This can be thought of as the neuron "allocating" phase-locked spikes to more than one phase. As a result, that portion of the overall spike total allocated to the first tone is decreased, *even though the overall spike count may increase.* Unlike **rate suppression,** which is bounded at low and high stimulus levels, synchrony suppression may occur anywhere within the tuning curve. Synchrony suppression is the neuronal analog of suppression of the hair cell AC response, which also can occur anywhere within the hair cell tuning curve (see Chapter 10).

Place Coding versus Temporal Coding of Complex Stimuli

The foregoing discussion has brought us to the point where we can finally consider how features of complex stimuli may be encoded. Complex stimuli mean stimuli having broad, continuous spectra, like

FIGURE 11-19 Frequency tuning curve sharpness versus characteristic frequency (CF) for afferent neurons in the gerbil. Sharpness of tuning has been quantified using the Q_{10dB} (A) or Q_{40dB} (B), respectively, calculated as the ratio of the CF to the bandwidth of the tuning curve (in Hertz) at 10 or 40 dB above CF threshold. Both measures increase with CF, although Q_{40dB} dips at mid-CFs. For mid-CFs tails become increasingly prominent, but the tuning curve tip is less than 40 dB, so that the tail is incorporated in the Q_{40dB} measure. SR, spontaneous firing rate. (From Ohlemiller, K. K., & Echteler, S. M. (1990). Functional correlates of characteristic frequency in single cochlear nerve fibers of the Mongolian gerbil. *Journal of Comparative Physiology, 167,* 329–338, by permission.)

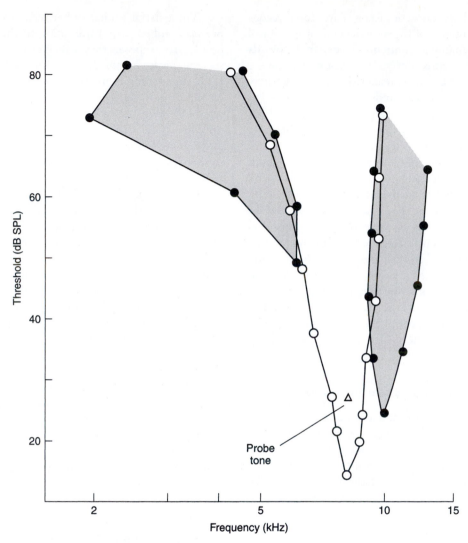

FIGURE 11-20 Typical suppression areas for an auditory neuron. These flank both sides of the tip, as well as the tail (not shown). The criterion for suppression was a 20% reduction in the response to a probe just above threshold at the characteristic frequency. SPL, sound pressure level.

those encountered in the real world. As meaningful complex stimuli that are somewhat stereotyped and can be synthesized for the laboratory, speech sounds are examined here. Speech sounds have been used in many studies of the auditory nerve (see Geisler, 1998, for summary). One approach has been to present vowels or consonant-vowel syllables and observe the extent to which large groups of neurons preserve the shape of the stimulus spectrum. If we were to put any stimulus through a microphone-amplifier-speaker system, we would consider the stimulus faithfully represented and transmitted by the system if the amplitude spectrum of the acoustic output closely matched that of the acoustic input (as determined by Fourier analysis). Because the cochlea appears organized around the principle of frequency analysis, it is reasonable to test the transmission of information by auditory nerve fibers in an analogous manner. One way to examine this is to measure the responses of many neurons to a particular stimulus and to plot normalized response versus CF. If the shape of the resulting "neurogram" resembles the amplitude spectrum of the stimulus, we might assert that the stimulus is faithfully represented. This type of analysis posits that the stimulus is encoded using a **rate–place code,** according to which each neuron indicates the prominence of its own CF in the stimulus spectrum by the magnitude of its firing rate. Figure 11-21 shows typical results for a vowel stimulus. The left column of Figure 11-21 shows the rate response of many neurons to the synthetic vowel /ɛ/ repeated many times at three different levels (38, 58, and 78 dB SPL). The vowel is represented by a tonal complex, and its amplitude spectrum is shown at the bottom of Figure 11-21. Three major formants appear as peaks in the spectrum. Because vowels can be well discriminated when pared down to contain only the first three formants, we are interested in whether the neural population response retains the formant peaks. In this experiment, neuronal rate responses were calculated from PSTHs over the duration of the stimulus, and the rate response of each neuron to the vowel is plotted at its CF. To make it possible to plot all the responses on the same axis, the rate response of each neuron has been normalized to its own maximum firing rate. Finally, the average normalized firing rate has been calculated for defined frequency bands, and the averaged points were joined by a solid line. Although the analysis framework may seem cumbersome, the key point is simple: Formant peaks are maintained in the neurogram at low levels, but they become less prominent with increasing stimulus level. At 78 dB SPL, they cannot be distinguished. The reasons for this include both compression and suppression. At higher levels, many neurons with CFs near the formants are firing at their maximum rate. Rate responses of some neurons tuned to the formants are suppressed by

adjacent tonal components falling at the boundaries of their frequency tuning curves. Rate-place coding schemes based on steady-state firing rates of neurons to their own CF appear severely limited.

From earlier discussions in this chapter, the results from this experiment are not surprising, and the reader may recognize that important factors have been left out. First, formant peaks at high stimulus levels would be expected to be retained by low-SR/high-threshold neurons, and research bears this out (Schalk & Sachs, 1980). Second, the initial portion of PSTHs exhibits greater spike rates, and onset spike rates have a wider dynamic range than steady-state spikes. If the analyses of Figure 11-21 were conducted using the initial portion of the PSTH, the formant peaks would be preserved at much higher levels (Smith, 1985). Real speech is highly dynamic, so this probably plays a role.

Finally, natural **place-coding** schemes probably combine both rate and temporal codes. Most spectral information in vowels lies below 5 kHz, where phase-locking is measurable. Assuming that coding of vowels is largely conducted by neurons with CFs less than 5 kHz, we can test whether a plot of strength-of-phase-locking versus CF reproduces the stimulus of the amplitude spectrum. Note that this analysis represents a fusion of place and temporal codes, because each neuron is assumed to represent its own CF by the *timing* of its spikes. The right column of Figure 11-21 shows the results of such an experiment for the same speech stimulus just considered. The actual response measure used, "average localized interval rate," is derived from the Fourier transform of the interval histogram of each neuron, but it can be thought of as analogous to normalized strength of phase-locking. Again, the idea being tested is whether the distribution of responses in this modified neurogram (only the average is shown) will reproduce the shape of the original stimulus spectrum, and whether formant peaks will be preserved at high intensities. In fact, the peaks are well preserved and show little effect of changes in stimulus level. Given that both phase-locking and spike rates saturate at high intensities (see Figure 11-11), why might phase-locking do a

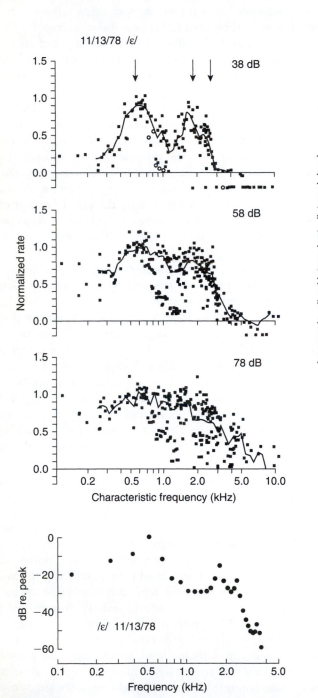

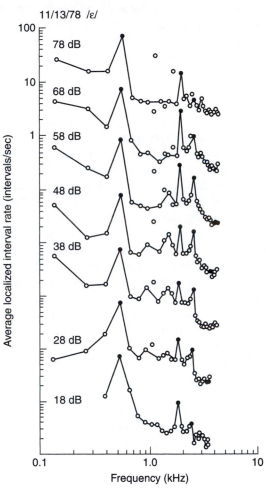

better job of preserving spectral peaks than rate responses? The key lies in differences between rate and synchrony suppression, and in the way spikes were included for analysis. Only spikes phase-locked to the CF of each neuron are included in Figure 11-21. Spikes phase-locked to other frequencies were ignored, even if they contributed to an overall increase in spike rate. Despite the impressive results that can be obtained using temporal measures, just how these are used by the brain is problematic. A combined temporal-place code requires that the central auditory system can somehow pick out only those spikes that are phase-locked to a neuron's own CF. As Chapter 15 explains, the timing precision of the auditory periphery is rapidly lost as one proceeds centrally. It is not clear how temporal codes are preserved or transformed in the brain.

GROSS MEASURES OF AFFERENT NEURONAL RESPONSES

Our earlier discussion of the electrical responses that can be recorded from the round window (or other remote location) in response to a tone burst (see Figure 10-11) focused on the summating potential (SP) and cochlear microphonic (CM), but ignored two early deflections that represent the neuronal contribution. Figure 11-22 shows a similar recording (although inverted, by virtue of the way it was obtained). The two early deflections (N_1 and N_2) are generally interpreted to represent the first and (at least in part) second synchronous spike of afferent neurons that respond to a tone burst or click (Ozdamar & Dallos, 1978). Subsequent spikes from all the participating neurons are generally not sufficiently synchronous to generate additional waves. These two deflections are collectively known as the **compound action potential** (CAP). The CAP may be isolated from the CM and SP by randomizing the phase of stimulus presentation (so that the CM cancels upon averaging) and high-pass filtering the response. Typically, the stimulus is repeated many times and the CAP is extracted from random electrical noise by averaging.

As discussed in Chapter 10, special recording configurations and masking paradigms are necessary to monitor restricted sets of hair cells with remote electrodes. That is fortunately not the case for the CAP. As long as stimulus levels are kept as low as possible, it is generally agreed that the CAP elicited by a tone burst will reflect the responses of neurons tuned to the stimulus frequency. As stimulus level increases, any tone burst will eventually enter the tail region of neurons tuned to higher frequencies, so that this assertion no longer holds. It follows that intensity curves for CAP amplitude reveal little about intensity curves for individual neurons. The CAP can be recorded from within the middle ear, or transtympanically. A plot of CAP threshold (i.e., the lowest level stimulus that elicits a detectable CAP) versus stimulus frequency provides a sensitive indicator of whether the organ of Corti is normal at each frequency location tested. Behavioral testing, evoked response audiometry, and CAP threshold testing generally yield similar results, although

FIGURE 11-21 Tests of speech-encoding abilities of auditory neurons using rate-place and modified temporal-place codes. In these "neurograms," each data point is the response of a single cat auditory neuron plotted at that neuron's characteristic frequency (CF). In all cases, the stimulus was the synthetic vowel /ɛ/ (amplitude spectrum shown at bottom) presented at levels shown indicated. In the left column, normalized rate responses have been plotted for three different presentation levels of the vowel. Formant peaks cannot be distinguished in the overall response profile (lines shows average) at high stimulus levels. In the right column, the average strength of phase-locking of neurons to stimulus components *at their own CF* has been plotted versus CF. This modified temporal-place code preserves formant peaks, nearly independent of stimulus level. The y-axis unit (average localized interval rate) refers to the Fourier transform of the interval histogram of the neurons and is closely related to strength of phase-locking. (From Sachs, M. B., & Young, E. D. (1980). Effects of nonlinearities on speech encoding in the auditory nerve. *Journal of the Acoustical Society of America, 68,* 858–875, by permission. Copyright 1980 American Institute of Physics.)

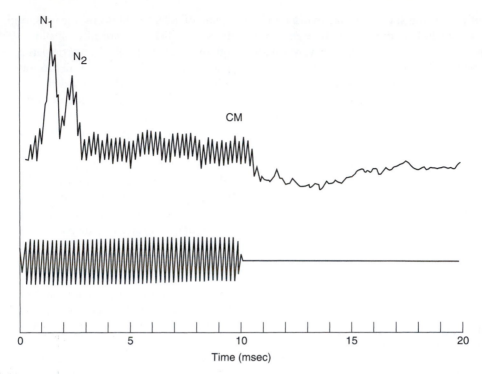

FIGURE 11-22   Signal recorded from the cochlear round window (top) in response to a tone burst (bottom). Negative changes are plotted upward. A slow offset response (summating potential), an oscillating response (cochlear microphonic [CM]), and two early peaks can be discerned. The peaks (N_1 and N_2) comprise the compound action potential, which reflects the nearly synchronous initial spikes generated by auditory neurons tuned to the stimulus. (From Moller, A. R. (2000). *Hearing: Its physiology and pathophysiology.* New York: Academic Press, by permission.)

offset on the *y*-axis because of their different sensitivities. Wave I of the auditory brainstem response (ABR) and N_1 of the CAP have similar latencies and are taken to represent equivalent events. The threshold for both may be artificially increased at high frequencies because neuronal density normally decreases in the base. "Threshold" has no absolute meaning in either case, because visual detection will depend on specific recording conditions and electrical noise level. Nevertheless, thresholds obtained using exactly the same procedures can be compared across experiments, laboratories, or clinics, and therein lies the utility of these methods.

N_1 of the CAP (as well as Wave I of the ABR) can be used to derive frequency tuning information under both normal and abnormal conditions. The strategy is analogous to using masking of the SP to

infer tuning of the hair cell DC response (see Chapter 10), although with an important difference. Hair cell responses and their gross potential analogs must be masked using simultaneous masker and probe. Recall that frequency tuning curves derived in this way will include two-tone suppression areas, which lie mostly outside the tuning curve. Thus, masking-derived tuning curves for the SP will be broader than their single hair cell counterparts. Neuronal responses show forward masking, whereby the response to one stimulus can be reduced or eliminated by the presentation of a prior stimulus (see Figure 11-8). This is purely masking by a "line busy" effect: Neurons that have just responded cannot respond as vigorously again until adaptation has subsided. Neuronal frequency tuning can therefore be examined by masking of the CAP using either a simultaneous or nonsimultaneous masker. As for hair cells, sharpness of tuning assessed using a simultaneous masker will be subject to the broadening effects of two-tone suppression. In a nonsimultaneous masking paradigm, a probe tone just above the CAP threshold at the frequency-place one wishes to test is paired with a preceding masking tone burst at various frequencies and levels. At each masker frequency, the goal is to identify the minimum masker level needed to reduce the response to the probe by some criterion amount. This process is selective for neurons that barely respond to both masker and probe. Iteration at many frequencies will outline the frequency tuning curve for a restricted set of neurons with CFs near the probe frequency. CAP tuning curves have been shown to mimic nearly all features of single neuron tuning curves (Figure 11-23).

ꙮ SUMMARY ꙮ

Radial afferent neurons constitute the output of the cochlea and is the basis of all we can know of our acoustic environment. Earlier steps in processing (basilar membrane, OHCs, and IHCs) merely set the stage for the neurons to perform their function. The characteristics and limitations of auditory neurons thus determine both the goals and tools of audiology, and in-depth understanding of these neurons will always make for more flexible and innovative practitioners.

Currently, the only therapy for sensorineural deafness that targets the inner ear is the cochlear implant. We have explored the responses of auditory neurons in some depth because it is the normal responses of these that an implant—or any other therapy—would ideally preserve or restore. Many aspects of afferent function are not mimicked by implants. These include traveling wave delays, sharp frequency tuning, staggering of thresholds by SR, the broader dynamic range of spike rates at stimulus onset, phase-locking, adaptation, and rate and synchrony suppression. All these influence normal perception. Overall, implants work quite well—even shockingly so, now that we have seen how much information is missing. This is testimony to the flexibility of the brain, including redundancy of coding strategies. Nevertheless, as technology progresses and improvements in implant performance or whole new therapies become possible, the full array of normal afferent response properties should guide new designs.

ꙮ KEY TERMS ꙮ

Action potential (spike)
Analog coding
Central nervous system
Characteristic frequency
Compound action potential
Critical band
Digital coding
Dynamic range
Forward masking

Frequency discrimination
Frequency resolution
Frequency tuning curve
Glutamate
Intensity response curve
Interval histogram
Modiolus
Period histogram

Peripheral nervous system
Phase-locking
Place coding
Poststimulus time histogram
Q_{10dB}
Q_{40dB}
Quanta
Radial afferent (type I)
Rate adaptation

Rate response
Rate suppression
Rate-place code
Refractory period
Sloping saturation
Spike probability
Spike rate
Spontaneous firing rate
Suppression areas
Synchrony suppression
Temporal coding

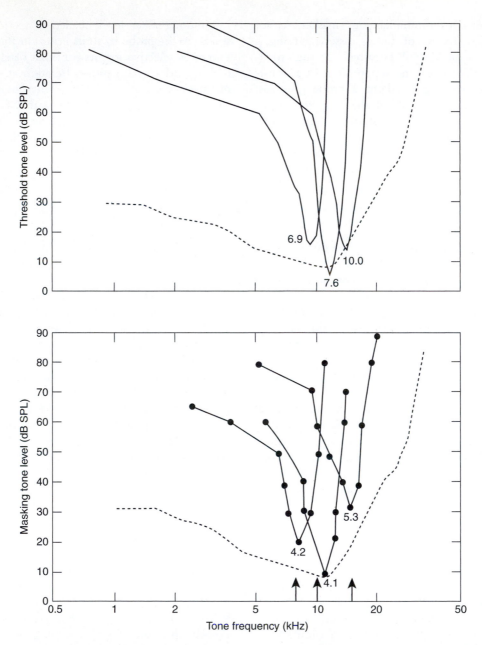

FIGURE 11-23 Comparison of frequency tuning curves of three single auditory neurons in a normal guinea pig (top) and compound action potential tuning curves obtained using masking (bottom). At each test frequency, the level of a simultaneous masker was adjusted to barely mask the compound action potential response to a tone burst presented just above threshold at three probe frequencies *(arrows)*. Q_{10}'s are shown. Single neuron and gross tuning measures are fairly similar. *Dashed lines* show CAP threshold versus stimulus frequency. SPL, sound pressure level. (From Harrison, R. V., Aran, J.-M., & Erre, J.-P. (1981). AP tuning curves from normal and pathological human and guinea pig cochleas. *Journal of the Acoustical Society of America, 69,* 1374–1385, by permission. Copyright 1981 Acoustical Society of America.)

⋖STUDY QUESTIONS⋗

1. Describe the typical innervation pattern of radial afferent neurons. How many hair cells does one neuron typically contact? How many neurons typically contact a single IHC?

2. What distinguishes low-SR neurons by their thresholds? The shape of their rate-intensity curve? How is this thought to be relevant to perception?

3. Describe how the IHC/afferent neuronal synapse is asymmetric and nonlinear.

4. Describe the relation between the IHC DC response and the afferent spike rate. How might synaptic nonlinearity enhance this?

5. How does the AC component of the IHC receptor potential cause neural phase-locking? Why does it decline at high frequencies?

6. Why is it said that an apparent gap exists between the dynamic range of auditory neurons and our perceptual abilities? How is it probably resolved?

7. What is the relation between spike rate adaptation and forward masking?

8. Why might we say that the synapse appears designed to emphasize changes in the acoustic environment?

9. How do neuronal frequency tuning curves change with increasing CF? What is the apparent relation between tuning curve tip width and critical bands? Is this more relevant to the notion of frequency *discrimination* or *resolution*?

10. Compare and contrast spike rate and synchrony suppression. How might these influence perception?

11. What are some possible limitations of rate-place coding?

12. How might characteristics of onset responses and the rate-intensity behavior of low-SR neurons help preserve rate-place coding?

13. What is the compound action potential. What is the relation between N_1 of the CAP and Wave I of the ABR?

⋖REFERENCES⋗

Arthur, R. M., Pfeiffer, R. R., & Suga, N. (1971). Properties of 'two-tone inhibition' in primary auditory neurones. *Journal of Physiology, 212,* 593–609.

Bobbin, R. P., & Thompson, M. H. (1978). Effects of putative neurotransmitters on afferent cochlear transmission. *Annals of Otology, Rhinology, and Otolaryngology, 87,* 185–190.

Cheatham, M. A., & Dallos, P. (1992). Two-tone suppression in inner hair cell responses: Correlates of rate suppression in the auditory nerve. *Hearing Research, 60,* 1–12.

Evans, E. F. (1978). Place and time coding of frequency in the peripheral auditory system: Some physiological pros and cons. *Audiology, 17,* 369–420.

Evans, E. F., Pratt, S. R., & Cooper, N. P. (1989). Correspondence between behavioural and physiological frequency selectivity in the guinea pig. *British Journal of Audiology, 23,* 151–152.

Geisler, C. D. (1998). *From sound to synapse.* New York: Oxford.

Harrison, R. V. (2001). The physiology of the cochlear nerve. In A. F. Jahn & J. Santos-Sacchi (Eds.), *Physiology of the ear* (pp. 549–573). San Diego, CA: Singular.

Harrison, R. V., Aran, J.-M., & Erre, J.-P. (1981). AP tuning curves from normal and pathological human and guinea pig cochleas. *Journal of the Acoustical Society of America, 69,* 1374–1385.

Javel, E., McGee, J. A., Horst, J. W., & Farley, G. R. (1988). Temporal mechanisms in auditory stimulus coding. In G. M. Edelman, W. E. Gall, & W. M. Cowan (Eds.), *Auditory function: Neurobiological bases of hearing* (pp. 515–558). New York: Wiley & Sons.

Johnson, D. H. (1974). *The response of single auditory nerve fibers in the cat to single tones: Synchrony and average discharge rate.* Unpublished doctoral dissertation, Massachusetts Institute of Technology, Boston.

Joris, P. X., & Yin, T. C. T. (1992). Responses to amplitude-modulated tones in the auditory nerve of the cat. *Journal of the Acoustical Society of America, 91,* 215–232.

Kiang, N.-Y. S., Watanabe, T., Thomas, E. C., & Clark, L. F. (1965). *Discharge patterns of single fibers in the cat's auditory nerve.* Cambridge, MA: MIT Press.

Klinke, R., & Oertel, W. (1966). Amino acids—putative neurotransmitter in the cochlea? *Experimental Brain Research, 30,* 145–148.

Liberman, M. C. (1978). Auditory nerve responses from cats raised in a low noise chamber. *Journal of the Acoustical Society of America, 63,* 442–455.

Liberman, M. C. (1980). Morphological differences among radial afferent fibers in the cat cochlea: An electron microscopic study of serial sections. *Hearing Research, 3,* 45–63.

Liberman, M. C. (1982a). Single neuron labeling in the cat auditory nerve. *Science, 216,* 1239–1241.

Liberman, M. C. (1982b). The cochlear frequency map of the cat: Labeling auditory-nerve fibers of known characteristic frequency. *Journal of the Acoustical Society of America, 72,* 1441–1449.

Lorente de Nó, R. (1937). Symposium: The neural mechanism of hearing. I. Anatomy and physiology. *The Laryngoscope, 47,* 373.

Moller, A. R. (2000). *Hearing: Its physiology and pathophysiology.* New York: Academic Press.

Moore, B. C. J. (1989). *An introduction to the psychology of hearing.* Boston: Academic Press.

Ohlemiller, K. K., & Echteler, S. M. (1990). Functional correlates of characteristic frequency in single cochlear nerve fibers of the Mongolian gerbil. *Journal of Comparative Physiology, 167,* 329–338.

Ohlemiller, K. K., Echteler, S. M., & Siegel, J. H. (1991). Factors that influence rate-versus-intensity relations in single cochlear nerve fibers of the gerbil. *Journal of the Acoustical Society of America, 90,* 274–287.

Ota, C. Y., & Kimura, R. S. (1980). Ultrastructural study of the human spiral ganglion. *Acta Oto-Laryngologica, 89,* 53–62.

Ozdamar, O., & Dallos, P. (1978). Synchronous responses of the primary auditory fibers to the onset of tone bursts and their relation to compound action potentials. *Brain Research, 155,* 169–175.

Rhode, W. S. (1971). Observations of the vibrations of the basilar membrane in squirrel monkeys using the Mössbauer technique. *Journal of the Acoustical Society of America, 49,* 1218–1231.

Sachs, M. B., & Abbas, P. J. (1974). Rate versus level functions for auditory-nerve fibers in cats. *Journal of the Acoustical Society of America, 56,* 1835–1847.

Sachs, M. B., & Young, E. D. (1980). Effects of nonlinearities on speech encoding in the auditory nerve. *Journal of the Acoustical Society of America, 68,* 858–875.

Schalk, T. B., & Sachs, M. B. (1980). Nonlinearities in auditory nerve fiber responses to bandlimited noise. *Journal of the Acoustical Society of America, 67,* 903–913.

Sellick, P. M., Patuzzi, R., & Johnstone, B. M. (1982). Measurement of basilar membrane motion in the guinea pig using the Mössbauer technique. *Journal of the Acoustical Society of America, 72,* 131–141.

Smith, R. L. (1977). Short-term adaptation in single auditory nerve fibers: Some post-stimulatory effects. *Journal of Neurophysiology, 40,* 1098–1112.

Smith, R. L. (1985). Cochlear processes reflected in the responses of the cochlear nerve. *Acta Otolaryngologica, 100,* 1–12.

Spoendlin, H. (1967). Innervation patterns in the organ of Corti of the cat. *Acta Otolaryngologica, 67,* 239–254.

Spoendlin, H. (1974). Neuroanatomy of the cochlea. In E. Zwicker & E. Terhardt (Eds.), *Facts and models in hearing* (pp. 18–32). Berlin: Springer-Verlag.

Spoendlin, H. (1981). Differentiation of cochlear afferent neurons. *Acta Otolaryngologica, 91,* 451–456.

Tasaki, I. (1954). Nerve impulses in individual auditory nerve fibers of guinea pig. *Journal of Neurophysiology, 17,* 97–122.

Viemeister, N. F. (1988). Psychophysical aspects of auditory intensity coding. In: G. M. Edelman, W. E. Gall, & W. M. Cowan (Eds.), *Auditory function-neurobiological bases of hearing* (pp. 213–241). New York: Wiley & Sons.

Zwicker, E., Flottorp, G., & Stevens, S. S. (1957). Critical bandwidth in loudness summation. *Journal of the Acoustical Society of America, 29,* 548–557.

◡‚SUGGESTED READING ∻

Brown, M. C. (2001). Functional neuroanatomy of the cochlea. In A. F. Jahn & J. Santos-Sacchi (Eds.), *Physiology of the ear* (pp. 529–548). San Diego, CA: Singular.

Gelfand, S. A. (1998). *Hearing: An introduction to psychological and physiological acoustics.* New York: Marcel Dekker.

Moore, B. C. J. (2003). Coding of sounds in the auditory system and its relevance to signal processing and coding in cochlear implants. *Otology and Neurotology, 24,* 243–254.

Pickles, J. O. (1988). *An introduction to the physiology of hearing.* New York: Academic Press.

Ulfendahl, M. (1997). Mechanical responses of the mammalian cochlea. *Progress in Neurobiology, 53,* 331–380.

Chapter

12

Cochlear Efferent Anatomy and Function

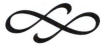

Dwayne D. Simmons, Ph.D.
Associate Professor of Otolaryngology
Washington University School of Medicine
St. Louis, Missouri

OVERVIEW

The function of the efferent **olivocochlear** system has remained controversial since its discovery as an anatomic pathway. Rasmussen (1946, 1953, 1960) first described the descending **(efferent)** innervation of the cochlea. This auditory brainstem pathway is defined by crossed and uncrossed components of the olivocochlear bundle. The uncrossed olivocochlear bundle projects to the **ipsilateral** ear, whereas the crossed olivocochlear bundle projects to the **contralateral** ear. The superior olivary complex, as the source of the olivocochlear bundle, is located in the ventral portion of the rostral medulla and caudal pons in a region of the brainstem known as the **trapezoid body.** The superior olivary complex is an auditory region dedicated to processing **binaural** acoustic signals. Its function within the ascending auditory system includes the detection of interaural time and intensity differences as the basis of spatial mapping. Descending efferent projections from the superior olivary complex influence otoacoustic emissions in both ears and play a role in the regulation of afferent fiber responses. Current studies of the efferent olivocochlear system are clarifying how the efferent system works to adapt the afferent system to background noise and provides protection to the ear from exposures to loud sounds. Clinically, understanding of the efferent olivocochlear system may ultimately provide benefit to those patients with auditory dysfunction in high-noise backgrounds and provide a window on central auditory status.

EFFERENT ANATOMY

In humans and mammals, olivocochlear efferent neurons have cell bodies located in a mostly ventral position in the hindbrain extending from the facial motor nucleus in the medulla to the lateral lemniscus in the midbrain (Figure 12-1). Within the brainstem, olivocochlear efferent axons form the olivocochlear bundle that travels through the facial genu and exits the brainstem along with the vestibular nerve before crossing over into the cochlear nerve. Olivocochlear efferents can be divided into two separate systems known as the **lateral** and **medial efferent systems.**

The lateral group of olivocochlear neurons is located in or near the **lateral superior olive.** Lateral olivocochlear neurons are defined by their dendrites extending into the lateral superior olive, rather than the location of cell bodies. In humans and primates, lateral olivocochlear neurons surround the lateral superior olive (see Figures 12-1B, C), whereas in most rodents, lateral olivocochlear neurons reside inside the lateral superior olive. Lateral olivocochlear neurons have small, unmyelinated fibers that project mostly, but not exclusively, to the ipsilateral cochlea via the uncrossed portion of the olivocochlear bundle (Figure 12-2). The medial group of olivocochlear efferent neurons resides in medial and ventral portions of the **periolivary** nuclei (see Figure 12-2). These neurons are scattered from the rostral periolivary regions that border the lateral lemniscus to caudal portions of ventral periolivary regions associated with the trapezoid body. Medial olivocochlear neurons have large, myelinated axons that project via crossed and uncrossed portions of the olivocochlear bundles. Across animals, roughly two-thirds of medial olivocochlear neurons send axons via the crossed olivocochlear bundles to the contralateral cochlea, whereas about one-third of neurons send axons via the uncrossed olivocochlear bundles to the ipsilateral cochlea.

Cochlear Projections of Efferent Neurons

Lateral and medial olivocochlear axons have different cochlear targets (see Figure 12-2). The majority of lateral olivocochlear axons terminate on the afferent auditory nerve fibers (spiral ganglion afferent fibers) just below inner hair cells, whereas medial efferent axons terminate on all three rows of outer hair cells. In the brainstem, lateral olivocochlear neurons project mostly to the ipsilateral (same side) cochlea. The projections of medial efferent axons are bilaterally organized, although the majority of axons originate from the contralateral side of the brainstem. Although the majority of medial efferent axons project to midfrequency regions of the cochlea (e.g., 2–10 kHz regions in the cat), medial efferent neurons projecting to the contralateral ear send most of their axons to high-frequency basal

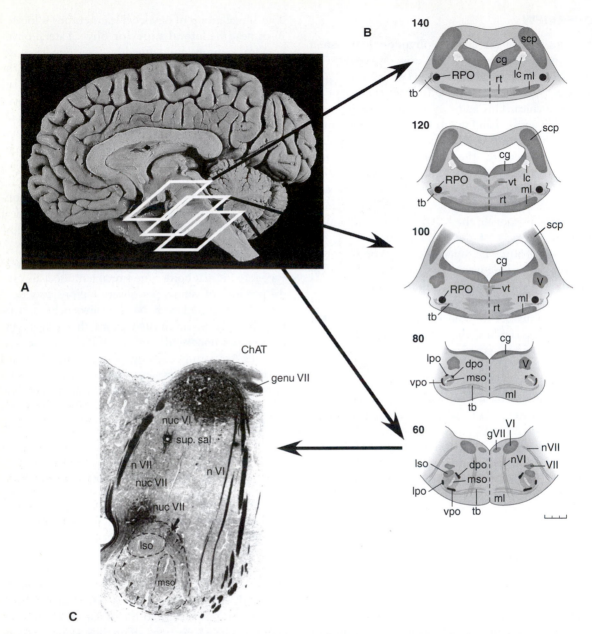

FIGURE 12-1   Midsagittal section (A) and coronal sections (B) of human brain illustrating the locations of the olivo-cochlear efferent system at various cross-section levels through the brainstem. Numbers next to sections in B are section numbers. (C) Cross section through the upper medulla that shows the location of the medial and lateral olivocochlear neurons. A marker (choline acetyltransferase [ChAT]) is used to identify neurons producing acetylcholine. Gg, central grey; dpo, dorsal periolivary nucleus; lc, locus coeruleus; lpo, lateral periolivary nucleus; lso, lateral superior olivary nucleus; ml, medial lemniscus; mso, medial superior olivary nucleus; nVI, abducens nerve; nVII, facial nerve; RPO, rostral periolivary nucleus; scp, superior cerebellar peduncle; tb, trapezoid body; vpo, ventral periolivary nucleus; V, trigeminal nucleus; nuc VI, abducens nucleus; nuc VII, facial nucleus; sup sal, superior salivatory nucleus; rt, reticulotegmental nucleus; vt, ventral tegmental nucleus; genu VII, genu of the facial nerve. (Adapted from Moore et al., 1999.)

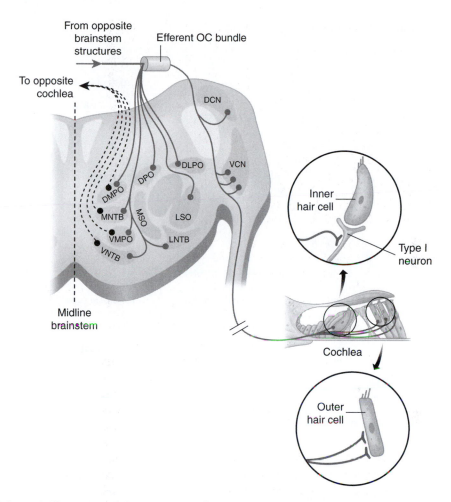

FIGURE 12-2 Schematic illustration of the projection of medial and lateral olivocochlear neurons to the inner and outer hair cells in the organ of Corti in the cochlea. DCN, dorsal cochlear nucleus; DLPO, dorsolateral posterior olive; DMPO, dorsomedial posterior olive, DPO, dorsal periolivary; LNTB, lateral nucleus of the trapezoid body; LSO, Lateral superior olive; MSO, medial superior olive; TB, trapezoid body; VCN, ventral cochlear nucleus; VNTB, ventral nucleus of the trapezoid body; VPO, ventral periolivary. (Adapted from Sahley et al., 1997.)

portions. In general, the apical 20% to 25% of the cochlear spiral receives little innervation from medial efferent axons. In cats, the innervation span of medial efferent axons can range from 0.55 to 2.8 mm, or roughly 2.2% to 11.2% of the cochlear spiral. Although medial efferent axons demonstrate frequency specificity in their responses, the broad terminal fields indicate that a comparatively greater range of the basilar membrane (cochlear partition) is influenced by medial efferent responses.

Efferent Neurotransmitters

Similar to motor neurons, **acetylcholine** is the primary neurotransmitter found in efferent cell bodies and in efferent nerve terminals. Despite its lack of complete specificity, histochemistry for the degradative enzyme for acetylcholine (acetylcholine sterase) has provided much of the early information on morphology of the efferent system. With the availability of an antibody to the synthesizing enzyme for acetylcholine (acetylcholine transerase),

Olivocochlear Efferent System

Medial olivocochlear system

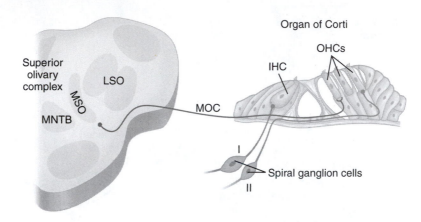

Cochlear location	Neurotransmitter	Receptor type
Base	Acetylcholine	Mixed nicotinic
Apex	ACh or GABA	Mixed nicotinic

Lateral olivocochlear system

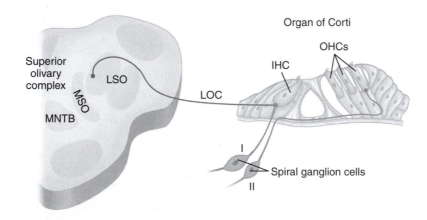

Cochlear location	Neurotransmitter	Receptor type
Base	ACh or GABA	Muscarinic/GABA?
Apex	ACh or GABA	Muscarinic/GABA?

FIGURE 12-3 Schematic illustrating the neurotransmitters used by the olivocochlear system. ACh, acetylcholine; GABA, γ-aminobutyric acid; IHC, inner hair cell; OHC, outer hair cell.

more accurate identification of **cholinergic** neurons is possible. Positive staining for the synthesizing enzyme has been used to identify inner ear efferent neurons in the brainstem and efferent terminals in the cochlea. In mammals, acetylcholine-containing neurons are found in two groups within the superior olivary complex: a group of large neurons located in ventral periolivary regions, and a group of smaller neurons located in or near the lateral superior olive. According to more recent studies, it is likely that all cholinergic cells in the lateral superior olive are lateral olivocochlear neurons, whereas only larger cholinergic cells in the ventral nucleus of the trapezoid body are medial olivocochlear neurons. Smaller cholinergic neurons in the ventral nucleus of the trapezoid body most likely send efferent projections to the cochlear nucleus.

Olivocochlear efferents in mammals are neurochemically heterogeneous. Both **γ-aminobutyric acid (GABA),** a major inhibitory neurotransmitter, and dopamine are found in some efferent cell bodies and terminals. Although GABA is more prominent than dopamine within olivocochlear neurons, the role of GABA in efferent function remains uncertain. Antibodies made directly against either GABA or its synthesizing enzyme show immunoreactivity in cell bodies located in the superior olivary complex and terminals located below hair cells in the cochlea. Consistent with a neurotransmitter role, cochlear efferent terminals demonstrate GABA uptake. The presence of GABA-positive fibers and terminals below inner and outer hair cells has led some to propose GABA as a neurotransmitter for both medial and lateral olivocochlear (OC) neurons. However, the presence of GABA-positive cell bodies is not well established in periolivary regions containing medial olivocochlear neurons, but they are clearly observed in the lateral superior olive by combinations of retrograde tracer labeling and immunocytochemistry. In addition, GABA-immunoreactive terminals found below outer hair cells (OHCs) are present mostly in apical regions of the cochlea where the medial olivocochlear innervation is minimal.

Another aspect of inner ear efferent neurochemistry is the presence of small neuroactive peptides (referred to as **neuropeptides**) such as calcitonin gene–related peptide (CGRP), enkephalins, and dynorphins. Among these, CGRP is colocalized with acetylcholine in most motor neurons and has been suggested to regulate acetylcholine receptor synthesis. In several mammalian species, CGRP appears to colocalize with cholinergic enzymes in lateral olivocochlear neurons, but not medial neurons. These studies appear to contradict the conclusions from studies performed within the inner ear. In the cochlea, lateral efferent synaptic transmission is mediated by acetylcholine and GABA receptors, whereas medial efferent synaptic transmission is mediated mostly by acetylcholine receptors. Figure 12-3 summarizes the current immunocytochemical data for acetylcholine, GABA, and CGRP in the rodent OC system. Extensive reviews of putative efferent neurotransmitters and neuropeptides in the inner ear have been published previously.

PHYSIOLOGY OF THE MEDIAL EFFERENT PATHWAY

It has been clear since the 1950s that electrical stimulation of the olivocochlear bundle increases cochlear thresholds, making the ear less sensitive to sounds. Since then, it has been shown that efferent fibers respond to sound, and thus form the effector arm of a sound-evoked reflex to the inner ear known as the efferent reflex (Figure 12-4). It is likely that all known effects of olivocochlear bundle stimulation can be attributed to the myelinated medial olivocochlear component, and that all physiologic recordings from the olivocochlear efferents have been from the medial olivocochlear fibers. Little is known about the physiology and function of lateral olivocochlear projections.

Activation of the medial olivocochlear system increases thresholds in the auditory periphery. Medial olivocochlear neurons project to each ear from both sides of the brainstem via the crossed olivocochlear bundles. Early animal studies took advantage of this anatomic pathway, especially that it could be stimulated electrically at the floor of the fourth ventricle. Galambos (1956) first demonstrated in cats that electrical stimulation of the crossed olivocochlear bundle alters the compound action potential (CAP) of the auditory nerve.

MOC reflex loop

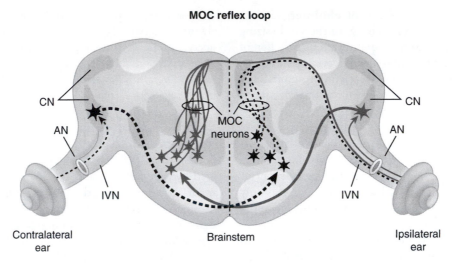

FIGURE 12-4   Schematic illustrating the neuronal circuitry underlying the sound reflex loop for the medial olivocochlear system (MOC). (Adapted from Liberman and Guinan, 1998.)

Galambos observed a reduction in the CAP amplitude in response to clicks in a quiet background. This gross neural response suggested an inhibitory role for crossed olivocochlear bundle stimulation. Electrical stimulation of the crossed olivocochlear bundle also reduces the discharge rate of single afferent fibers in response to low- or moderate-intensity sound stimulus. Maximal suppression in afferent fiber discharge rate occurs some 40–90 milliseconds after the onset of electrical stimulation. The suppression of afferent fiber discharge rate from electrical stimulation of the olivocochlear bundle can range from 1–25 dB sound pressure level (SPL), corresponding to a reduction in spike activity of between 10% and 95% and a shift in threshold of 12–14 dB.

Similar to the middle-ear-muscle acoustic reflex, the medial olivocochlear reflex is driven by sounds in either the ipsilateral or contralateral ear. The reflex is maximally stimulated from binaural noise. The ipsilateral responsive loop of this reflex is stronger than the contralaterally responsive loop. The thresholds for activation of the medial olivocochlear reflex are low, roughly 10–20 dB above the threshold for hearing. The sound frequencies most strongly affected by the medial olivocochlear path-

way are in the mid- to high-frequency regions. This frequency specificity mimics the density of medial olivocochlear terminals along the cochlear spiral: efferent terminals are rare in apical regions. We would expect the region of peak effectiveness to be somewhat lower in humans than in animals, from which all data have been collected to date. The reflex mechanism involves modulation of outer hair cell function.

The threshold-elevating effects of olivocochlear bundle stimulation arise subsequent to release of acetylcholine from medial olivocochlear terminals on outer hair cells. In the absence of medial olivocochlear stimulation, outer hair cells act like tiny motors, amplifying the vibration along the organ of Corti in response to sound. This motion results in the increased bending of the sensory hair bundles on inner hair cells. Activation of medial olivocochlear synapses on outer hair cells changes their response properties so as to decrease their contribution to the amplification of motion. Acetylcholine release by olivocochlear axons increases outer hair cell conductance and decreases the normal electromechanical contribution of the outer hair cells to the enhancement of vibration of the cochlear partition, especially at low sound pressure levels, by mechanisms that are still unclear. Activation of the medial olivocochlear system effectively turns down the gain on the outer hair cell amplifiers. This reduced gain causes the sound levels required to stimulate the auditory nerve to be elevated by as much as 30 dB when the medial olivocochlear system is activated electrically.

FUNCTIONAL SIGNIFICANCE OF THE EFFERENT-MEDIATED REFLEX

A number of hypotheses have been suggested for the functional significance of the medial olivocochlear reflex system. These hypotheses have included the following ideas:

1. The medial olivocochlear reflex system serves as an automatic gain control to extend the dynamic range of hearing.

2. It reduces the effects of **masking** arising from increases in auditory–nerve steady-state responses to continuous background noise.

3. It mediates selective attention by allowing the central processor to suppress auditory input when, for example, attending to a visual stimulus or when attending to one component of a complex acoustic signal.

4. It acts to protect the ear from damage caused by intense sounds.

Efferent-Mediated Protection

The idea that the olivocochlear efferents might reduce the threshold shift subsequent to noise exposure appeared in the literature in the mid-1960s. In a study showing that addition of loud sound to the contralateral ear reduced the **temporary threshold shift** (TTS) in the ipsilateral ear, Ward (1970) concluded that the effect was probably due to middle-ear muscle contractions, but speculated that an effect of the olivocochlear efferents was also a logical possibility, because both middle-ear muscles and the olivocochlear efferents are binaural reflexes to the auditory periphery. One of the first experimental tests of the hypothesis of olivocochlear-mediated protection was performed by Trahiotis and Elliott (1970). In an animal study concentrating on the effects of chronic section of the olivocochlear bundle on psychophysical performance, they also tested the degree of TTS after a 10-minute exposure to BBN at 107 dB SPL. They found no significant differences between control and de-efferented cats with respect to the degree of TTS. Little else was done in this area until the pioneering experiments from the Johnstone laboratory in the 1980s investigating TTS in guinea pigs.

In a series of experiments in the 1990s, anesthetized guinea pigs were exposed to a 10 kHz tone at intensities in excess of 100 dB SPL for 1 minute. The TTS was assessed by comparing the "thresholds," before and after the exposure, for the CAP recorded from the round window in response to short tone pips at different test frequencies. The degree of TTS was significantly reduced in animals in which the olivocochlear bundle was stimulated electrically at high rates (e.g., 250–400 shocks/sec) during pure tone oversimulation.

Slow versus Fast Effects of Efferent Stimulation: How Protection Is Produced

It has been known since the 1960s that activation of the olivocochlear bundle increases cochlear thresholds to tones presented in quiet (that is, in the absence of masking noise). This "classic" efferent effect has been demonstrated via measures of CAP, intracellular recordings from inner hair cells, and activity of single auditory nerve fibers. These studies have shown that the time course of classic efferent effects is on the order of 60 milliseconds. However, more recently, it was discovered that there are also "slow" effects that have time constants nearly 1,000 times slower than "classic" effects. Delivery of a 60-second train of shocks to the olivocochlear bundle suppresses the CAP nearly 50%. However, during the shock train, the CAP amplitude slowly declines by a further 20%, and most dramatically, the CAP amplitude remains depressed after the cessation of the shock train and does not return to preshock values until almost 100 seconds later. The slow and fast effects are differentially distributed

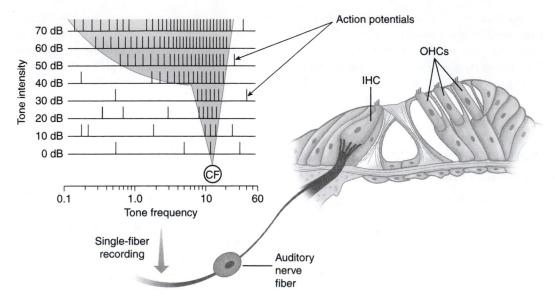

FIGURE 12-5   Tuning curve of a single auditory nerve fiber. The tuning curve outlines the response area *(shaded portion),* which comprises all the frequency and intensity combinations at which a pure tone excites this fiber. The characteristic frequency (CF) is the frequency to which the fiber is most sensitive. IHC, inner hair cells; OHCs, outer hair cells. (Adapted from Liberman and Guinan, 1998.)

along the cochlear partition. Whereas fast effects are largest in the 6 to 12 kHz region of the cochlea, slow effects are quite small in the 6- to 10-kHz cochlear regions and peak in the 14 to 17 kHz region. These slow effects are possibly mediated by lateral efferent neurons.

Antimasking Effects of Olivocochlear Efferents

Frequency resolution is one component of frequency selectivity, and it corresponds closely to the physiologic mechanisms of frequency selectivity measured in auditory neurons. Human and nonhuman subjects have the ability to detect a particular frequency component of a complex stimulus in the presence of other frequency components, all presented simultaneously. The extent to which a subject is able to filter one stimulus out from another on the basis of frequency defines frequency resolution. It is analogous to tuning in a radio receiver so that the filter in the input circuit receives the de-

sired station and rejects all others. The resolution tells us how good it is at passing one station while rejecting others that are close to it in frequency. In the auditory system, resolution bandwidths are a measure of the fundamental frequency filtering properties of the auditory system. However, conditions exist during which the filtering is overwhelmed or masked, making audibility (or discrimination) more difficult. Masking is defined as: (1) the process by which the threshold of audibility for one sound is raised by the presence of another (masking) sound; and (2) the amount by which the threshold of audibility of a sound is increased by the presence of another (masking) sound. Threshold refers to the amount of stimulus energy that can be just detected. The masked threshold is the threshold for the signal measured in the presence of a masker. At threshold, the masker alone and the signal-plus–masker stimuli are discriminable.

To understand how **antimasking** properties of the olivocochlear system arise, we must first consider the physiologic bases for masking at the level of the auditory nerve. A single auditory nerve fiber responds to sound by increasing the rate at which it produces action potentials above its spontaneous rate (SR) (see Chapter 11). In Figure 12-5, action potential traces represent the trains of action potentials as they might appear on an oscilloscope screen while a tone is swept across sound frequencies at sound pressure levels ranging from 0 to 70 dB SPL. In this way a "response area" is constructed, loosely bounded by the frequency tuning curve (see Chapter 11). At low sound pressures, there is a narrow range of frequencies to which it will respond. The frequency to which an auditory nerve fiber is most sensitive is called the characteristic frequency (CF) (see Chapter 11). Addition of noise can increase the thresholds of auditory nerve fiber in two fundamentally different ways; these two mechanisms have been called **excitatory masking** and **suppressive masking.**

Excitatory Masking Figure 12-6 illustrates a high-frequency noise "masker" on the response of the high-CF neuron to a "signal" presented at CF. In the absence of noise, the signal is within the frequency tuning curve of the neuron. The noise band contains energy at frequencies and levels to which the nerve responds. In the presence of noise, the fiber responds vigorously for the duration. Noise-driven excitation increases the fiber's threshold to tones so that the signal no longer elicits a response when the noise is on. The excitation of the fiber by the steady noise is like increasing its background discharge rate. Thus, for a tone signal to cause a response (increase rate), its level must be higher than normal. This phenomenon is much like a line-busy effect; that is, auditory nerve fibers become fatigued by continuous stimulation by noise, and when fatigued, they are less responsive to an additional tran-

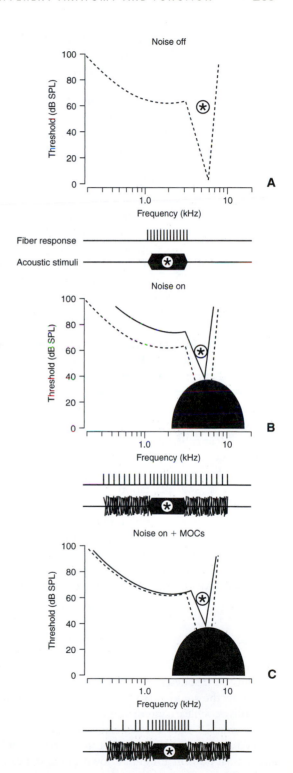

FIGURE 12-6 Antimasking effects of the medial olivocochlear reflex. Effects are schematized for a high-characteristic-frequency (CF) fiber responding to a high-frequency signal without versus with background noise (A vs B) and without versus with medial olivocochlear system (MOC) activation (B vs C). (Adapted from Liberman and Guinan, 1998.)

sient signal such as a tone burst. This rate adaptation probably involves the depletion of neurotransmitter from the synapse (see Chapter 11).

Suppressive Masking The effects of a low-frequency noise band on the responses of the same high-CF fiber to the same high-frequency signal illustrate suppressive masking. In the absence of noise, the fibers respond to the signal. The high-CF fiber does not respond to this low-frequency noise band; however, the inner ear shows striking nonlinearity whereby sound energy placed just below a fiber's response area can increase thresholds near the CF. Suppressive masking shrinks the high-CF response area such that the signal is now outside the tuning curve (TC). Suppressive masking also underlies the phenomenon of the upward spread of masking by low-frequency maskers.

Antimasking Effects of the Medial Olivocochlear System in Normal Ears The high-frequency noise band has energy within the response area of the auditory nerve fiber, and thus will excite the fiber and increase its thresholds to tones via excitatory masking. Addition of the noise with the medial olivocochlear reflex inactivated greatly increases the background discharge rate of the auditory nerve fiber and decreases the response to the signal, because of line-busy and adaptation effects of the steady noise-driven discharge. The medial olivocochlear reflex decreases the steady response to noise by auditory nerve fibers, thereby increasing the response to the signal transient, because the degree of adaptation is reduced (see Figure 12-6). The signal is now easier to detect. Notably, the medial olivocochlear system

does not suppress noise more effectively than the signal, because the noise is broadband, whereas the signal is narrow-band. Rather, the important difference is that the noise is continuous, whereas the signal is transient. The medial olivocochlear reflex acts to minimize the response to long-lasting stimuli (which become "noise" if present for well beyond the time required to decode and react to them), while maximizing the response to novel stimuli. The medial olivocochlear system will not aid in the detection or discrimination of continuous tones in continuous noise. The medial olivocochlear reflex also cannot contribute large antimasking effects for low-frequency noise, because the medial olivocochlear effects are small in the low-frequency regions of the cochlea.

Antimasking Effects of the Medial Olivocochlear System in Impaired Ears Sensorineural hearing loss involving OHC pathology will severely limit the medial olivocochlear antimasking effects because the medial olivocochlear system acts directly through outer hair cells. The medial olivocochlear-mediated attenuation of auditory nerve fiber responses arises via the medial olivocochlear synapses on outer hair cells that reduce the gain of the "cochlear amplifier." Thus, as outer hair cells are progressively damaged or lost, the outer hair cell–based amplification mechanism is reduced and cochlear thresholds are increased. As the amplification is reduced, the ability of the medial olivocochlear system to modulate the amplification is also reduced. With complete loss of outer hair cells, the medial olivocochlear system becomes completely ineffectual.

⌒SUMMARY⌒

Rasmussen first described the efferent olivocochlear system in the middle part of the twentieth century. The olivocochlear system resides in brainstem nuclei associated with the superior olivary complex, located in the ventral portion of the rostral medulla and caudal pons in a region known as the trapezoid body. The efferent olivocochlear pathway has

crossed and uncrossed components. The uncrossed olivocochlear bundle has fibers that project to the ipsilateral ear, whereas the crossed olivocochlear bundle has fibers that project to the contralateral ear. Descending efferent projections from medial regions of the superior olivary complex influence otoacoustic emissions in both ears and play a role in the regulation of afferent fiber responses. Current studies of the efferent olivocochlear system are clarifying how the efferent system works to adapt the afferent system to background noise and provides protection to the ear from exposures to loud sounds. Auditory dysfunction in high-noise backgrounds may be one of the clinical manifestations of a defective efferent olivocochlear system.

∿ KEY TERMS ∿

Acetylcholine	Efferent	Lateral superior olive	Periolivary
Antimasking	Excitatory masking	Masking	Suppressive masking
Binaural	GABA	Medial efferent system	Temporary threshold
Cholinergic	Ipsilateral	Neuropeptides	shift
Contralateral	Lateral efferent system	Olivocochlear	Trapezoid body

∿ STUDY QUESTIONS ∿

1. Where are the cell bodies of medial and lateral olivocochlear neurons located?

2. Olivocochlear axons travel across or in which cranial nerves (tracts)?

3. What are the crossed and uncrossed projections of olivocochlear axons?

4. How do medial and lateral olivocochlear neurons differ with respect to their terminations?

5. What are the primary neurotransmitters used by olivocochlear neurons.

6. When the olivocochlear system is stimulated, what are the effects on the periphery?

7. How does the medial olivocochlear reflex differ from the middle-ear-muscle acoustic reflex?

8. What role does the olivocochlear system play in masking noise?

∿ REFERENCES ∿

Galambos, R. (1956). Suppression of auditory nerve activity by stimulation of efferent fibers to cochlea. *Journal of Neurophysiology, 19*(5), 424–437.

Guinan, J. J. (1996). The physiology of olivocochlear efferents. In P. Dallos, A. N. Popper, & R. R. Fay (pp. 435–502). *The Cochlea.* New York: Springer-Verlag.

Liberman, M. C., & Guinan, J. J. J. (1998). Feedback control of the auditory periphery: Anti-masking effects of middle ear muscles vs. olivocochlear efferents. *Journal of Communication Disorders, 31*(6), 471–482, quiz 483, 553.

Moore, J. K., Simmons, D. D., & Guan Y-L. (1999). The human olivocochlear system: Organization and development. *Audiology and Neuro-otology, 4,* 311–325.

Rasmussen, G. L. (1946). The olivary peduncle and other fiber projections of the superior olivary complex. *Journal of Comparative Neurology, 84,* 141–219.

Rasmussen, G. L. (1953). Further observations of the efferent cochlear bundle. *Journal of Comparative Neurology, 99*(1), 61–74.

Rasmussen, G. L. (1960). Efferent fibers of the cochlear nerve and the cochlear nucleus. In G. L. Rasmussen & W. G. William (Eds.), *Neural mechanisms of the auditory and vestibular systems* (pp. 105–115). Springfield, IL: Charles C. Thomas.

Sahley, T. L., Nodar, R. H., & Musiek, F. E. (1997). *Efferent Auditory System: Structure and Function.* San Diego: Singular.

Trahiotis, C., & Elliott, D. N. (1970). Behavioral investigation of some possible effects of sectioning the crossed olivocochlear bundle. *Journal of the Acoustical Society of America, 47*(2), 592–596.

Ward, W. D. (1970). Temporary threshold and damage-risk criteria for intermittent noise exposures. *Journal of the Acoustical Society of America, 48,* 561–574.

⤳SUGGESTED READING⤳

Evans, M. G. (1996). Acetylcholine activates two currents in guinea-pig outer hair cells. *Journal of Physiology, 491*(pt 2), 563–578.

Eybalin, M. (1993). Neurotransmitters and neuromodulators of the mammalian cochlea. *Physiological Reviews, 73*(2), 309–373.

Le Prell, C. G., Bledsoe, S. C., Bobbin, R. P., & Puel, J. (2001). Neurotransmission in the inner ear: Functional and molecular analyses. In A. F. Jahn & J. Santos-Sacchi (Eds.), *Physiology of the ear* (pp. 575–611). New York: Singular Publishing.

Moore, J. K. (2000). Organization of the human superior olivary complex. *Microscopy Research and Technique, 51*(4), 403–412.

Simmons, D. D. (2002). Development of the inner ear efferent system across vertebrate species. *Journal of Neurobiology, 53*(2), 228–250.

Warr, W. (1991). Organization of olivocochlear efferent systems in mammals. In D. B. Webster (Ed.), *Mammalian auditory pathways: Neuroanatomy* (pp. 383–396). New York: Raven Press.

Warr, W. B. (1975). Olivocochlear and vestibular efferent neurons of the feline brain stem: Their location, morphology and number determined by retrograde axonal transport and acetylcholinesterase histochemistry. *Journal of Comparative Neurology, 161,* 159–181.

Warr, W. B., & Guinan, J. J. (1979). Efferent innervation of the organ of corti: Two separate systems. *Brain Research, 173,* 152–155.

White, J. S., & Warr, W. B. (1983). The dual origins of the olivocochlear bundle in the albino rat. *Journal of Comparative Neurology, 219*(2), 203–214.

Yao, W., & Godfrey, D. A. (1998). Immunohistochemical evaluation of cholinergic neurons in the rat superior olivary complex. *Microscopy Research and Technique, 41*(3), 270–283.

Chapter

13

Otoacoustic Emissions

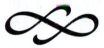

Dwayne D. Simmons, Ph.D.
Associate Professor of Otolaryngology
Washington University School of Medicine
St. Louis, Missouri

A remarkable property of the inner ear is its great sensitivity. From early on it was recognized that such sensitivity could not arise solely from passive responses to sound. Rather, some active amplification mechanism would be required to enhance the vibration of inner ear structures in response to low-level acoustic stimuli. This mechanism has been linked to outer hair cell (OHC) motility and receptor potential and is termed the cochlear amplifier (see Chapters 9 and 10). One of the major discoveries over the past several decades was that the normal ears of humans and other vertebrate animals produce audiofrequency sounds or echoes in response to sounds and, in some cases, spontaneously as well. Metabolic energy is required for the generation of **otoacoustic emissions (OAEs)**. The discovery of low-level emissions provided the first evidence for the presence of an active amplification mechanism within the inner ear. Since their discovery, OAEs have been reported to be present in all classes of terrestrial vertebrates, suggesting that they reflect a fundamental property of normal hearing. Because OAEs can be recorded noninvasively, they provide an important tool to hearing researchers. These emissions can be measured by placing a sensitive microphone in the ear canal. In humans and animals, OAEs are widely used to study cochlear function and the efferent system. The origin of OAEs is ascribed to processes associated with the mechanical motion of the OHCs, and efferent olivocochlear pathways can modulate OAEs. In clinical settings, OAEs are often used for diagnostic screening of frequency-dependent cochlear function or middle ear damage. OAEs are sensitive to subtle changes in cochlear function that are not revealed in the standard audiogram. With OAEs, clinicians have acquired a sensitive new tool for use in screening the various types of hearing loss.

WHAT ARE OTOACOUSTIC EMISSIONS?

OAEs are echoes within the ear canal that are generated from distortions within the cochlea, either spontaneously or in response to acoustic stimulation. These **cochlear echoes** are subaudible (low-level) sounds and can be recorded from the external ear canal using sensitive low-noise microphones. David Kemp (1978) was the first to publish measurements of OAEs. Kemp found that when a click is directed into the ear, it is followed by a cochlear echo with a peak latency between 5–15 milliseconds. Although much of the early research on OAEs was concerned with replicating Kemp's original observations, subsequent work has not only confirmed Kemp's findings, but also extended them to nearly all vertebrate species. Clinically, the measurement of OAEs is increasingly the first line of assessment for hearing disorders and lends itself extremely useful in assessing newborn hearing.

Recordings of OAEs are made via an ear canal probe that is inserted deeply into the ear canal (Figure 13-1). Having the probe seal the ear canal is an essential part of OAE measurement. A good seal enables any oscillatory movement of the eardrum to maximize OAE collection and minimize any ambient noise. The tympanic membrane motions responsible for OAEs are subatomic in scale. Usually click stimuli of about 84 dB SPL evokes a robust OAE response only if hearing threshold is 20 dB hearing level or better. A probe device containing both a sound source (an earphone) and a microphone occludes the ear when inserted. A click or other acoustic stimulus is presented to the ear, and the sound pressure is measured over time. If the probe is inserted into a **Zwislocki coupler** (a metal cavity that has the same impedance characteristics as the human ear), there is a damped oscillation (the passive impulse response of the coupler). In the human ear, in addition to the damped oscillation (6 milliseconds), there is a much smaller oscillation occurring after a latency of roughly 6 to 7 milliseconds. The initial oscillations are the passive impulse responses of the ear. The later and smaller oscillations constitute the cochlear echo of the evoked OAE. Unlike other audiometric tests, it is not necessary for the stimulus to be near to threshold levels to detect abnormal function using OAEs. **Spontaneous otoacoustic emissions (SOAEs)** were the first type to be discovered. Since Kemp's classic description of OAE in 1978, SOAEs have been studied extensively in normal and pathologic ears of infants, children, and adults. Sometimes these SOAEs can be at high levels.

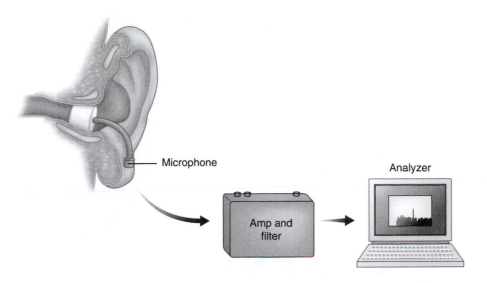

FIGURE 13-1 Schematic of basic instrumentation for measuring spontaneous emissions.

The SOAE in Figure 13-2 was recorded from a young boy who was not aware of the high-level emission. Importantly, middle ear status affects OAEs and can prevent their detection.

The field of OAE research has grown enormously since OAEs were discovered in the late 1970s. The increasing availability of various commercial devices for measuring OAEs makes it important that the clinician or other hearing professional have a basic understanding of OAEs. It is important to keep in mind that the widespread clinical use of OAEs is just beginning and our knowledge of all the strengths and weaknesses of OAE clinical application is incomplete.

From Where Do Otoacoustic Emissions Originate?

The exact source of OAEs is debatable. Detectable OAE sound pressure is produced by extremely small vibrations of the eardrum (tympanic membrane). For example, an eardrum oscillation of only 10 nm (roughly the equivalent of the diameter of a hydrogen atom) can create an OAE intensity of 34-dB SPL. To understand how OAEs are generated, we need to review some basics of cochlear micromechanics.

Fluid motions across the cochlear partition (scala vestibuli and scala tympani) displace the basilar membrane, but only the portion of the basilar membrane that is tuned to the frequency of stapes vibration (see Chapter 9). Recall that von Békésy originally demonstrated that the basilar membrane is stiff near the cochlear base and more compliant nearer the apex. Thus, near the base, where stiffness is high, stiffness governs the resultant vibration. Toward the apex, where stiffness is lower, the mass and inertial force acting on the system limit vibration. Because a **stiffness-limited system** always starts to move before a mass-limited system, basal regions will move first followed by apical portions that are more mass-limited. This means that a pressure difference across the cochlear partition causes a transverse wave of deflection that travels up the cochlea (i.e., from base to apex). Sound-induced displacements of cochlear fluids interact with the stiffness and mass of the basilar membrane to produce a progressive basal-to-apical traveling wave on the membrane. The maximal or peak displacement of the basilar membrane is the place where, for a given stimulus frequency, the force of inertia equals and cancels the elastic restoring force, that is, resonance. Because the inertial forces increase with frequency, the place along the basilar membrane at

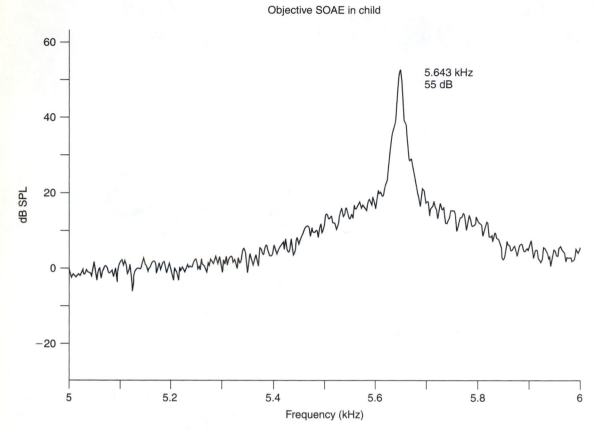

FIGURE 13-2 Waveform of a spontaneous otoacoustic emission from a normal-hearing 2.5-year-old boy. SOAE, spontaneous otoacoustic emissions; SPL, sound pressure level.

which this peak in the traveling wave occurs tuned as a function of distance along the basilar membrane (Figure 13-3).

Traveling waves produced by high-frequency sounds have peak displacement amplitude near the cochlear base, and traveling waves produced by low-frequency sounds come to a peak displacement near the cochlear apex. The traveling wave envelope corresponds to the excitation intensity applied to the organ of Corti as a function of distance along the length of the cochlea. The basilar membrane motion is converted to fluid motion across hair cell stereocilia, leading to receptor cell stimulation and then neural excitation. However, basilar membrane motion by itself leads only to passive, broadly tuned traveling waves caused by high levels of viscous

damping by cochlear structures as can be found, for example, in a deaf or cadaver ear. The sharpness of the peak of the traveling wave is achieved by the addition of active mechanisms associated with the OHC motility (see Chapter 10). These active mechanisms provide additional mechanical energy that directly opposes the viscous drag caused by cochlear structures. If the active mechanisms provide energy that exceeds viscous drag, then excitation will be increased above that delivered by the stimulus (amplification) and sharpen the peak displacement of the traveling wave.

OAEs provide clear signs of the reaction of the cochlea to sound and activation of active processes thought to be critical to the exquisite sensitivity and frequency discrimination of normal hearing.

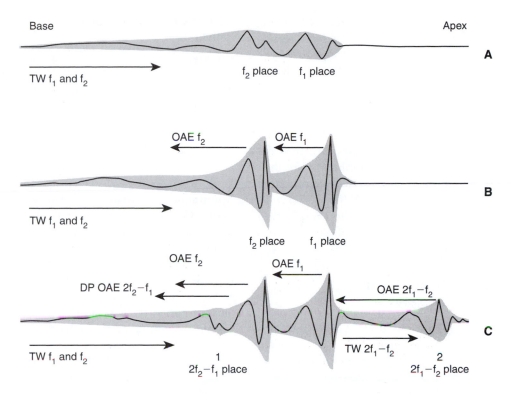

FIGURE 13-3 Schematic illustration of the sources of distortion product otoacoustic emissions. In response to two tones with frequencies f_1 and f_2 such that $f_2/f_1=1.2$, traveling waves (TW) with peaks at the places where these frequencies are represented are produced. (A) The passive mechanical response of the basilar membrane (BM) to input f_1 and f_2 if there were no amplification. (B) Amplification of the BM response produced by the active OHC process for f_1 and f_2 generates recordable emissions at these frequencies. (C) Nonlinear interactions of amplified mechanical responses create distortion that is propagated basally to the $2f_2-f_1$ place and apically to the $2f_1-f_2$ place. The distortion signals are propagated forward to the auditory nervous system and backward through the middle ear into the ear canal. (Adapted from Kemp, 2002.)

OAEs reflect active mechanisms also known as the "cochlear amplifier" that are preneural (i.e., before the afferent nerve synapses with hair cells) and occur along the cochlear partition (see Chapters 9 and 10). The cochlear amplifier is essential to the high sensitivity of hearing and to the formation of a sharp (roughly 0.25 octave resolution) tonotopic "image" of the acoustic environment along the length of the cochlea. As Figure 13-3 indicates, OAEs are a by-product of this cochlear amplifier. They arrive in the ear canal as a result of basilar membrane motion that escapes from the cochlear amplifier mechanism and travel away from the sensory hair cells back to the base of the cochlea. There, the motion of the basilar membrane exerts a

differential oscillating fluid pressure on the oval and round windows, causing vibration of the ossicles and eardrum and hence giving rise to OAEs. Thus, OAEs are a by-product of normal cochlear function that involve nonlinearities and irregularities of cochlear amplification added to the traveling wave.

OAEs can be generated only if the cochlear amplifier is present and operational. Thus, OAEs are sensitive indicators of the functional state of cochlear amplification. When, for example, the OHCs are missing or selectively damaged, not only is hearing sensitivity significantly compromised, but there are no OAEs. That OAEs are independent of eighth nerve activity is shown by experiments where OAEs are still measured when eighth nerve responses are blocked. In addition, OAEs are vulnerable to noxious agents, such as ototoxic drugs, intense noise, and hypoxia, which are known to affect the cochlea in general and OHCs in particular. For these and other reasons, the OHCs are strongly implicated and are widely accepted as the generators of OAEs. However, current debate centers on the details of the underlying processes: Are they direct manifestations of OHC motility, or are they reflections of energy in the traveling wave with a contribution from OHCs? If OHCs do serve to produce a positive feedback in the transduction process, then the occurrence of spontaneous OAEs is not that surprising.

What Are the Various Types of Otoacoustic Emissions?

OAEs are typically measured in terms of their frequency and level components. They are detected within the ear canal using narrowband filtering, which usually involves spectral analysis of the signal. OAEs may be classified as either spontaneous or evoked sounds that can be recorded from the closed ear canal (Table 13-1). SOAEs occur in the absence of external stimulation; that is, they require no external stimulus to elicit a response. Evoked OAEs occur during or after external sound stimulation. Evoked OAEs may be further subdivided into three classes, each requiring a different type of external stimulus. **Transient-evoked otoacoustic emissions (TEOAEs)** are obtained in response to brief stimuli such as clicks or tone bursts. **Distortion product otoacoustic emissions (DPOAEs)** are produced by pairs of pure tones. Stimulus-frequency otoacoustic emissions (SFOAEs) are generated by presentation of continuous tonal stimuli. Whereas SOAEs and SFOAEs are based on spectral averaging, in which a number of fast Fourier transforms (FFTs) of the waveforms are summed and then averaged, TEOAEs and DPOAEs are detected using standard stimulus-locked averaging. Consequently, the spectral analysis of TEOAEs and DPOAEs is performed on the average time waveform.

TABLE 13-1 Classification of Otoacoustic Emissions

Category	Type	Stimulus
Spontaneous	Spontaneous	None
Evoked	Transient	Clicks or tone bursts
	Distortion product	Pairs of pure tones
	Stimulus frequency	Swept pure tones

Spontaneous Otoacoustic Emissions Spontaneous OAEs are continuous frequency responses with narrow bandwidths near 1 Hz. They are recorded by coupling a sensitive, miniature microphone to the external ear canal. Noise from the ear canal is amplified, high-pass filtered, and delivered to a spectrum analyzer or FFT software for spectral analysis to detect a typical SOAE frequency. An SOAE is a definite, tonelike narrowband frequency response that is at least 3 dB above the noise floor (Figure 13-4). Generally, SOAEs have a substantial latency or time lag that characterizes the acoustic response. The latency can vary from 2–20 milliseconds or more after stimulation with an acoustic click. These SOAEs may appear at 1–5 or more frequencies between 0.5 and 9.0 kHz, but typically are concentrated in the frequency region from 1 to 3 kHz. Frequencies below 0.5 kHz are not typically measured because of the filters used to eliminate low-frequency physiologic noise during recording. The amplitude of SOAEs range from about −25-dB SPL up to 20-dB SPL, with the majority falling between −10- and +10-dB SPL. Audible SOAEs up to 50-dB SPL have been reported in, for example, dogs and occasionally humans. In human ears, SOAEs have not been recorded in the presence of hearing loss greater than 25–30 dB, although they may be detected in some ears with mild sensorineural hearing loss. Although SOAE frequencies are relatively stable over short periods, they are vulnerable to adverse metabolic conditions.

Most normal-hearing adults and infants produce measurable SOAEs in the absence of external stimulation. The prevalence of SOAEs is less than evoked emissions and SOAEs may be sex and ear

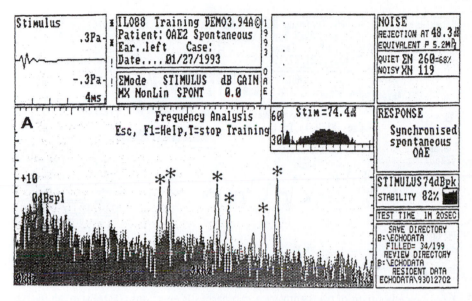

FIGURE 13-4 Typical recordings of spontaneous otoacoustic emissions (SOAEs; *asterisks*) from a normal-hearing ear.

dependent. However, estimates of the prevalence of SOAEs depend on the instrumentation and data collection procedure used to obtain them. Approximately twice as many women as men exhibit SOAEs, and they are more often observed in right ears than in left ears. Several studies have reported genetic differences in the prevalence of SOAEs. Infants, children, and young adults have the same prevalence of SOAEs; however, newborn and infant ears have typically higher frequency SOAEs (between 3 and 4 kHz). For subjects older than 60 years, the prevalence of SOAEs appears to decrease. To date, there has been little, if any, correlation between SOAEs and the sensation of tinnitus.

Transient-Evoked Otoacoustic Emissions
TEOAEs are complex acoustic responses that can be recorded in nearly all persons with normal hearing. The TEOAEs are usually elicited by wide-band clicks of about 48-dB SPL and displayed primarily as a combined cross- (emission) and difference-power (noise) spectrum of averaged response waveforms. After a brief stimulus such as a click or tone burst, a frequency dispersive waveform can be obtained (Figure 13-5). Generally, the spectrum of a TEOAE elicited from a normal ear reflects the spectrum of the stimulus. Thus, TEOAEs obtained in response to clicks are expected to have broad response spectra, and those obtained in response to tone bursts are quite frequency specific. In addition to the sensitive low-noise microphone used for recording SOAEs, the probe contains a miniature sound source for delivering the stimulus. Responses to multiple stimuli are averaged to extract the TEOAE signal from background noise. In a typical TEOAE recording, the ear canal sound pressure is amplified by a factor of 100–10,000 and high-pass filtered at 300–400 Hz. The TEOAE signal is then digitized at a rate of 40–50 kHz and averaged using routines similar to auditory-evoked potentials. Typical measurement parameters in available commercial devices (all either manufactured or licensed by Otodynamics Ltd., United Kingdom) include signal-to-noise ratio, absolute TEOAE level in decibels SPL, and percentage reproducibility of the two averaged response waveforms. It needs to be emphasized that the measured response will be determined by the evoking stimulus and recording parameters, as well as the status of the middle ear and ear canal.

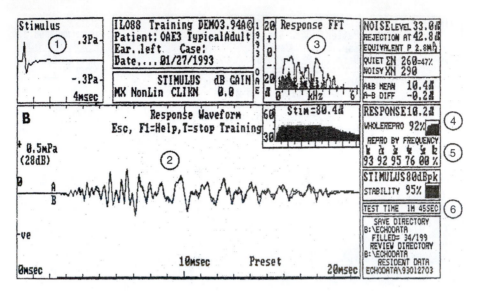

FIGURE 13-5 Typical measurement of transiently evoked otoacoustic emissions (TEOAEs) in adults. (1) Stimulus, (2) response to two separate trials (A and B), (3) fast Fourier transform (FFT) of the response showing the background noise (black) and the responses (white), (4) overall reproducibility of the response, (5) reproducibility as a function of frequency, and (6) test time.

TEOAEs are sensitive to cochlear loss because the recording is made during the interval of silence between stimulus presentations. In addition, TEOAEs are highly sensitive to cochlear pathology and in a frequency-specific way. Frequencies at which hearing thresholds exceed 20–30 dB hearing loss are typically absent in the TEOAE response. Because of their sensitivity to cochlear dysfunction, TEOAEs have found widespread application in newborn hearing screening. Healthy infant ears typically produce strong OAE levels of 15-dB SPL to more than 30-dB SPL. Little signal processing is required to extract these responses from noise, and fully validated frequency-specific measurements can often be made in a few seconds. This contrasts with recordings of the auditory brainstem response (ABR), which require electrodes and must be extracted from the relatively much stronger electroencephalographic (EEG) background signal over a longer period of signal averaging. Although TEOAEs have high sensitivity and speed, they cannot be used for high-frequency hearing assessment.

Unfortunately, high-frequency TEOAEs emerge quickly and are lost in the stimulus portion of the recording.

Distortion Product Otoacoustic Emissions In addition to using short-duration stimuli, robust OAEs can be generated in response to two simultaneous, tone stimuli (f_1 and f_2). These DPOAEs have nonlinear characteristics: They do not grow in proportion to the input, and they give rise to distortion products. In the cochlea, distortion products result from the intermodulation of two pure tones (Figure 13-6). The distortion product is a tonal signal that is not present in the eliciting pure-tone stimuli (see Figure 13-3). By convention, the lower frequency tone is referred to as the f_1 primary, and its corresponding level, L_1; the higher frequency tone is the f_2 primary with a corresponding level, L_2. The largest DPOAEs recorded in all mammals occur at $2f_1 - f_2$, although DPOAEs are present at other frequencies including other cubic (e.g., $2f_2 - f_1$, $3f_1 - 2f_2$) and quadratic distortion products (e.g.,

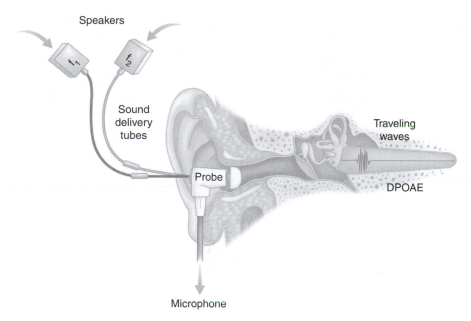

FIGURE 13-6   (See Color Plate) Schematic of basic instrumentation for measuring distortion product emissions (DPOAE).

$f_2 - f_1$). The intensity of the cubic difference product ($2f_1 - f_2$) is routinely used as an indicator of cochlear status. The levels of $2f_1 - f_2$ DPOAE vary systematically with parameters of the simultaneously applied primary tones (f_1, f_2) including absolute frequencies, frequency separation (f_2/f_1), absolute level of primaries (L_1 and L_2), and the level difference ($L_1 - L_2$). Typically, the level of the cubic difference tone is plotted as a function of one of the primary frequencies in the **DP-gram** (see Figure 13-8). Although TEOAEs are absent in some animals such as gerbils, all animals appear to produce DPOAEs. In humans, the level of the $2f_1 - f_2$ DPOAE is greatest when the f_2/f_1 ratio is roughly 1.22 and when $L_1 - L_2 = 0$ dB at high stimulus levels, increasing to $L_1 - L_2 = 30$ dB or more at low stimulus levels. Healthy ear canal $2f_1 - f_2$ DPOAE levels may be greater than 20-dB SPL. However, typical DPOAEs are smaller (i.e., 5- to 15-dB SPL) and are usually 60- to 70-dB SPL less than stimulus levels. A significantly reduced or absent DPOAE suggests hearing loss caused by either middle ear or cochlear pathologic factors.

The probe typically contains a miniature microphone and two miniature speakers to measure DPOAEs (see Figure 13-6). The probe is tightly sealed into the ear canal. In contrast with TEOAEs, DPOAEs are measured in the presence of the primary tones. Typical DP-gram measurement consists of a series of DPOAE measurements at $2f_1 - f_2$ with the stimulus frequency swept between 1 and 6 kHz (Figure 13-7). General agreement exists that DPOAEs are most easily detected if the ratio of primary stimulus frequencies is between 1.2:1 and 1.3:1. The relative level of the intensities has a significant effect on the DPOAE response, and it is generally agreed that the level of f_1 may be equal to or greater than the level of f_2 to advantage. No advantage has been noted by reducing the level of f_1 below that of f_2. The frequency sweep is repeated and the data are averaged. As more data are collected, the noise contamination will decline in value, revealing the DPOAE data standing above the noise level. The protocols typically used for clinical testing of DPOAEs are given in Figure 13-8.

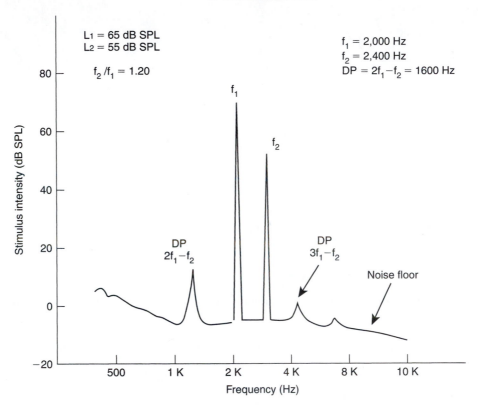

DPOAE measurement

L₁ = 65 dB SPL
L₂ = 55 dB SPL

$f_2/f_1 = 1.20$

f_1 = 2,000 Hz
f_2 = 2,400 Hz
DP = $2f_1 - f_2$ = 1600 Hz

FIGURE 13-7 Generic representation of spectra of ear canal sound pressure from the ear of a normal-hearing adult. Shown are the stimulus frequencies (f_1 and f_2) and the cubic distortion products (DPs) ($2f_1 - f_2$ and $3f_1 - f_2$). Sound levels (L_1 and L_2) for stimulus frequencies (f_1 and f_2) differ by 10-dB sound pressure level (SPL).

A wide range of frequencies of stimulation readily produces DPOAEs, although they are more difficult to measure reliably below 1,000 Hz because of noise. Unlike TEOAEs, DPOAE measurement does not depend on the time delay of DPOAE for its detection, so the technique is effective at higher frequencies. However, higher levels of stimulation are needed to keep recording times short, because each frequency band has to be measured separately. This means that DPOAEs are a little less sensitive to slight cochlear disorders leading to only 10 to 20 dB hearing loss. DPOAEs give you high-frequency assessment but compromise on sensitivity to gain speed.

The combination of TEOAE followed by DPOAE provides a comprehensive view of cochlear status not afforded by either technique alone (high sensitivity, speed, and high-frequency effectiveness).

Is It Possible to Suppress Otoacoustic Emissions?

OAEs are not only valuable in analyzing the integrity of individual ears, they can also be used to evaluate interactions between the two ears by studying OAE suppression after presentation of additional stimuli to the same, opposite, or both ears. A number of studies have described suppression of SOAEs, TEOAEs, and DPOAEs in humans by contralateral sound stimuli. Efferent suppression effects observed in humans are consistent with suppression of both cochlear emissions and auditory nerve activity observed in animal

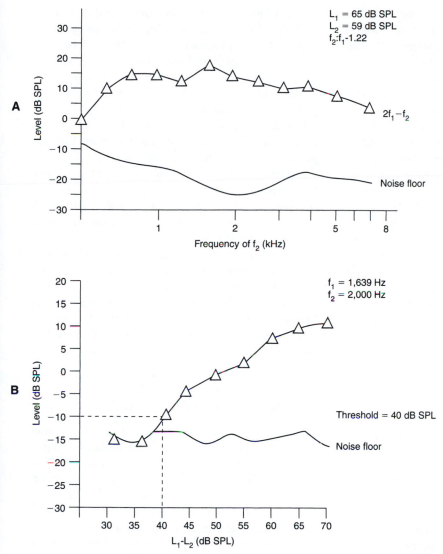

$L_1 = 65$ dB SPL
$L_2 = 59$ dB SPL
$f_2:f_1$-1.22

A — $2f_1-f_2$

Noise floor

Frequency of f_2 (kHz)

$f_1 = 1,639$ Hz
$f_2 = 2,000$ Hz

B

Threshold = 40 dB SPL

Noise floor

L_1-L_2 (dB SPL)

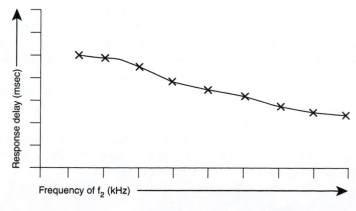

C

Frequency of f_2 (kHz)

FIGURE 13-8 The effect of f_1 and f_2 frequency and relative level on DPOAE amplitude. (A) shows a DP-gram, a plot of $2f_1-f_2$ amplitude versus stimulus frequency (typically either by f_2 or the geometric mean of f_1 and f_2). (B) shows dependence of $2f_1-f_2$ on the relative level of f_1. The response is largest when f_1 is ~10 dB more intense than f_2. This probably reflects the fact that the f_2 place on the basilar membrane (where the two responses interact nonlinearly) is less sensitive to f_1. (C) shows that the latency of the response will be greater for low-frequency f_2, due to traveling wave delay.

studies. The mechanical motion of the OHCs is controlled, in part, through the efferent auditory pathways via the olivocochlear system. Because descending medial efferent fibers preferentially terminate on OHCs, the prevailing view is that the dynamic properties of OHCs are modulated, at least in part, by the descending medial efferent system (see Chapter 12). Efferent suppression of TEOAEs is characterized as a reduction in emission amplitude and/or a time change or phase shift. Animal studies show that direct stimulation of medial efferents (via bipolar electric currents) causes a 20% to 66% reduction in the $(2f_1 - f_2)$ DPOAEs. A direct cochlear infusion of acetylcholine (together with acetylcholinesterase inhibitor eserine) mimics the effects of direct medial efferent stimulation, by producing small but significant reductions in the $2f_1 - f_2$ DPOAEs. The 4- to 6-dB contralateral sound-activated suppression of the DPOAE is reversed by surgical interruption of the medial efferent fibers crossing the midline of the brainstem. Such experiments further support the notion that the OHCs are dynamic, force-generating, "mechanical effectors" responsible for the generation of nonlinearities (like DPOAEs) within the cochlea.

What Are Some of the Clinical Applications of Otoacoustic Emissions?

OAEs are now a valuable part of the test battery approach for determining an auditory site of lesion. Clinical applications have focused on TEOAEs and DPOAEs in the evaluation of cochlear function, screening for hearing loss in newborns, and monitoring changes in cochlear function. Emissions are generally absent in ears that exhibit partial or complete hearing loss. In general, OAEs are sensitive to cochlear pathology, so clinical applications are evolving. Increasingly, OAEs are considered a "site-of-lesion" test. For example, they have been used to detect cochlear dysfunction associated with eighth nerve tumors and to detect cochlear dysfunction accompanying meningitis.

OAEs are well suited for hearing screening that involves difficult-to-test subjects including infants who cannot respond to the tester. Because of porta-bility, industrial settings and schools lend themselves well to OAE hearing screening. They can be useful in monitoring progressive hearing loss, ototoxicity, middle ear surgery, and noise-induced hearing loss. However, the absence of DPOAEs may indicate inner or middle ear pathology. This should be investigated with tympanometry. The presence of DPOAEs with hearing loss does not prove but is consistent with a retrocochlear function. Electrophysiologic confirmation of auditory function should be undertaken in cases where there is risk for neurologic involvement, for example, after serious jaundice in newborns. In general, infants with known risk factors for hearing impairment should receive both OAE and ABR tests.

In summary, the presence of true OAE activity means that some degree of normal cochlear function is present. However, middle ear as well as cochlear pathology can block OAEs. It is also important to remember that no precise relation to the threshold of hearing has been determined. The decibel level of OAE responses is not clinically informative.

Are There Clinical Advantages of Otoacoustic Emission Testing?

OAE measurement techniques have several distinct advantages over more traditional audiologic tests. First, these techniques are objective; that is, no behavioral responses are required from the patient. Second, OAE tests are efficient and can be accomplished in a few minutes. Third, OAE measurements are noninvasive: Signal delivery and OAE response detection are accomplished via a small probe that is held in place by a soft, disposable ear tip. Fourth, OAE measurements are extremely sensitive to the overall status of cochlear function, and they are useful in site-of-lesion testing to distinguish sensory (i.e., cochlear) from neural hearing loss. And finally, it has been suggested that deficits in the contralateral suppression of OAEs may provide yet another objective, noninvasive clinical test for an exploration of the active, nonlinear micromechanics of the OHCs and the clinical neurologic evaluation of auditory brainstem pathways, specifically in general and descending efferent fiber pathways.

Newborn Screening

The early identification of children with hearing impairment is an important public health objective in the United States. Each year in the United States, approximately 1.5 to 3 per 1,000 children are born with significant hearing impairment. With an annual birth rate of approximately 4 million infants, this prevalence rate translates into as many as 33 children born with hearing impairment each day. Up until recently, many of these children were not identified until the second year of life or later, despite advances in the technology available for the early detection of hearing impairment. Currently, many infants have their hearing tested before leaving the hospital in the first days of life. The tests are simple and inexpensive. They take only a few minutes to perform and are noninvasive and painless. Newborn hearing screening is important. The consequences of a late diagnosis of hearing impairment are significant delays in spoken language and literacy. Without appropriate and timely identification and intervention, early childhood hearing impairment interferes with the development of oral/aural communication, impedes academic performance, and results in long-term vocational consequences. Finding hearing loss early helps to prevent such consequences.

A National Institutes of Health Consensus Conference held in March of 1993 recommended hearing screening of all newborns, termed *universal newborn hearing screening.* Access to the largest possible number of newborns is necessary to promote early identification of hearing impairment for all infants and subsequent referral for diagnosis and intervention. The best opportunity for achieving this goal appears to be provided by the development of hearing screening programs for newborns in hospital nurseries or in birthing centers before discharge. Screening programs are typically referred to as Early Hearing Detection and Intervention (EHDI). This title is popular because detecting a hearing loss is just the first step.

Hospitals routinely screen infants for some specific problems, such as PKU (phenylketonuria). Children born with this rare genetic disorder cannot metabolize a part of protein in food. Interestingly, hearing loss occurs more often in infants than any of the other problems that are screened for at birth. Approximately 1 to 3 per 1,000 infants are born with permanent hearing loss.

Based on a review of published data, a physiologic response implemented with objective response criteria best meets the above requirements. Acceptable approaches include: (1) ABR, (2) TEOAE or DPOAE, or (3) a combination of OAE and ABR. Future research may yield additional objective, physiologic measures that could advance universal newborn hearing screening. For the ABR test, sounds are played to the infant's ear. Adhesive bandage-like electrodes are placed on the infant's head and detect electrical activity evoked by the sound. Hearing loss is detected when there is an absence of evoked electrical activity. For the EOAE test, a miniature earphone and microphone are placed in the ear, sounds are played, and a response is measured. If an infant hears normally, an echo is reflected back into the ear canal and picked up by the microphone. When an infant has a hearing loss, no echo can be measured on the EOAE test.

When an infant's results of the newborn hearing-screening test are abnormal, this does not necessarily mean there is hearing loss. It is possible that an infant with normal hearing does not respond positively to the newborn hearing-screening test. Several common reasons include obstructed ear canal, middle ear fluid, and movements and/or crying during the test. Most infants pass the follow-up hearing testing. In the United States, between 20 and 100 infants per 1,000 (or 2–10%) do not pass the initial screening test. Only 1 to 3 infants per 1,000 (less than 1%) actually have hearing loss. Therefore, the majority of infants referred for follow-up testing will demonstrate normal hearing.

Although rare, sometimes hearing loss is not detected by the initial hearing screen. Some mild hearing losses or losses that affect only some frequencies may not be picked up by the initial screening tests. In addition, some infants have hearing loss that is not present at birth. These infants are born with normal hearing, but hearing loss develops after the newborn period. This condition may result from certain illnesses or from some genetic causes. Hearing loss after the newborn period may also happen because of the use of certain medications or as a result of trauma or disease.

If the results of the screening test are abnormal, the first step is to rescreen using additional techniques. A diagnostic ABR test is done. Recall that ABR was discussed earlier, but that was a screening version of the test. A diagnostic ABR is a more thorough test of infant hearing than the ABR screening. A diagnostic ABR is a test that helps determine how much hearing loss is present for these different frequencies. The goal of this test is to find

Continues

the lowest sound levels that produce a response for low-, middle-, and high-frequency sounds.

If an infant is tested before 2 months of age, testing usually can be done while the infant is sleeping naturally. If an infant is older or very active, a liquid medicine may be used to make your baby sleepy. This will ensure that the infant's movements do not interfere with the test. If the infant passes the ABR test, no further testing is needed.

However, babies should continue to be watched for hearing loss that occurs after the newborn period.

If diagnostic testing shows that an infant has a hearing loss, it is essential that appropriate services begin as soon as a diagnosis of hearing loss is made. The Joint Committee on Infant Hearing and the American Academy of Pediatrics recommend that services should begin before 6 months of age, if at all possible.

⌁SUMMARY⌁

One of the major discoveries over the past several decades was that the normal ears of humans and other vertebrate animals produce audiofrequency sounds or echoes in response to sounds and, in some cases, spontaneously as well. These echoes have been linked to the ear's great sensitivity. Both the ear's sensitivity and the production of acoustic echoes or OAEs result from an active amplification mechanism that enhances the vibration of inner ear structures in response to low-level acoustic stimuli. This mechanism has been linked to OHC motility and receptor potential and is termed the *cochlear amplifier*. Metabolic energy is required for the generation of OAEs. Since their discovery, OAEs

have been reported to be present in all classes of terrestrial vertebrates, suggesting that they reflect a fundamental property of normal hearing. Because OAEs can be recorded noninvasively, they provide an important tool to hearing researchers. In humans and animals, OAEs are widely used to study cochlear function, as well as the efferent system where stimulation of efferent olivocochlear pathways can modulate OAE responses. OAEs are sensitive to subtle changes in cochlear function that are not demonstrated in the standard audiogram. Clinicians typically use OAEs for diagnostic screening of frequency-dependent cochlear function or middle ear damage.

⌁KEY TERMS⌁

Cochlear echo
DP-gram
Distortion product otoacoustic emissions (DPOAEs)

Otoacoustic emission (OAE)
Spontaneous otoacoustic emissions (SOAEs)

Stiffness-limited system
Transient otoacoustic emissions (TEOAEs)

Zwislocki coupler

⌁STUDY QUESTIONS⌁

1. Define OAEs.
2. How are OAEs classified, and what stimuli are used to generate OAEs?
3. How do OAEs originate? Provide evidence to support your arguments.

4. What are the clinical advantages of OAE testing over more traditional audiologic tests?
5. How does stimulation of the olivocochlear system affect OAEs?

⌣SUGGESTED READING〰

Anderson, S. D., & Kemp, D. T. (1979). The evoked cochlear mechanical response in laboratory primates. A preliminary report. *Archives of Oto-rhino-laryngology, 224*(1-2), 47–54.

Berlin, C. I., Hood, L. J., Hurley, A., & Wen, H. (1994). The First Jerger Lecture. Contralateral suppression of otoacoustic emissions: An index of the function of the medial olivocochlear system. *Otolaryngology and Head and Neck Surgery, 110*(1), 3–21.

Berlin, C. I., Hood, L. J., Hurley, A. E., Wen, H., & Kemp, D. T. (1995). Binaural noise suppresses linear click-evoked otoacoustic emissions more than ipsilateral or contralateral noise. *Hearing Research, 87*(1-2), 96–103.

Berlin, C. I., Hood, L. J., Wen, H., Szabo, P., Cecola, R. P., Rigby, P., & Jackson, D. F. (1993). Contralateral suppression of non-linear click-evoked otoacoustic emissions. *Hearing Research, 71*(1-2), 1–11.

Brownell, W. E. (1990). Outer hair cell electromotility and otoacoustic emissions. *Ear and Hearing, 11*(2), 82–92.

Burns, E. M., Campbell, S. L., & Arehart, K. H. (1994). Longitudinal measurements of spontaneous otoacoustic emissions in infants. *Journal of the Acoustical Society of America, 95*(1), 385–394.

Gold, T. (1948). Hearing II. The physical basis of the action of the cochlea. *Proceedings of the Royal Society of London. Series B: Biological Sciences, 135,* 492–298.

Hall III, W. H. (2000). *Handbook of otoacoustic emissions.* San Diego: Singular.

Harris, F. & Probst, R. (2002). Otoacoustic emissions and audiometric outcomes. In Robinette, M. S. & Glattke, T. J. (Eds.), *Otoacoustic emissions—clinical applications* (2nd ed.) (pp. 213–242). New York: Thieme.

Kemp, D. T. (1978). Stimulated acoustic emissions from within the human auditory system. *Journal of the Acoustical Society of America, 64(5),* 1386–1391.

Kemp, D. T. (1979). Evidence of mechanical nonlinearity and frequency selective wave amplification in the cochlea. *Archives of Oto-rhino-laryngology, 224*(1-2), 37–45.

Kemp, D. T. (1998). *Otoacoustic emissions: Basic science and clinical applications.* San Diego: Singular Publishing Group.

Kemp, D. T. (2002). Otoacoustic emissions, their origin in cochlear function, and use. *British Medical Bulletin, 63,* 223–241.

Kujawa, S. G., Glattke, T. J., Fallon, M., & Bobbin, R. P. (1992). Intracochlear application of acetylcholine alters sound-induced mechanical events within the cochlear partition. *Hearing Research, 61,* 106–116.

Margolis, R. (2002). Influence of middle ear disease on otoacoustic emissions. In Robinette, M. S. & Glattke, T. J. (Eds.), *Otoacoustic emissions—Clinical Applications* (2nd ed.) (pp. 192–212). New York: Thieme.

Mathis, A., Probst, R., De Min, N., & Hauser, R. (1991). A child with an unusually high-level spontaneous otoacoustic emission. *Archives of Otolaryngology—Head and Neck Surgery, 117*(6), 674–676.

Musiek, F. E. (1999). Central auditory tests. *Scandinavian Audiology Supplementum, 51,* 33–46.

Ohlms, L. A., Lonsbury-Martin, B. L., & Martin, G. K. (1991). Acoustic-distortion products: Separation of sensory from neural dysfunction in sensorineural hearing loss in human beings and rabbits. *Otolaryngology and Head and Neck Surgery, 104*(2), 159–174.

Penner, M. J., & Zhang, T. (1997). Prevalence of spontaneous otoacoustic emissions in adults revisited. *Hearing Research, 103*(1-2), 28–34.

Prieve, B. (2002). Otoacoustic emissions in neonatal screening. In Robinette, M. S. & Glattke, T. J. (Eds.), *Otoacoustic emissions—Clinical applications* (2nd ed.) (pp. 348–374. New York: Thieme.

Probst, R., Lonsbury-Martin, B. L., & Martin, G. K. (1991). A review of otoacoustic emissions. *Journal of the Acoustical Society of America, 89*(5), 2027–2067.

Puel, J. L., & Rebillard, G. (1990). Effect of contralateral sound stimulation on the distortion product 2F1-F2: Evidence that the medial efferent system is involved. *Journal of the Acoustical Society of America, 87*(4), 1630–165.

Robinette, M. S., Cevette, M. J. & Webb, T. M. (2002). Otoacoustic emissions in differential diagnosis. In Robinette, M. S. & Glattke, T. J. (Eds.), *Otoacoustic emissions—Clinical applications* (2nd ed.) (pp. 297–324). New York: Thieme.

Ruggero, M. A., Kramek, B., & Rich, N. C. (1984). Spontaneous otoacoustic emissions in a dog. *Hearing Research, 13*(3), 293–296.

von Békésy, G. (1960). *Experiments in hearing.* New York: Acoustical Society of America Press.

Chapter

14

Neuroanatomy of the Auditory System

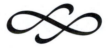

Dwayne D. Simmons, Ph.D.
Associate Professor of Otolaryngology
Washington University School of Medicine
St. Louis, Missouri

The human brain is remarkable in its complexity. Our brains analyze and store information about the external and internal environments and guide our behavior. There are approximately 50 to 100 billion neurons in the human brain, and each of these neurons may communicate directly with as many as 2,000 other neurons. These numbers effectively translate into trillions of points of contact where information is exchanged. Although remarkably robust in many respects, the nervous system is nonetheless susceptible to malfunction in countless ways. Nearly everyone faces significant neurologic, psychological, or psychiatric problems at least once in their lifetime. All health practitioners, whether generalists or specialists, encounter patients who have major neurologic or psychiatric disorders, or both. This chapter describes the human nervous system in anatomic, functional, and developmental terms. There are merits to these approaches as tools to learn about the nervous system; therefore, the goal of this chapter is to introduce you to all three approaches. Hopefully, you will come to understand that a combination of anatomic, functional, and developmental views is necessary to understand the way the brain and especially the auditory nervous system work, as well as some of the pathologies that you will see as audiologists and educators.

NERVE CELLS AND TISSUES

The nervous system is composed of billions of nerve cells, or neurons, and a variety of supportive cells collectively called glia. Neurons have a cell body with many short extensions and a longer extension or axon that is covered by supporting glial cells. The **gray matter** of the nervous system comprises the masses of neuronal cell bodies, whereas the **white matter** of the nervous system represents the collection of neuronal axons and glial myelin sheaths. Nerve cell bodies and axons are surrounded by glial cells. There are between 10 and 50 times more glial cells than neurons in the nervous system. Glial cells are the connective tissue cells within the gray and white matter, and they serve as supporting elements, providing firmness and structure to the brain. The two major classes of glial cells, the oligo-

dendrocyte in the central nervous system (CNS) and Schwann cells in the peripheral nervous system (PNS), form the myelin sheaths that insulate axons. Astrocytes form a third major class of glial cell that is involved in establishing the blood–brain barrier that prevents toxic substances in the blood from entering the brain. Other types of glial cells also serve as scavengers, removing cellular debris after injury or neuronal death.

Two essential properties of nervous tissue are the capacity to react to various physical and chemical agents (i.e., irritability) and the ability to transmit resulting excitation from one cell to another (i.e., conductivity). In signaling the reception of a stimulus from either outside or inside the body, various forms of energy are transduced into electrical energy by specialized cellular structures called **receptors.** Patterns of electrical activity, or nerve impulses, are transmitted from receptors to nerve centers, where they evoke in other nerve cells additional patterns of signals, which are then integrated and distributed to muscles, glands, or both. The pattern of integrated nervous activity results in appropriate sensations and responses. For humans, the nervous system provides the structural and chemical basis of conscious experience; it furnishes the mechanisms for behavior and its regulation, and it is central for the expression of our personality.

Neurons are the cells of the nervous system primarily involved in its special functions. The sensory, integrative, and motor functions of nerve cells depend mainly on irritability and conductivity. The electrical impulses propagated along the axon, called *action potentials,* are rapid and transient all-or-none nerve impulses, with amplitude of 100 millivolts (mV) and duration of about 1 millisecond (see Chapters 5 and 11). They sweep like a wave along axons to transfer information from one place to another in the nervous system. Action potentials are conducted without failure or distortion, at rates between 1 and 100 m/sec. In addition, however, some nerve cells possess secretory capabilities similar to those of the endocrine system, which conducts its integrative function by means of blood-borne chemical agents called *hormones.* Some nerve cells and their corresponding accessory structures give rise to specialized sensory receptors that receive stimuli from the body surface or environment, receive stimuli from internal organs, or receive stimuli from muscles, tendons, and joints. Other nerve cells connect with the peripheral effector organs such as muscles forming neuromotor systems. Still other nerve cells collect into large central masses and assume the task of correlation and integration.

A typical neuron has four morphologically defined regions: cell body (soma), dendrites, axon, and presynaptic terminals (see Chapter 5). The cell body consists of a nucleus and a surrounding cytoplasm (perikaryon). Axons, which constitute the "output wiring" of the neurons, may convey electrical signals along distances that range from as short as 0.1 mm to as long as 2 m. The size, shape, and other peculiarities of the nerve cell body and the number and mode of branching of its processes are all subject to variation, which results in many morphologically distinguishable types of nerve cells. Functional specializations correlate with this morphologic diversity. To ensure high-speed conduction of action potentials, a fatty, insulating sheath called *myelin* surrounds large axons. Their processes to other nerve cells, or to epithelial, muscular, or glandular cells, also anatomically and functionally relate neurons. At synapses, which are points of contact between neurons, action potential impulses pass usually in only one direction by means of chemical transmitters or by electrical coupling. The cell transmitting a signal is called the *presynaptic cell,* and the cell receiving the signal is the *postsynaptic cell.* Specialized swellings on the branches of the axon serve as the transmitting site in the presynaptic cell. The countless neurons are anatomically independent but functionally interrelated at synapses.

From the number of processes that arise from the cell body, neurons are typically classified into three large groups: pseudo-monopolar, bipolar, and multipolar. Pseudo-monopolar and bipolar neurons are commonly sensory neurons. Pseudo-monopolar neurons have a single primary process, exiting from the cell body that splits (bifurcates) into two or more processes, both of which function as axons. One axon will be directed peripherally to the receptor organ, whereas the other is directed centrally. Bipolar neurons have an oval-shaped cell body that gives rise to two processes: a dendrite that conveys information

from the periphery to the cell body, and an axon that carries information from the cell body to the CNS. Multipolar neurons predominate in the CNS. These neurons have a single axon and several highly branched dendrites that emanate from all parts of the cell body. The size and shape of the cell body and length of their processes vary greatly. A **motor neuron** may receive about 10,000 contacts, whereas a Purkinje neuron in the **cerebellum** may receive 150,000 contacts.

Neurons are classified by their function into sensory, motor, and interneuronal neurons. Primary sensory (or afferent) neurons carry information into the CNS both for perception and for motor coordination. Primary sensory neurons may have specialized receptors to detect environmental signals. Motor neurons carry commands to muscles and glands. Relay or projection neurons have long axons and relay information over great distances, from one brain region to another. **Interneurons** constitute by far the largest class, consisting of all the cells in the nervous system that are not specifically sensory or motor. Local interneurons have short axons and process information within local circuits.

MAJOR DIVISIONS OF THE NERVOUS SYSTEM

The nervous system can be anatomically, functionally, and developmentally subdivided in a number of ways. Anatomically, the nervous system can be divided into a CNS and PNS. Functionally, the nervous system can be subdivided into an **autonomic** and a **somatic nervous system.** Developmentally, the nervous system is encephalized (enlarged) at one end that becomes further subdivided into a **forebrain, midbrain,** and **hindbrain.**

Anatomic Subdivisions

The nervous system is generally considered to have two major anatomic components. The CNS consists of the brain and **spinal cord** and is surrounded by a tough protective set of membranes or **meninges.** Figure 14-1 shows the brain, spinal cord, and spinal nerves of an adult human. The meninges consists of an outermost plastic-like membrane called the *dura*

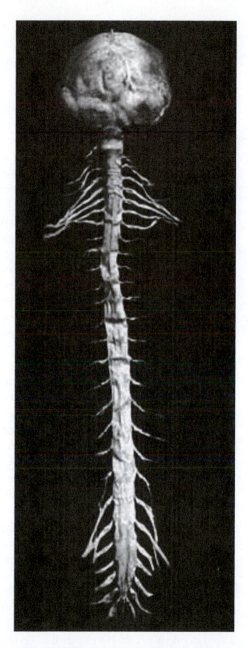
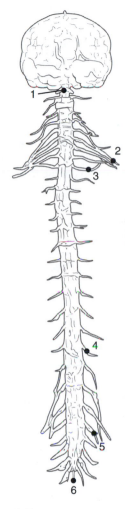

1. Foramen magnum level
2. Brachial plexus
3. 1st thoracic nerve
4. 1st lumbar spinal ganglion
5. 1st sacral nerve
6. Filum terminale

FIGURE 14-1   Human brain and spinal cord with spinal nerves. A tough, plastic-like covering, dura mater, completely surrounds the brain and extends from the foramen magnum where the spinal cord connects to the brainstem to its blind ending at the level of the sacral vertebra (filum terminale).

mater, a middle membrane called the *pia mater,* and an innermost membrane directly adjacent to brain tissues called the *arachnoid.* The brain and spinal cord are further enclosed by a bony skull and vertebral

(spinal) column, respectively. The PNS consists of 12 pairs of cranial nerves, 31 pairs of spinal nerves, and associated sensory structures. The PNS lies mostly outside of the brain and spinal column and functions to keep the other body tissues and organs in communication with the CNS.

The brain includes the **cerebrum,** cerebellum, and the **brainstem** as its principal constituents. The brain is linked to the external world by 12 pairs of cranial nerves and by massive connections with the spinal cord. The human brain is a relatively small structure weighing about 1,400 g and constituting up to 2% of the total body weight. The gray and white matter that comprise the brain have a consistency similar to gelatin and are less dense than cerebrospinal fluid. In fact, within the skull, the brain actually floats in the fluid-filled space contained within the dura mater. Thus, the dura mater and its fluid serve to protect, as well as to cushion, the brain from damage. The cerebrum consists of paired, highly corrugated, **cerebral hemispheres** and three deep-lying structures: basal ganglia, hippocampus, and amygdala. The cerebrum shown in Figure 14-2 is ovoid, is broader behind than in front, and is divided along its antero-posterior axis. The cerebral hemispheres are mirror image duplicates and consist of a convoluted gray cortex, an underlying white matter, and a collection of deeply located neuronal masses, known as the *basal ganglia*. The cerebral hemispheres are partially separated from each other by a major groove called the longitudinal (interhemispheric) **fissure.** The surface convolutions consist of shallower grooves *(sulci)* that separate elevated regions *(gyri).* The smaller sulci vary among individuals, but larger sulci (e.g., central and lateral) are consistent in position across individuals, and thus can be used as boundaries to divide the cortex into defined regions. In the front *(anterior* and *rostral)* and rear *(posterior* and *caudal)* portions of the cerebrum, the separation of the hemispheres is complete, but in the central region, the longitudinal fissure extends only to the interconnecting fibers of the corpus callosum (Figure 14-3).

Each cerebral hemisphere is subdivided into lobes separated by fissures and sulci. The four major lobes of the brain are named for the bones of the skull that overlie them: frontal, parietal, temporal, and occipital. Each of these lobes can be further subdivided into a number of functionally distinct regions that include major modalities associated with different senses (vision, hearing, touch, taste, and smell) and regions involved in controlling movement (motor areas). Primary sensory areas receive information from peripheral receptors with only a few synaptic relays interposed. Primary motor areas contain neurons that project directly to the spinal cord to activate somatic motor neurons. These primary cortical regions are associated with nearby secondary and tertiary regions depending on the level of information processing. Surrounding these primary, secondary, and tertiary areas are large regions of cortex, called *association areas,* that contain higher order neurons whose function is mainly to integrate diverse information.

The largest of all of the lobes, the **frontal lobe,** contains the primary and secondary motor areas—notably, primary motor, premotor, and prefrontal cortical areas. The precentral **gyrus** contains the primary motor area and a cortex that mediates voluntary movements of the limbs and trunk. In the dominant hemisphere, the inferior frontal gyrus is known as **Broca's speech area,** a region concerned with the motor mechanisms of speech formulation. The **parietal lobe** resides between the frontal and **occipital lobes** and on top of the **temporal lobe.** The parietal lobe most notably receives somatic (body and skin) sensory information. The primary somatic sensory cortex is found on the postcentral gyrus. The temporal lobe is ventral and lateral to the frontal and parietal lobes and is bounded by the Sylvian fissure (also known as the lateral **sulcus).** The temporal lobe contains most notably the primary auditory cortex (superior temporal gyrus) and major language association regions such as **Wernicke's area.** The occipital lobe is just above the cerebellum at the caudal end of the cerebrum. It contains the primary visual cortex.

The cerebrum is also divided into two less well-distinguished lobes: insular and limbic lobes. Neither the insular nor the **limbic lobe** is a true lobe. The insular lobe occupies the medial wall of the lateral sulcus and is not visible on the surface of the brain (see Figure 14-3). The insular lobe is defined by the cingulate sulcus, which begins below the rostrum of the corpus callosum and arches in front of the genu of the corpus callosum, about a fingerbreadth distant from it. Above the splenium of the corpus callosum, the cingulate sulcus turns abruptly upward to reach the superior margin of

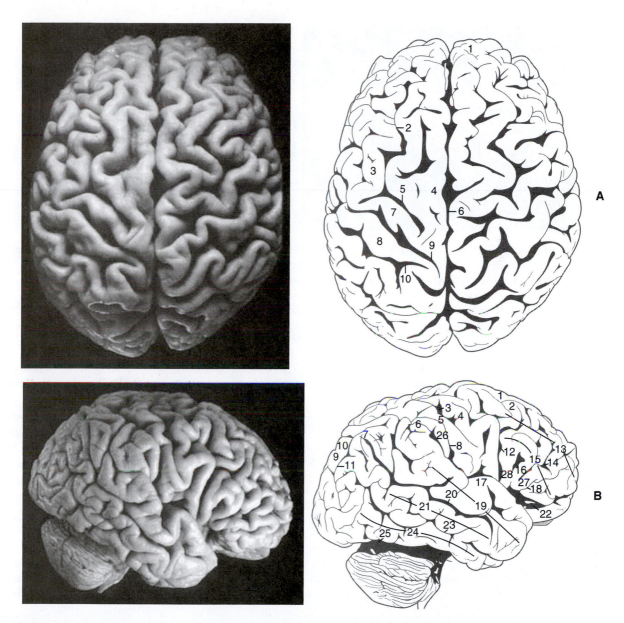

FIGURE 14-2 (A) Dorsal view of cerebral hemispheres. (1) Frontal pole. (5) Precentral sulcus. (6) Longitudinal cerebral fissure. (7) Precentral gyrus. (8) Postcentral gyrus. (9) Central sulcus. (10) Postcentral sulcus. (11) Occipital pole. (B) Lateral view of cerebral hemispheres. (1) Superior frontal gyrus. (3) Central sulcus. (4) Precentral gyrus. (5) Postcentral gyrus. (7) Angular gyrus. (8) Postcentral sulcus. (9) Parieto-occipital sulcus. (10) Parietal lobe. (17) Transverse temporal gyrus. (19) Superior temporal gyrus. (20) Superior temporal sulcus.

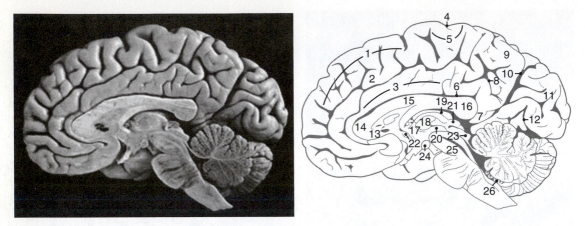

FIGURE 14-3 Midsaggital view of cerebral hemispheres. (1) Medial frontal gyrus. (2) Cingulate sulcus. (3) Cingulate gyrus. (4) Central sulcus. (6) Callosal sulcus. (7) Isthmus of cingulate gyrus. (10) Parieto-occipital sulcus. (11) Cuneus. (12) Calcarine sulcus or fissure. (13) Rostrum of corpus callosum. (14) Genu of corpus callosum. (15) Trunk of corpus callosum. (16) Splenium of corpus callosum. (17) Choroid plexus in interventricular foramen. (21) Pineal body. (22) Anterior (rostral) commissure. (23) Tectum of midbrain. (24) Mamillary body. (25) Medial longitudinal fasciculus. (26) Choroid plexus of 4th ventricle.

the hemisphere. Although poorly understood, insular cortex is associated with cognition.

The limbic lobe is not a distinct area, but rather consists of the medial portions of the frontal, parietal, and temporal lobes that form a continuous band of cortex overlying the rostral brainstem and **diencephalon.** The basal ganglia, hippocampus, and amygdala are considered a part of the limbic band. This band is considered a unit because it forms a complex circuit of interconnected neurons that play a role in learning, memory, and emotions.

Both the cerebrum and cerebellum overlie brainstem structures. The term *brainstem* is generally used to refer to the **medulla, pons,** and midbrain. The brainstem rests on the rostral (superior) end of the spinal cord and like the spinal cord is organized around the embryologic **neural tube.** At the core of the brainstem lies the **reticular formation,** so named because of its "reticulated" (forming a network) appearance that is produced by the diffuse arrangement of cell bodies, axons, and dendrites. The brainstem and its reticular formation core are involved in primitive behavioral and vegetative functions, such as regulation of respiration and heartbeat, sleep and waking, and orientation reflexes.

The spinal cord lies within the vertebral column, sheltered by the bony vertebrae to which it is attached by ligaments (Figure 14-4). It begins at the foramen magnum, a large opening in the occipital bone at the base of the skull, and extends a variable

FIGURE 14-4 (A) The arches and processes of three thoracic vertebrae (6 through 8) have been removed to display a portion of the spinal cord. The spinal nerve roots are shown, together with associated ganglia and the meningeal membranes of the spinal cord. In the upper part of the preparation, the dura mater and pia mater have been stripped away to expose the dorsal nerve tracts. The spinous process and part of the arch of the 9th thoracic vertebra have been removed to show the fatty tissue and venous plexus of the epidural space. The 10th thoracic vertebra has been left intact. (B) The cut surface of the cervical spinal cord is slightly flattened (on both anterior and posterior aspects). In this unstained preparation, the gray matter of the cord is not easily recognized. The epidural fat, the subdural space, and the arachnoid trabeculae are seen. The subarachnoid space is a wide interval that in alive individuals is filled by cerebrospinal fluid and is continuous at the foramen magnum with the cranial subarachnoid space.

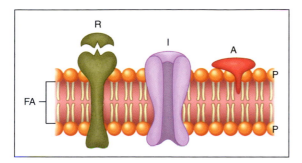

FIGURE 4-1 An artist's rendition of the lipid bilayer common to most cell membranes. Each lipid molecule possesses a hydrophilic phosphate head group (P) and hydrophobic fatty acid chains (FA). This structure makes the membrane impermeable to most ions and molecules. Proteins are commonly found embedded in the membrane that serve as receptors (R), ion channels (I), and anchoring points (A) used to stabilize the cell within the extracellular environment. Proteins such as these allow the cell to control its intracellular environment by making the membrane selectively permeable to desirable ions and molecules (page 47).

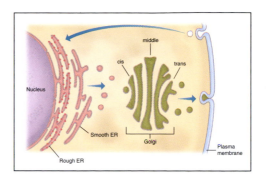

FIGURE 4-2 The membrane system of the cell includes the nuclear envelope, rough and smooth endoplasmic reticulum (ER), the Golgi apparatus, and the plasma membrane. These membrane-bound structures are functionally connected and communicate with one another by direct physical connections and through budding vesicles. The unidirectional flow of macromolecules through this system allows the orchestrated modification, folding, and packaging of raw peptides that is required to make them fully functional and delivered to the correct cellular location. Molecules may also be engulfed by the cell membrane and fuse with the ER for proper modification before use by the cell (page 48).

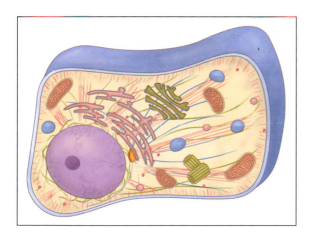

FIGURE 4-4 The individual cell requires a diverse and complex array of organelles for both structural and metabolic support at the cellular, tissue, and organismal levels. Through the coordinated efforts of these organelles, the cell can control its internal environment, manufacture needed molecules, become motile, interact with other cells to form tissues, and even alter these processes as changes in the extracellular environment dictate (page 54).

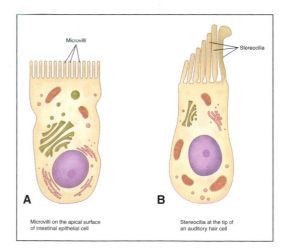

FIGURE 4-5 Certain cells possess specializations that impart unique functional attributes to the cell. (A) Finger-like extensions of membrane, called *microvilli,* increase the apical surface area of epithelial cells in the small intestine to enhance the absorption of water and molecules as they pass through the gut. (B) The stereocilia found on top of sensory hair cells in the inner ear activate cellular signaling mechanisms when deflected in the proper direction, allowing for exquisite sensitivity to auditory signals (page 55).

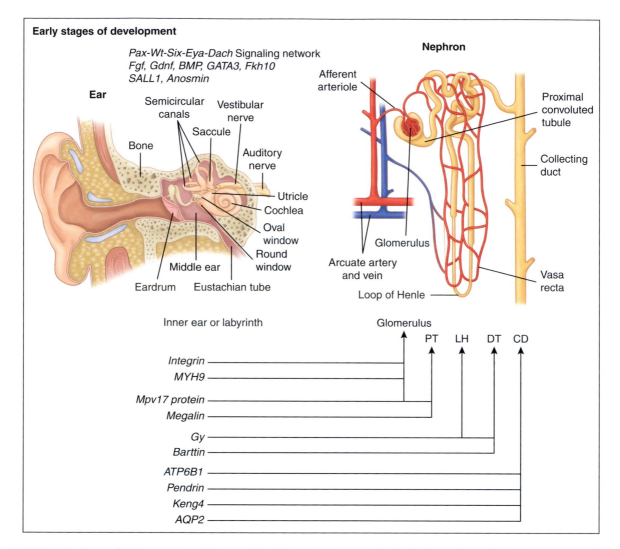

FIGURE 6-7 Ear and kidney genetic linkages. CD, Collecting duct; DT, distal tubule; LH, loop of Henle; PT, proximal tubule. (Adapted from Izzedine et al., 2004.) (page 88)

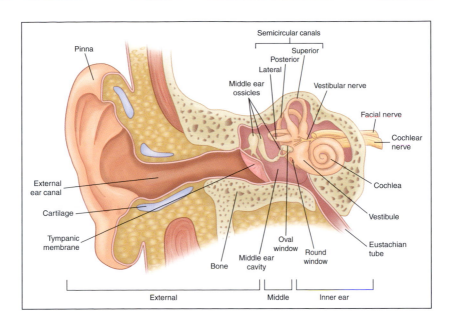

FIGURE 7-1 The human peripheral auditory system has three divisions: external, middle, and inner ears. The external ear consists of the pinna (or auricle) and the external ear canal (or external auditory meatus). The tympanic membrane (or eardrum) closes off the medial end of the external ear canal. The middle ear is an air-filled cavity that contains the three middle-ear ossicles: malleus (M), incus (I), and stapes (S). The middle-ear cavity is connected to the nasopharynx by the Eustachian tube. The inner ear (or membranous labyrinth), which is housed within the petrous portion of the temporal bone, includes the cochlea, vestibule (containing the saccule and utricle), and three semicircular canals (lateral, posterior, and superior). The cochlea contains the end organ for hearing. Its sensory cells are innervated by the cochlear branch of the 8th cranial nerve. The vestibule and three semicircular canals contain the end organs for balance and motion detection, respectively. Sensory cells in these end organs are innervated by the vestibular branch of the 8th cranial nerve. There are two openings from the middle to the inner ear: the oval window into which is fitted the footplate of the stapes, and the round window, covered by the round window membrane (page 94).

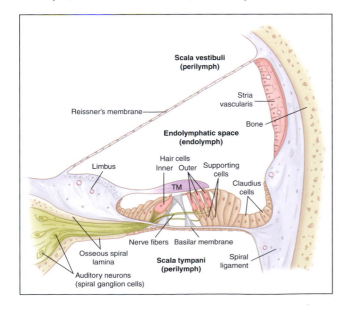

FIGURE 8-4 Schematic view of a portion of the membranous cochlea. C, Claudius cell; IS, inner sulcus cell; TM, tectorial membrane. (Adapted from Davis, et al., 1953, by B.A. Bohne, 2004.) (page 113)

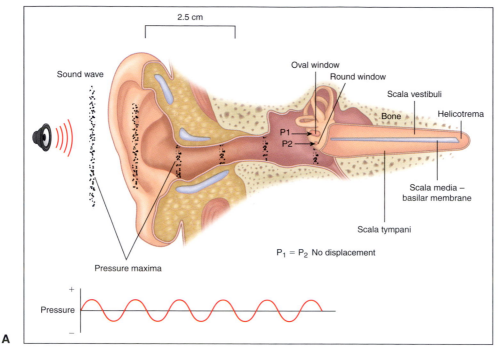

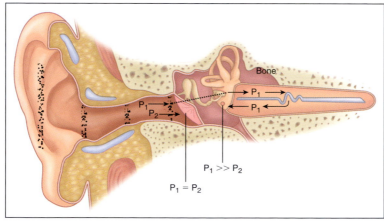

FIGURE 9-2 Schematic representation of sound transmission to the basilar membrane. (A) Without a middle ear, the positive pressures (P_1 and P_2) in a sound wave will strike both the oval window and the round window nearly simultaneously. Because the cochlear fluids are nearly incompressible, pressing inward on each window will cause no net movement of fluid and no displacement of the basilar membrane. (B) The middle ear transmits and amplifies the pressure gradient (P_1) to the stapes and oval window, and protects the round window from airborne sound (that is, P_2 is much smaller than P_1). In this case, the inward "push" of the stapes causes a displacement of fluid toward the round window membrane, which serves as a pressure relief valve. The net result is a displacement of the basilar membrane (page 126).

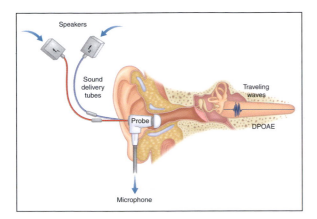

FIGURE 13-6   Schematic of basic instrumentation for measuring distortion product emissions (DPOAE) (page 221).

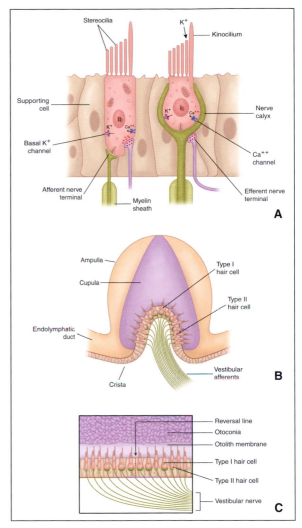

FIGURE 16-2   Vestibular receptors and their locations in the labyrinth. (A) Type I and II vestibular receptor hair cells. (B) Semicircular canal ampulla. Hair cells are located in the crista, with stereocilia embedded in the cupula membrane. Type I and II hair cells are located in the central and peripheral regions of the crista, respectively. (C) Hair cells are located in the otolith macula, with stereocilia embedded in otolith membrane and otoconia secured on top (page 288).

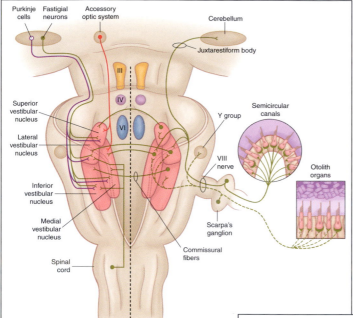

FIGURE 16-6   Sensory afferents to the vestibular nuclei. Four vestibular nuclei (superior, lateral, medial, inferior) receive primary afferent information from the ipsilateral labyrinth. Other signal inputs arise from the spinal cord, commissural fibers, cerebellum, accessory optic nuclei, and cortical pathways (not shown) (page 293).

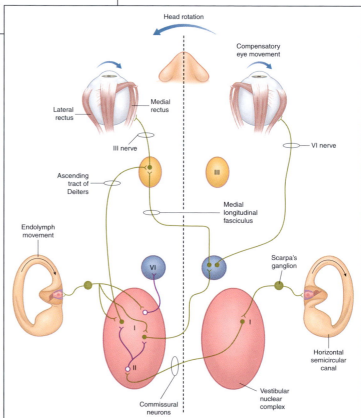

FIGURE 16-7   Horizontal vestibulo-ocular reflex to rotational head motion (page 297).

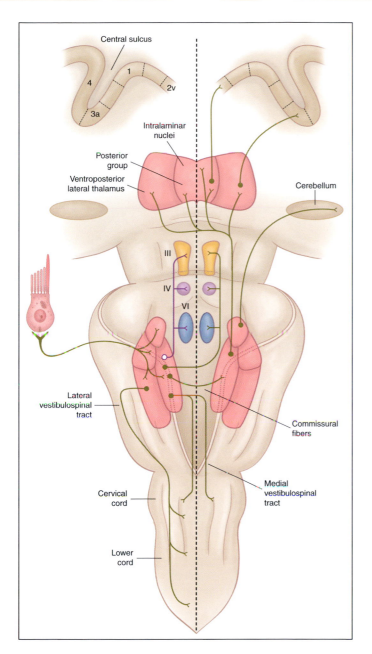

FIGURE 16-8   Vestibular nuclei efferent projections to the major systems. Separate paths for the lateral vestibulospinal tract, medial vestibulospinal tract, commissural fibers, vestibulo-ocular reflex, and vestibulo-thalamo-cortical systems are shown (page 300).

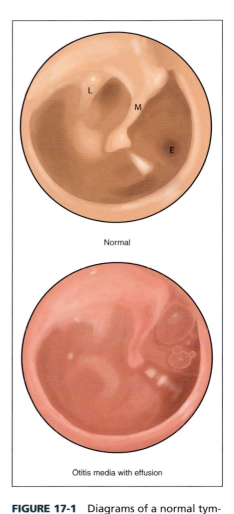

FIGURE 17-1   Diagrams of a normal tympanic membrane (top) and during an episode of otitis media with effusion. The normal membrane is sufficiently translucent that some underlying structures can be clearly seen: (L) the long process of the incus, (M) the chorda tympani, manubrium of the malleus, and (E) the opening to the eustachian tube. The ear with otitis may show considerable redness, distention of the membrane, and the presence of fluid, ranging from clear to amber. Underlying structures are not typically as visible as they are in the normal state (page 315).

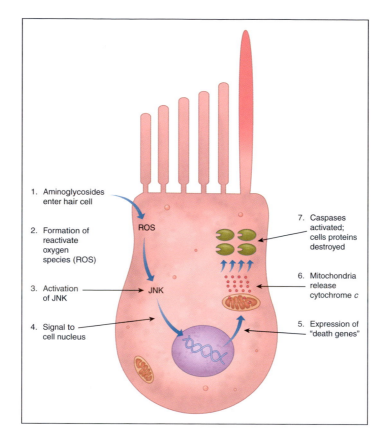

FIGURE 22-2 Programmed cell death pathway in hair cells. JNK, c-Jun N-terminal kinase; ROS, reactive oxygen species (page 405).

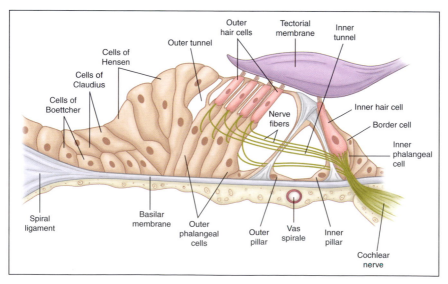

FIGURE 22-4B Morphology of supporting cells in the vestibular organs versus cochlea (page 409).

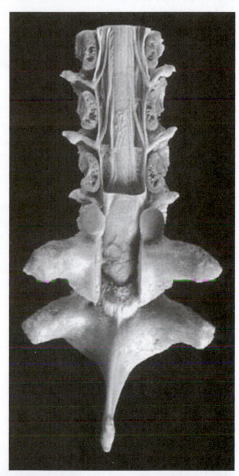

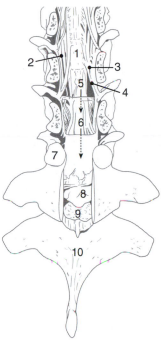

A

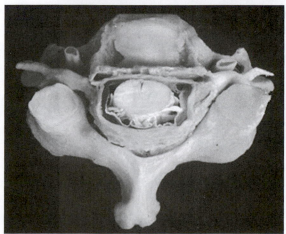

1. Pia mater
2. Denticulate ligament
3. Motor root of 7th thoracic nerve
4. Sensory root of 7th thoracic nerve
5. Subarachnoid space
6. Subdural space
7. Superior articular process of 9th
   thoracic vertebra

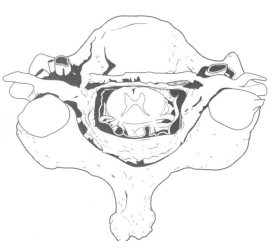

B

length, depending on the age of the subject, down the vertebral canal. The 31 pairs of spinal nerves in humans correspond to the 31 spinal cord segments. The segments are arbitrarily determined from the arrangements of the spinal roots. Humans have 8 cervical, 12 thoracic, 5 lumbar, 5 sacral, and 1 coc-cygeal segment.

The spinal cord is the major input-output structure for the limbs and trunk. Figure 14-4A shows a dorsal (back) view of the adult spinal cord, surrounded by meninges and enclosed by vertebrae. The spinal cord widens at cervical and lumbar seg-ments and narrows at thoracic segments. Spinal nerves at cervical segments form the brachial plexus. In cross section, the spinal cord contains a central region of gray matter, which contains neu-

ronal cell bodies, dendrites, and synapses. Sensory regions occupy the dorsal horn, and motor regions are located in the ventral horn (see Figure 14-4B). The surrounding white matter contains numerous axonal tracts that carry ascending sensory informa-tion and descending motor signals. The spinal cord communicates with the rest of the rest of the body via peripheral spinal nerves, which are part of the PNS. The spinal nerves make their exit from the vertebral canal by passing through the intervertebral foramina. They are all mixed nerves; that is, they contain sensory, motor, and autonomic compo-nents. Each spinal nerve is formed by the coales-cence of a dorsal (posterior) and a ventral (anterior) root. The fibers comprising the dorsal roots emerge laterally from the dorsal surface of the spinal cord as

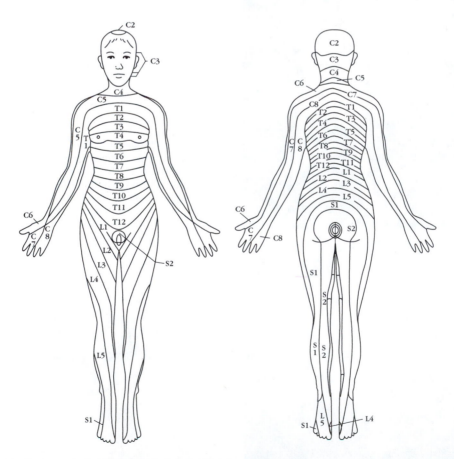

FIGURE 14-5 Dermatomes reflecting sensory innervation by spinal nerves.

a series of rootlets, whereas the fibers comprising the ventral roots emerge from the ventral surface of the cord. The dorsal and ventral rootlets that go to make up a single pair of spinal nerves originate from a single segment of the spinal cord. Motor neurons whose cell bodies lie in the ventral horn send axons through the ventral spinal roots. Sensory neurons have their cell bodies in dorsal root ganglia, and their central axons enter the spinal cord through the dorsal roots.

An appreciation of the topographic relation between the spinal cord segments and their corresponding somatic segments is of clinical importance, because spinal cord disease is recognized and localized by the motor or sensory deficits or disorders that appear in the periphery, that is, in the area of distribution of the spinal nerves. The area of skin supplied by a single dorsal root is called a *dermatome*. Actually, the dermatomes of adjacent roots overlap significantly, so that at least two, and sometimes three, roots supply a single patch of skin (Figure 14-5).

Functional Subdivisions

If you have a close call on a highway or hear a sudden, loud noise, you have felt the result of the autonomic nervous system—the part of the PNS that innervates the internal organs, blood vessels, and glands. The autonomic nervous system governs the involuntary actions of visceral (smooth and striated) muscles involved in digestion, vascular, and heart functions. Major divisions of the autonomic nervous system include **sympathetic** and **parasympathetic systems** (Figure 14-6). The autonomic nervous system also includes the less well-known enteric division that specifically innervates the digestive organs. The sympathetic system responds to stimulation through energy expenditure, and the parasympathetic system counters these responses. Sympathetic responses include vasoconstriction, increase in blood pressure, dilation of pupils, accelerating heart rate, and glandular secretion of sweat. These responses fall into the "flight, fight, or fright" category of behavior. The parasympathetic system counteracts sympathetic stimulation by slowing heart rate, constricting pupils, and reducing blood pressure.

The CNS component of the autonomic nervous system arises from the prefrontal region of the cerebral cortex, as well as from the hypothalamus, **thalamus,** hippocampus, brainstem, cerebellum, and spinal cord. Afferent (ascending) and efferent (descending) tracts connect these regions to visceral muscles and organs under autonomic control. The PNS components of the autonomic nervous system include paired sympathetic ganglia running adjacent to the spinal column, nerve plexuses, and visceral ganglia. Parasympathetic neurons are located in different nuclei throughout the brainstem, as well as a few in the sacral spinal cord. Their axons travel to the target organ and synapse in ganglia in or near the organ wall. Postganglionic fibers finally innervate the target organ. Examples of these ganglia include the ciliary and otic in the head and diffuse networks of cells in the walls of the heart, gut, and bladder. Sympathetic neurons are found in the intermediolateral column and in the thoracic spinal cord. They also travel to ganglia before reaching the target organ, but the sympathetic ganglia are often far from the target.

In contrast with the autonomic nervous system, the somatic nervous system is largely responsible for modulating the action of the skeletal (somatic) muscles involved in the voluntary control of speech and volitional movements. The precentral region of the CNS controls most somatic muscles through descending motor tracts of the brainstem and spinal cord. The somatic nervous system also includes the cranial and spinal nerves and their sensory ganglia that relay sensory information important for peripheral action.

The somatic motor system may be further subdivided into **pyramidal** and **extrapyramidal systems.** The pyramidal system arises from pyramidal neurons of the motor strip of the cerebral cortex and is largely responsible for initiation of voluntary motor behavior (Figure 14-7). The extrapyramidal system arises mostly from premotor regions of the frontal lobe and is responsible for the resting tone and movement supportive of voluntary behavior.

The primary motor pathway is also called the *corticospinal pathway*. It starts in the **precentral gyrus,**

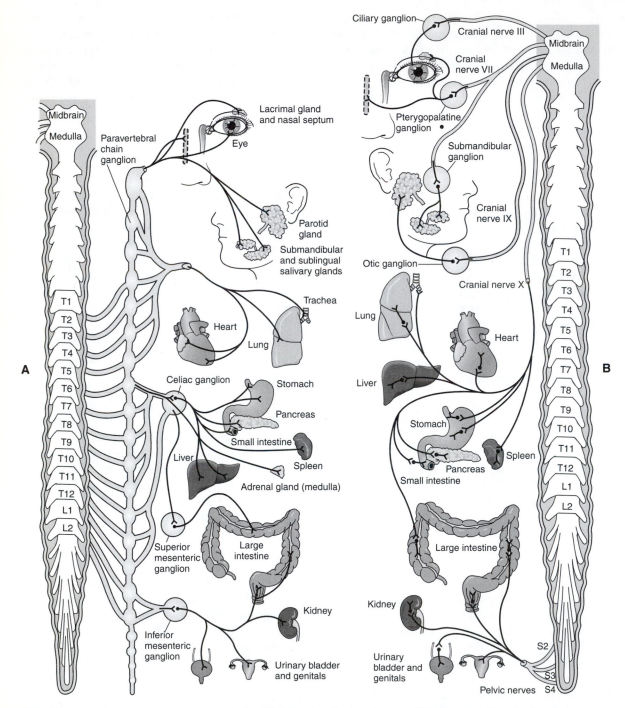

FIGURE 14-6 The autonomic nervous system: (A) the sympathetic system and (B) the parasympathetic system.

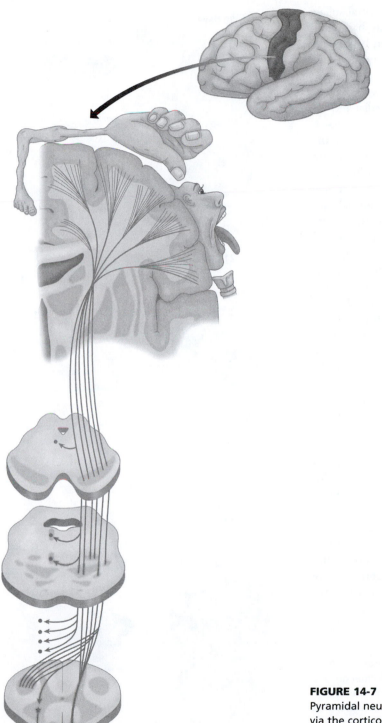

FIGURE 14-7 Primary (pyramidal) motor pathway. Pyramidal neurons in the precentral gyrus send axons via the corticospinal tracts to terminate on motor neurons in the ventral horn of the spinal cord.

the fold of cortex just anterior to the central sulcus (see Figure 14-7). The precentral gyrus has many names, including primary motor cortex, Brodmann area 4, and M1. The topographic organization of the precentral gyrus is such that motor control of the face originates from lateral regions, whereas the trunk and limbs originate from more medial and superior regions. The corticospinal tract originates as the axons of pyramidal neurons in layer V of the (mainly) primary motor cortex. Once the axons leave the pyramidal cells, they enter the white matter just below. At this point, all of these axons are called the *internal capsule.* At the midbrain, the internal capsule coalesces into a tight bundle called the *cerebral peduncles,* or the "stalks" of the cerebrum. The peduncles make up the floor of the midbrain and contain all of the descending axons going to the brainstem or spine. In the medulla, the fibers come together again as the pyramids. The pyramids were actually named as landmarks on the surface of the brainstem; on a human brainstem, you can clearly see them as two ridges running down the ventral midline. The pyramids run the entire length of the medulla, as large, uninterrupted axonal tracts on the ventral surface. At the caudal-most end of the medulla, about at the point where you have to start calling it cervical spinal cord, the fibers in the pyramids cross. The crossing event is called the *decussation* of the pyramids. By the time the decussation is completed, the corticospinal fibers reside in this new location, now called the *lateral corticospinal tract.* From this position, they dive into the gray matter of the spinal cord at their target levels. Those fibers controlling the arms, for example, get off in the cervical levels of the cord. Once in the ventral horn, they synapse either on interneurons (most common) or directly on the motor neurons that innervate the limbs and distal muscles.

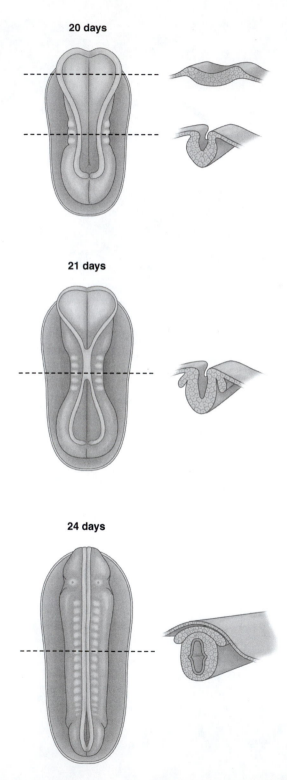

FIGURE 14-8   Formation of the nervous system. The ectoderm forms the neural plate. An ectodermal groove forms and gradually the neural folds meet in the midline to form the neural tube. The neural tube closes first near the middle of the embryo and proceeds rostrally and caudally. The peripheral nervous system develops from neural crest cells.

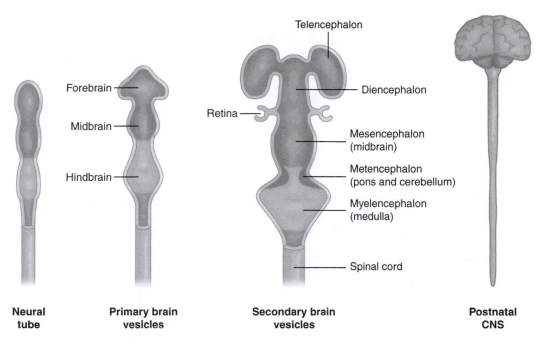

FIGURE 14-9 Development of primary and secondary brain vesicles. CNS, central nervous system.

Developmental Subdivisions

The CNS and PNS are derived from a dorsally located, thickened plate of ectoderm, known as the neural plate, which first appears late in the third week of gestation (Figure 14-8). This dorsal plate ectoderm eventually grows to form a neural groove, which is bounded on each side by an elevated neural fold that ultimately fuses to form the neural tube. First, the ectoderm in the dorsal midline of the embryo thickens, forming the neural plate. After the neural plate enlarges dorsally, the neural groove forms at day 19, and gradually the neural folds meet in the midline to form the neural tube and overlying ectoderm. Around day 22, the neural tube closes first near the middle of the embryo and proceeds rostrally and caudally, reflecting the gradient of nervous system development. The neural tube differentiates into the brain and the spinal cord by day 28. Neural crest develops into the PNS. By the time the neural tube closes, three primary brain vesicles are evident. From these vesicles the brain develops. The posterior (caudal) portion of the neural tube remains relatively small in diameter to form the spinal cord. The anterior (rostral) portion of the neural tube enlarges and shows the first signs of primary brain vesicles.

Early during embryonic brain development, the anterior portion of the embryo greatly expands and becomes what is known as the encephalon (Figure 14-9). Three distinctive subdivisions of the developing brain are apparent as soon as the neural tube closes, and each subdivision undergoes elaborate, and sometimes unique, development as growth continues. The three basic subdivisions of the brain are the **prosencephalon** (forebrain), the **mesencephalon** (midbrain), and the **rhombencephalon** (hindbrain), which develop within the embryonic encephalon. Each of these embryonic brain regions undergoes further differentiation.

At 25 days, the neural tube forms. By 40 days, the three-vesicle stage is present. The three vesicles form the forebrain, midbrain, and hindbrain. Between 40 and 100 days, the brain has reached the five-vesicle stage: telencephalon, diencephalon, mesencephalon, **metencephalon,** and myelencephalon (see Figure 14-9). By the end of the 12th

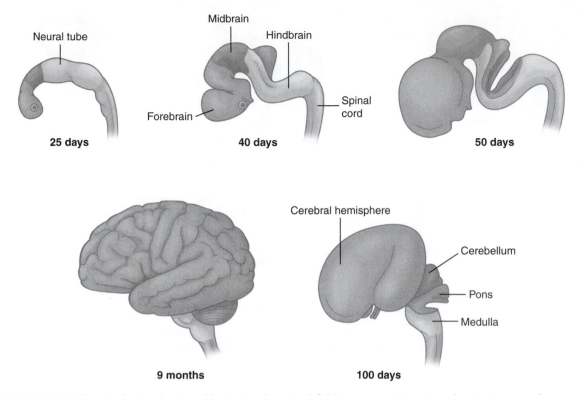

FIGURE 14-10   The developing brain and brainstem bend and fold in stereotypic patterns beginning as early as 5 weeks and continuing well into the fetal period.

week, the prosencephalon differentiates into a telencephalon and diencephalon. The telencephalon, or "extended" brain, includes the cerebral hemispheres, the white matter immediately beneath it, the basal ganglia, and the olfactory tract. The rhinencephalon consists of olfactory-associated structures that develop within the telencephalon. These include the olfactory bulb, tract, and striae; pyriform area; intermediate olfactory area; paraterminal area; hippocampal formation; and fornix. The prosencephalon also contains the diencephalon that is the next descending area and includes the thalamus, hypothalamus, pituitary gland, and optic tract. The midbrain or mesencephalon is the highest level within the brainstem. The mesencephalon includes several midbrain structures, the cerebral aqueduct, and cerebral peduncles. At birth, the metencephalon is the most visible besides the cerebral hemispheres (Figure 14-10). The metencephalon includes the pons and cerebellum. Finally,

the myelencephalon refers to the medulla oblongata, the lowest level of the encephalon.

CENTRAL AUDITORY PATHWAYS
Principles of Pathway Organization

A few basic principles govern the organization of the nervous system. The PNS relays information to the CNS and executes motor commands generated in the brain and spinal cord. The simplest behaviors involve the integrated activity of several distinct sensory, motor, and motivational pathways in the CNS. The major functional pathways of the CNS are interconnected by relay nuclei. These nuclei are not just relay stops; they also function to process, integrate, and modify incoming information before relaying the information to other areas. These relay centers receive both ascending information from lower brain centers or peripheral receptors and descending information from higher brain centers. The two basic types of neurons in relay centers are projection neurons and local interneurons. Projection (principal) neurons transmit the output of the nucleus; these neurons have long axons that leave the nucleus to communicate with cells in other regions of the CNS. Local interneurons have axons that are confined to the area of the relay nucleus itself. They mediate local excitatory and inhibitory synaptic interactions and receive synaptic input from descending and ascending axons. One of the most prominent multisensory relay structures in the brain is the thalamus, a collection of functionally distinct nuclei. Nearly all sensory information that goes to the cerebral cortex is first processed within the thalamus. The cerebral cortex, in turn, sends recurrent axons back to the thalamus.

Each functional pathway represents topographic maps of peripheral areas and may be further divided into distinct subsystems that perform specialized tasks. The spatial arrangement of the receptors in the peripheral sense organs (retina, cochlea, skin) is preserved in a topographic fashion throughout the CNS. In this way, an orderly neural map of the specific sensory field is retained at each successive level of processing. These sensory maps are somewhat distorted, in that the regions of greatest interest or sensitivity are given a disproportionate representation in the cortex.

Finally, many pathways cross over (decussate) to the opposite (contralateral) side of the brain or spinal cord. As a result, sensory events on one side of the body are processed by the cerebral hemisphere on the opposite side; likewise, voluntary movements on one side of the body are initiated or controlled by the contralateral hemisphere. Although pathways cross at different anatomic levels in different systems, a general rule of thumb is that the second-order neuron within a pathway is the one that projects to centers on the contralateral side of the brain or spinal cord. Structures that contain overdecussating axons are termed *commissures*.

Ascending Auditory Pathways

Auditory information from the cochlea travels through brainstem relay centers to eventually reach the thalamus where information is then re-layed to the primary auditory cortex. Auditory information is conveyed to the brain via two types of pathways: a primary auditory pathway, which exclusively carries messages from the cochlea (Figure 14-11), and a nonprimary pathway (also called the *reticular sensory pathway*), which carries all types of sensory messages. The auditory nerve leaves the inner ear via the internal auditory meatus, where it joins with the vestibular nerve to form the eighth cranial nerve or vestibulocochlear nerve. The vestibulocochlear nerve enters the brain at the lateral aspect of the upper medulla near the caudal pons. The axons of the auditory nerve constitute the first-order neurons of the ascending central auditory pathways. Auditory nerve fibers from the apex of the cochlea occupy the middle portions of the nerve trunk, with more basal fibers spiraling and coursing peripheral to the apical ones. This basic spatial (cochleotopic) arrangement of cochlear fibers continues into the **cochlear nuclei** and is reflected by the **tonotopic organization** of the nerve. Cochlear nuclei receive first-order projections from the ipsilateral spiral ganglion. These nuclei are located in the upper portion of the medulla, where they encircle the superior and lateral surface of the inferior cerebellar peduncle. Auditory nerve fibers bifurcate as they enter the cochlear nuclei giving rise to an ascending branch to the ventral cochlear nuclei and a descending branch that terminates in the dorsal cochlear nuclei. The **cochleotopy** of the auditory nerve is continued in the cochlear nuclei. Fibers arising from progressively more basal locations of the cochlea (i.e., higher frequency regions) bifurcate and arborize in progressively more dorsal regions of the ventral and dorsal cochlear nuclei.

The primary auditory pathway is actually two pathways, one via the dorsal **acoustic stria** and the other via the ventral acoustic stria (see Figure 14-11). Both of these primary pathways carry information from the cochlea, and each relay nucleus does specific work of decoding and integration. Second-order neurons from the dorsal cochlear nuclei cross to the opposite side via the dorsal acoustic stria and ascend in the contralateral **lateral lemniscus.** These fibers terminate either within nuclei of the

FIGURE 14-11 Auditory pathways. The primary auditory pathways are direct (only three to four relays), fast (with large myelinated fibers), and end in the primary auditory cortex. In humans, the primary auditory cortex is located in the temporal area within the lateral sulcus. LF, Low frequency; HF, high frequency; AVCN, anterior ventral cochlear nucleus; PVNC, posterior ventral cochlear nucleus; DCN, dorsal cochlear nucleus; MSO, medial superior olive; LSO, lateral superior olive; MNTB, medial nucleus of trapezoid body; DNLL, dorsal nucleus of the lateral lemniscus; VNLL, ventral nucleus of the lateral lemniscus; ICC, inferior central colliculus; IC, inferior colliculus; MG, medial primary; AI, auditory primary; AII, auditory secondary. (Adapted from Phillips, 2001.)

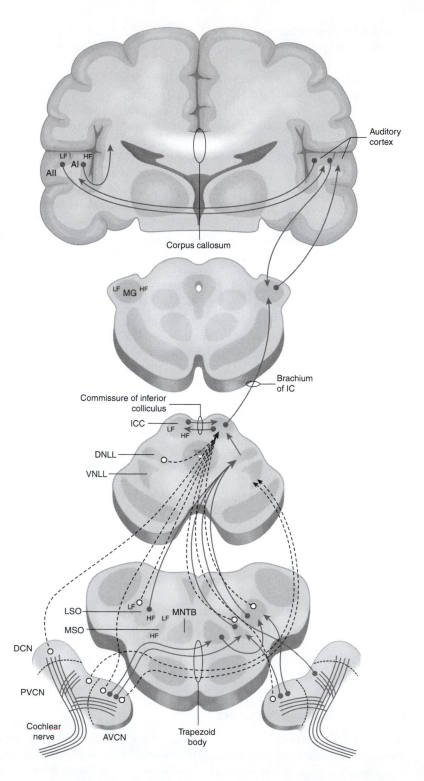

lateral lemniscus or the **inferior colliculus** of the midbrain. Second-order neurons from the ventral cochlear nuclei project via the ventral acoustic stria to the **superior olivary complex.** Within the trapezoid body, the fibers of the ventral acoustic stria **decussate** to synapse with the nuclei of the contralateral superior olivary complex. Thus, superior olivary nuclei receive bilateral projections from cochlear nuclei on both sides of the brainstem. The superior olivary complex is located in the rostral third of the medulla and the caudal third of the pons and is responsible for processing binaural cues of directional hearing. Two prominent nuclei with the superior olivary complex are the **lateral superior olive** and the **medial superior olive.** The medial superior olive is more sensitive to interaural timing differences, whereas the lateral superior olive is more sensitive to interaural intensity differences. From the superior olivary complex, third-order neurons ascend in the lateral lemniscus.

The lateral lemniscus is a fiber tract that carries information from the cochlear nuclei, superior olivary nuclei, and other pontine auditory relay centers to the midbrain inferior colliculus. The inferior colliculi appear as two prominent swellings on the dorsal surface of the caudal half of the midbrain. Communication also exists between the colliculi of the two sides via the commissure of the inferior colliculus. Several fibers may pass the inferior colliculus and follow a more direct path to the **medial geniculate** body of the thalamus. The brachium of the inferior colliculus is the fiber tract that projects from the inferior colliculus to the medial geniculate nucleus of the thalamus. Fibers ascending from the inferior colliculus terminate primarily in the pars principalis of the medial geniculate. The medial geniculate body is the last subcortical relay station for all ascending auditory pathways. Although the medial geniculate has three principal regions—ventral, medial, and dorsal divisions—it is often divided into two, pars principalis and ventral.

The auditory (geniculotemporal) radiations project from the medial geniculate to the transverse temporal gyrus on the temporal cortex of the same side. Also referred to as Heschl's gyrus, this cortical area corresponds to Brodmann cytoarchitectural areas **41** and **42.** Area 41 is the primary auditory cortex. Area 41, which consists of a portion of the anterior and posterior temporal gyri, is actually obscured from view within the central sulcus. Area 42, which is an auditory association area (Wernicke's area), is adjacent to area 41 on parts of the posterior transverse and superior temporal gyri.

Descending Auditory Pathways

Several descending auditory pathways have been demonstrated coming from cortical areas to the medial geniculate and to the inferior colliculus, as well as from inferior colliculi to the superior olivary complex. However, the most well-studied descending pathway is the olivocochlear bundle, sometimes referred to as Rasmussen's bundle because Rasmussen originally characterized it in 1946. The **olivocochlear pathway** is made up of neurons derived bilaterally from regions of the medial and lateral regions of the superior olivary complex. Olivocochlear neurons project via the olivocochlear bundle and then enter the inner ear along the vestibular branch of the vestibulocochlear nerve (see Figure 14-11). Crossing via the bundle of Oort, efferent olivocochlear fibers enter the cochlea where they terminate directly on outer hair cells and indirectly with inner hair cells via synapses on the afferent fibers of spiral ganglion neurons.

Olivocochlear neurons give rise to at least two efferent systems. Neurons surrounding lateral regions of the lateral superior olivary give rise to projections that mostly terminate on the afferent fibers below inner hair cells, whereas neurons in ventral and medial locations of the superior olivary complex terminate directly on the outer hair cells. Lateral olivocochlear neurons send the majority of their projections to the ipsilateral cochlea, whereas the majority of medial olivocochlear neurons have projections to the contralateral cochlea. Finally, most of the lateral olivocochlear neurons cause unmyelinated axons, in contrast with medial olivocochlear neurons, which tend to be heavily myelinated. These differences among olivocochlear neurons suggest that they may have fundamentally different functions.

Auditory Neuropathy

Sensorineural hearing loss is the most common type of permanent hearing loss. A less common type of hearing loss is auditory neuropathy, or auditory dyssynchrony. With this type of hearing disorder, the cochlea appears to receive sounds normally. However, neural signals leaving the cochlea become disorganized, disrupted, or incorrectly processed.

The first identification of auditory neuropathy was reported in the 1980s by a University of California at Irvine neurologist Arnold Starr and colleagues. Auditory neuropathy is diagnosed by abnormal auditory nerve and brainstem responses (ABRs), with outer hair cell function (as determined by otoacoustic emissions [OAEs] and cochlear microphonic), and defects in speech processing. Auditory neuropathy may be inherited genetically, caused by trauma, or by disease. Although the underlying causes of this disorder are probably complex and multifaceted, common features that coincide with auditory neuropathy include varying degrees of hearing loss, difficulty understanding speech especially in noise, and hearing that can fluctuate daily and even hourly. In addition, persons with auditory neuropathy will manifest other conditions that affect coordinated activities such as writing, talking, or running.

Auditory neuropathy is commonly associated with a lack of oxygen (anoxia) at birth; hyperbilirubinemia requiring blood transfusion, associated with severe jaundice during the newborn period; infectious diseases such as mumps; immune disorders; nonsyndromic recessive neuropathy; and neurologic disorders such as Charcot–Marie–Tooth syndrome and Friedreich's ataxia (see Chapter 6). There are large individual differences among children with this hearing disorder. For some, hearing may improve over time. This is most common when the cause of the disorder is hyperbilirubinemia.

Depending on what method is used for newborn hearing screening (OAEs or ABRs), some children with auditory neuropathy may pass an initial hearing screening conducted in the hospital. This may delay the identification of auditory neuropathy. Parents and physicians may not suspect hearing loss right away if an infant's response to sound changes from day to day. As children get older,

more hearing information becomes available. Ongoing testing may show poorer than expected speech understanding and great difficulty hearing in noisy backgrounds. A wide variety of hearing loss degrees and hearing loss shapes can be seen. Children with auditory neuropathy may also have hearing responses that fluctuate or worsen over time.

Published reports of patients with auditory neuropathy indicate that they are extremely heterogeneous in underlying medical diagnosis, age, severity, and test results, and that only a small number have undergone the detailed investigations that would enable a more precise diagnosis of the location of their pathologies. It is likely that some patients diagnosed with auditory neuropathy in reality have CNS dysfunction and not strictly PNS neuropathy. A more comprehensive evaluation of patients may be necessary to serve patients adequately, including potential candidates for cochlear implants, and to increase knowledge of auditory pathologies. Medical treatment of auditory neuropathy currently is unavailable. Management typically involves the use of hearing aids or cochlear implants. Audiologists vary in their opinions about using hearing aids for a child with auditory neuropathy. Some children benefit from hearing aids. However, many children get limited hearing aid benefit or no benefit at all. At this time, there is no reliable way to predict who will and will not benefit. Hearing aids must be set carefully to prevent damage to the parts of the ear that receive sounds normally. Some professionals have recommended the use of personal frequency-modulated speaker systems to improve listening in noisy backgrounds.

Previously, it was thought that children with auditory neuropathy would not be good cochlear implant candidates. It is now known that some children benefit more from a cochlear implant than from hearing aids. Children with some types of genetically inherited auditory neuropathy may benefit more from cochlear implants than children with other causes of the disorder. More will be known as future genetic and hearing science research becomes available.

Tinnitus

Tinnitus is the medical term for "ringing in the ears." Although ringing is the most common sensation reported, tinnitus may also present as hissing, whistling, or a pulsatile click or chirp, which may suggest clues as to its origin. Tinnitus is not related to an external auditory stimulus, but rather is an internally generated phenomenon. Approximately one in five people in the United States has tinnitus, though not all would say they "suffer" from the disorder. Even though some 83% of people with tinnitus hear ringing constantly, without intermission, three-fourths of tinnitus patients report that they eventually habituate to the ringing and are not bothered by it.

The causes of tinnitus are quite varied. The most prevalent cause is exposure to loud noise, either acutely or long term. Other causes include: stress or anxiety; high or low blood pressure; medications, including antibiotics, antidepressants, and aspirin; tumors; diabetes; thyroid problems; sinus and respiratory infections; ear wax buildup; and head trauma. Tinnitus generally can be classified on the basis of its nature and expression as either "objective" or "subjective," and either "pulsatile" or "nonpulsatile." These descriptors offer clues to the pathogenesis of the tinnitus. Pulsatile tinnitus commonly appears due to the movement of blood through vessels in the vicinity of the middle or outer ear, or both. Glomus tumors of the middle ear can also cause pulsatile tinnitus, especially if the tumor is in contact with the tympanic membrane (Weissman & Hirsch, 2000) (see Chapter 17). However, this type of tinnitus may also be caused by the spasmodic contraction of muscles in or near the middle ear or palate. These types of tinnitus are considered objective and can be heard by outside observers with the aid of a microphone. Other types of tinnitus consist of a nonpulsatile or constant ringing sensation and are more likely subjective in nature, unable to be heard by an outside listener. In older adults, most tinnitus appears to be a consequence of hearing loss, and the pitch of the tinnitus is often related to the frequency of the hearing loss. In young children, tinnitus is often the first sign of hearing loss and should always be referred for proper medical attention.

The origin or source of tinnitus is often attributable to malfunction of neurons of the central or peripheral auditory system. Most commonly, tinnitus is believed to involve damage to the nerve endings at the base of sensory hair cells in the cochlea. However, higher nervous system centers have been implicated, including the brainstem cochlear nucleus and auditory cortex.

Treatments for tinnitus are quite varied. When a specific cause such as infection, tumor, or ear wax impaction can be identified, then removal of the inciting circumstances often offers relief. However, if a specific cause is not found, then relief is unlikely. Hearing aids and other masking devices have offered some relief in hiding sensations of tinnitus. Other attempts include concentration and relaxation exercises, counseling for emotional and psychological problems, and tinnitus retraining therapy, which attempts to retrain the brain to consider tinnitus-related neuronal activity as representing a neutral or nonsignificant stimulus such as background noise.

∽ SUMMARY ∾

There are approximately 50 to 100 billion neurons in the human brain, and each of these neurons may communicate directly with as many as 2,000 other neurons. Although remarkably robust in many respects, the nervous system is nonetheless susceptible to malfunction in countless ways. The human nervous system can be described in anatomic, functional, and developmental terms. A combination of anatomic, functional, and developmental views is necessary to understand the way the brain and especially the auditory nervous system work. The vertebrate nervous system is generally considered as having two major anatomic components. The CNS consists of the brain and spinal cord and is surrounded by a tough protective set of membranes or meninges. The PNS consists of 12 pairs of cranial nerves, 31 pairs of spinal nerves, and associated sensory structures. The PNS lies mostly outside of the brain and spinal column and functions to keep the other body tissues and organs in communication with the CNS. Functionally, the autonomic nervous system governs the involuntary actions of visceral (smooth and striated) muscles involved in digestion, vascular, and heart functions. Major divisions of the autonomic nervous system include sympathetic and parasympathetic systems. In contrast with the autonomic nervous system, the somatic nervous system is largely responsible for modulating the action of the skeletal (somatic) muscles involved in the voluntary control of speech and volitional movements. Three distinctive subdivisions of the developing brain are apparent as soon as the neural tube closes, and each subdivision undergoes elaborate, and sometimes unique, development as growth continues. The three basic subdivisions of the brain are the prosencephalon (forebrain), the mesencephalon (midbrain), and the rhombencephalon (hindbrain), which develop within the embryonic encephalon. Each of these embryonic brain regions undergoes further differentiation. Auditory information from the cochlea travels through brainstem relay centers to eventually reach the thalamus where information is then relayed to the primary auditory cortex. Auditory information is conveyed to the brain via two types of pathways: a primary auditory pathway, which exclusively carries messages from the cochlea, and a nonprimary pathway (also called the reticular sensory pathway), which carries all types of sensory messages. Several descending auditory pathways have been demonstrated coming from cortical areas to the medial geniculate and to the inferior colliculus, as well as from inferior colliculi to the superior olivary complex.

✌KEY TERMS✌

Acoustic stria	Fissure	Mesencephalon	Rhombencephalon
Area 41	Forebrain	Metencephalon	Somatic nervous
Area 42	Frontal lobe	Midbrain	system
Autonomic nervous	Gray matter	Motor neuron	Spinal cord
system	Gyrus	Neural tube	Sulcus
Brainstem	Hindbrain	Occipital lobe	Superior olivary
Broca's speech area	Inferior colliculus	Olivocochlear pathway	complex
Cerebellum	Interneuron	Parasympathetic system	Sympathetic system
Cerebral hemispheres	Lateral lemniscus	Parietal lobe	Temporal lobe
Cerebrum	Lateral superior olive	Pons	Thalamus
Cochlear nuclei	Limbic lobe	Precentral gyrus	Tonotopic
Cochleotopy	Medial geniculate	Prosencephalon	organization
Decussate	Medial superior olive	Pyramidal system	Wernicke's area
Diencephalon	Medulla	Receptor	White matter
Extrapyramidal system	Meninges	Reticular formation	

✌STUDY QUESTIONS✌

1. What are the major lobes of the cerebral hemispheres?

2. What are the borders of the parietal lobe?

3. Describe the formation of the CNS.

4. At the pons-medulla border, what sensory and motor information is present?

5. Describe the pathway for sound localization in the brainstem.

6. Describe the cortical areas associated with the speech/language pathway.

⌇SUGGESTED READING⌇

Berlin, C. I., Hood, L., Morlet, T., Rose, K., & Brashears, S. (2003). Auditory neuropathy/dys-synchrony: Diagnosis and management. *Mental Retardation and Developmental Disabilities Research Reviews, 9*(4), 225–231.

Rapin, I., & Gravel, J. (2003). Auditory neuropathy: Physiologic and pathologic evidence calls for more diagnostic specificity. *International Journal of Pediatric Otorhinolaryngology, 67*(7), 707–728.

Rasmussen, G. L. (1953). Further observations of the efferent cochlear bundle. *Journal of Comparative Neurology, 99,* 61–74.

Rasmussen, G. L. (1960). Efferent fibers of the cochlear nerve and the cochlear nucleus. In Rasmussen, G. L., & W. G. William (Eds.), *Neural mechanisms of the auditory and vestibular systems* (pp. 105–115). Springfield, IL: Charles C. Thomas.

Rasmussen, G. L. (1964). The olivary peduncle and other fiber projections of the superior olivary complex. *Journal of Comparative Neurology, 84,* 141–219.

Starr, A., Isaacson, B., Michalewski, H. J., Zeng, F. G., Kong, Y. Y., Beale, P., Paulson, G. W., Keats, B. J., & Lesperance, M. M. (2004). A dominantly inherited progressive deafness affecting distal auditory nerve and hair cells. *Journal of the Association for Research in Otolaryngology, 5*(4), 411–426.

Starr, A., Michalewski, H. J., Zeng, F. G., Fujikawa-Brooks, S., Linthicum, F., Kim, C. S., Winnier, D., & Keats, B. (2003). Pathology and physiology of auditory neuropathy with a novel mutation in the MPZ gene (Tyr145>Ser). *Brain, 126*(pt 7), 1604–1619.

Starr, A., Picton, T. W., Sininger, Y., Hood, L. J., & Berlin, C. I. (1996). Auditory neuropathy. *Brain, 119*(pt 3), 741–753.

Weissman, J. E., & Hirsch, B. E. (2000). Imaging of tinnitus: A review. *Radiology, 216,* 342–349.

Chapter
15

Functional Organization
of the Auditory Central Nervous System

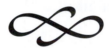

Kevin K. Ohlemiller, Ph.D.
Associate Professor of Otolaryngology
Washington University School of Medicine
St. Louis, Missouri

Chapter 14 introduced the auditory central nervous system (ACNS) and explored some aspects of its functional organization. This chapter considers in greater detail how spectral and temporal aspects of sounds, as well as the location of their source, may be encoded and represented by the ACNS. Unlike the simple stimuli used in the clinic and laboratory, real-world stimuli are quite complex. They have elaborate spectra and vary along temporal dimensions of rise and fall times, duration, and the manner of amplitude and frequency modulation (AM and FM, respectively). Throughout the ACNS, one can find neurons that appear to encode almost any spectral or temporal stimulus feature examined. Rarely, however, can we be sure that a given neuron and others like it are essential for the perception of a given feature. Nevertheless, a number of functional organizational principles within the ACNS have withstood repeated examination. The principles presented here have emerged from a consensus of human and animal observations.

The brain is not a single homogeneous structure, but rather includes distinct components connected by axonal "wiring." The space between components is crammed with bundles of axons and is generally referred to as *white matter* for the myelin insulation that covers each axon. Axons connect the two cerebral hemispheres with each other, the cerebellum, and with a host of distinct **nuclei** (i.e., clusters of neuronal cell bodies, the brain's *gray matter*) in the thalamus and brainstem. It is these interconnected islands of cells in **cortex,** thalamus, and brainstem whose properties are examined in this chapter (Figure 15-1). Often, the cells in neighboring "processing" subunits have different shapes and densities, so that with appropriate staining, they can be distinguished by ordinary light microscopy. Different cortical regions can also be distinguished in this manner. Moreover, any point on the cortex can be further functionally divided into layers that differ in the number and shape of the cells they contain and in their connections.

Historical Highlights

1861–1876	Paul Broca and Carl Wernicke demonstrate link between injury to temporal cortical areas and deficits in speech perception, and spatial separation of speech perception and production areas in the brain. D. Ferrier first identifies cortical areas associated with hearing.
1907	Lord Rayleigh formulates duplex theory of sound localization.
1911	Santiago Ramón y Cajal delineates subdivisions of the inferior colliculus by cytoarchitecture.
1929	D. Rioch recognizes subdivisions of auditory thalamus based on cytoarchitecture.
1942	C. Woolsey and E. Walzl demonstrate existence of multiple cortical fields and tonotopic organization of auditory cortex.
1943	R. Galambos and H. Davis publish first microelectrode studies of central auditory neurons.
1967–1974	Lesion studies by B. Masterton, D. Neff, and others demonstrate role for superior olivary complex in sound localization.
1966–1969	J. Rose, J. Goldberg, and others reveal binaural properties of neurons in the inferior colliculus and superior olive.
1972-1980	A. Graybiel distinguishes lemniscal/nonlemniscal auditory pathways. M. Merzenich, D. Andersen, and others further refine distinct tonotopic and nontonotopic pathways.
1983	N. Suga demonstrates organization of *mustached* bat's auditory cortex for echolocation, as well as the existence of combination-sensitive neurons.
1988–1994	C. Schreiner, J. Mendelson, M. Sutter, and others demonstrate secondary organization for spectral analysis within primary auditory cortex.
1988–1994	M. Reichle, R. Zatorre, and others apply positron emission tomography to speech, producing the first detailed information regarding cortical organization for speech perception.

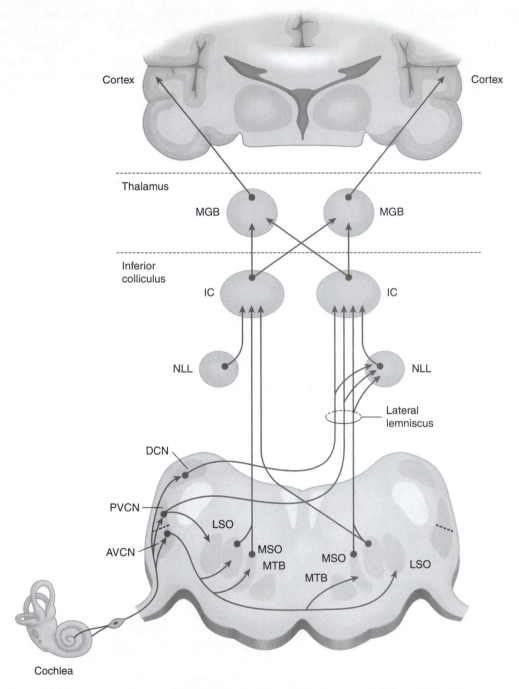

FIGURE 15-1 Simplified schematic organization of the auditory central nervous system. AVCN, anteroventral cochlear nucleus; DCN, dorsal cochlear nucleus; IC, inferior colliculus; LSO, lateral superior olive; MGB, medial geniculate body; MSO, medial superior olive; PVCN, posteroventral cochlear nucleus; NLL, nucleus of the lateral lemniscus; MTB, medial nucleus of the trapezoidal bundle. (Adapted from Pickles, 1982.)

Presented in extensive detail, the names and properties of all ACNS components would be daunting. The names of structures often seem non-intuitive, and the physiologic methods used to identify neural codes draw increasingly from linear and nonlinear systems analysis (e.g., Barbour & Wang, 2003; Escabi & Read, 2003). One goal of this chapter is to impart a basic understanding of how the ACNS functions, since this ultimately dictates the requirements of optimal cochlear implant and hearing aid design. Another goal is to help clinicians navigate the literature on central auditory processing disorders and related clinical techniques. We also hope to engage your interest in the fascinating puzzle that is the ACNS.

ORGANIZATIONAL AND FUNCTIONAL THEMES OF THE AUDITORY CENTRAL NERVOUS SYSTEM

The major theme of this chapter is the "representation" of sounds by the brain. Yet what is represented is simply one possible version of our acoustic surroundings. We do not hear the world as it really is, but rather, a highly filtered version of it. Just as we cannot perceive all wavelengths of light, we do not hear all frequencies. Other animals, including other mammals, do not see or hear the same world we do, because their retinas and cochleas detect somewhat different wavelengths of light and sound. Moreover, even as the brain creates visual illusions as a means of simplifying and interpreting the visual world, it "edits" sounds in ways we are not aware. For example, when an incoming sound is interpreted as speech, the brain ignores some spectral and temporal features that are not deemed to carry essential information. Similarly, the brain localizes sound sources by comparing the intensity and timing differences at the two ears, but we are often not aware of these characteristics—We unconsciously interpret them as location.

Representation implies the translation of real-world acoustic features into neuronal responses. For a unique stimulus to be unambiguously represented, it presumably must initiate a unique spatiotemporal pattern of neuronal activity across the ACNS. Theoretically, if we knew the code perfectly, we could work backward and recreate the stimulus. But we do not know the code perfectly. In fact, we can only guess what should be measured. Should we be more concerned with spike rates or interspike intervals? How far apart in time can spikes occur and still contribute to the same percept? What part of poststimulus time histogram (PSTH) contains the most significant spikes? How much of the code can be discerned by observing only one neuron at a time? Do we obtain meaningful responses if the subject is asleep or if the stimuli hold no significance for reward or survival? Finally, when we think about representation, we may unconsciously build in an "observer" who interprets the pattern. But where in the brain is the observer? The "you" that is (hopefully) conscious of these written words is somewhere in your brain—a gelatinous mass in the dark, cramped space that is the cranial cavity. The feeling of immediacy of the physical world is an illusion, although a useful and compelling one. Is the conscious "you" separable from the acoustic image of the world presented by your ACNS, as if you were listening to a radio? We are only just beginning to understand the link between ACNS function and perception. The following sections define some concepts and dimensions along which the ACNS may be usefully divided.

Channels

Channels are a somewhat loose notion that may be seen under other names (e.g., *modules, streams, pathways*). The idea is that, at every level within the ACNS, there is parcellation of neurons according to broad perceptual aspects of a stimulus. Each level has regions that are clearly tonotopically organized and those that are not. Nontonotopic regions appear likely to possess another—often obscure—organizational structure and probably serve a different function. Although there remains disagreement as to the division of jobs across pathways, candidates include "what" versus "where" aspects of stimuli and dedication of circuits to specialized functions such as communication, including speech. Functional divisions may align with long-recognized anatomically separable pathways, including *tono-topic/polysensory/diffuse, lemniscal/nonlemniscal, and core/belt* (Moller, 2000; Eggermont, 2001; Read et al., 2002; Rauschecker, 1998; Kaas & Hackett, 1998; Hu, 2003). These overlapping schemes are considered in more detail in this chapter.

Multidimensional Tuning

Chapter 11 examines tuning of neurons in the frequency domain, as characterized by frequency tuning curves. But "tuning" can refer to a preference for part of any stimulus continuum. One may also define tuning for temporal characteristics such as rise/fall time, duration, AM rate, FM rate, or AM/FM sweep direction. Cochlear neurons do not show band-pass tuning for any of the latter. Except for frequency, they show preferences that would be considered high- or low-pass tuning, or no preference at all. For example, cochlear neurons exhibit low-pass tuning for sinusoidal AM rate and no preference for stimulus duration. By contrast, at all levels of the ACNS (but especially inferior colliculus [IC] and higher), one may find neurons with band-pass tuning for one or more of these parameters. A single ACNS neuron may be tuned for any combination of stimulus frequency, stimulus rise time, duration, AM rate, or other characteristics (Figure 15-2). That ACNS neurons are tuned for such characteristics, whereas peripheral neurons are not, indicates that this tuning arises from the way ACNS neurons are connected together and serves a purpose. The majority of ACNS neurons probably simultaneously code for several stimulus features. In all likelihood, no neuron does only one job or analyzes just one stimulus attribute.

FIGURE 15-2 Tuning of cells in the central nucleus of the inferior colliculus of the *big brown* bat for tone duration. Data are shown from four neurons, each tuned to a different duration. Stimulus frequency and level are given in each graph. (Reprinted with permission from Casseday, J.H., Ehrlich, D., & Covey, E. (1994). Neural tuning for sound duration: Role of inhibitory mechanisms in the inferior colliculus. *Science, 264,* 847–850. Copyright 1994, AAAS.)

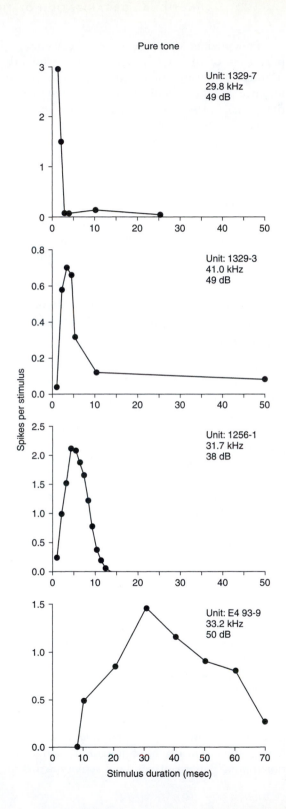

Multidimensional tuning greatly complicates the study of the ACNS. The most common tool used to classify response types in the ACNS is the frequency tuning curve, obtained in the same manner as for cochlear neurons. Because neurally mediated **lateral inhibition** is prominent in the ACNS, inhibitory areas are often measured as part of this process. Obtaining inhibitory areas usually entails presenting a low-level probe tone at the characteristic frequency (CF), preceded by tone bursts at various other frequency/level combinations to determine those that inhibit the response to the probe. Excitation/inhibition areas determined in this manner have value, in that they aid the classification of neurons, and have some predictive value as to what kinds of stimuli a given neuron will respond to. However, as investigators have tested how well frequency tuning curves predict responses to complex stimuli, substantial gaps have also been found. All excitatory or inhibitory influences may not be equally effective or grow similarly with intensity, making it impossible to predict their net effect. Changing probe tone intensity, stimulus repetition rate, or the delay between the conditioning and probe tones can change the shape of the curve. Stimulus parameters that can change the shape of the tuning curve constitute "tuning dimensions" beyond frequency tuning. Ignoring these dimensions may mean missing essential aspects of coding and representation.

Multidimensional Responses

An experimenter studying the ACNS must decide in advance what constitutes a "response." Typically, a short-latency increase in spike rate over the spontaneous firing rate is accepted as a response. But the shape of the PSTH varies across neurons (Figure 15-3), and for a given neuron, may vary with both stimulus frequency and level. Moreover, although phase-locking and temporal modulation-following are quite limited in ACNS neurons, they do occur, so that either spike rate or spike synchrony to the stimulus may be measured (Figure 15-4). Synchronous activity may also be found among neurons in different cortical fields, or in neurons within the same field. Whether this synchrony is vital to perception is unclear. What is clear is that measuring spike rate in single neurons over a fixed time window may overlook other equally important codes.

Dynamic Changes in Tuning

No matter what index of response is applied, careful study of many ACNS neurons would demonstrate that their tuning is not fixed. Throughout the ACNS, spectral and temporal tuning can be modified by level of alertness, by emotional and motivational state, and by learning (Suga, Xiao, Ma, & Ji, 2002; Edeline, 2003; He, 2003). Nonlemniscal (nontonotopic) collicular and thalamic auditory centers interconnect extensively with nonauditory centers that integrate context variables (i.e., the importance and meaning of a stimulus) and pass this information to cortex. Descending pathways from auditory cortex to auditory thalamus and colliculus may, in turn, shift tuning to particularly meaningful ranges and suppress responses to stimuli deemed less important (Figure 15-5). This process operates as a loop, such that modified information is passed back to cortex in what may constitute a progressive "focusing" operation. Spectral and temporal parameters of particularly salient stimuli may become overrepresented (i.e., may excite a greater proportion of neurons in a given region). This overrepresentation may enhance detection and allow finer discrimination, and may be temporary or persistent. Surprisingly, even the temporal modulation-following ability of auditory cortex—a feature that might be expected to be based on fundamental physical constraints—can be improved by learning paradigms (Bao, Chang, Woods, & Merzenich, 2004).

Maps

From previous chapters we know the main organizational principle of the cochlea: In the cochlea, distance along the basilar membrane and frequency tuning are inseparably linked. Tonotopy is also the most prominent organizing theme for the ACNS, so that the organizational foundation of the auditory system, like the visual and somatosensory systems,

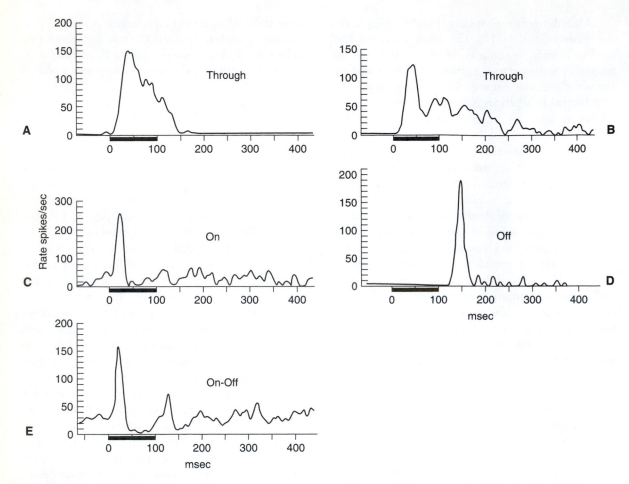

FIGURE 15-3 Variability of response pattern to tones across auditory cortical neurons. Poststimulus time histograms from five neurons, obtained in response to tones presented at times indicated *(bars)*. Patterns of response include onset (C), offset (D), onset-offset (E), and different types of tonic ("through") responses (A, B). (Reprinted from *Brain Research,* 42, Abeles, M., & Goldstein, M.H. Responses of single units in the primary auditory cortex of the cat to tones and tone pairs, 337–352, Copyright 1972, with permission from Elsevier.)

mirrors the spatial layout of the peripheral receptors. Of course, unlike the one-dimensional character of frequency representation in cochlea, the brain is three-dimensional. Thus, for example, instead of referring to the 1.5 kHz *place* in the cochlea, we might refer to the 1.5 kHz *lamina* in a particular region of the auditory brainstem or thalamus (Figure 15-6), or the 1.5 kHz *iso-frequency band* in an auditory cortical field. ACNS structures that show an orderly progression of frequency tuning are said to contain a frequency **map.** More generally, when any structure exhibits an orderly progression of tuning along any stimulus continuum (e.g., AM rate, sound source location), that stimulus feature is said to be *mapped.* Reversals and discontinuities of tonotopic gradients provided the first indications in early microelectrode studies that ACNS structures can be subdivided. For those regions that do not appear to contain a frequency map, the question always remains whether any other type of map exists.

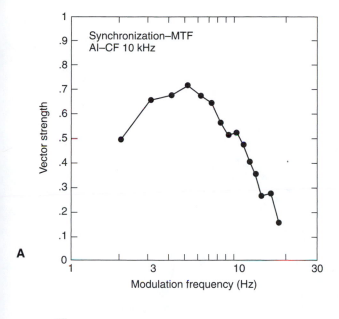

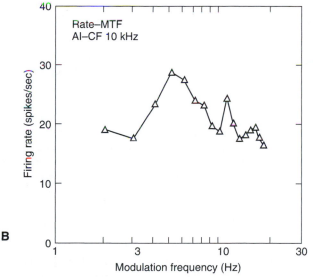

FIGURE 15-4 Tuning of a neuron in primary auditory cortex of the cat for amplitude modulation rate. Tuning was examined both for spike synchronization to the modulator (A) and firing rate (B). In both cases, the best modulation frequency was 5 to 6 Hz. CF, characteristic frequency. (Adapted from Schreiner and Langner, 1988.)

The most common pattern appears to be "clustering," whereby small patches of neurons are similarly tuned for a particular parameter, but there is no clear progression of tuning across the region.

Maps may have evolved as a way to simplify "wiring" of the ACNS during development, and they may also simplify the architectures needed for lateral inhibition, whereby neighboring neurons tuned to slightly different parameter values inhibit each other's responses. This presumably serves as a way to sharpen tuning. Whether maps are somehow essential to representation and perception is an open question.

ACNS frequency maps, where they are present, may not be allocated in a way that closely reflects the cochlear frequency map. Recall that the cochlear map is log-linear, with little apparent expansion of any frequency band in most mammals. But for most animals and humans, some bands actually are more important than others (e.g., echolocation frequencies in bats, wing-beat frequencies of aerial predators, communication frequencies). If increased space can lead to improved frequency resolution, it might be advantageous to devote more space to especially important frequencies. In fact, some species (e.g., echolocating bats; Suga, 1988) and structures (e.g., the lateral and medial superior olive in most mammals; see Figure 15-6) show permanently skewed frequency maps that reflect the needs of function and survival. Also, as mentioned earlier, learning can lead to expansion of portions of a frequency map (Edeline, 2003; Suga et al., 2002).

Parallel-Hierarchical Organization

The ACNS is composed of several processing levels from the brainstem nuclei, to the midbrain (IC), to the auditory thalamus (medial geniculate body [MGB]), and cortex (see Figure 15-1). Cortex also appears to contain multiple processing levels, in that "primary" areas receive most of their excitatory input from the thalamus, whereas other areas may receive their major excitatory input from primary areas (e.g., Kaas & Hackett, 1998; Rauschecker, 1998). Each processing level represents an opportunity to

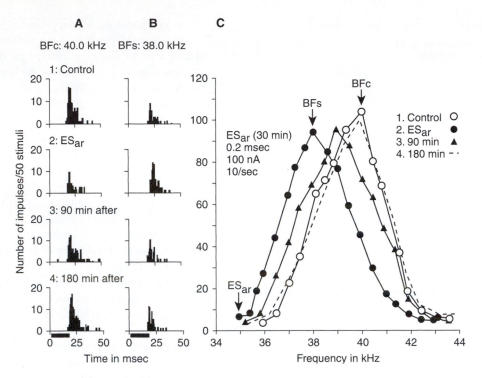

FIGURE 15-5 Plasticity of frequency tuning in auditory cortex of a *big brown* bat. The neuron from which the recordings are taken was originally tuned to ~40.0 kHz, identified in (C) as the "control" best frequency (BFc) based on the number of spikes elicited across test frequencies. Electrical stimulation (ESₐᵣ) of the neighboring 35.0 kHz region of cortex caused the BF to shift to ~38.0 kHz (BFs in C). Over the subsequent 180 minutes, the BF shifted back near 40.0 kHz. Histograms in (A) and (B) show that more spikes are elicited by a 38.0 kHz stimulus after the electrical stimulus. Cortical electrical stimulation mimics the effects of acoustic stimulation in behavioral training wherein a tonal stimulus at a particular frequency signals a reward or an aversive stimulus. Temporary shifting of tuning toward the frequency of an especially meaningful stimulus probably enhances discrimination. (Used with permission from Ma, X., & Suga, N. (2001). Plasticity of bat's central auditory system evoked by focal electric stimulation of auditory and/or somatosensory cortices. *Journal of Neurophysiology, 85*, 1078–1097.)

recombine information from a lower level, so that new selectivities and response properties are created. What types of changes might we notice in neuronal preferences and responses as we ascend the hierarchy? Actually, differences from one level to the next are surprisingly subtle. For example, although binaural sensitivity first arises within the superior olivary complex within the brainstem, the complexity of binaural responses changes little as we ascend further (Middlebrooks, Xu, Furukawa, & Mickey, 2001). Tuning for periodic modulation rate first arises in mammals at the level of the IC, but it does not become more refined at higher levels. Instead, the range

of frequencies over which neurons can follow periodic modulations is progressively reduced (Schreiner & Langner, 1988; Palmer & Summerfield, 2002). "Complexity" of tuning similarly does not appear to increase at higher ACNS levels. It has been suggested that neuronal architectures for the representation of speech and other complex stimuli rely on neurons that act as "AND" logic elements (Suga, 1988; Rauschecker, 1998). Such neurons might require multiple components of a complex sound (e.g., multiple frequency bands, such as the formants in a vowel) to elicit a response. Such a requirement for combinations of acoustic components has been

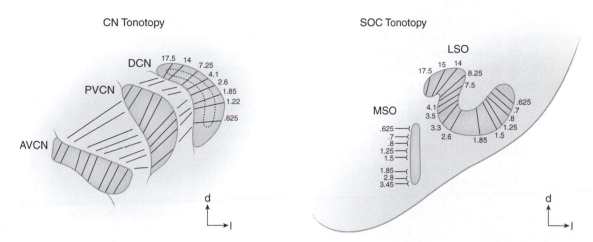

FIGURE 15-6 Schematic frequency map of the gerbil cochlear nucleus (CN, left) and superior olivary complex (SOC, right). The three major divisions of the CN have been aligned to emphasize that they all contain a complete frequency map. The frequency maps of the medial superior olive (MSO) and lateral superior olive (LSO) are heavily skewed toward low and high frequencies, respectively. This is in keeping with the different functions of these nuclei. The MSO detects binaural temporal differences at low frequencies, whereas the LSO detects binaural spectral differences at higher frequencies. AVCN, anteroventral cochlear nucleus; DCN, dorsal cochlear nucleus; PVCN, posteroventral cochlear nucleus. (From Müller, M. (1990). Quantitative comparison of frequency representation in the auditory brainstem nuclei of the gerbil, *Pachyuromys duprasi. Experimental Brain Research, 81*, 140–149. With kind permission of Springer Science and Business Media.)

called **combination sensitivity** (Suga, 1988). Hypothetically, the convergence of such neurons onto neurons at higher processing levels could create "super-adder" neurons, requiring several acoustic elements such as those that define phoneme combinations. Through a series of such convergences, moreover, one could hypothetically create "detector" neurons for entire words or phrases. Combination-sensitive neurons can indeed be found, and they appear to serve echolocation and communication in bats (Suga, 1988; Ohlemiller, Kanwal, Butman, & Suga, 1994) and communication in primates (Rauschecker, 1998). However, they may be found in IC, auditory thalamus, and cortex, and their tuning properties do not necessarily become more complex with ACNS level.

There is not just one hierarchy, but several. As stated earlier, starting in the brainstem and continuing through all higher levels, each ACNS structure is composed of several divisions. These are thought to correspond to partly segregated analysis of different types of information at each level, so that we can identify distinct pathways that run from brainstem to cortex. Each pathway or stream can, in turn, be subdivided, such that different sets of stimulus attributes are processed in *parallel* by neurons tuned to different values of each attribute.

Finally, as we considered, hierarchical processing does not imply one-way flow of information. The tuning properties of cortical neurons at higher levels are constantly adjusted via efferent feedback loops that run through the MGB and IC. In fact, more neurons may mediate the transfer of information *from* cortex than *to* cortex (He, 2003). In attempting to find "ultimate recipient" neurons of the ACNS, we are presented with a loop. There are no ultimate recipients.

Divergence and Convergence

Divergence and **convergence** refer to the nature of connections between and within ACNS structures, whereby new channels and new kinds of tuning are created. The most significant divergence within the ACNS occurs in the brainstem within the cochlear nucleus (CN). Each cochlear neuron bifurcates after entering the CN and, ultimately, contacts several kinds of neurons in three major subdivisions. Thus, information pertaining to a single frequency is distributed to several types of cells that code for additional stimulus characteristics. The "design" of the CN becomes especially important when it is considered that all the response properties of neurons of the entire remainder of the ACNS must be established there. Other than binaurality, information not present at the level of the CN cannot be added by later stages.

A good example of neuronal convergence is the combining of input from both ears that occurs in brainstem auditory nuclei. This convergence makes possible the necessary cues needed for sound source localization in the horizontal plane. These cues are not possible using either ear alone. An essential aspect of convergence is that the neurons whose axons project onto a given neuron may be either excitatory or inhibitory, depending on the neurotransmitter they release.

The general role of convergence in the ACNS appears to be refinement of tuning and creation of new selectivities. Refinements of frequency tuning often include narrowing of tuning and elimination of the "tail" of tuning curves (Figure 15-7). Tuning of ACNS neurons may be similar to that of cochlear neurons at low levels, near the tip of the tuning curve, but is often much sharper at higher levels. For any neuron, this is accomplished by convergence of inhibitory inputs from neurons tuned to higher and lower frequencies. For example, if the neuron has a CF of 1.0 kHz, it might receive inhibitory inputs from neurons tuned to 0.5 and 1.5 kHz. Thus, a 1.0 kHz stimulus would excite this neuron, but as the stimulus frequency is moved upward or downward, we would rapidly encounter frequencies that not only do not excite the neuron, but even decrease its background (spontaneous) activity level. (Recall that this does not occur in cochlear neurons.) Lateral inhibition can produce quite narrow

excitatory tuning curves. This inhibition is often accomplished by local *inhibitory interneurons* whose axons project only within a region, instead of from one region to another. This allows any neuron projecting *into* a given region to exert both excitatory and inhibitory influences, by virtue of contacting its "target" neurons either directly, or indirectly through inhibitory neurons.

Through simple convergence arrangements, we can create a variety of neurons with surprisingly complex selectivities. Consider, for example, the response to FM of neuron 4 in Figure 15-8. This neuron is excited by neuron 2 (and so tuned to the same frequency), but inhibited by neurons 1 and 3, which are tuned to lower and higher frequencies, respectively. Thus, the excitatory areas for neurons 1 and 3 constitute the inhibitory areas of neuron 4. Either an upward or downward sweeping FM tone ending at 1.0 kHz will first pass through an inhibitory sideband. For an FM sweep, any excitatory input to this neuron will be preceded by inhibition. As a result, the neuron may not respond to FM, or at least not as well as it would respond to a simple tone at 1.0 kHz. Another property that may emerge in this same neuron is stimulus-level tuning. Note that the triangular inhibitory areas show increasing overlap with the center excitatory area at higher stimulus levels. A loud tone at the CF will therefore engage both excitatory and inhibitory influences. As a result, a loud CF tone may not excite this neuron as effectively as a tone at moderate levels. This neuron may therefore have a nonmonotonic input-output curve, and thus be tuned to a specific stimulus level. Repetition and minor tweaking of this arrangement could create an array of neurons tuned to different stimulus levels. Now imagine that the inhibitory input from either neuron 3 is removed or is changed to excitation. Neuron 4 will now respond to downward FM, but not upward FM. Of course, the response strength of a real neuron will depend on a complex balance of many excitatory

FIGURE 15-7 Comparison of frequency tuning curve shape in cat auditory nerve (AN; A) and inferior colliculus (IC; B). Note loss of tails and overall narrower tuning in collicular neurons. SPL, sound pressure level. (Reprinted from *Neuroscience Research, 21*, Suga, N., Sharpening of frequency tuning by inhibition in the central auditory system— Tribute to Yasuji Katsuki, 287–299, Copyright 1995, with permission from Elsevier.)

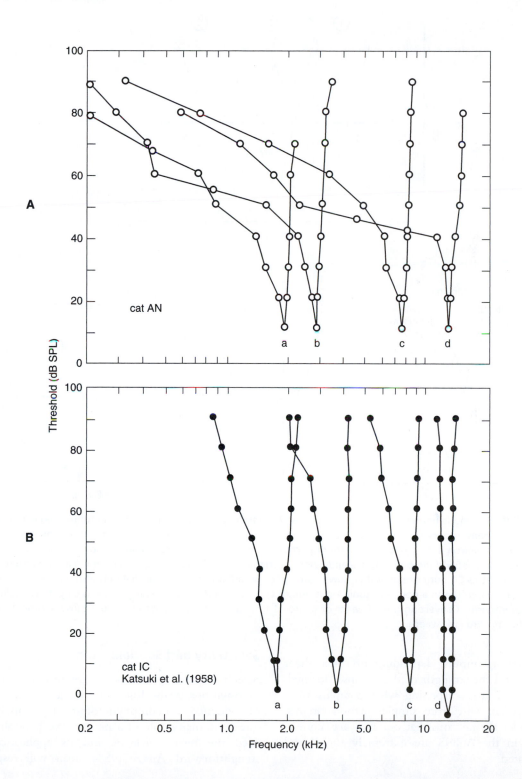

A

cat AN

a   b   c   d

B

cat IC
Katsuki et al. (1958)

a   b   c   d

Threshold (dB SPL)

Frequency (kHz)

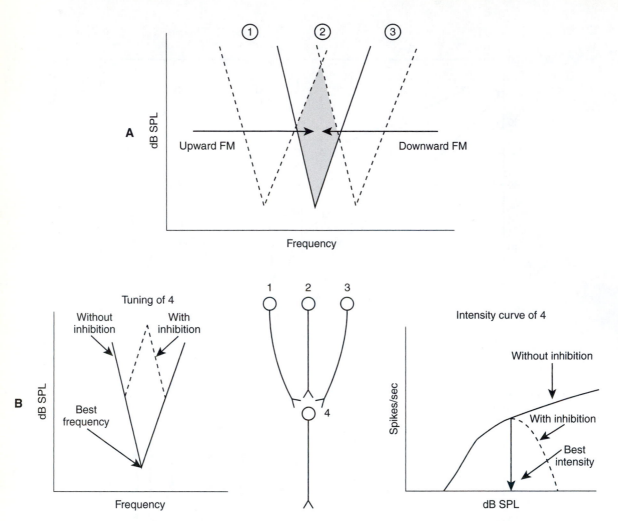

FIGURE 15-8 Schematic neuronal circuit showing how sharp tuning, FM selectivity, and level tuning can hypotheti-cally arise from convergence of only a few neurons onto a single neuron. Neurons 1 and 3 inhibit neuron 4, whereas neuron 2 excites neuron 4. Neurons 1 and 3 are respectively tuned to frequencies higher and lower than neuron 2 (A). Because of *sideband inhibition* above and below its characteristic frequency (CF), neuron 4 may respond to low intensity tones at its CF, but not upward or downward FM or broadband noise. Neuron 4 may also display a closed excitatory area (B, left) and a nonmonotonic input-output curve (*dashed line* in B, right). Thus, it may show tuning to a particular intensity. Converting the influence of neuron 1 from inhibitory to excitatory would cause neuron 4 to be selective for upward FM sweeps.

and inhibitory inputs, depending on their sheer numbers and the strength of the synapses formed. Nevertheless, it is surprising what complex filter properties can arise from simple cartoon circuits. No wonder the neurons that one may actually en-counter in the ACNS are extremely varied and complicated.

Selectivity and Specialization

Selectivity and specialization are related, but not synonymous, terms. Together, they define the kinds of evidence a neurophysiologist might apply to guess the major role of a neuron. We have already used the term *selectivity*, and its application is straightforward. An ACNS neuron will respond more robustly to some stimuli than others. In general, the more inhibitory inputs a neuron receives, the fewer types of broadband stimuli that will elicit a response. The notion of specialization goes further, however, requiring (1) that simple stimuli such as tones elicit no response, and (2) combination sensitivity, that is, a **facilitative** response to a combination of two or more stimulus elements (the logical "AND" unit we considered previously).

Because combination sensitivity requires specialized circuitry, it is taken as an indication of purposeful neuronal specialization when it is found. When the apparent specialization fits well with a known behavior, a strong case can be made. Extensive work by N. Suga in echolocating bats (particularly *mustached* bats) has shaped much of the discussion about what types of neuronal specializations exist and how they may be used by humans and animals (Suga, 1988) (Figures 15-9, 15-10, and 15-11). Echolocating bats emit *biosonar pulses* and compare the timing and spectral distribution of the outgoing pulse with the echo returned from the target. Because echolocation is a means of finding food, the bat's ACNS is organized around this function. The principles underlying determination of an insect's flight velocity and distance require fine spectral and temporal comparisons of pulse and echo. This problem was solved evolutionarily by the creation of combination-sensitive neurons that respond only to particular combinations of simultaneous "constant frequency" tones (CF/CF neurons), or to combined downward-sweeping frequency-modulated tones separated by precise time intervals (FM-FM neurons). The mustached bat's auditory cortex contains several areas in which the majority of neurons are either CF/CF or FM-FM. Moreover, there are orderly maps in most of these regions for specific CF/CF ratios or FM-FM delays.

Few investigations of combination-sensitive neurons have enjoyed the advantage of such a clear correspondence between apparent neural specialization and the dictates of behavior in an "auditory specialist" animal like the bat. Additional claims of specialization in primates (Rauschecker, 1998) and even bats (Ohlemiller et al., 1994) have relied on a reasonable correspondence between the acoustic elements required to excite neurons and the elements present in the communication sounds. As an example, many animal communication repertoires include calls with frequency-modulated harmonics, such as the one shown in Figure 15-11 (top right). In the *mustached* bat, variants of this call will excite FM-FM neurons in a combination-sensitive manner. These calls generally will not drive CF/CF neurons effectively, because these receive more prominent inhibitory input (see Figure 15-9). CF/CF neurons will respond in a combination-sensitive manner to some narrowband communication sounds, however. Do the responses of FM-FM and CF/CF neurons to bat communication sounds contribute to the representation of these in the bats' ACNS? That is less clear than in the case of echolocation, because the "fit" between the filter properties of these neurons and the properties of the sounds is not as obvious and could be a coincidence. However, the *mustached* bat possesses a diverse communication repertoire. A type of economy may exist in using neurons specialized for echolocation to represent them.

Brain regions that appear to be specialized for complex functions such as communication are usually heterogeneous in the types of neurons they contain. Not all the neurons in these areas may be particularly selective or show obviously tailored specializations. Demonstrations of selectivity and apparent specialization can support a role for particular neurons in an auditory task, but they typically are not "proof." Evidence must also show that the neurons (or rather, the area that contains them) are active during the task. This might be achieved by recording from many individual neurons or small groups of neurons in a behaving subject. Electroencephalography (EEG) and magnetoencephalography (MEG) are effective tools for identifying cortical areas involved in specific tasks (e.g., Pantev & Lütkenhöner, 2000). Two additional methods, positron emission tomography (PET) and functional magnetic resonance imaging (fMRI), which rely on the detection of increased metabolic activity in active brain regions, allow investigators to monitor the activity of whole cortical fields and subcortical structures with resolution of a few millimeters (e.g., Rauschecker, 1998; Read et al., 2002; Palmer & Summerfield, 2002). Lesion studies may also show that an area of interest is necessary for the

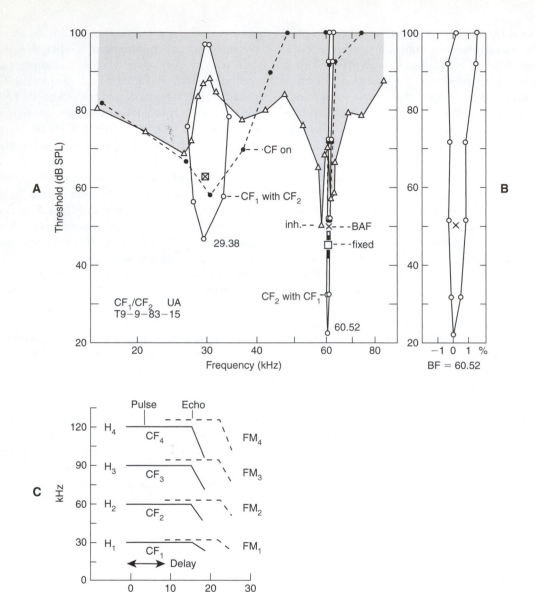

FIGURE 15-9 (A) Excitatory and inhibitory frequency tuning curves of a CF$_1$/CF$_2$ neuron in auditory cortex of a *mustached* bat. The neuron showed a selective facilitated response to simultaneous constant frequency (CF) tones near 30 and 60 kHz, thus demonstrating combination sensitivity. (B) Facilitated tuning to the 60 kHz component on an expanded scale. Under natural conditions, the lower frequency would be prominent in the bat's biosonar pulse, and the higher frequency would be prominent in the returning echo (see C). Such pulse/echo frequency comparisons yield target velocity information. Other specialized cortical neurons show responses to different CF/CF combinations. Prominent inhibitory areas (*gray shading* in A) typically prevent responses to broadband stimuli. Dashed curves denoted "CF on" show tuning to low and high frequency components when presented alone. Under these conditions, thresholds are higher and tuning is broader. BAF, Best amplitude for facilitation; BF, best frequency; SPL, sound pressure level. (Used with permission from Suga, N. & Tsuzuki, K. (1985). Inhibition and level-tolerant frequency tuning in the auditory cortex of the mustached bat. *Journal of Neurophysiology, 53*, 1109–1145.)

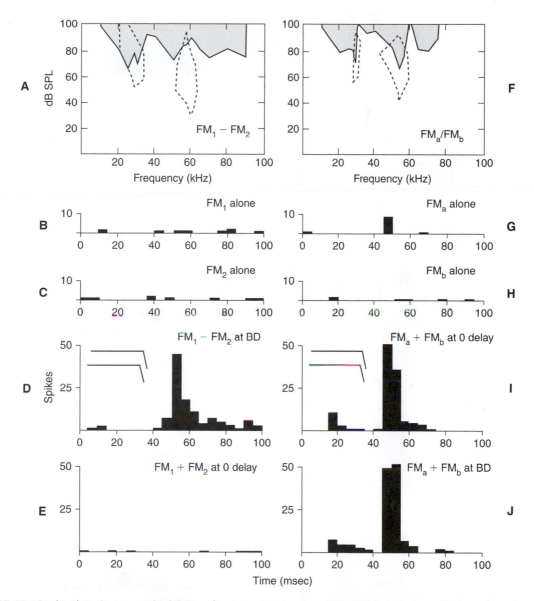

FIGURE 15-10 (A–E) Excitatory and inhibitory frequency tuning in an FM_1-FM_2 neuron in auditory cortex of a *mus-tached* bat. Frequency-modulation (FM)-FM neurons respond selectively and facilitatively to combined downward FM sweeps at the end of the biosonar pulse and its returning echo at particular pulse-echo delays (best delay (BD) 2.4 milliseconds for this neuron), thus providing information about target distance. FM-FM neurons are somewhat broadly tuned, with little inhibition at low intensities. Pulse-echo frequency combinations that are effective in echolocation are generally greater than one octave. (Best starting frequencies were 28.6 and 60.5 kHz in this case.) (F–J) Nearly harmonic FM-FM combinations presented simultaneously were also effective in exciting the neuron. (F) Tuning for simultaneous FM sweeps (FM_a/FM_b). Combination sensitivity for harmonics appears better suited to rep-resentation of communication sounds than echolocation (see Figure 15-11). (Used with permission from Ohlemiller, K.K, Kanwal, J.S., Butman, J.A., & Suga, N. (1994). Stimulus design for auditory neuroethology: Synthesis and manipu-lation of complex communication sounds. *Auditory Neuroscience, 1,* 19–37.)

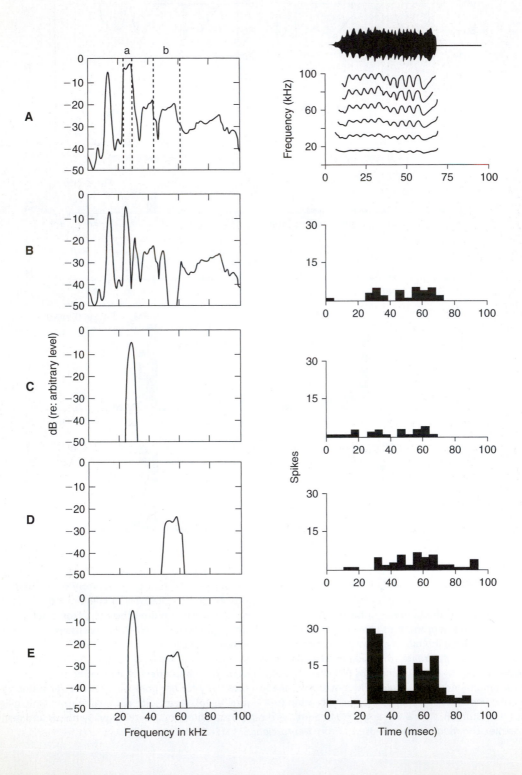

posited perceptual task. Such evidence comes from experimental lesions in animals (e.g., Heffner & Heffner, 1990), as well as clinical cases wherein an accident or stroke has by chance damaged the area.

Conversion from Temporal Coding to Place Coding

Chapter 11 considers probable place and temporal codes used by cochlear neurons. A place code conveys information by virtue of the spatial distribution of neurons that are most active, whereas a temporal code conveys information by the precise timing of spikes. Information encoded temporally may include stimulus phase (for frequencies less than ~5.0 kHz), the phase and magnitude of periodic AM and FM (for modulation frequencies up to ~300 Hz), and the onsets and offsets of stimuli (via adaptation effects on instantaneous spike rates). The cochlea transmits temporal information to the brainstem with high fidelity. A high degree of fidelity is maintained in the CN and in the superior olive, where binaural comparisons are first made. This is possible through special synaptic structures and fast-acting membrane ion channels that are unique to the auditory system (Trussell, 1997). As information ascends within the ACNS, however, there is a reduction in temporal fidelity of spikes, due to variability in neuronal conduction times and temporal dispersion of converging excitatory signals. As a result, phase-locking is nonexistent above the lower brainstem. The maximum frequency at which neuronal spike times can follow periodic modulation declines to less than 120 Hz at the level of the IC and less than 40 Hz in cortex (Palmer & Summerfield, 2002). At the level of the IC and above, temporally coded information derived from stimulus phase and periodic AM and FM (including phase-locking codes for speech formant structure and AM coding of period-

icity pitch; see Chapter 11) must somehow be recoded using a place code.

Despite loss of temporal acuity, ACNS neurons exhibit short latencies and reduced variance in spike times, compared with central neurons in other sensory systems. This enables spikes entrained to stimulus onsets and offsets to be sufficiently synchronous so that timing cues related to phoneme identification (such as voice-onset times) appear retained in primary auditory cortex (e.g., Steinschneider, Schroeder, Arezzo, & Vaughan, 1990).

Shift from Tonic to Phasic Responses

Recall from Chapter 11 that PSTHs of cochlear neurons demonstrate **tonic** responses that are fairly homogenous across neurons. Tonic means that as long as the stimulus is on, the spike rate will be increased above the spontaneous firing rate. PSTHs of ACNS neurons, by contrast, show **phasic** responses. The spike rate may be only transiently increased at the beginning (and possibly after the end) of a stimulus (see Figure 15-2).

Binaural Interactions

Humans have two ears. The most obvious advantage of this is for sound localization (how binaural comparisons of timing/phase and intensity make this possible is considered later in this chapter). It is worth considering, however, whether there are other perceptual advantages of having two ears (that is, *perceptual enhancement*). In fact, absolute thresholds and difference limens (DL) for frequency and intensity are all improved when the same stimulus is presented to the two ears (Yin, 2001). For localization, binaural interaction exploits interaural differences in timing or intensity. These interactions occur in specific brainstem nuclei that mediate localization. Neurons

FIGURE 15-11 Combination-sensitive response of the FM-FM neuron from Figure 15-10 to a bat communication sound containing FM harmonics (top right). The frequency spectrum of the original call is shown in A. Eliminating frequency bands FM$_a$ and FM$_b$ (see Figure 15-10F) eliminated the response (B). Reducing the call to only bands FM$_a$ and FM$_b$ yielded essentially the same response as the original call (E). Either frequency band alone was ineffective (C, D). (Used with permission from Ohlemiller, K.K, Kanwal, J.S., Butman, J.A., & Suga, N. (1994). Stimulus design for auditory neuroethology: Synthesis and manipulation of complex communication sounds. *Auditory Neuroscience, 1,* 19–37.)

in the midbrain and higher centers often show binaural interactions of opposite sign. Most are "IE" neurons, meaning that they are inhibited by sounds in the ipsilateral ear and excited by sounds in the contralateral ear. These interactions translate into a best source location in the horizontal plane. The types of interactions that mediate binaural perceptual enhancements (improved sensitivity, frequency, and intensity DLs) are likely to be of the same sign (EE). Although such neurons are found, they are not predominant, and the physiologic bases of such enhancements currently are unclear.

THE COCHLEAR NUCLEUS AS AN ESSENTIAL HUB

Armed with broad anchoring principles, let us consider specific ACNS structures, starting in the lower brainstem. The CN merits emphasis as the requisite hub and site of initiation for all coding transformations that occur in the ACNS (Cant & Morest, 1984; Rhode & Greenberg, 1992). Given that cochlear neurons are fairly homogenous, it falls to the CN to generate the properties that make possible the tremendous variety of response characteristics in the ACNS. Perhaps it is surprising how *few* major cell types the CN appears to contain. Separate consideration of the CN also provides an opportunity to emphasize the close link between neuronal structure and function.

The CN contains three main divisions: anteroventral (AVCN), dorsal (DCN), and posteroventral (PVCN), each of which contains a complete tonotopic map. Each type I (radial) afferent neuron entering the brain from the cochlea gives rise to two main processes, an ascending and descending branch (Figure 15-12). The ascending branch makes contact with cells in the PVCN on its way to the DCN. The descending branch contacts cells in the AVCN. Some researchers contend that the major function of the PVCN is stimulus identification, while that of the AVCN and DCN is localization, so that segregation of information channels arises immediately within the ACNS (Eggermont, 2001). Evidence for this includes that fact that the largest projections of the PCVN bypass the superior olive (a localization center), as well as

good evidence that the neurons in DCN are highly sensitive to pinna effects on the sound spectrum (Young & Davis, 2001). Steep "notches" in the stimulus spectrum caused by the shape of the pinna are thought to be the major cue for sound-source elevation. The DCN, however, also receives nonsensory and polysensory input, as well as indirect feedback from auditory cortex, so integration of stimulus context and meaning may be a significant role for this structure (Ryugo, Haengelli, & Doucet, 2003). The major neuronal types in the CN are described below (see Figure 15-12).

Spherical Bushy Cells   Spherical bushy cells of the AVCN receive strong input from a small number of cochlear afferents via large-current synapses directly on the cell body. A combination of a few strong inputs and postulated constant (tonic) inhibition imparts superior phase-locking to these cells over cochlear neurons, at least for stimulus frequencies less than 1.0 kHz. The PSTHs of their responses to tones look much like those of cochlear neurons. These neurons appear important for conveying spike timing information to higher centers and project to brainstem nuclei involved in localization.

Globular Bushy Cells   Globular bushy cells of the AVCN receive weak input from many ($\sim$20) cochlear afferents directly on their cell bodies. This arrangement, combined again with inhibitory influences, somehow also endows these cells with superior phase-locking over cochlear neurons at low-stimulus frequencies (Figure 15-13). Thus, two quite different architectures produce enhancement of phase-locking in spherical and globular bushy cells over the cochlear neurons that drive them. The PSTHs of globular cell responses to tones also resemble those of cochlear neurons, but tend to include a "notch" of reduced activity soon after the onset peak. These neurons also project to brainstem nuclei involved in localization.

Stellate Cells   Stellate cells of the AVCN and PVCN receive weak excitatory input from many cochlear neurons out on their dendritic tree, and they have membrane conductances that lend an un-

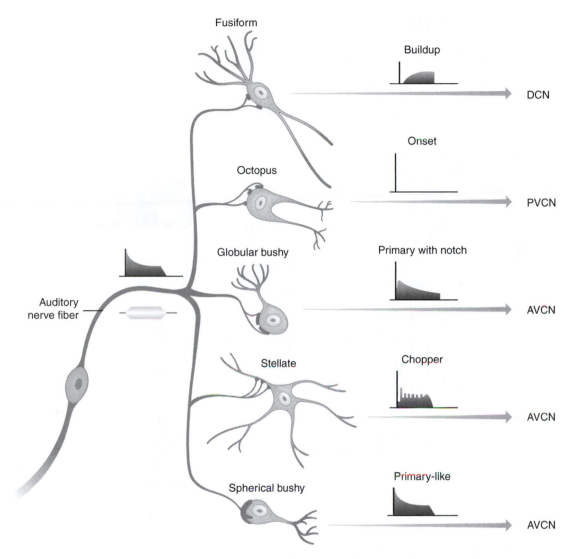

FIGURE 15-12 Schematic showing divergence of input from an individual cochlear neuron as its axon enters the cochlear nucleus to drive five major cell types having different morphologies and response patterns. Names above the poststimulus time histograms at right are the generally accepted names of these response patterns. These different patterns reflect the type of synapse formed (excitatory versus inhibitory), the number of afferent contacts, the shape of the postsynaptic cell, and the types of channels in the cell membrane. AVCN, anteroventral cochlear nucleus; DCN, dorsal cochlear nucleus; PVCN, posteroventral cochlear nucleus. (Adapted from Cant and Morest, 1984.)

usual shape to their PSTH. This includes rhythmic peaks that superficially look like phase-locking, but rather are completely unrelated to the phase of incoming spikes. This pattern has earned them the name *chopper* cells. Not surprisingly, these cells exhibit poor phase-locking. The projections of these cells bypass brainstem nuclei involved in localization, targeting instead the ventral nucleus of the lateral lemniscus and IC. By virtue of their wide dynamic range and lateral inhibitory influences, these cells appear to retain the capacity to code for spectral peaks (such as formants) in complex stimuli. It has

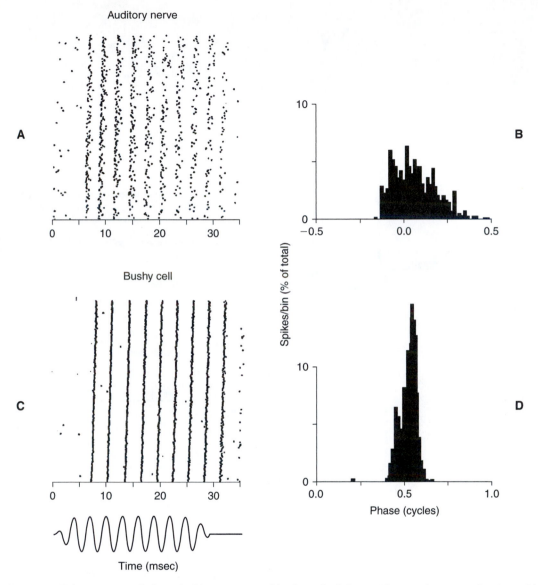

FIGURE 15-13 Enhancement of phase-locking in a typical bushy cell of the cochlear nucleus over that in cochlear neurons. (A, C) Raster displays of individual spike times over many stimulus presentations. (B, D) Phase histograms. Spikes are more narrowly distributed over the stimulus cycle for the bushy cell. (Reprinted from *Neuron, 21*, Joris, P.X, Smith, P.H., & Yin, T.C.T., Coincidence detection in the auditory system: 50 years after Jeffress. 1235-1238, Copyright 1998, with permission from Elsevier.)

therefore been proposed that they participate in analysis of spectral shape. Herein lies the origin of the term *lemniscal pathway*, because clear tonotopy and apparent organization for spectral analysis demarcate this principally monaural projection route.

Octopus Cells Dendrites of octopus cells of the PVCN extend across frequency lamina, so that these cells are poorly frequency tuned. However, because of strong convergent input, they respond to tones with a first spike that has a precise latency and show strong phase-locking. Octopus cells project to brainstem nuclei involved in localization. Generally, there is a tendency for neurons anywhere in the ACNS to show high fidelity with regard to timing or frequency, but not both. The timing precision of octopus cells, which arises from the convergence of neurons tuned to many frequencies, is a case in point.

Fusiform Cells   Fusiform cells of the DCN show narrow frequency tuning and are readily inhibited by broadband sounds. As a class they are heterogeneous. A typical PSTH profile is a "buildup" profile, whereby the spike rate increases over the course of a tone burst. These cells bypass brainstem nuclei involved in horizontal sound localization, instead projecting to the contralateral IC. Nevertheless, they may play a role in localizing sound sources in the vertical plane. This has been suggested based on recordings in cats, where it has been noted that the frequency tuning curves of fusiform cells contain sharp regions of inhibition that often match the spectral shaping influence of the cat's pinna. Such a match in not always evident, however, causing investigators in this area to propose a broader role for these cells in complex spectral analysis.

The preceding list omits several subtypes, and a clear functional picture of the CN is still emerging. We can summarize, however, by noting that cells of the CN include both those that retain and enhance the cycle-by-cycle structure of the stimulus and those that appear to be designed to suppress it, emphasizing instead the beginning and end of the stimulus and perhaps its amplitude.

LOCALIZATION PATHWAYS

How we locate sound sources is the best understood functional aspect of ACNS architecture (Irvine, 1992; Yin, 2001; Yin & Chan, 1988; Joris, Yin, & Smith, 1990; Joris, Smith, & Yin, 1998). Localization has been amenable to investigation, partly because the anatomy and physiology of certain brainstem nuclei seem unequivocally based around long-predicted requirements of localization. Most ACNS neurons appear spatially tuned to some degree. This spatial tuning is nearly always superimposed on other types of tuning. The basis of interaural comparisons resides in the

spectral and temporal properties of the stimulus. These comparisons are carried out in the brainstem **lateral superior olive** (LSO) and **medial superior olive** (MSO), respectively (Figure 15-14). Based on the location of the source, the sound is expected to be louder in one ear than the other. For low-frequency, steady-state stimuli, one ear will experience a phase lag relative to the other ear. For transient, noisy stimuli, the wave front of the sound will impinge on one ear before the other. All of these cues will be most pronounced for sounds located to the far left or right of the listener, and least pronounced for sounds coming from the midline. Localization of sound sources in the vertical direction relies, in part, on a somewhat different set of cues. The pinna alters the spectrum of sounds, depending on their elevation, so that sources are localized vertically by the shape of their spectrum. By contrast with azimuth localization, vertical localization can be performed monaurally.

The Duplex Theory of Sound Localization

The idea that interaural time differences are used to localize low-frequency stimuli in the horizontal plane and interaural intensity differences are used to localize high-frequency stimuli horizontally, known as the **duplex theory,** was put forth by Lord Rayleigh (aka J. W. Strutt) more than a century ago (see Yin & Chan, 1988; Yin, 2001). Based on the typical dimensions of the human head, Rayleigh realized that frequencies less than about 700 Hz would not cast an acoustic "shadow," and thus could not be localized using interaural intensity cues. From observations of binaural beat phenomena, he reasoned that the ear must be sensitive to the phase of tones. As discussed in Chapter 2, low-frequency sounds have longer spatial wavelengths. It is therefore for lower frequencies that the width of the head causes the two ears to "sample" the stimulus at different phases. This spatial sampling equates to a constant interaural time difference (again based on average head dimensions) of about 800 microseconds, so that the phase difference sensed by the two ears will depend on frequency. As the stimulus frequency increases, however, there will come a point where the two ears sample the stimulus at exactly one cycle, that is, at the same phase. That is typically 1.4 kHz. In fact, because there

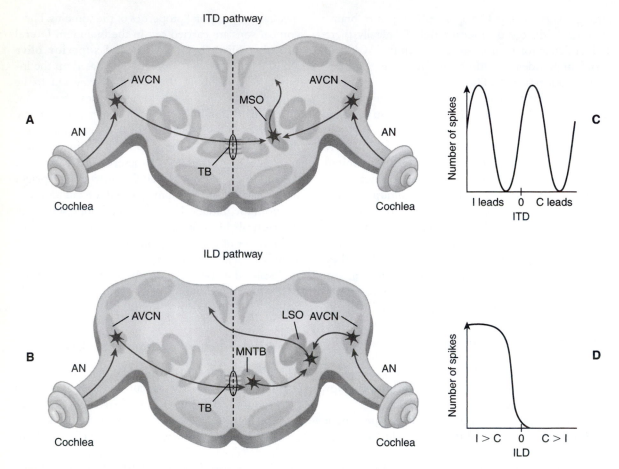

FIGURE 15-14 Schematic of separate pathways for coding interaural time differences (ITD) and interaural level differences (ILD) within the medial superior olive (MSO; A) and lateral superior olive (LSO; B). Sensitivity to ITD depends on simultaneous convergent excitation from the two ears. Tuning for ITD (C) shows a cyclic character, because a tonal stimulus will repeat a given ITD at multiples of the stimulus period. Tuning for ILD (D) will favor one ear, based on the convergence of contralateral inhibition and ipsilateral excitation in the LSO. Initial excitation from the contralateral ear undergoes a "sign change" to inhibition in medial nucleus of the trapezoid body (MNTB). AN, auditory nerve; AVCN, anteroventral cochlear nucleus; TB, trapezoid bundle. (Adapted from Joris et al., 1990.)

are two zero-crossings per cycle, phase cues become increasingly ambiguous for frequencies greater than about 700 Hz, well below the 4.0 to 5.0 kHz phase-locking limit of cochlear neurons. The duplex theory holds rigidly only for tonal stimuli. Most real-world stimuli are transient and noisy, however. For brief stimuli, the absolute time difference for any sound to traverse the head, which is not dependent on frequency, becomes an important cue. Another typical real-world stimulus condition involves amplitude modulation of high frequencies. Such stimuli may

also be localized using interaural phase cues, in this case, the phase of the modulating frequency. Note that this must be coded by neurons tuned to high frequencies. Timing "channels" in the brainstem are skewed toward lower frequencies, but do contain a complete frequency map (see later).

Sound frequencies that are optimal for localization based on timing/phase complement those best suited to interaural intensity cues. Such intensity cues are based on the physical laws governing *diffraction,* that is, the bending of sound around objects

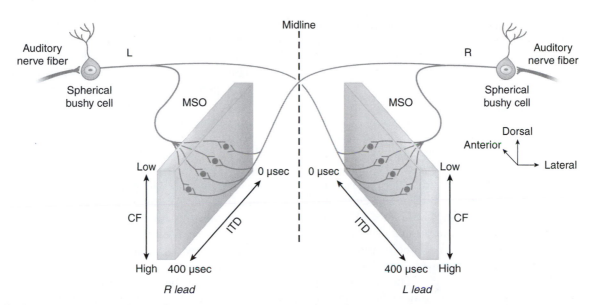

FIGURE 15-15   Schematic representation of delayed convergence of inputs from the two ears to each medial superior olive (MSO). Interaural time differences (delays) vary along the interaural time difference (ITD) axis. Variation in tuning to different ITDs occurs within each frequency lamina, so that ITD analysis is carried out at many frequencies. Converging inputs are from spherical bushy cells in the cochlear nucleus. (From Yin, T. C. T. (2001). Neural mechanisms of encoding binaural localization cues in the auditory brainstem. In D. Oertel, R. R. Fay, & A. N. Popper (Eds.), *Integrative functions in the mammalian auditory pathway* (pp. 99–159). New York, NY: Springer. With kind permission of Springer Science and Business Media.)

as if they weren't there. Diffraction occurs only when the object is smaller than the wavelength of the sound. Given the typical human head width (~23 cm), diffraction will occur for frequencies less than about 1.4 kHz. For progressively higher frequencies, acoustic shadowing becomes progressively more pronounced. Maximum differences (source at 90 degrees right or left) are less than 10 dB for frequencies below about 2 kHz, but they can exceed 20 dB for frequencies above 6.0 kHz. Interaural intensity "channels" in the brainstem are skewed toward higher frequencies, although they may contain a complete frequency map.

The Jeffress Coincidence Model and the Medial Superior Olive

L. A. Jeffress (1948) anticipated the type of simple neuronal circuitry needed to code for interaural time differences more than a half century ago. He proposed that the brainstem contains a *coincidence detection* cir-

cuit, containing cells that receive precisely timed excitatory input from the two ears. Unless excitation from both ears arrives at the same time, the neurons will not fire. If the hypothetical auditory center resides on one side of the midline, the travel time for excitation from the two ears will differ: It will take the signal longer to arrive from the opposite side of the head. Therefore, only if the ipsilateral side of the head receives a *delayed* signal will the two signals reach the postsynaptic cell at the same time. This scheme has an appealing simplicity, because it does not require elaborate synaptic machinery. Yet, the real beauty of this idea is that it may be correct: Without any direct knowledge of the architecture of the ACNS, Jeffress presaged the properties of neurons in the MSO (Figure 15-15). The wiring of this nucleus is consistent with a delay line based on distance, although the expected orderly map of *characteristic delays* (interaural delays that maximally excite MSO neurons) is not yet well supported. Delay tuning appears superimposed on a complete tonotopic map so that any given neuron is tuned for both frequency and interaural delay. Although the **Jeffress model** includes no role for inhibition, evidence for inhibition has nevertheless been found. Its role currently is unclear.

Lateral Superior Olive

Neurons that principally code for interaural intensity differences are found in the LSO. Sensitivity of these neurons to intensity disparities arises from the opposing signs of the inputs from the two ears. Ipsilateral stimuli excite the cells through a direct projection from spherical bushy cells of the AVCN on the same side. However, contralateral stimuli inhibit them. This inhibition comes about through an intermediary nucleus, the medial nucleus of the trapezoid bundle (MNTB). The neurons of the MNTB receive tonotopic input from globular bushy cells of the AVCN on the opposite side and perform a "sign inversion" so that excitation becomes inhibition. The cells that drive the major *(principal)* cells of the LSO are, therefore, the same cells that provide high-fidelity timing information to the MSO. In fact, principal cells of the LSO tuned to low frequencies phase-lock well to their own CFs, while responses of high-CF principal cells entrain well to low frequency modulations (AM or FM) of carriers near their CFs. Thus, the LSO may use interaural timing information to some extent.

Localization versus Binaural Enhancement in Higher ACNS Centers

Why auditory neurons of the thalamus and cortex are tuned for source location is a paradox. Presumably, the rapid localization of a potentially threatening sound source placed a premium on minimizing neuronal deliberations and on keeping this analysis at as low a level in the ACNS as possible. Indeed, the neuronal capacity for sound localization appears "complete" at the level of the IC, and the results passed on to the superior colliculus for coordination of motor responses. The need for further analysis at higher levels may have to do with the need to discern how many sources in the environment we need to monitor, fusing those we decide to moni-

tor, and suppressing those we do not (Middlebrooks et al., 2001). Thus, it may not really be possible to divorce sound source identity from location.

Do binaural pathways involved in sound-source fusion and perceptual enhancement overlap with those subserving location? It is difficult to know, because neurons that prefer nearly the same stimulus in both ears (i.e., no timing or level differences), and thus might be candidates for serving binaural functions other than localization, may instead be tuned to the midline, where binaural disparities will be minimal. One clue comes from *binaural beats,* in which simultaneous tones of different frequencies presented to the two ears generate the perception of a *difference frequency* (literally, the difference of the two frequencies) that may appear to lateralize (to come from inside the head, but to one side of the midline) or to localize outside the head (Yin, 2001). Unlike monaural beats, this phenomenon is observed only for frequencies less than about 600 Hz. This corresponds roughly with the limits of phase and timing cues for localization, so that binaural beats may be mediated by localization pathways. In addition, the "cocktail party effect (i.e., our ability to detect speech or other complex signals in noise) has been shown to depend on the interaural timing disparities of the modulating envelope. This again suggests involvement of pathways specialized for timing in a nonspatial task. From the brainstem to the cortex, there are more than a dozen points of *decussation* (midline crossing), so that some of these may specifically mediate aspects of perception other than localization.

SEPARATE FUNCTIONAL PATHWAYS ASCENDING FROM THE INFERIOR COLLICULUS

The IC is the final brainstem processing center for information en route to auditory thalamus and cortex. The IC represents the major point of divergence for hypothesized channels mentioned earlier, namely, *tonotopic, polysensory,* and *diffuse* pathways, or alternately, lemniscal and nonlemniscal pathways (Moller, 2000; Eggermont, 2001) (Figure 15-16). Although some evidence places the origin of these separate pathways as low in the ACNS as the CN (Egger-

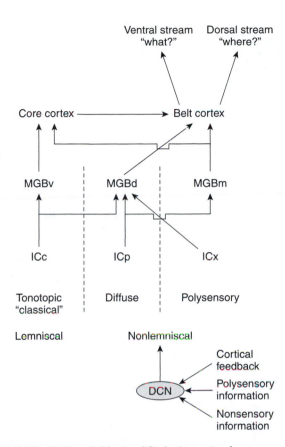

FIGURE 15-16 Highly simplified schematic of connections of major auditory pathways ascending from inferior colliculus (IC) to auditory cortex. Three major divisions of the IC are associated with *tonotopic* (lemniscal or "classic"), *diffuse,* and *polysensory* pathways. These pathways remain partially segregated through auditory thalamus. In cortex, diffuse and polysensory paths may converge onto "belt" cortical areas, whereas tonotopically organized thalamus projects mostly to "core" cortex. Belt cortex receives both parallel input from thalamus and serial input from core cortex. Belt areas may be divided into ventral (potentially specialized for stimulus identification and meaning) and dorsal areas (specialized for stimulus localization). Segregation of channels has been suggested to begin at the cochlear nucleus, where the dorsal division receives substantial nonsensory and polysensory "integrative" input, as well as feedback from cortex. DCN, dorsal cochlear nucleus; ICc, central division of the IC; ICp, pericentral division of the IC; ICx, external division of the IC; MGBv, ventral division of the thalamus; MGBd, dorsal division of the thalamic medial geniculate body; MGBm, medial division of the thalamic medial geniculate body.

mont, 2001; Ryugo et al., 2003). At the level of auditory cortex, proposed **core, belt,** and **parabelt** divisions recombine segregated information from lower centers and may also be serially connected (Kaas & Hackett, 1998; Rauschecker, 1998; Read et al., 2002; Moller, 2000; Eggermont, 2001). This architecture may redistribute the incoming information into new functionally distinct pathways within cortex. At all levels of the ACNS, there are structures and regions that exhibit clear tonotopic organization, as well as those that do not. Within the tonotopic regions, one can generally observe strong responses to simple tones and little habituation to repeated stimulation. Within nontonotopically organized regions, neurons may not respond well to simple tones and may readily habituate. Clues as to what these areas may be doing have come from physiologic recordings, tracing of connectivity patterns, lesion experiments, and functional imaging.

Tonotopic Pathway

The main components of the tonotopic or "classic" pathway (Moller, 2000) are taken to be the central nucleus of the IC, the ventral nucleus of the MGB of the thalamus, and two-to-five tonotopically organized auditory cortical fields, including primary auditory cortex.

Central Nucleus of the Inferior Colliculus   The ICc receives input from CN, superior olive and lateral lemniscus, as well as the contralateral ICc. The ICc contains a single, well-defined frequency map. Superimposed on this map, apparently unsystematically, one may find cells with many types of frequency tuning curves and preferences for particular FM or AM rates or directions. There is, however, some evidence that tuning for AM rate is topographically organized (Schreiner & Langner, 1988). Most of the response properties within the ICc appear to be "handed up" from lower levels, with some modifications arising through local circuits. One exception is binaural responses, which appear to be shaped by competing inputs from lower levels. This convergence corresponds to a puzzling "reprocessing" of interaural timing and intensity information used in the superior olivary complex and even adds new delay lines (Yin, 2001). It is clear that the ICc is involved in spatial analysis of the sound source, but how this works currently is unclear. There is no consensus on the existence of an orderly map of auditory space in mammalian ACNS, although such a map has been found in the ICc analog of owls. Spatial analysis in the ICc may include motion of the source and context variables, so that tuning for fixed source locations is not the major organizing principle.

Instead of localization, the primary purpose for the delay lines that are created within the ICc may be general temporal processing. Delay lines inserted into converging monaural inputs could hypothetically create neurons that are tuned for specific stimulus durations or AM and FM rates.

Thalamic medial geniculate body, ventral nucleus The **thalamic medial geniculate body,** ventral nucleus (MGBv) is the major thalamic relay to the auditory cortex. It also receives an equal or greater number of descending projections, so that the thalamus is not simply a passive relay, nor the cortex a passive recipient. Rather, MGBv neurons probably inherit their essential response properties from their presynaptic neurons in the ICc, and these are modified "on the fly" by feedback from the cortex. As with the counterparts of MGBv in other lemniscal centers, neurons are narrowly tuned and arranged in frequency lamina. Reports have described an orthogonal organization, whereby neurons in the anterior half of MGBv show shorter latencies and narrower frequency than those in the posterior half. Overall, few clear distinctions exist between the response properties of neurons in the MGBv and ICc.

Tonotopic Auditory Cortex Depending on species, auditory cortex may include up to 15 fields. In primates, 3 of 15 well-characterized fields show clear tonotopic organization and are generally referred to as core areas (Figure 15-17). Although primary auditory cortex (AI) is the best-studied area across species, other consensus core areas include an anterior auditory field and other rostrally located areas. These areas predominantly contain neurons that respond well to tones and receive major input from the MGBv. In general, AI is organized such that high frequencies are represented anteriorly and low frequencies posteriorly (Figure 15-18). Within iso-frequency bands, early studies demonstrated the existence of interleaved *binaural bands,* whereby alternating cortical patches are driven preferentially by the ipsilateral ear, contralateral ear, or both equally. This implies a role for AI in sound localization, a notion that has been supported by demonstrations in animals of frequency-specific deficits in localization after narrowly confined cortical lesions (Heffner & Heffner, 1990). The majority of auditory cortical neurons are broadly tuned for location of the sound source (typically contralateral) (Middlebrooks et al., 2001). The basis of this tuning is interaural timing and intensity differences, just as for the superior olive, although the contribution of facilitative interactions appears to be greater in the cortex. Although sound source location is clearly one of the features analyzed by AI, it does not appear to add any capabilities not already present at the level of the IC. Thus, AI is proposed to be involved in spatial segregation of multiple sound sources.

Another organizational principle within iso-frequency bands of AI may be that of a frequency gradient for inhibition (Schreiner, 1998). This may, in turn, impart variation in yet other response properties of neurons located along iso-frequency bands, including FM direction preference, intensity curve shape, and the shape of the stimulus spectrum around the CF (see Figure 15-8). Although there is no clear map for any single stimulus attribute, neurons near the middle of an iso-frequency band may have the most symmetric tuning, lowest thresholds, and shortest latencies (see Figure 15-18).

Notions of "simple" or "general" analyses in core auditory cortex do not preclude influences of learning and plasticity or polysensory input. Findings of plasticity in both spectral and temporal domains and expanded representation after learning have come from both tonotopic and nontonotopic cortex (Suga et al., 2002; Bao et al., 2004). This is in keeping with that the nontonotopic medial division of the MGB, which may mediate auditory learning (Edeline, 2003), projects broadly within cortex (see

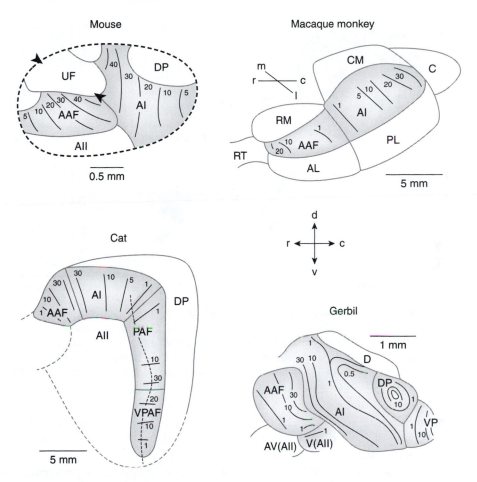

FIGURE 15-17 Schematic illustration of auditory cortex in four species. Typical arrangement includes two to four tonotopically organized core areas surrounded by nontonotopic belt areas, which are differently named in each species (reflecting different investigators and different brain topologies). Homology of areas has been shown among species for tonotopic areas AI and AAF (anterior auditory field) and belt area AII. (Copyright 2001 from Frisina, R.D., Walton, J.P. (2001) Neuroanatomy of the central auditory system. In: J.F. Willott (Ed.), *Handbook of Mouse Auditory Research: From Behavior to Molecular Biology* (pp. 243–277). New York: CRC Press. Reproduced by permission of Routledge/Taylor & Francis Group, LLC.)

Figure 15-16). In addition, recent functional imaging studies in humans have demonstrated activation of primary auditory cortex by visual stimuli (Pekkola et al., 2005). Interestingly, this activation was more robust for lip movements, as in speech, than for more general visual stimuli.

The characteristics of cortex vary not only along the surface of the brain, but also with depth. Cortex contains six layers (I–VI, beginning at the surface)

that differ in the size and shape of the cells they contain, as well as in their connections (Linden & Schreiner, 2003). The main "relay" input layer to the cortex from the auditory thalamus is in the middle layers (III–IV). The remaining layers project to other cortical areas (locally or at some distance, including the opposite hemisphere) or back to thalamus and colliculus. Superficial layers receive inputs that may reflect behavioral context and relevance of the

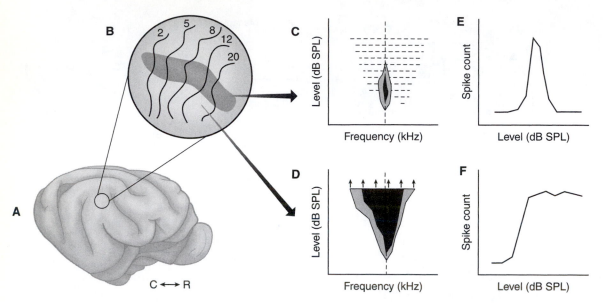

FIGURE 15-18 Schematic view of cat's brain (A) with indicated location of primary auditory cortex (AI). (B) Expanded AI with iso-frequency contours running orthogonal to the frequency axis. (C, E) Response trends for neurons located near the middle of each iso-frequency band. Neurons in this region tend to show narrow tuning, closed excitatory areas, and nonmonotonic input-output curves. Neurons located more dorsally and ventrally (toward the edges of AI) may show less extensive inhibition (D) and monotonic input-output curves (F). SPL, sound pressure level. (Adapted from Phillips, 2001.)

stimulus. A recording electrode inserted perpendicular to the cortical surface will record superficially similar tuning properties of neurons at different depths. Response properties that may change with cortical depth include response threshold, tuning bandwidth, and the nature of binaural interactions. It follows that yet undiscovered maps in cortex may be specific to particular cortical layers.

Nontonotopic Pathways

Because fewer general organizational principles have received wide recognition in the nontonotopic (nonlemniscal or polysensory/diffuse) pathways, these will be considered somewhat briefly.

Nonlemniscal Colliculus and Thalamus Nonlemniscal colliculus is taken to include the thin cell layer that surrounds the ICc. This outer peel of the ICc comprises two nuclei, known as IC external (ICx) and IC pericentral (ICp) (see Figure 15-16). Within the thalamus, nonlemniscal pathways include the dorsal and medial divisions of the MGB

(MGBd and MGBm, respectively), which receive major input from the ICx and ICp. Beyond weak responses to simple tones, characteristics reported for neurons in these regions include low spontaneous firing rates and a preference for changing temporal patterns. Plasticity and modulation by stimulus context are generally more robust than for lemniscal areas.

Belt and Parabelt Auditory Cortex Belt and parabelt auditory cortical areas are proposed to conduct higher "levels" of processing beyond those occurring in core areas. These may include integration of stimulus acoustic features, location, other sensory information, and context, so that the acoustic information stream is attached to specific objects in the environment. The number, names, and positions of proposed belt auditory cortical areas vary with species (see Figure 15-17). As their name suggests, these tend to surround core areas. Predominant input to belt areas comes from core cortical areas, and MGBd and MGBm of the thalamus. Parabelt areas also receive strong input from the MGBd and

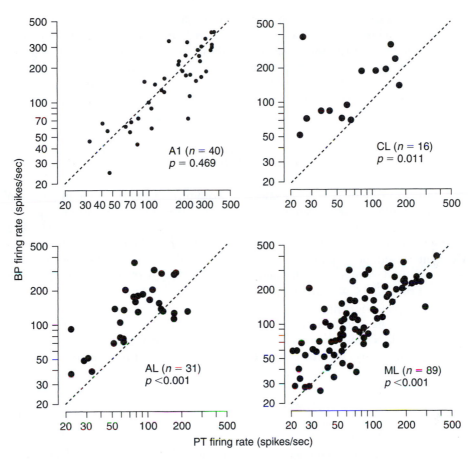

FIGURE 15-19 Preference for broadband stimuli (x-axis) versus tones (y-axis) in primary auditory cortex (AI; top left) and belt areas CL, AL, and ML in the rhesus monkey. Primary cortex shows no preference, whereas belt areas respond better to noise. These belt areas may be specialized for complex spectral analysis. Names of brain regions refer to their lateral location to AI (anterolateral, mediolateral, caudolateral) in this species. (Used with permission from Rauschecker, J.P., & Tian, B. (2003). Processing of band-passed noise in the lateral auditory belt cortex of the rhesus monkey. *Journal of Neurophysiology, 91*, 2578–2589.)

MGBm, but their strongest cortical connections are with other belt areas (Kass & Hackett, 1998).

Superimposed on the functional organization of cortical core, belt, and parabelt divisions may be the theme of *ventral* and *dorsal* streams, which may, respectively, interpret "what" (What is the object?) versus "where" (Where is the object?) aspects of stimuli (Rauschecker, 1998; Read et al., 2002). In this regard, the ACNS is proposed to mirror the organization of the visual system. Although core cortical areas may participate in both identification and localization, neurons in different belt and parabelt

areas show specializations that appear more appropriate either to the analysis of complex acoustic patterns or to location of the source. As an example, Figure 15-19 compares the preference of neurons in four cortical areas in rhesus monkeys for noise stimuli versus tones. Belt areas CL, AL, and ML (which respectively correspond to areas C, AL, and PL in Figure 15-17B) clearly prefer broadband stimuli, indicating facilitative interactions of components contained within the noise. Similar comparisons of these same areas for FM sweeps (Tian & Rauschecker, 2004) show facilitative responses to

FM in belt areas. This is in keeping with the notion of specialization for complex acoustic features in belt cortex. Based on preferences for stimulus bandwidth and FM sweep rate, it has been proposed that area AL participates in stimulus identification, whereas area CL is more involved in localization. PET and fMRI studies in humans similarly support a spread in activity from core to ventral belt/parabelt areas when tonal stimuli are replaced with those containing AM and FM or elements of communication sounds (Read et al., 2002). By contrast, stimuli associated with moving sound sources or localization tasks promote spreading of activity to dorsal belt/parabelt.

✌SUMMARY✍

Consideration of how to treat cochlear dysfunction should take into account what information provided by the cochlea is preserved in the ACNS, and how it is parceled out. Moreover, possible future interventions for central auditory dysfunction will rely explicitly on our understanding of the functional architecture of the ACNS. We have seen that both rate and temporal spike codes in cochlear neurons are captured and re-encoded by different sets of neurons within the CN, and then processed somewhat independently by functional and anatomic channels extending to multiple levels within the cortex. The surprising tolerance of the brain to corrupted code (as is typically the case with a cochlear implant) in identification tasks does not obviate the need to better imitate the natural code. The ability to identify a sound also is not a complete substitute for full appreciation of sound qualities, such as musical timbre and harmony. Through better understanding of how such qualities arise, clinicians and basic scientists can continue to close the gap between normal and assisted hearing.

✌KEY TERMS✍

Cochlear nucleus
Combination sensitivity
Core/belt/ parabelt
Cortex

Divergence/ convergence
Duplex theory
Facilitation
Inferior colliculus
Jeffress model

Lateral inhibition
Lemniscal/ nonlemniscal
Map
Medial/lateral superior olive

Nucleus
Thalamic medial geniculate body
Tonic/phasic

✌STUDY QUESTIONS✍

1. Defend the following claim: "We don't hear the world as it really is."

2. What is meant by multidimensional tuning?

3. What kinds of maps are well-supported in the ACNS? What others have been proposed?

4. What types of response properties and neuronal abilities change as one ascends the hierarchy within the ACNS?

5. Explain the term *parallel-hierarchical* as it applies to the ACNS.

6. How have observations of combination-sensitive neurons supported notions about the involvement of specialized neurons in perception?

7. Contrast the general response property neurons in lemniscal and nonlemniscal pathways.

8. Where do binaural interactions first arise within the ACNS? Contrast the general principles that underlie the operation of the centers that conduct analysis of interaural time and level differences.

9. Describe the duplex theory of sound localization and relate the operation of the medial superior olivary complex to the Jeffress model.

10. What kinds of evidence might be brought to bear on questions regarding the function of a particular cortical area in hearing?

⚘REFERENCES⚘

Abeles, M., & Goldstein, M. H. (1972). Responses of single units in the primary auditory cortex of the cat to tones and tone pairs. *Brain Research, 42,* 337–352.

Bao, S., Chang, E. F., Woods, J., & Merzenich, M. M. (2004). Temporal plasticity in the primary auditory cortex induced by operant perceptual learning. *Nature Neuroscience, 7,* 974–981.

Barbour, D. L., & Wang, X. (2003). Auditory cortical responses elicited in awake primates by random spectrum stimuli. *Journal of Neuroscience, 23,* 7194–7206.

Cant, N. B., & Morest, D. K. (1984). The structural basis for stimulus coding in the cochlear nucleus of the cat. In C. I. Berlin (Ed.), *Hearing science: Recent advances* (pp. 371–421). San Diego: College Hill.

Casseday, J. H., Ehrlich, D., & Covey, E. (1994). Neural tuning for sound duration: Role of inhibitory mechanisms in the inferior colliculus. *Science, 264,* 847–850.

Edeline, J.-M. (2003). The thalamo-cortical receptive fields: Regulation by the states of vigilance, learning and the neuromodulatory systems. *Experimental Brain Research, 153,* 554–572.

Eggermont, J. J. (2001). Between sound and perception: Reviewing the search for a neural code. *Hearing Research, 157,* 1–42.

Escabi, M. A., & Read, H. L. (2003). Representation of spectrotemporal sound information in the ascending auditory pathway. *Biological Cybernetics, 89,* 350–362.

Frisina, R. D., & Walton, J. P. (2001). Neuroanatomy of the central auditory system. In J. F. Willott (Ed.), *Handbook of mouse auditory research: From behavior to molecular biology* (pp. 243–277). New York: CRC Press.

He, J. (2003). Corticofugal modulation of the auditory thalamus. *Experimental Brain Research, 153,* 579–590.

Heffner, H. E., & Heffner, R. S. (1990). Role of primate auditory cortex in hearing. In W. C. Stebbins, & M. A. Berkley (Eds.), *Comparative perception: Complex signals* (Vol. 2, pp. 279–310). New York: Wiley Interscience.

Hu, B. (2003). Functional organization of lemniscal and nonlemniscal auditory thalamus. *Experimental Brain Research, 153,* 543–549.

Irvine, D. (1992). Physiology of the auditory brainstem. In A. N. Popper & R. R. Fay (Eds.), *The mammalian auditory pathway: Physiology* (pp. 153–231). New York: Springer.

Jeffress, L. A. H. (1948). A place theory of sound localization. *Journal of Comparative Physiology and Psychology, 41,* 35–39.

Joris, P. X, Smith, P. H., & Yin, T. C. T. (1998). Coincidence detection in the auditory system: 50 years after Jeffress. *Neuron 21,* 1235–1238.

Joris, P. X., Yin, T. C. T., & Smith, P. H. (1990). Mechanisms of azimuthal sound localization in the central nervous system of the cat. *Nederlands Akoestisch Genootschap, 104,* 25–35.

Kaas, J. H., & Hackett, T. A. (1998). Subdivisions of auditory cortex and levels of processing in primates. *Audiology & Neuro-otology, 3,* 73–85.

Kiang, N.-Y. S. (1975). Stimulus representation in the discharge patterns of auditory neurons. In D. B. Tower (Ed.), *The nervous system: Human communication and its disorders* (pp. 81–96). New York: Raven Press.

Linden, J. F., & Schreiner, C. E. (2003). Columnar transformations in auditory cortex? A comparison to visual and somatosensory cortices. *Cerebral Cortex, 13,* 83–89.

Ma, X., & Suga, N. (2001). Plasticity of bat's central auditory system evoked by focal electric stimulation of auditory and/or somatosensory cortices. *Journal of Neurophysiology, 85,* 1078–1097.

Middlebrooks, J. C., Xu, L., Furukawa, S., & Mickey, B. J. (2001). Location signaling by cortical neurons. In D. Oertel, R. R. Fay, & A. N. Popper (Eds.), *Integrative functions in the mammalian auditory pathway* (pp. 319–357). New York: Springer.

Moller, A. R. (2000). *Hearing: Its physiology and pathophysiology.* New York: Academic Press.

Müller, M. (1990). Quantitative comparison of frequency representation in the auditory brainstem nuclei of the gerbil, *Pachyuromys duprasi. Experimental Brain Research, 81,* 140–149.

Ohlemiller, K. K, Kanwal, J. S., Butman, J. A., & Suga, N. (1994). Stimulus design for auditory neuroethology: Synthesis and manipulation of complex communication sounds. *Auditory Neuroscience, 1,* 19–37.

Palmer, A. R., & Summerfield, A. Q. (2002). Microelectrode and neuroimaging studies of central auditory function. *British Medical Bulletin, 63,* 95–105.

Pantev, C., & Lütkenhöner, B. (2000). Magnetoencephalographic studies of functional organization and plasticity of the human auditory cortex. *Clinical Neurophysiology, 17,* 130–142.

Pekkola, J., Ojanen, V., Autti, T., Jääskeläinen, I. P., Möttönen, R., Tarkiainen, A., & Sams, M. (2005). Primary auditory cortex activation by visual speech: An fMRI study at 3T. *NeuroReport, 16,* 125–128.

Phillips, D. P. (2001). Introduction to the central auditory nervous system. In A. F. Jahn, & J. Santos-Sacchi (Eds.), *Physiology of the ear* (pp. 613–638). San Diego: Singular.

Pickles, J. O. (1982). *Introduction to the physiology of hearing.* New York: Academic Press.

Rauschecker, J. P. (1998). Parallel processing in the auditory cortex of primates. *Audiology & Neuro-Otology, 3,* 86–103.

Rauschecker, J. P., & Tian, B. (2003). Processing of band-passed noise in the lateral auditory belt cortex of the rhesus monkey. *Journal of Neurophysiology, 91,* 2578–2589.

Read, H. L., Winer, J. A., & Schreiner, C. E. (2002). Functional architecture of auditory cortex. *Current Opinion in Neurobiology, 12,* 433–440.

Rhode, W. S., & Greenberg, S. (1992). Physiology of the cochlear nuclei. In A. N. Popper, & R. R. Fay (Eds.), *The mammalian auditory pathway: Physiology* (pp. 94–152). New York: Springer.

Ryugo, D. K., Haengelli, C. A., & Doucet, J. R. (2003). Multimodal inputs to the granule cell domain of the cochlear nucleus. *Experimental Brain Research, 153,* 477–485.

Schreiner, C. E. (1998). Spatial distribution of responses to simple and complex sounds in the primary auditory cortex. *Audiology & Neuro-otology, 3,* 104–122.

Schreiner, C. E., & Langner, G. (1988). Coding of temporal patterns in the central auditory nervous system. In G. M. Edelman, W. E. Gall, & W. M. Cowan (Eds.), *Auditory function: Neurobiological bases of hearing* (pp. 337–361). New York: Wiley & Sons.

Steinschneider, M., Schroeder, C. E., Arezzo, J., & Vaughan, H. G. (1990). Tonotopic features of speech evoked activity in primate auditory cortex. *Brain Research, 519,* 158–168.

Suga, N. (1988). Auditory neuroethology and speech processing: Complex sound processing by combination-sensitive neurons. In G. M. Edelman, W. E. Gall, & W. M. Cowan (Eds.), *Auditory function: Neurobiological bases of hearing* (pp. 679–720). New York: Wiley & Sons.

Suga, N. (1995). Sharpening of frequency tuning by inhibition in the central auditory system: Tribute to Yasuji Katsuki. *Neuroscience Research, 21,* 287–299.

Suga, N., & Tsuzuki, K. (1985). Inhibition and level-tolerant frequency tuning in the auditory cortex of the mustached bat. *Journal of Neurophysiology, 53,* 1109–1145.

Suga, N., Xiao, Z., Ma, X., & Ji, W. (2002). Plasticity and corticofugal modulation for hearing in adult animals. *Neuron, 36,* 9–18.

Tian, B., & Rauschecker, J. P. (2004). Processing of frequency-modulated sounds in the lateral belt cortex of the rhesus monkey. *Journal of Neurophysiology, 92,* 2993–3013.

Trussell, L. O. (1997). Cellular mechanisms for preservation of timing in central auditory pathways. *Current Opinion in Neurobiology, 7,* 487–492.

Yin, T. C. T. (2001). Neural mechanisms of encoding binaural localization cues in the auditory brainstem. In D. Oertel, R. R. Fay, & A. N. Popper

(Eds.), *Integrative functions in the mammalian auditory pathway* (pp. 99–159). New York: Springer.

Yin, T. C. T., & Chan, J. C. K. (1988). Neural mechanisms underlying interaural time sensitivity to tones and noise. In G. M. Edelman, W. E. Gall, & W. M. Cowan (Eds.), *Auditory function: Neurobiological bases of hearing* (pp. 385–430). New York: Wiley & Sons.

Young, E. D., & Davis, K. A. (2001). Circuitry and function of the dorsal cochlear nucleus. In D. Oertel, R. R. Fay, & A. N. Popper (Eds.), *Integrative functions in the mammalian auditory pathway* (pp. 160–206). New York: Springer.

∼SUGGESTED READING∼

Aitkin, L. (1986). *The auditory midbrain.* Clifton, NJ: Humana Press.

Casseday, J. H., Fremouw, T., & Covey, E. (2001). The inferior colliculus: A hub for the central auditory system. In D. Oertel, R. R. Fay, & A. N. Popper (Eds.), *Integrative functions in the mammalian auditory pathway* (pp. 238–318). New York: Springer.

Nelken, I. (2001). Feature detection by the auditory cortex. In D. Oertel, R. R. Fay, & A. N. Popper,

(Eds.), *Integrative functions in the mammalian auditory pathway* (pp. 358–416). New York: Springer.

Smith, P. H., & Spirou, G. A. (2001). From cochlea to cortex and back. In D. Oertel, R. R. Fay, & A. N. Popper, (Eds.), *Integrative functions in the mammalian auditory pathway* (pp. 6–71). New York: Springer.

Webster, D. B., A. N. Popper, & R. R. Fay (Eds.) (1991). *The mammalian auditory pathway: Neuroanatomy.* New York: Springer-Verlag.

Chapter 16

Vestibular System Function: From Physiology to Pathology

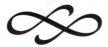

Asim Haque, Ph.D.
Washington University School of Medicine
St. Louis, Missouri
University of Mississippi School of Medicine
Jackson, Mississippi

J. David Dickman, Ph.D.
Professor of Neurobiology
Washington University School of Medicine
St. Louis, Missouri

Motion detection and our sense of position in space are determined by receptors of the vestibular system that lie in close proximity to the cochlea within the inner ear. Information gathered by the receptors is transmitted to the brain, where central vestibular structures process and integrate sensory information from vestibular, visual, and somatosensory receptors together with motor information from the cerebellar and cerebral cortices. Although not considered to be a cognitive sense, the vestibular system is responsible for many crucial functions, including the fine control of visual gaze, posture, autonomic reflexes, spatial orientation, and navigation. Most vestibular functions are conducted at a subconscious level; however, unusual motions such as experienced during air flight, amusement rides, or boat travel can result in acute disorienting awareness through **dizziness** or **vertigo.** Vestibular dysfunction can also be quite debilitating, ranging from relatively benign conditions such as **motion sickness** to more severe conditions such as a loss of balance or visual stability. In fact, dizziness, whether of vestibular or other origins, is one of the most common complaints presented to clinicians. Malfunction of the vestibular system cannot be easily reported by patients, as is true for the primary sensory systems. Fortunately, a number of diagnostic measures are available to assess vestibular system integrity, and more is being learned through research regarding vestibular system influence for many vital sensory and motor behaviors. Because of the intricate associations of auditory and vestibular structures, as well as common developmental origins, it is imperative that the audiology professional be aware of the basic anatomy, physiology, and pathology of vestibular function. This chapter discusses the peripheral receptor apparatus, the central vestibular processing centers, clinical measures of vestibular function, and common vestibular disorders. The primary focus is on the structure and function of the vestibular system as related to the salient aspects of clinical care.

VESTIBULAR SYSTEM STRUCTURE

In everyday life, two types of motion, rotational and linear, are experienced. In addition, our position in space relative to gravity is constantly detected. Rotational motions (angular acceleration) are experienced by head turns, whereas linear motions (linear acceleration) are experienced by translations (walking, falls, or vehicular travel) and by head tilts relative to gravity. Detection of motion and spatial position begins with the vestibular receptors lying in the inner ear. These receptors transduce and encode this information into neural signals that are sent to the brain, where it is processed into a uniform signal regarding direction and speed of motion, as well as the position of the head in space. In the brain, signals from vestibular receptors combine with information from other systems that detect motion such as muscle proprioceptors and visual receptors, as well as motor information from the cerebellum and cortex. Central processing of these multimodal signals occurs very rapidly to ensure adequate coordination of visual gaze and postural responses (balance), autonomic responses, and awareness of spatial orientation.

Peripheral Vestibular Labyrinth

The vestibular labyrinth of the inner ear is located in the temporal bone lateral and posterior to the cochlea (Figure 16-1). It consists of two parts: The *bony labyrinth* houses and protects the more fragile sensory structures contained inside the *membranous labyrinth.* Five separate receptor structures are represented in the vestibular portion of the membranous labyrinth. These include three **semicircular canals** and two **otolith** organs. The five vestibular receptor organs on each side of the head complement each other in function. The three semicircular canals, including the horizontal, anterior, and posterior canals, lie in three different head planes and respond to rotational head movements. The two otolith organs, including the **utricle** and **saccule,** perceive linear motions of the head and the orientation of the head relative to gravity. Each of the semicircular canals and otolith organs are spatially aligned so as to be maximally sensitive to movements in specific directions (see Figure 16-1). For example, the horizontal semicircular canal and the utricle both lie in a plane roughly equivalent to that of the head held during normal walking posture. In humans,

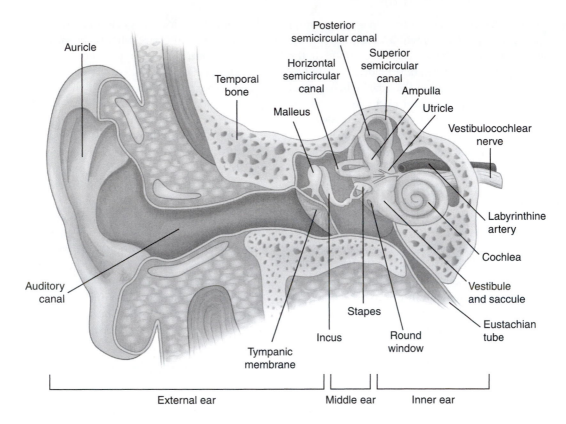

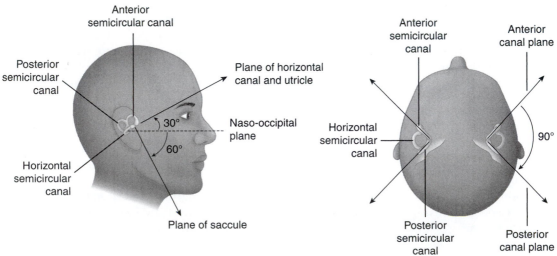

FIGURE 16-1 The external, middle, and inner ear containing the vestibular labyrinth in the temporal bone. The orientation of the semicircular canals and otolith organs within the head are shown.

that plane lies about 30 degrees elevated from the naso-occipital axis. The angle of elevation for these two receptor organs varies among species but reflects each animal's natural head position during normal body motion. In contrast, the vertical canals and the saccule lie in vertical head planes, nearly orthogonal to horizontal semicircular canal. Each of the canals on one side of the head works in opposite fashion to their counterparts in the contralateral ear. Together, receptors inside the semicircular canals and otolith organs can respond to head motion in any spatial direction.

The membranous labyrinth consists of a series of fluid-filled tubes and sacs where the mechanics of motion detection and transduction occur. Surrounding the membranous labyrinth is a fluid called **perilymph.** It is similar to cerebrospinal fluid, with a high sodium (150 mM) and low potassium (7 mM) content. Inside the membranous labyrinth, where the vestibular receptors lie, is a very different fluid called **endolymph,** which is similar to an intracellular solution with high potassium (150 mM) and low sodium (16 mM) concentrations. Endolymph is important, because it is the high potassium concentration that drives transduction of the motion detection mechanoreceptors. The three semicircular ducts of the membranous labyrinth connect to the utricle, where each duct ends with a single enlarged sac, termed the *ampulla* (see Figure 16-1). The sensory receptors for the semicircular canals are contained in a specialized epithelium within the ampulla. For the otolith organs, the sensory receptors are contained in the basal epithelium. The utricle is aligned coplanar to the horizontal semicircular canal and is connected to the endolymphatic sinus and saccule by a small duct. The sensory neuroepithelium of the saccule is oriented nearly vertically in the head and is also connected to the endolymphatic sinus and the cochlea. The endolymphatic sinus empties into the endolymphatic sac, which exits the temporal bone and terminates next to the dura of the brain. The delicate balance between the disparate ionic constituencies of endolymph and perilymph is carefully maintained by specialized secretory cells within the membranous labyrinth and the endolymphatic sac.

The blood supply to the labyrinth is primarily via the labyrinthine artery, a branch of the *anterior inferior cerebellar artery.* In addition, the smaller stylomastoid artery supplies portions of the semicircular canals. These vessels enter the labyrinth through the internal acoustic meatus, where any interruption of blood supply can lead to symptoms of labyrinthine-associated disease.

Vestibular Sensory Receptors

Vestibular sensory receptors are mechanoreceptor cells called *hair cells* because of the many **stereocilia** that project from the apical portion of the receptor cell (Figure 16-2). Each hair cell contains between 50 and 100 stereocilia and a single longer kinocilium, which are interconnected by small filaments. The stereocilia are oriented in a number of rows of ascending height, where the tallest stereocilia lie next to the lone kinocilium. There are two types of hair cells that differ in their morphology, afferent terminations, and channel currents (see Figure 16-2). **Type I hair cells** are amphora-shaped. They are completely surrounded by a unique calyceal afferent terminal, which exhibits an exclusive inward-rectifying potassium current. **Type II hair cells** are cylindrically shaped and are innervated by simple synaptic boutons from the vestibular afferent fibers. The hair cells are innervated by primary afferent neurons that make up part of the **vestibulocochlear nerve.** The somas of these bipolar afferents lie in Scarpa's ganglion nestled in the internal acoustic meatus, a small, shelflike opening through which axons from the ganglion pass into the brainstem. Both types of hair cells exhibit excitatory synapses on VIIIth nerve afferents, and both receive vestibular efferent input from the brainstem. The efferent innervation is little understood, but it is believed to be involved in controlling receptor sensitivity.

For each of the semicircular canals, the receptor hair cells lie in a specialized patch of neuroepithelium, termed the **crista,** that runs along the base of the ampulla. Type I hair cells are concentrated near the central regions of the cristae, whereas type II hair cells are more numerous in the peripheral zones. The crista is completely covered

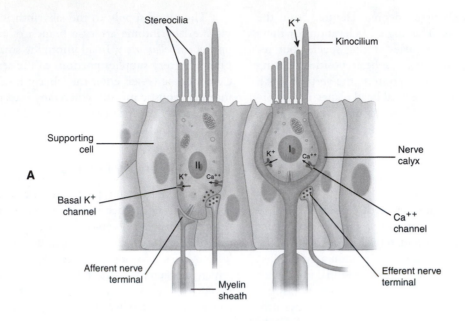

A

Stereocilia

K⁺

Kinocilium

Supporting cell

Nerve calyx

Basal K⁺ channel

Ca⁺⁺ channel

Afferent nerve terminal

Myelin sheath

Efferent nerve terminal

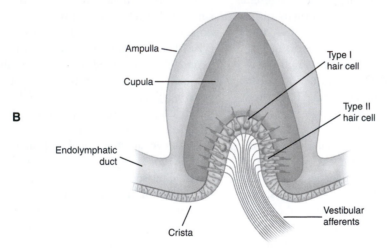

B

Ampulla

Cupula

Endolymphatic duct

Crista

Type I hair cell

Type II hair cell

Vestibular afferents

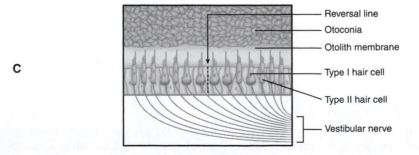

C

Reversal line

Otoconia

Otolith membrane

Type I hair cell

Type II hair cell

Vestibular nerve

by a gelatinous membrane, termed the **cupula,** that forms a fluid-tight partition across the ampulla. The stereocilia of the hair cells are embedded in the gelatinous cupula (see Figure 16-2). During rotational head movements, endolymph in the membranous semicircular duct is displaced (lags behind) because of inertia and viscous drag, which, in effect, pushes the cupular partition in a direction opposite to that of the head turn. Cupular movement causes the stereocilia and kinocilium to flex toward or away from each other, which causes either excitatory or inhibitory responses (see later). In each of the three semicircular canals, all of the hair cells have the same spatial polarization. Thus, it is the anatomic plane of the membranous duct in the head that causes the directional selectivity of each semicircular canal.

Linear accelerations are detected by receptor hair cells in the otolith organs, which lie in a specialized neuroepithelium termed the **macula** (see Figure 16-2). The stereocilia of the otolith hair cells extend into a gelatinous coating above the macula that is covered by thousands of calcium carbonate crystals, termed **otoconia** (derived from Greek, meaning "ear stones"). The otoconia, being much more dense than the surrounding endolymph, are not displaced by normal endolymph movements, but instead are moved only during linear motion or changes in head position relative to gravity (*linear accelerations*) because of their inertia. Thus, the otolith organs are inertial transducers of linear acceleration. When otoconia are displaced, they produce a subsequent movement of the gelatinous membrane and bending of the embedded hair cell stereocilia.

Mechanoelectric Transduction Motion detection begins with the receptor hair cells, which are directionally selective to stereocilia displacement. With movements of the stereocilia *toward* the kinocilium, hair cell membranes are **depolarized,** and the innervating vestibular afferent fibers increase their firing rate (Figure 16-3). However, if the stereocilia are deflected *away* from the kinocilium, the hair cell is **hyperpolarized,** and the afferent fibers decrease their firing rate. This works through *mechanoelectric transduction* of specific potassium (K^+) channels in the apical portion of the kinocilium. When the stereocilia are deflected toward the kinocilium, potassium channels open, allowing K^+ to enter the hair cell (due to concentration gradients from the endolymph), which depolarizes the cell membrane. Depolarization produces opening of Ca^{2+} channels at the base of the hair cell, which results in synaptic vesicle release of the excitatory neurotransmitter (*aspartate* or *glutamate*). Transmitter release from the hair cell then binds with receptors in the postsynaptic vestibular afferent terminal. Depolarization of the afferent follows, leading to an increase in the neural firing rate. When the kinocilium and stereocilia are returned to their normal position, voltage-sensitive potassium channels at the base of the hair cell open and release K^+, thereby repolarizing the membrane to its resting potential. When the stereocilia are deflected away from the kinocilium, more potassium channels (as well as Ca^{2+} channels) close and further release of K^+ through the basolateral potassium channels occurs, resulting in cell hyperpolarization. When the head is stationary, vestibular primary afferent fibers have a high spontaneous firing rate (~90 spikes/sec). The high rate allows for bidirectional response of the afferents so that silencing of the neural response to most natural head motions does not occur.

Morphologic Polarization of Hair Cells Because the hair cells are directionally selective, one might expect that their orientation on the cristae and maculae is important for signaling

FIGURE 16-2 (See Color Plate) Vestibular receptors and their locations in the labyrinth. (A) Type I and II vestibular receptor hair cells. (B) Semicircular canal ampulla. Hair cells are located in the crista, with stereocilia embedded in the cupula membrane. Type I and II hair cells are located in the central and peripheral regions of the crista, respectively. (C) Hair cells are located in the otolith macula, with stereocilia embedded in otolith membrane and otoconia secured on top.

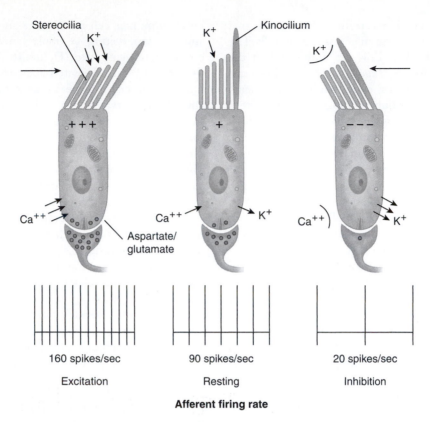

FIGURE 16-3 Directional selectivity of vestibular hair cells. At rest, hair cells maintain some transmitter release, producing a high spontaneous firing rate in the innervating afferent fibers. Stereocilia displacement toward the kinocilium opens channels that depolarize the cell and increase the afferent firing rate. Stereocilia displacement away from the kinocilium hyperpolarizes the cell and decreases the afferent firing.

movement direction. This is, in fact, the case. For example, all hair cells in the horizontal semicircular canal cristae are arranged similarly, with their kinocilium lying closest to (i.e., pointing toward) the utricle (Figure 16-4). Horizontal head rotations that produce endolymph movement toward the utricle cause deflections of the stereocilia toward the kinocilium, and all of the hair cells in the horizontal semicircular canal are depolarized. Because all hair cells in each of the semicircular canals have the same anatomic orientation, the geometry of the canals determines directional selectivity. In the utricle, hair cells are polarized such

that the kinocilia are always lying toward an imaginary *reversal line* that curves through a central region of the macula termed the **striola** (see Figure 16-4). In the saccule, all of the hair cell kinocilia are oriented away from the reversal line. The utricle primarily encodes linear motion in the horizontal head plane, and the saccule encodes primarily vertical motion. However, because both maculae have curved surfaces and because the reversal lines course through the epithelium, directional selectivity is constantly provided from a subpopulation of hair cells for linear motions along any direction in three-dimensional space.

Hair cell morphological polarization

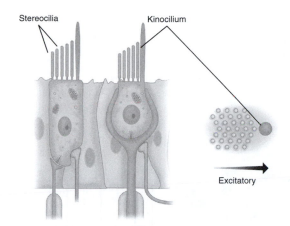

A

Excitatory

Semicircular canal cristae

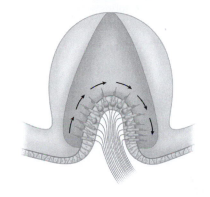

B

Otolith maculae

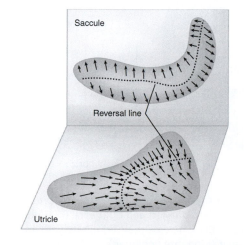

C

SEMICIRCULAR CANAL FUNCTION

Remember that the membranous semicircular ducts are fluid-filled tubes with a partition (the cupula) in the middle. In addition, hair cells of the semicircular canals on one side of the head are oppositely polarized to those of the complementary canal in the contralateral ear. While the head is stationary, no rotational acceleration is being imparted to the semicircular canals and no endolymph flow occurs (Figure 16-5). The afferents from the complementary canals on both sides of the head have equivalent firing rates. When the head turns, the horizontal semicircular canals turn with it, leaving the endolymph fluid behind (lagging the duct) because of inertial forces and viscous drag between the fluid and the walls of the duct. This lag in endolymph movement relative to the skull and semicircular duct causes the cupula partition to be deflected. Cupula deflection, in turn, produces stereocilia deflection on the hair cells. With a leftward head turn, such as to look over one's left shoulder, the relative endolymph movement in the left horizontal canal pushes the cupula partition toward the utricle, which produces stereocilia deflection toward the kinocilium, resulting in increased discharge of the left VIIIth nerve afferents (see Figure 16-5). Conversely, endolymph movement in the right-side horizontal canal retracts the cupula from the utricle. This causes stereocilia deflection away from the kinocilium, and the hair cells will be hyperpolarized, producing decreased firing rates in right VIIIth nerve fibers. With a rightward head turn, the opposite activation pattern in the hair cells and afferents will be produced. The functional coupling of the two horizontal semicircular canals also applies to pairs of vertical semicircular canals. For

FIGURE 16-4 Morphologic polarization of hair cells. (A) Each hair cell is directionally polarized according to the location of the kinocilium at an eccentric location of the apical surface. (B) All hair cells in the semicircular canal cristae have identical polarization directions. (C) Hair cells in the otolith maculae have different polarization directions, relative to an imaginary reversal line that courses through the central receptor epithelium.

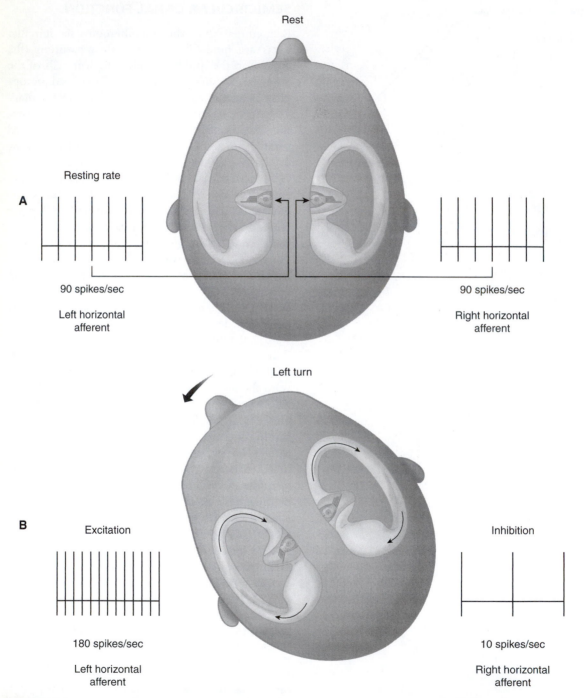

FIGURE 16-5 Horizontal semicircular canal response to head rotation. (A) At rest, no rotational motion is present, the cupula is stationary, and afferent fibers have equivalent firing rates for both the left and right ears. (B) With a leftward head turn, all of the left canal hair cells are excited and afferent fibers increase their firing rate with an excitatory response. Conversely, right horizontal canal afferents decrease their firing rate (inhibited).

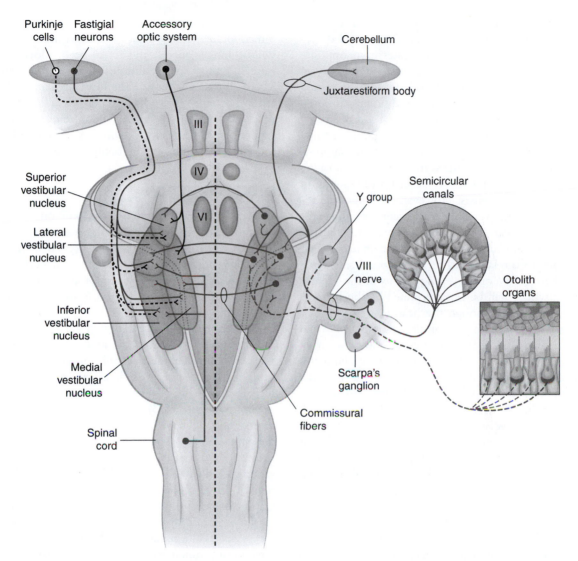

FIGURE 16-6 (See Color Plate) Sensory afferents to the vestibular nuclei. Four vestibular nuclei (superior, lateral, medial, inferior) receive primary afferent information from the ipsilateral labyrinth. Other signal inputs arise from the spinal cord, commissural fibers, cerebellum, accessory optic nuclei, and cortical pathways (not shown).

example, the left posterior semicircular canal lies in roughly the same plane as the right anterior semicircular canal. When the head is pitched down at an angle of about 45 degrees between the nose and the ear, the discharge from afferents of the left anterior semicircular canal increases and the discharge from the right posterior semicircular canal decreases.

Neural information carried on vestibular afferent fibers from both the left and right semicircular canals is transmitted into the brain (Figure 16-6). Many central vestibular neurons receive information from semicircular canal receptors on both sides of the head. Through these bilateral convergent signals, central vestibular neurons are able to interpret head rotation based on the relative firing rates of canal afferents in the left versus right ears. Neural information is constantly being evaluated by the central neurons, whose baseline set point is determined by the high spontaneous firing rate of vestibular afferents even when the head is stationary. Thus, small differences in the afferent discharge rates from opposite ears can be determined, increasing the sensitivity of the system. During a leftward head turn, central vestibular neurons receive increased firing rate information from the left horizontal canal and decreased firing rate information from the right horizontal canal. Similar conditions exist when the head is pitched or rolled, with the vertical semicircular canals being stimulated by the rotational accelerations in their respective planes. However, the opposing responses from the vertical canals occur with the anterior semicircular canal in one ear and the coplanar posterior semicircular canal of the opposite ear. Damage to the labyrinth or vestibulocochlear nerve can change the normal resting activity in the afferent fibers, which will be misinterpreted by the brain as head turns, even though the head is stationary. For example, an occluding lesion of the VIIIth nerve can result from a number of sources, such as an acoustic neuroma tumor, which often reduces or eliminates the discharge rates of the afferent fibers on one side. In this case, the **vestibular nuclei** neurons will receive higher firing rate information from the intact vestibular nerve compared with the lesion side, which would be interpreted as a head turn *away* from the lesioned ear. Clinical diagnoses of vestibular pathology relies on the knowledge of bilateral labyrinth function.

Because of the mechanics of the semicircular canal system (endolymph flow and cupula elasticity), as well as the transduction properties of synaptic processing, angular accelerations are integrated into a *head velocity* signal. It is the head velocity that is actually encoded by semicircular canal afferents. However, afferents do not respond equally to all head motion speeds and are band limited in their *frequency response* functions. Slow head rotations (e.g., less than 1–2 degrees/sec) produce little response. Instead, afferents are most responsive to rotation speeds between 10 and 150 degrees/sec, which encompasses the range of most natural human head movements. Another important property of the semicircular canal system is that it experiences adaptation to continuous rotational motion. If

one undergoes constant velocity rotation in a single direction for 30 to 60 seconds, the canal afferents will no longer encode the actual head velocity, but instead return to prestimulus spontaneous firing levels. This occurs because the head angular acceleration becomes zero during periods of constant rotational velocity. In these circumstances, people report that they are not moving, even though high rotation speeds are actually being delivered.

OTOLITH FUNCTION

Linear motion or changes of head position with respect to gravity cause otoconial displacement because of inertia (greater density of the crystals than surrounding endolymph) and consequent deflection of stereocilia in otolithic hair cells. Otolith hair cells do not respond to rotational motion. Similar to semicircular canal receptors, otolith hair cells are either depolarized or hyperpolarized with stereocilia deflection toward or away from the kinocilium. However, as described earlier, the hair cells on the maculae are morphologically polarized differently depending on their location with respect to the reversal line in the striola (see Figure 16-3). Hair cells on one side of the reversal line will be depolarized, whereas hair cells on the opposite side of the reversal line will be hyperpolarized. Because of the striola curvature, only certain groups of cells will be affected by any specific direction of linear motion or head tilt. In fact, a topographic coding of movement direction is represented by the activation of hair cells in particular regions of the maculae. The innervating VIIIth nerve fibers are directionally tuned to linear motion, because each afferent innervates only hair cells from a small region on the macular neuroepithelium. Unlike semicircular canal afferents, otolith afferents have broad frequency-response functions. They respond to static head positions, slow head movements, fast head movements, and even fast vibrations with high fidelity.

CENTRAL VESTIBULAR NUCLEI

Four major vestibular nuclei in humans lie in the rostral medulla and caudal pons of the brainstem (see Figure 16-6). The *medial vestibular nucleus* lies adjacent to the fourth ventricle and runs extensively through a rostrocaudal extent of the brainstem. It contains smaller homogenous cells that are densely packed. The lateral vestibular nucleus has cells that differ greatly in size, including the giant Deiters' neurons, and lies lateral to the medial vestibular nucleus. The superior vestibular nucleus lies dorsally in the central pons and lateral to the medial nucleus. The inferior vestibular nucleus is ventral to the other vestibular nuclei and runs in the caudal pons and rostral medulla. Each of the vestibular nuclei differ in their cytoarchitecture and their afferent and efferent connections. The central processing of motion and positional information for control of compensatory movement reflexes largely occurs in vestibular nuclei neurons. Additional processing of spatial orientation and navigational information also begins in these cells, with further task-specific integration occurring in the cerebellum and thalamocortical networks. The major efferent outputs for the vestibular nuclei include the **oculomotor nuclei** for the extraocular muscles, the cerebellum, the contralateral vestibular nuclei, the spinal cord, the reticular formation, and the thalamus.

Inputs to the Vestibular Nuclei

A number of signals converge into vestibular nuclei neurons (see Figure 16-6). The first of these multisensory signals arises from vestibular primary afferents innervating the semicircular canal and otolith receptors. All vestibular afferents bifurcate on entering the brain. Afferent fibers from the semicircular canals project primarily to the superior and medial vestibular nuclei, although projections to the lateral and inferior vestibular nuclei also exist. The otolith organs project primarily to the lateral, medial, and inferior vestibular nuclei. Saccular afferents have a unique projection to an additional region, known as the y group, whose cells project to the vertical eye muscle motor neurons of the contralateral oculomotor nucleus. The termination of vestibular afferent fibers onto individual nuclei neurons is highly ordered. Central neurons in the superior and medial vestibular nuclei appear to receive information from only one semicircular canal pair (either horizontal

or vertical canals) and otolith receptors. Convergence of afferent information from orthogonal canal pairs appears to be rare for these cells. Vestibular neurons in the lateral and inferior nuclei primarily receive information from several canal pairs and otolith receptors. This specificity of receptor input produces the observed directional selectivity of central neurons to particular head movements in space. Because many vestibular nuclei neurons receive inputs from both semicircular canal and otolith afferents, their responses can encode both the angular and linear components of head movements. The combined processing capability of the central neurons is impressive. These cells distribute information concerning both the direction and speed of the head movement, as well as the position of the head with respect to gravity to many different regions of the brain.

The vestibular labyrinth is the only sensory organ in the body with direct primary afferent projections to the cerebellum. Vestibular afferents project to the nodulus, uvula, and fastigial nucleus, with smaller projections to the anterior vermis, posterior vermis, and flocculus. In addition, there are reciprocal projections to and from the cerebellum from neurons in all four vestibular nuclei, with major connections between the nodulus, uvula, flocculus, fastigial nucleus, and dentate nucleus (see Figure 16-6). The cerebellovestibular fibers consist of Purkinje cell axons (inhibitory) from the nodulus, uvula, flocculus, and cerebellar vermis, as well as axons from fastigial nucleus neurons (excitatory). The reciprocal connections between the cerebellum and the vestibular nuclei comprise important regulatory mechanisms for the control of eye movements, head movements, and posture. One class of these connections has been shown to be crucial for *adaptive motor learning* in the vestibulo-ocular reflex (VOR; see later).

Commissural vestibulovestibular fibers arise from each of the vestibular nuclei, but they appear to be most prominent from the superior and medial nuclei (see Figure 16-6). There are generally two types of commissural fibers. Many fibers form reciprocal connections with the analogous contralateral nucleus (medial vestibular nucleus neurons project to contralateral medial nucleus cells), whereas other commissural fibers project to different nuclei. Both excitatory and inhibitory vestibulovestibular fibers exist, but the majority appear to contain the inhibitory neurotransmitters γ-aminobutyric acid (GABA) or glycine. These commissural fibers are thought to provide the required informational exchange between vestibular nuclei neurons, which comprise the comparative processing of complementary semicircular canal pairs. Commissural fibers also play a major role in *vestibular compensation,* a process by which the loss of unilateral vestibular receptor function (as can occur through trauma or disease) is restored centrally.

Spinovestibular fibers arise from all levels of the spinal cord and project primarily to the medial and lateral vestibular nuclei. Visual motion information also reaches vestibular nuclei neurons through the *accessory optic system.* Vestibular nuclei neurons receive input from the reticular formation, primarily from cells relaying information regarding proprioception. Finally, several parallel pathways arising from different cortical regions send descending projections directly to the vestibular nuclei. It is thought that these *corticovestibular fibers* help regulate fine gaze and postural control, as well as suppress the normally compensatory vestibular nuclei-mediated reflexes during volitional movements.

VESTIBULAR GAZE STABILIZATION

One of the primary vestibular functions is to provide *gaze stabilization* when the head moves. During normal head, trunk, or body movements, it is often necessary to maintain visual stabilization on an object of interest. For example, we might wish to maintain a stable gaze on a street sign while driving or walking. Gaze stabilization actually involves a combination of rotational and translational head and eye movements that work together to maintain fixed visual acuity on a single point in space. The vestibular system provides this capacity by eliciting compensatory eye, neck, spinal, and limb movements through an immense network of neural connections and muscle motor coordination. Gaze stabilization is actually composed of several vestibular-mediated components, including

contributions from *VOR, VCR,* and *cervicocollic reflexes* (CCR), as well as head inertia responses. Of these, the most well understood are the VOR mechanisms (see later for detailed examination). The VOR and other components of gaze stability are said to be *compensatory* because they work together to produce a total response that is equal in magnitude and opposite in direction to the perceived head motion. In fact, gaze stabilization has been shown to be completely compensatory (essentially perfect) in humans for most natural behaviors. The result is a stable visual image during many types of head motion.

Rotational Vestibulo-ocular

Special neurons in the vestibular nuclei are responsible for the generation of visual stability during head motion. These cells receive sensory information from the vestibular receptors, visual motion information, neck proprioceptors, cerebellum, and probably cortical inputs. These cells integrate this information to produce a signal that is appropriate to control the motor neurons innervating the six pairs of oculomotor muscles for each eye. Essentially, three types of vestibular-induced eye movements exist: horizontal, vertical, and torsional. To elicit conjugate movements of both eyes, each of the six pairs of eye muscles must be controlled in unison. Specifically, the vertical semicircular canals (anterior and posterior canals) and the saccule are primarily responsible for controlling vertical eye movements, whereas the horizontal canals and the utricle predominantly control horizontal eye movements. Torsional eye movements appear to be controlled, to some degree, by all of the vestibular organs. The simplest description of neural connectivity and eye movement control for the VOR may be understood by examining the basic horizontal VOR (Figure 16-7). Primary horizontal semicircular canal afferents project to specific neurons in the vestibular nuclei (type I cells). These central nuclei neurons, in turn, project an excitatory signal through the **medial longitudinal fasciculus** (MLF) to the *contralateral* **abducens nucleus.** Abducens motor neurons project through cranial nerve VI to innervate the lateral **rectus muscle.**

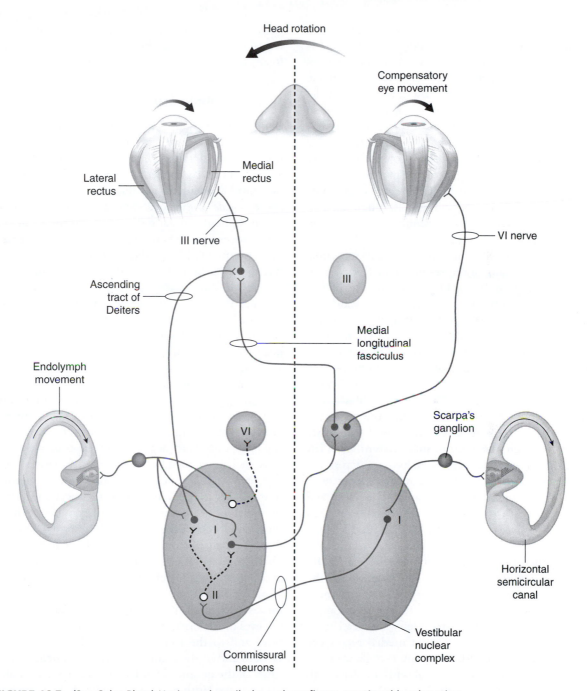

FIGURE 16-7   (See Color Plate) Horizontal vestibulo-ocular reflex to rotational head motion.

Other abducens interneurons also send excitatory projections back across the midline to the oculomotor nucleus, where a subdivision of motor neurons project through cranial nerve III to innervate the *ipsilateral* medial rectus muscle. Vestibular nuclei neurons also project excitatory signals directly to the medial rectus subdivision of the ipsilateral oculomotor nucleus through the ascending tract of Deiters. Inhibitory signals also project from other vestibular nuclei neurons to the ipsilateral oculomotor and abducens nuclei. Finally, vestibular commissural fibers provide indirect (through type II vestibular nuclei neurons) inhibitory information from the contralateral nuclei.

To illustrate the function of the rotational VOR, let us examine the results of a leftward head turn (see Figure 16-7). Deflection of the cupula causes deflection of the stereocilia toward the kinocilium, depolarizing the left horizontal semicircular canal hair cells. This increased receptor potential causes synaptic neurotransmitter release to the primary vestibular afferents, which increase their neural firing rate. Excitatory responses in the afferents are transmitted to the left vestibular nuclei neurons. At the same time, these central vestibular neurons receive a decreased inhibitory signal through the commissural system. The left vestibular nuclei neurons then project across the midline to excite the right abducens motor neurons. Abducens interneurons are also excited and project back to the left oculomotor neurons. Together, a conjugate contraction of the right lateral rectus and left medial rectus muscles occurs, resulting in a rightward eye movement. The VOR response stabilizes the object of interest on the retina for greatest visual acuity. Similar matching bilateral connections for the other sets of eye muscles also exist, so that with a leftward head turn, the left lateral rectus and right medial rectus eye muscles are inhibited. The same organizational principles apply to the vertical semicircular canals and the motor neurons in the trochlear and oculomotor nuclei that allow vertical and torsional responses. Interestingly, the eye muscle pulling directions line up approximately with their semicircular canal counterparts (e.g., the medial and lateral recti align with the horizontal canals, and so forth).

Linear Vestibulo-ocular

Linear motions also produce a VOR response, although the eye movements and neural mechanisms involved differ depending on the direction and type of linear acceleration. For example, side-to-side head movements produce oppositely directed and *conjugate* (eyes move same direction) horizontal eye movement. Similar responses occur for up-down head movements, where oppositely directed vertical eye movements are produced. These responses are due to activation of the otolith receptors, with connections to the extraocular motor neuron pools that are similar to those described earlier for the rotational VOR. However, unlike the rotational VOR where distance of the visual target relative to the head is unimportant, the amplitude of the linear VOR depends on viewing distance. This is true because the vergence angle (angle between the two lines of sight for each eye) varies as a function of the inverse of the distance to the visual object. For far visual targets (greater than ~2 m away) the vergence angle is nearly zero degrees. However, for near objects, such as a pencil held close to one's nose, a large vergence angle accrues. To maintain visual acuity on near objects, the eyes must converge together during linear motion. Let us review an example of how these factors affect the linear VOR response. During fore-aft translation, as one moves closer to a nearby object directed straight ahead, the eyes must move *disconjugate* toward each other (increase in vergence) as one moves closer to the visual target. When one moves backward, the vergence angle decreases and the eyes move apart. Fixating on an object that is upward and to the right requires both eyes to move upward and to the right, but at different degrees because of the geometric differences in vergence angle for each eye. With roll tilts of the head, the compensatory eye movement is termed *counter-roll* and is actually a torsional eye movement in the direction opposite to the roll tilt. Volitional torsional movement of the eye is not possible, yet torsional **nystagmus** (see later) can be produced by large head tilts or by experimental stimulation using linear acceleration directed along the utricular plane (e.g., as experienced in a centrifuge of linear sled). As one can appreciate, the characteristics that describe the linear VOR are quite complex and are still being investigated. Consequently, it is the angular or rotational VOR that is most often tested clinically as a diagnostic for vestibular integrity (see later).

VESTIBULOSPINAL AND VESTIBULOCOLLIC NETWORK

The vestibular system influences muscle tone and produces reflex postural adjustments of the head and body through two major descending pathways to the spinal cord. These include the lateral vestibulospinal tract (LVST) and the medial vestibulospinal tract (MVST; Figure 16-8). The fast-acting VCR serves to stabilize the head in space and participates in gaze control. The neural pathway for the VCR includes the primary vestibular nerve afferent, a vestibulospinal neuron (in the vestibular nuclei), and a cervical motor neuron. A reticulospinal pathway also exists that receives input from the vestibular system, but much less is known concerning its function.

Medial Vestibulospinal Tract

Responses to motion of the head and neck arise primarily through the neurons in the MVST. Vestibular nuclei neurons of the MVST mainly in the medial vestibular nucleus (MVN) receive input from vestibular receptors, the cerebellum, and somatosensory information from the spinal cord. MVST output fibers descend through the MLF to terminate bilaterally in the cervical spinal cord (see Figure 16-8). The fibers of MVST neurons carry both excitatory and inhibitory signals to innervate neck flexor and extensor motor neurons in the spinal cord, with a precise connectivity pattern. If, for example, while walking, one trips and falls forward, MVST neurons will receive pitch rotation signals from the vertical semicircular canals, forward

linear motion signals from the utricle, and downward linear acceleration signals from the saccule. Together, these changing head position signals are processed by MVST neurons to elicit excitatory signals to the dorsal neck flexor muscles. At the same time, inhibitory signals are sent to the ventral neck extensor muscles. The result is a neck movement upward, opposite to the falling motion, to protect the head from impact.

Lateral Vestibulospinal Tract

Neurons in the lateral and inferior vestibular nuclei project to all levels of the ipsilateral spinal cord to comprise the LVST. A specific topographic organization for lateral vestibular nuclei neurons that project to the spinal cord exists. LVST cells in the rostral region project to the cervical cord, central neurons project to the thoracic cord, and cells in the caudal region of the nucleus project to the lumbosacral cord. These neurons receive substantial input from the vestibulocerebellum and proprioceptive inputs from the spinal cord. Many neurons that comprise the LVST receive convergent afferent fibers from several semicircular canal pairs and otolith receptors. Other LVST neurons are more specific in their vestibular receptor inputs. Fibers of the LVST course through the lateral medulla dorsal to the inferior olivary complex, then through the ventral cord (see Figure 16-8) to terminate directly on spinal motor neurons and interneurons in laminae VII, VIII, and IX. Axons of many LVST neurons give off collaterals in different segments of the cord so that coordination of different muscle groups for postural control is possible. The LVST neurons contain either acetylcholine or glutamate as a neurotransmitter and exert an excitatory influence on extensor muscle motor neurons. How the specific coordinated actions of vestibular neurons that comprise the LVST provide postural stabilization and complex muscle group control is not completely understood. However, if one tilts the body sideways, LVST fibers exert excitatory extension of the contralateral axial and limb musculature. At the same time, ipsilateral flexor muscles will be activated and ipsilateral extensor muscles inhibited.

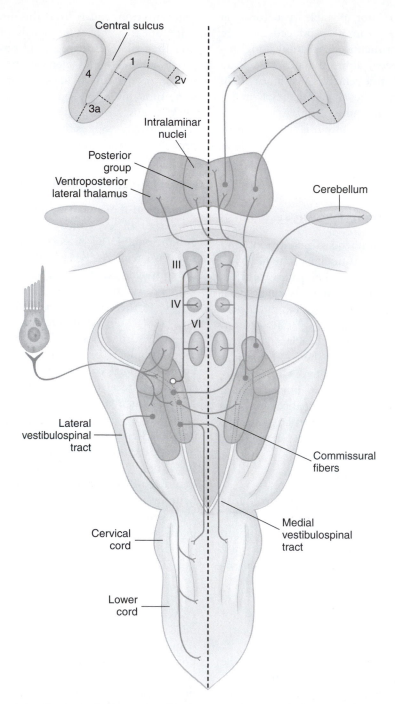

FIGURE 16-8 (See Color Plate) Vestibular nuclei efferent projections to the major systems. Separate paths for the lateral vestibulospinal tract, medial vestibulospinal tract, commissural fibers, vestibulo-ocular reflex, and vestibulo-thalamo-cortical systems are shown.

These actions serve to stabilize the body's center of gravity to preserve upright posture.

VESTIBULO-THALAMO-CORTICAL NETWORK

Vestibular Thalamus

The cognitive perception of motion, spatial orientation, and navigation through space arise through convergent information from the vestibular, visual, and somatosensory systems at the thalamocortical level. Neurons in the superior, lateral, and inferior vestibular nuclei project bilaterally to the thalamus (see Figure 16-8). Three thalamic regions, including the **ventral posterolateral nucleus, posterior nuclear group,** and **intralaminar nuclei,** are known to respond to vestibular stimulation. In humans, electrical stimulation of these areas produces sensations of movement and sometimes dizziness. These three different thalamic regions comprise separate parallel pathways of vestibular information and likely serve different functions. In addition, neurons in the anterior dorsal thalamus serve a fascinating function in providing specific information regarding heading direction. Each of these cells is tuned to respond only when the animal faces a specific direction in space, with different neurons tuned to different directions. These cells can learn to change their heading tuning relative to visual landmarks and depend entirely on vestibular input to function. If vestibular information from the labyrinth is deprived, these cells loose their tuning and the ability to acquire new direction specificity. How thalamic neurons perform perceptual, orientation, and navigation functions is only beginning to be understood.

Vestibular Cortex

Vestibular information carried to the cortex may be much more broadly placed than once thought. Classically, two primary cortical areas were known to respond to motion stimulation (see Figure 16-8). The first is **area 2v,** which lies at the base of the intraparietal sulcus just posterior to the hand and mouth areas of the postcentral gyrus. Electrical stimulation of this area in humans produces sensations of moving, spinning, or dizziness. Area 2v neurons respond to head movements in a manner similar to that for vestibular nucleus neurons and receive a direct projection from the posterior group in the thalamus. These cells also receive visual motion signals through the optokinetic system and proprioceptive signals from muscles and joints, and it is currently thought that these cells are involved with motion perception. This notion is consistent with the connections of area 2v, which is believed to have a reciprocal exchange of information with areas 5 and 7 of the parietal cortex, which are also involved with spatial orientation. Lesions of the parietal cortical areas result in confusion regarding spatial awareness. The second cortical region, known as **area 3a,** lies at the base of the central sulcus, adjacent to the motor cortex (see Figure 16-8). Area 3a neurons receive input from ventral posterolateral thalamus neurons and the somatosensory system. These cells do project to area 4 of the motor cortex; thus, it is believed that area 3a cells are involved with integrative motor control of the head and body. In addition, recent studies have shown that perception of motion through space involves vestibular signals in visual processing areas such as the **medial superior temporal** (MST) cortex near the tip of the superior temporal gyrus. Many of the MST neurons encode visual motion information called *optic flow,* and they also respond to concurrent body motion through vestibular signals. How motion perception and heading direction are deciphered by cortical processing is a matter of intense ongoing research.

VESTIBULAR TESTING

Although it is difficult to noninvasively assess the functionality of the vestibular labyrinth and receptors directly, it is possible to indirectly assess function by vestibular laboratory testing. The most common diagnostic evaluations include examination of vestibular-mediated secondary responses such as the VOR or postural responses to vestibular stimulation.

As discussed earlier in this chapter, prolonged rotation or intense vestibular stimulation will induce a nystagmus (Figure 16-9). During head rotation, a slow-phase eye movement response occurs that opposes the motion both in direction and speed. Then, when the eyes reach a limit, a fast-phase saccadic eye movement occurs in the same direction as head motion that resets the eyes in the orbit. The fast-phase is used by clinicians to describe the direction of nystagmus (e.g., right or left beating). If one rotates in a single direction for several complete turns, then stops, a postrotatory nystagmus on cessation of rotational motion occurs. Here, the nystagmus manifests in the opposite manner to that seen during rotation, with slow-phase movements occurring in the same direction as the previous rotation and fast-phase movements in the opposite direction. In addition to direction, nystagmus can also be classified according to plane of elicitation (horizontal, torsional, or vertical), intensity, and evoking maneuvers. Finally, nystagmus is also present under pathologic conditions. In fact, nystagmus is the only objective sign of vertigo. Clinically, the primary method used to diagnose and monitor vestibular pathology is to measure the VOR, nystagmus, and postural responses elicited by caloric, rotational motion, linear motion, posturography, or head-shake testing.

Eye Movement Testing Methods

Observation of eye movements is currently performed using electronystagmography (ENG), ocular videography, or magnetic-search coil techniques. Because the retina and cornea have different electric charges, surface electrodes attached to the periorbital region will transduce a potential change whenever the eyes move. A limiting factor of using ENG is that only horizontal and vertical eye movements can be measured, because torsional eye movements exert no potential difference between the front and back of the eye. A more robust, yet more expensive, method involves the use of infrared cameras mounted on glasses or goggles. Images are computer analyzed to determine eye movement component, direction, and speed. Videography is widely used but suffers from poor resolution of fast eye movement components, and torsional measures are possible but less accurate.

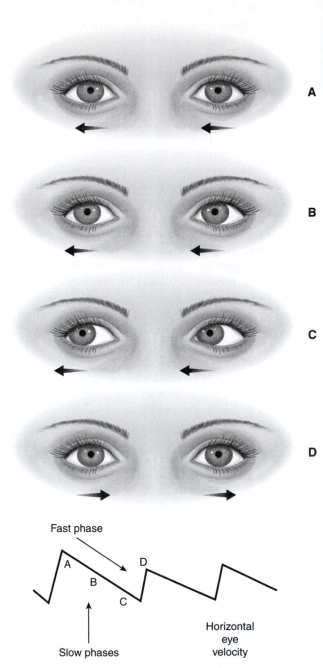

FIGURE 16-9 Mechanism of nystagmus. (A) Eyes at rest. (B) For a leftward head turn, eyes begin to move to the right to maintain visual gaze. (C) Eyes reach resetting point in orbit. (D) Eyes return to center position rapidly (fast phase). Bottom trace shows measured horizontal eye velocity where *A to C* represent the slow-phase response and *D* represents the fast phase of nystagmus.

Currently, the most robust method involves the use of miniature coils imbedded in a contact lens that is placed on the cornea. The wearer sits within a magnetic field where any eye (or head) movement can be measured by computer data acquisition systems. Eye and head movements can be acquired rapidly, accurately, and in three dimensions (horizontal, vertical, and torsional) for absolute measures of eye/head position and velocity.

Vestibular Testing Methods

Several diagnostic batteries are used to assess vestibular function, including caloric, rotational, evoked, posturography, and head-shake testing. These may be performed using the eye movement monitoring equipment discussed earlier, or direct visual unaided observation by the clinician.

Caloric testing involves the administration of either warm or cold water (or air) to irrigate the external auditory canal. The basis for the test is heat transfer, which induces a response through two mechanisms. The first is to produce an endolymph shift caused by a temperature gradient: increase under application of warmer temperatures (40°C) or decline using colder temperatures (30°C). The second mechanism is heat transfer to the VIIIth nerve afferents directly. Because the horizontal semicircular canal lies closest to the middle ear, convective and conductive heat transfer affects the endolymph and nerve here preferentially, and deflection of the cupula can be induced. In healthy individuals, application of warm water to one side results in a horizontal nystagmus, which beats (fast phases) are directed to the same side. Conversely, irrigation with cold water produces contralateral beating nystagmus. A mnemonic may be helpful: COWS—*Cold* water produces fast phases to the *Opposite* side, *Warm* water produces fast phases to the *Same* side. The extent of nystagmus elicited with caloric irrigation should be equivalent from both ears in healthy individuals. However, if a unilateral lesion exists in the vestibular pathway, deficits in the elicited nystagmus will be apparent by a reduction in the response of the affected ear.

Rotational chair testing involves the patient sitting on a rotary chair with sinusoidal or long-duration vestibular stimuli delivered via computer control. Different frequencies ranging from low (0.05 Hz) to high (2 Hz) are tested, and subsequent eye movements are noted. Of interest is the slow-phase velocity of the VOR, which should oppose the direction of rotary motion. Gains for the response are calculated by dividing the peak VOR slow-phase eye velocity with the peak speed of rotational motion (chair velocity). An ideal VOR gain would be one (unity), which would indicate a perfect compensatory response (in the opposite direction) for a given rotational movement. Another measurement made is the timing relation between the slow phase and the slow movement of the chair. This difference is called the *phase lag*. Ideally, phase lag should be 180 degrees, which indicates that when the chair is at the apex of its movement, the eyes should be at the extreme opposite position. The gain and phase test responses are plotted as a function of stimulus frequency, similar to that of an audiogram. Differences between normal and lesioned conditions can then be noted.

Head-thrust testing is a simple procedure that can be done in the clinic or even at the bedside. It involves grasping the patient's head with both hands and rapidly rotating the head to one side. The test can be performed in any direction to examine the response from specific semicircular canals. Nystagmus should be induced in healthy individuals. Absent or altered nystagmus should be taken as a sign of pathology.

Vestibular-evoked myogenic potentials (VEMPs) detect the sensitivity of the otolith organs to sound. Specifically, the saccule is sensitive to loud clicks, typically 95-dB hearing level (HL) or louder. Electrodes can be placed on the neck muscles, such as the sternocleidomastoid, with the patient sitting. The VCR response, the portion of vestibulospinal reflex primarily responsible for neck stabilization, can be monitored by recording electromyogenic potentials. In addition, click-evoked VOR responses have also been noted, especially in conditions such as superior canal dehiscence (SCD; see later).

Posturography involves monitoring vestibular interaction with postural control mechanisms. Because proprioception and visual cues are integrated with vestibular signals to facilitate truncal stability, removal of these other extravestibular signals can test the integrity of the vestibular system.

The simplest way to examine the system is the *Romberg test,* during which the patient stands with their feet together. The patient is then asked to close his or her eyes, thus removing visual input. This test can also be performed on a foam mat, which minimizes proprioceptive input. If the patient cannot balance properly or is unable to alter the direction of a fall during Romberg testing by head turning, a peripheral vestibular abnormality can be suspected. Further tests should be performed, including neuroimaging studies to rule out sites of lesions.

VESTIBULAR PATHOLOGY

Symptoms of acute vertigo, dizziness, and dysequilibrium occur in approximately 10% of patients treated by general practitioners and nearly 20% of patients treated by otolaryngologists and neurologists, totaling nearly 7 million clinical visits annually. Causes of dizziness can be classified as due to problems in the periphery (benign paroxysmal positional vertigo, vestibular neuritis, **Ménière's disease,** ototoxicity, trauma), problems in the central regions (strokes, vestibular schwannomas, migraines), or systemic/metabolic conditions (presyncope, anemia, hypo/hyperglycemia, medication-related, hyperventilation, or other neurologic causes). Of these causes, nearly 50% of dizziness cases is attributable to peripheral vestibulopathies. Because elderly adults are highly susceptible to falls resulting in serious, yet preventable, injuries, including those precipitated by vestibular deficits, it is imperative that proper identification and treatment of vestibular dysfunction be made. Ultimately, it is the imbalance between the two labyrinths that is the cause of vertiginous symptoms.

Because of the nature of vestibular pathology, often patients will have difficulty describing their symptoms, using such words as *dizziness* or *light-headedness. Dizziness* is a nonspecific term that generally denotes some form of spatial disorientation and may or may not involve feelings of movement. Many conditions may produce dizziness, which may not be of vestibular origin. Dizziness is seldom a warning sign of a life-threatening condition (except due to central causes, such as cerebellar hemorrhage or infarction). Vertigo, in contrast, is a specific sensation of motion (the patient or the environment) when no real motion is taking place. Acute onset of vertigo can be categorized as follows: (1) attacks of vertigo (episodic), (2) sustained vertigo, and (3) positional vertigo. Incidentally, one can induce vertigo by spinning rapidly in place and then abruptly stopping. An account of vertigo can be suggestive of a peripheral or even a central vestibular lesion. **Oscillopsia** is the perception that a stationary object is in motion and is most often a sign of bilateral peripheral vestibulopathy. Light-headedness is more indicative of a vascular problem, such as that accompanying postural changes (e.g., orthostatic hypotension) or exercise, as well as anxiety/hyperventilation or metabolic abnormalities, such as improper glucose control.

As is the case with most medical conditions, the most important aspect of an evaluation of a patient with a vestibular deficit is obtaining a thorough history. Without usage of the tests described in the previous section, a patient's description of their condition can oftentimes lead to a diagnosis. Obtaining a complete history from a patient includes the following items:

- Onset of symptoms and description of initial event
- Precipitating and exacerbating factors
- Related symptoms
- Severity
- Temporal pattern
- Usage of any medications
- Other disease processes

Benign Paroxysmal Positioning Vertigo

Benign paroxysmal positioning vertigo (BPPV), first described by Austrian physician Robert Bárány in the early twentieth century, is the most common vestibular abnormality treated in neuro-otology clinics, with approximately 160,000 cases diagnosed per year in the United States. It is characterized by brief episodes of vertigo (less than 30 seconds), which usually follow changes in head and body position. As its name implies, BPPV is a benign condition that invariably remits spontaneously. This condition can manifest after trauma to the skull, excessive bedrest, assuming unusual postures with the head supine, sequelae to viral or ischemic labyrinthitis, or as a result of ongoing inner ear disease such as Ménière's disease. In nearly half of the cases, however, the exact cause remains unknown. In addition, those patients suffering from migraines are predisposed to development of BPPV.

Pathophysiology   BPPV is caused by otoconia (calcium carbonate) crystals detaching from the utricular macula and entering the semicircular canal system. Because the specific gravity of otoconia is higher than that of the endolymphatic fluid contents, these particles will sink to the lowest position possible. Because of its location below the utricle when the head is supine (such as during sleep), the posterior (inferior) semicircular canal is the most vulnerable to entrapment of otoconia, resulting in a condition termed *canalolithiasis*. When the patient moves in the plane of the afflicted canal, the "clump" of crystals has a "plunger effect" as it moves in the canal, thereby displacing the cupula and causing vertigo.

Clinical Features   Diagnosis of BPPV is dependent on noting the characteristic fatigable paroxysmal positional nystagmus of a patient elicited by performing the Dix–Hallpike test whereby the patient is moved from the sitting to the head-hanging position. The canal of involvement is identified by direction of the positionally provoked nystagmus, most often the posterior semicircular canal, though it can affect any of the canals. Usually, the nystagmus is torsional with the upper pole of the eye beating toward the ground. In the majority of patients, the nystagmus dissipates with repeated positioning.

Treatment   For most cases of BPPV, treatment involves repositioning the head (Epley maneuver) such that the otoconia particles are shifted from the canal to the utricle, much like a child's toy. This maneuver involves several steps from the sitting to head-down and back to the sitting position. BPPV caused by ongoing inner ear disease, such as Ménière's disease, is less easily treated and has a higher rate of occurrence, perhaps because of increased blockage or macular damage of the otoliths.

Superior Canal Dehiscence Syndrome

Sound-induced eye and head movements via the vestibular labyrinth were first investigated by Tullio (1929), who observed in pigeons that when a semicircular canal was opened, sound propagated more readily through that canal. In humans, Tullio's phenomenon is characterized by dizziness caused by sound or pressure stimulus, or both. Recently, Minor, Schessel, and Carey (2004) have shown that this condition is caused by an opening in the bone overlying one of the canals. Most patients afflicted with this condition describe vertigo or oscillopsia as a result of loud noises or pressure stimuli. Findings of temporal bone surveys suggest that approximately 2% of individuals have a dehiscence or extremely thin bone overlying the labyrinth either below the middle cranial fossa or at the superior petrosal sinus.

Pathophysiology   The cause of SCD is dehiscence or opening of the bone above the superior semicircular canal. Because of its anatomic position, the superior canal is the uppermost organ of the labyrinth in the temporal bone. The dehiscent bone above the canal acts as a third mobile window in the cochleovestibular system. As a result, positive pressure on the tympanic membrane and oval window causes flow of endolymph in the superior canal such that subsequent excitation in hair cell activity and vestibular nerve afferents occurs together with outward bulging of the dehiscence. Consequently, the superior canal becomes excitable not only during head movement, but also when exposed to loud noise, as well as during the Valsalva maneuver against pinched nostrils (performed by attempting to forcibly exhale while keeping the mouth and nose closed, such as during descent of an airplane to equalize middle ear pressure).

Clinical Features Responses to tones at frequencies of 500 to 2,000 Hz with intensities of 100- to 110-dB HL, pure-tone audiometry, VEMPs, as well as computed tomography (CT) imaging are useful in the diagnosis of SCD. With the loud-tone tests, vertical-torsional nystagmus will be evident. An air-bone gap with normal bone conduction (some may be even better than threshold) thresholds is normally observed, indicating a dissipation of acoustic energy through the dehiscence. In addition, VEMP responses for the affected ear will be seen. Recent data suggest that some individuals may have minimal vestibular problems such as vertigo or oscillopsia, but have more auditory manifestations.

Treatment For patients with debilitating vestibular symptoms, surgical procedures can be performed to close the dehiscence. Currently, the two procedures being used involve either resurfacing of the superior canal with fascia and cortical bone or plugging of the membranous labyrinth with bone dust and fascia such that the lumen of the canal is occluded.

Ménière's Disease

Ménière's disease is an inner ear disorder characterized by episodic vertigo, roaring tinnitus, low-frequency hearing loss, and aural fullness. Because of its episodic nature, it can be quite debilitating, with nearly one-third of those afflicted having overwhelming disability. It is estimated that nearly 100,000 new cases are diagnosed yearly in the United States. Unfortunately, Ménière's disease can pose a significant challenge to clinicians in controlling the symptoms, as well as effectively treating the disorder.

Pathophysiology Although the exact cause of Ménière's disease remains unknown, the most widely accepted theory is endolymphatic hydrops.

This condition is the result of overdistension of the membranous labyrinth due to excessive buildup of endolymph resulting from overproduction or impaired resorption processes, or both. Numerous causative factors have been linked to endolymphatic hydrops, including autoimmune dysfunction, endocrine disturbance, fibrosis, altered glycoprotein metabolism, altered electrolyte balance, viral infections, as well as vascular, genetic, and nutritional conditions. The episodic vertigo experienced is attributed to hyperfunctioning transients in the resting discharge of vestibular hair cells.

Clinical Features The course of Ménière's disease varies among patients. Some patients experience symptoms briefly for a few months, which then abate forever; others have cycles of exacerbation and remission for life. Because of the nature of symptoms, Ménière's disease is generally characterized in two phases: early and late. The early phase has symptoms that are episodic in nature, and the disease is nearly always unilateral. The late phase is more chronic, with symptoms persisting much of the time. In addition, two subtypes of Ménière's disease have been noted, one with mostly auditory involvement, whereas the other displays mostly vestibular dysfunction. Involvement of the contralateral ear, which is a major setback in dealing with the disease, occurs anywhere from 30% to 60% of the time. Some patients experience sudden episodes of falling without loss of consciousness (Tumarkin's crisis or drop attacks), which can be dangerous because of possible head injuries or bone fractures. Many patients describe these episodes as feeling as if they were pushed to the ground by some external force. These spells are thought to originate specifically in the otolith organs. Pure-tone audiograms generally serve as the best indicator of inner ear condition and document fluctuating hearing loss.

Treatment Because the exact cause is not known, management of Ménière's disease has been aimed at vestibular suppression of episodic vertigo. However, much of the treatment strategies vary with differences in the causative theories regarding this condition. Current treatment includes antihistamines, neuroleptics, antiemetics, and sedatives for acute attacks, as well as diuretics, steroids, vasoactives, and aminoglycosides for maintenance therapy, though there is also a significant placebo effect seen in treatment. In addition, intratympanic gentamicin injections are advocated by many to knock out partial populations of hair cells in the various vestibular organs (with minimal hearing loss in the process) such that the amount of hyperfunction within the system is reduced. For more serious vertigo, drastic measures such as endolymphatic sac surgery, vestibular neurectomy, or even vestibular organ ablation are indicated. Because animal models of endolymphatic hydrops fail to show signs of vertiginous episodes, such as unsteady gait or postural imbalances similar to those seen in clinical Ménière's disease, stringent treatment therapies have been difficult to develop, much less quantify.

Vestibular Neuritis

Also referred to as acute unilateral (idiopathic) vestibular paralysis, vestibular neuritis presents with acute onset of vertigo, nausea, vomiting, and postural imbalance. An attack can occur acutely at any time, and most patients improve gradually over a period of weeks or sometimes months.

Pathophysiology   An exact cause for the vertigo is unknown, though inflammation caused by viral infection, such as an occasional finding of herpes zoster, has been noted, as have ischemic causes due to vascular insufficiency, such as that of the anterior vestibular artery. The resulting imbalance in tonic vestibular activity results in vertigo. Trauma such as that from pressure changes (barotrauma) or from blunt blows to the head (labyrinthine concussion) or perilymphatic fistulas should be ruled out as the cause of vertigo.

Clinical Features   Typically, spontaneous nystagmus of peripheral origin is horizontal with a torsional component and does not change with gaze (opposite that of centrally originating vertigo). A simple head-thrust test of the horizontal VOR can result in abnormal nystagmus. Most patients with a peripheral deficit will be able to stand, whereas those with vertigo of central origin will have difficulty standing without support. The diagnostic hallmark for vestibular neuritis is unilateral hyporesponsiveness to caloric testing (the eye positions remain unaltered when the ears are irrigated with warm or cold water). Generally, audiometric testing is normal, unless cochlear involvement has occurred resulting in labyrinthitis, marked by moderate-to-severe ipsilateral sensorineural hearing loss. A recent viral infection, including those of the respiratory system, may be noted on examination.

Treatment   Recovery involves a combination of possibly incomplete labyrinthine function, increased reliance on visual and proprioceptive cues for postural balance, and central vestibular compensation to offset the tonic imbalance. Pharmacotherapy includes antihistamines, anticholinergics, antidopaminergics, corticosteroids, and GABAergic agents. These agents do not eliminate the vestibular imbalance, yet reduce the vertiginous symptoms. In addition, these agents should be used only for short-term duration, because some amount of dizziness is necessary to allow proper central compensatory processes to occur. Many clinicians have also noted the benefits of exercise, which also increases the process of vestibular compensation.

Ototoxicity

Numerous drugs, including aminoglycoside antibiotics, loop diuretics, aspirin, nonsteroidal anti-inflammatory agents, antineoplastics, antimalarials, and chemical solvents are known to be ototoxic to the labyrinth. They cause functional impairment and cellular degeneration of the inner ear tissues including the neuroepithelium. Usage of ototoxic drugs is prevalent, especially in developing countries, where the goal is to eradicate some underlying disease process and concerns about hearing and balance are secondary. Often, auditory and vestibular monitoring is unavailable to track labyrinthine status.

Pathophysiology The exact mechanisms of ototoxicity remain unknown, but are thought to occur by activation of cell death pathways of hair cells, damage to hair cell membrane channels, and damage of supporting cells.

Clinical Features Most instances of ototoxicity will involve bilateral labyrinthine involvement; therefore, asymmetries in vestibular function will generally not be evident. For aminoglycoside injury, vestibular involvement initially presents with a headache, followed by signs of nausea, vomiting, vertigo, and nystagmus. Chronic effects include difficulty walking and ataxia. It is vital that the clinician obtain a thorough patient history, including medications taken.

Treatment Although no single treatment has been clinically proved to prevent ototoxic effects, possible preventative therapies under investigation include the use of antioxidants and glutathione to prevent excess free radical formation, iron chelation therapy to prevent iron-catalyzed free radical formation, and the use of salicylates to attenuate gentamicin-induced hearing loss.

Motion Sickness

Motion sickness occurs when there is a sensory mismatch among vestibular, visual, and proprioceptive input. For example, if one reads a book while in a car that goes over many bumps, one may feel nauseous, yet sight is redirected out the window, and much of the queasiness subsides. When the apparent mismatch between the visual input and the somatosensory/vestibular input is resolved, one feels fine. In addition, optokinetic stimuli such as that seen in flight simulation video games where the visual field elicits a feeling of movement can also cause sickness because of the mismatch between visual and vestibular signals. Vertical oscillatory motion (heave) or roll oscillations at frequencies of 0.2 Hz or less are most likely to cause motion sickness, with higher frequencies offering little problem.

✍ SUMMARY ✍

Our ability to sense position, to coordinate movements, and to move our eyes so as to maintain a constant visual field as we or our heads move is critical to our survival. The vestibular system is primitive and also complex. Its function is not just to sense gravity or movement, but also to integrate sophisticated input from a number of sensory systems and to control those systems in such a manner that the world is held constant as we move. It is easy to overlook the importance of good vestibular function, but anyone who has experienced vertigo, even after getting off an amusement park ride, can understand how debilitating functional deficits in the vestibular system can be.

This chapter has reviewed the structures and some of the pathways involved in normal and abnormal vestibular function, and it has described some disorders that are seen clinically. An understanding of the vestibular system is crucial for audiologists, not just because the vestibular system is the next-door neighbor to the cochlea and shares plumbing (endolymph and perilymph) and electricity (VIII cranial nerve), but also because many disorders of hearing also affect the vestibular system. And for many patients so afflicted, the hearing loss, although important, is far less troublesome than the vestibular deficits, which can be devastating. Effective rehabilitation of the patient requires clinical and therapeutic attention to both systems.

❧KEY TERMS❧

Abducens nucleus

Caloric testing

Crista

Cupula

Depolarized

Dizziness

Endolymph

Hyperpolarized

Macula

Medial longitudinal fasciculus

Medial vestibulospinal tract

Ménière's disease

Motion sickness

Nystagmus

Oculomotor nucleus

Oscillopsia

Otoconia

Otolith

Perilymph

Rectus muscles

Rotational chair testing

Saccule

Semicircular canals

Spinovestibular fibers

Stereocilia

Striolar

Type I and II hair cells

Utricle

Vertigo

Vestibular-evoked myogenic potentials

Vestibular nuclei

Vestibulocochlear nerve

❧STUDY QUESTIONS❧

1. During surgery to remove an acoustic neuroma, the VIIIth nerve on the left side of the head is transected. What effects would you expect to see immediately? What long-term problems might the patient have?

2. You are administering a caloric test. When warm water is introduced in the right ear, what direction and type of nystagmus would you expect in a normal patient? If a labyrinthine lesion on the right ear is present, how would the nystagmus differ for right and left ear irrigations of warm water?

3. A patient is presented during ENT rounds with symptoms including, unsteadiness when standing in the dark, nausea, dizziness, and nystagmus. CT and magnetic resonance imaging scans were unremarkable. The patient has been undergoing a lengthy treatment for tuberculosis with aminoglycosides. How would the vestibular system be affected?

4. Outline the VOR for a common horizontal rotational head movement. What are the neural pathways involved and what type of eye movement response will occur?

5. Describe three ways one can measure eye movement in patients. What are the disadvantages of each?

❧REFERENCES❧

Minor, L. B., Schessel, D. A., & Carey, J. P. (2004). Meniere's disease. *Current Opinion in Neurology, 17,* 9–16.

Tullio, P. (1929). *Das Ohr und die Enstehung der Sprache und Schrift.* Berlin: Urban & Schwarzenberg.

❧SUGGESTED READING❧

Fernandez, C., & Goldberg, J. M. (1971). Physiology of peripheral neurons innervating semicircular canals of the squirrel monkey. II. Response to sinusoidal stimulation and dynamics of peripheral vestibular system. *Journal of Neurophysiology, 34,* 661–675.

Fernandez, C., & Goldberg, J. M. (1976). Physiology of peripheral neurons innervating otolith organ in the squirrel monkey. I. Response to static tilts and to long-duration centrifugal force. *Journal of Neurophysiology 39,* 970–984.

Hudspeth, A. J. (2005). How the ear's works work: Mechanoelectrical transduction and amplification by hair cells. *Comptes Rendus Biologies, 328,* 155–162.

Hullar, T. E., Della Santina, C. C., Hirvonen, T., Lasker, D. M., Carey, J. P., & Minor, L. B. (2005). Responses of irregularly discharging chinchilla semicircular canal vestibular-nerve afferents during high-frequency head rotations. *Journal of Neurophysiology, 93,* 2777–2786.

Lysakowski, A., & Goldberg, J. M. (1997). A regional ultrastructural analysis of the cellular and synaptic architecture in the chinchilla cristae ampullares. *Journal of Comparative Neurology, 389,* 419–443.

Zakir, M., & Dickman, J. D. (2006). Regeneration of vestibular otolith afferents following ototoxic damage. *Journal of Neuroscience, 26,* 2881–2893.

Part

III

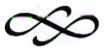

Pathology of Hearing

Chapter

17

Pathology of the Middle Ear

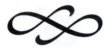

Brian T. Faddis, Ph.D.
Assistant Professor of Otolaryngology
Washington University School of Medicine
St. Louis, Missouri

No textbook on the anatomy and physiology of hearing would be complete without some discussion of the disease processes that affect hearing. This chapter will discuss conductive hearing loss and some recent advances in our understanding of the underlying mechanisms. Basic knowledge in this area will not only enable the reader to understand how and why these diseases affect hearing, but to recognize abnormalities and refer patients for appropriate medical attention.

MANIFESTATIONS OF MIDDLE EAR DISEASE

Hearing loss can be characterized by the extent of hearing loss, the type of loss (conductive, sensory, or neural), the location of the damage, or the cause of the hearing loss. Types of hearing loss are commonly divided into two broad categories: conductive or sensorineural. Some texts prefer to further divide sensorineural losses as strictly sensory (hair cell damage) or strictly neural (auditory nerve damage). The causes of hearing loss are so abundant and varied we cannot discuss them here. These varied causes include genetic, congenital, infectious, traumatic, toxic, occupational, and personal noise exposure, as well as medical causes.

Conductive hearing loss is the result of defects in the external or, more commonly, the middle ear. The mechanics of middle ear structures such as the tympanic membrane and ossicles are sensitive to conditions such as fluid or bone growth, which might impede their natural movement. Ear infections and **otosclerosis** are two conditions that constitute the prevalent causes of conductive hearing loss in children and adults, respectively. Patients referred to otolaryngologists commonly report one or more of a distinct set of symptoms that may be indicative of middle ear disease. These include tinnitus (see Chapter 14), hearing loss, **otalgia, otorrhea,** and vertigo (see Chapter 16). The following sections describe some of these symptoms in brief detail and suggest possible causes for their appearance.

Otalgia

Otalgia is the medical term for ear pain. In children, most ear pain is, in fact, otogenic and is typically caused by ear infections. Children are particularly susceptible to both **otitis media** (infection of the middle ear) and **otitis externa** because of the horizontal positioning and wider lumen of their Eustachian tubes and their propensity for swimming pools. The pain associated with either type of otitis can be rather excruciating, which is why this disease is the leading cause of visits to the pediatrician. Ear wax impaction is another common cause of ear pain in children and adults. Tonsillitis and orthodontic treatments are examples of nonotogenic causes of ear pain in children.

The majority of otalgia complaints in adults, in contrast, may not be otogenic. Rather, adult ear pain is more commonly associated with disorders affecting the larynx, pharynx, tonsils, and muscles of mastication. The temporomandibular joint (TMJ), for example, is a common site of referred ear pain due to teeth clenching and grinding and orthodontic treatments. Many of the more important otologic diseases of adulthood, such as **cholesteatoma,** otosclerosis, Ménière's disease, and acoustic neuroma, are not associated with pain at all.

Otorrhea

Otorrhea means fluid drainage from the ear. Fluid can arise from the ear canal, middle ear cavity, or cranial cavity. With the rare exception of a cerebrospinal fluid (CSF) leak, ear drainage almost always results from an infectious condition. Acute drainage preceded by pain is usually indicative of acute otitis media with drainage released after rupture of the tympanic membrane. Painless drainage may be the result of a more chronic otitis media, and sustained drainage of months or years may be the result of a cholesteatoma. The color, odor, chronicity of the drainage, and associated symptoms or trauma are clues to the cause and origin of otorrhea. A yellowish color and thicker fluid almost always signifies infection. Although odor may also signify infection, it is also associated with the bone destruction that results from cholesteatoma. CSF is clear, thin, and odorless, but may be tinged with blood in cases of trauma that result in temporal bone fracture. In any case, fluid drainage from the ear is cause for medical attention.

Vertigo

The term *vertigo* refers to the sensation of movement, usually spinning or whirling, that results from disturbances in equilibrium. When the patient is perceived to be moving, he or she is experiencing subjective vertigo. When the environment is perceived to be moving, the vertigo is referred to as objective. Vertigo can result from problems occurring in the inner ear, vestibular nerve, brainstem, or cerebellum (see Chapter 16). It is not uncommon for vertigo to be accompanied by other ear-related symptoms, such as hearing loss, tinnitus, or ear pressure, that last for minutes to days.

COMMON DISEASES OF THE MIDDLE EAR

Some or all of the preceding symptoms may be associated with each of the following common middle ear disorders: acute otitis media, chronic otitis media, cholesteatoma, otosclerosis, and glomus tumors of the middle ear. As each disorder is reviewed in the following subsections, keep in mind how the pathology of these diseases might affect the mechanical function of the middle ear (see later).

Acute Otitis Media

Acute otitis media is a common disorder in children, affecting more than 70% of all children by the age of 3. It represents an acute purulent infection and is characterized by edema (swelling), hyperemia (increased blood flow), hemorrhage (bleeding), and fever. To the patient, however, the most critical symptom is pain caused by the inflammation and pressure on the tympanic membrane (Figure 17-1). This pain may reach excruciating levels and often does not

resolve until the tympanic membrane ruptures, relieving the pressure and allowing the middle ear cavity to drain. Fortunately, most tympanic membrane ruptures heal spontaneously, but the middle ear **effusion** (fluid buildup in the middle ear) may take weeks or months to resolve. In some cases, the effusion persists indefinitely and may be asymptomatic or cause a mild-to-moderate hearing loss.

Infants and young children are more predisposed to acute otitis media because of differences in the anatomy of the Eustachian tubes in this population. These tubes in young children are shorter, wider, and more horizontally positioned, allowing easier access for bacteria-laden secretions in the oropharynx to reach the middle ear (Mencher, Gerber, & McCombe, 1997). Children with Eustachian tube malfunction, in which the tubes are chronically open, are particularly susceptible to otitis media. But as important as Eustachian tube closure is to middle ear health, blockage of the tube may prevent proper recovery from otitis media by not allowing middle ear effusions to drain. Blockage of the tube can be perpetuated by allergies and exposure to cigarette smoke (even secondhand) and pool water chlorine.

In adults and children, acute otitis media is quite responsive to antibiotic treatment. Many pediatricians believe that antibiotics are overused for otitis media, and studies have shown that most cases will resolve spontaneously, without antibiotics. Tympanostomy tubes, short tubes placed through the tympanic membrane, are recommended for young children whose chronic effusions are unresponsive to conventional therapy and have resulted in a hearing loss greater than 15 dB, when speech/language impairments are noticeable, or when performance at school has become compromised. Tympanostomy tubes are usually extruded after about 1 year, and the tympanic membrane heals spontaneously in most cases.

Chronic Otitis Media

Chronic otitis media or otitis media with effusion exhibits few of the same symptoms as acute otitis. It is less likely to be painful or produce a discharge,

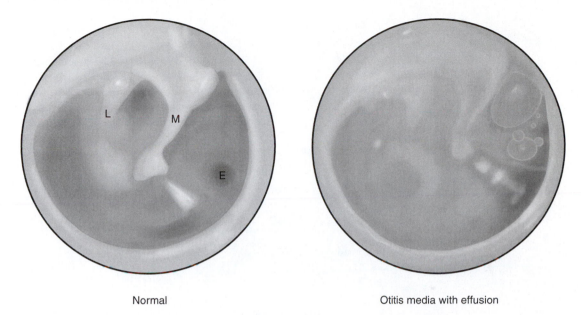

Normal   Otitis media with effusion

FIGURE 17-1 (See Color Plate) Diagrams of a normal tympanic membrane (left) and during an episode of otitis media with effusion. The normal membrane is sufficiently translucent that some underlying structures can be clearly seen: (L) the long process of the incus, (M) the chorda tympani, manubrium of the malleus, and (E) the opening to the Eustachian tube. The ear with otitis may show considerable redness, distention of the membrane, and the presence of fluid, ranging from clear to amber. Underlying structures are not typically as visible as they are in the normal state.

even though it may be associated with a low-grade or recurrent infection. Chronic otitis media is typically only intermittently responsive to antibiotic therapy. The causes of persistent middle ear effusion are unclear but have been associated with malfunction of the Eustachian tube and the concurrent presence of sinusitis. The onset of the chronic condition also typically follows an episode of acute otitis media. Adhesions that develop within the confines of the middle ear and the presence of bacteria can lead to substantial tissue damage, especially bone erosion. The most common symptom of these outcomes is hearing loss (Roland, Marple, & Meyerhoff, 1997).

Cholesteatoma

Cholesteatome refers to a cyst caused by invasion of skin cells into the middle ear. As explained in earlier discussions of middle ear anatomy, the skin found on the lateral (outside) surface of the tympanic mem-

brane is shed much like any other skin, and the shed debris is removed by a unique outward migration of the tympanic membrane and ear canal epithelium. However, sometimes the tympanic membrane is retracted too deeply into the middle ear space, forming a pocket from which the shed debris cannot escape via epithelial migration. As the shed debris accumulates, it becomes an excellent medium for bacterial growth. The growing mass expands through the normal tympanic membrane and invaginates into the middle ear space. This type of cholesteatoma is known as a *primary acquired cholesteatoma*. Congenital cholesteatomas, in contrast, can occur behind an intact tympanic membrane in patients without a history of trauma or otitis (Rash, 2004). In either type, as the cholesteatoma expands, it contacts the bony ossicles, otic capsule, and walls of the middle ear. Contact between cholesteatoma and bone leads to erosion of the bone caused by pressure of the cholesteatoma and factors released by resident bacteria. Involvement of the ossicles leads to conductive

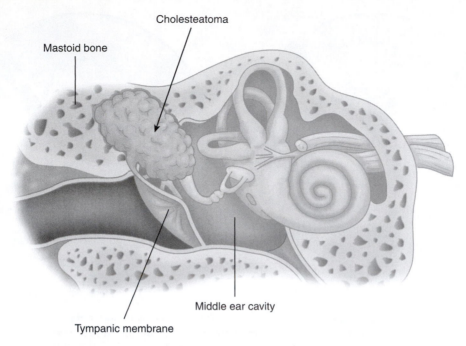

Cholesteatoma

Mastoid bone

Middle ear cavity

Tympanic membrane

FIGURE 17-2   Cross-sectional diagram of the middle ear cavity with a cholesteatoma present. This growing mass starts typically on the internal surface of the tympanic membrane and extends to fill the middle ear space and mastoid bone. Tissue destruction is common wherever the cholesteatoma is in contact with bony structures, enhancing the conductive hearing loss caused by reduced tympanic membrane movement. Erosion may eventually affect inner ear structures, as well as extend intracranially.

hearing loss. Once the otic capsule is eroded, the membranous labyrinth is easily penetrated, resulting in sensorineural hearing loss and vertigo. In advanced cases, the cholesteatoma can erode completely through the temporal bone and penetrate the cranial cavity (Figure 17-2).

The pathogenesis of acquired cholesteatoma is not well understood, and several theories have been proposed to try and explain the initial formation. The epithelial invasion theory suggests that keratinizing epithelium invades the middle ear space via a perforation of the tympanic membrane with subsequent enlargement of the mass caused by epithelial proliferation. Another theory suggests that cholesteatomas start as hyperplastic or rapidly dividing basal epithelial cells that grow into the middle ear space. Another similar theory suggests that some epithelial cells first transform into metaplastic cells

and the mass expands much like a cancer. The cause of congenital cholesteatoma is similarly controversial. The most accepted theory describes the cholesteatoma as developing from residual epithelial rests (masses) in the middle ear that are normally resorbed during fetal development (Kazahaya & Potsic, 2004). However, the cholesteatoma develops, and whether it is congenital or acquired, its growth leads to the same devastating results.

Bacteria present within the cholesteatoma can cause recurrent (chronic) otitis media with effusion that is only intermittently responsive to antibiotic therapy. In some cases, severe infections such as mastoiditis or meningitis can occur (Holt, 2003). Currently, cholesteatomas can be eradicated only by surgical removal, and in many instances, the disease reappears and surgery must be repeated, often several times.

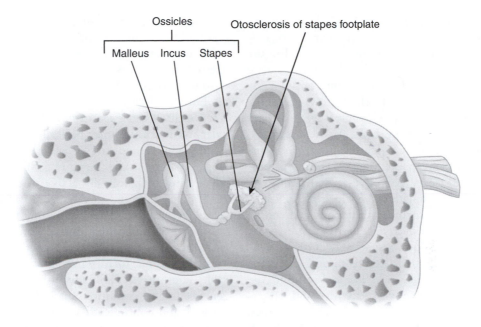

FIGURE 17-3 Diagram of conductive apparatus of the middle ear affected by otosclerosis. In otosclerosis, free movement of the ossicular chain may be impeded by the abnormal growth of spongy bone on the ossicles. This form of otosclerosis commonly freezes the stapes footplate to the oval window. This condition most commonly freezes the stapes footplate to the oval window. I, Incus; M, malleus; S, stapes.

Otosclerosis

Otosclerosis is a disorder of temporal bone metabolism. In this disease, the normally hard quiescent labyrinthine temporal bone is replaced by lesions of excessive vascular spongy bone. These lesions primarily affect the oval window, extending to the stapes footplate (Figure 17-3). This results in an effective immobilization of the footplate in the oval window, which is known as true otosclerosis, and results in a conductive hearing loss. Sometimes, the lesions affect primarily the cochlea or otic capsule, leading to sensorineural hearing loss and even complete deafness. In fact, many of the first cochlear implants were done on patients who had been deafened by otosclerosis.

In about 10% of the U.S. population, otosclerosis is often inherited as an autosomal dominant genetic disorder. However, only 10% of those affected will exhibit hearing loss, thus otosclerosis is detected in only 1% of the population. Approximately two-thirds of those affected are females, and three-fourths of those afflicted will develop otosclerosis in both ears (Holt, 2003; Roland et al., 1997). Hearing loss in the typical patient is first noticed at about 30 to 40 years of age and progresses slowly. Most patients benefit from hearing amplification devices, and a common and successful surgical procedure to replace the lesioned stapes with a prosthesis that attaches to the ossicular chain is a popular choice in more advanced stages of the disease.

Glomus Tumors of the Middle Ear

Glomus tumors arise from paraganglionic tissues found within the temporal bone; hence, they are also commonly referred to as *paragangliomas*. These tissues, sometimes called *glomus bodies,* are found along large vessels and nerves and serve as baroreceptors, capable of sensing changes in oxygen pressure. Glomus tumors are rare, but they are still the most common neoplasms of the temporal bone and are typically named by their site or origin. Glomus tympanicum tumors arise within the middle ear, whereas glomus jugulare tumors arise within the jugular vein in the vicinity of the jugular foramen. They are both slow-growing, highly vascular tumors that spread along pathways of least resistance. Depending on their relative spread and involvement, symptoms of glomus tumors can include cranial nerve palsies, hearing loss, and pulsatile tinnitus (see Chapter 14). Symptoms are most commonly unilateral, and hearing loss may be conductive, sensorineural, or both, depending on the involvement of middle ear structures, inner ear structures, or both, respectively (Forest, Jackson, & McGrew, 2001). Glomus tumors can grow large, filling the middle ear space and invading the mastoid and skull base with extensive and irregular pattern of bone erosion (Lowenheim, Koerbel, Ebner, Kumagami, Ernemann, & Tatagiba, 2006). Aided by high-resolution computed tomography scans, surgical excision is now the recommended treatment for glomus tympanicum tumors. Radiation therapy is often used in conjunction with surgery. Although surgery is also the treatment of choice for glomus jugulare tumors, larger tumors of this variety present special challenges because of spread and involvement of adjacent tissues and nerves. Often, radiation therapy is required after a less than total surgical resection of the tumor.

BACTERIAL BIOFILMS IN CHRONIC MIDDLE EAR DISEASE

The chronic or recurrent nature of those middle ear diseases associated with bacterial infection suggests the presence of a new adversary in medical research: **bacterial biofilms.** These biofilms are colonies of bacteria embedded in a polysaccharide matrix secreted by the bacteria themselves. The biofilm appears designed to enhance bacterial survival under adverse conditions and has raised problems in all types of industrial applications. It also hampers effective medical treatment of many chronic diseases, including cystic

fibrosis, urinary tract infections, tonsillitis, and sinusitis. Otitis media and cholesteatoma also fall into this category and recently have been suggested to involve biofilm infections (Chole & Faddis, 2002, 2003; Post, Stoodley, Hall-Stoodley, & Ehrlich, 2004).

Bacteria can exist in two different states. The planktonic form is metabolically active and replicating. This is the form we associate with acute infections. The sessile form is a hibernating form that is not metabolically active or replicating and exhibits a pronounced resistance to antibiotics that are effective against the planktonic form. The sessile form typically inhabits the biofilm proper, encased in its matrix, but can be activated to revert to a planktonic form when conditions are favorable. Thus, these biofilms may be able to monitor environmental conditions, including antibiotic exposure, and continue to support a chronically recurring infection for years or decades. Creating treatments aimed at eradicating biofilms is now one of the most active areas of both medical and industrial research.

EFFECTS OF DISEASE ON MECHANICS OF THE MIDDLE EAR

The primary function of the middle ear is to match the impedance of an airborne signal with the fluid environment of the inner ear. The most important mechanisms that enable this impedance matching are the area ratio of the tympanic membrane to the oval window and the lever action of the ossicles (see Chapter 7). Free movement of these middle ear structures is crucial for creating the necessary increased force to the oval window. Any physical obstruction that limits the mobility of middle ear structures could result in a hearing loss. It is easy, therefore, to appreciate how the fluid formed in otitis media, the growing cholesteatoma mass, or the immobilizing bone deposition seen in otosclerosis all lead to a conductive form of hearing loss. Fortunately, most of these circumstances are reversible by pharmacologic or surgical intervention, followed by a return to normal or near-normal hearing.

❧ SUMMARY ❧

This chapter examines some of the symptoms and characteristics of several common middle ear diseases. Otitis media is one of the most common ailments faced by humans. Acute infections can be painful and result in tympanic membrane perforation and purulent discharge from the middle ear. Chronic infections may exist that are not painful but involve fluid collection in the middle ear space that produces a conductive hearing loss. Cholesteatoma, a mass of keratinizing epithelial debris and bacteria, grows into the middle ear space and erodes adjacent bony structures leading to hearing loss that is conductive or sensorineural in nature. Because the cholesteatoma provides a good environment for bacteria, they are often associated with chronic otitis media. Otosclerosis is a genetic disorder of bone metabolism that results in a conductive hearing loss in the majority of cases, but may cause sensorineural deafness when the otic capsule is involved. Bacterial biofilms were presented as a novel explanation of the chronicity observed in many otolaryngologic diseases.

❧ KEY TERMS ❧

Bacterial biofilm

Cholesteatoma

Effusion

Glomus tumor

Otalgia

Otitis externa

Otitis media

Otorrhea

Otosclerosis

❧ STUDY QUESTIONS ❧

1. Name and describe the common symptoms associated with ear disease.

2. Explain why children are more susceptible than adults to ear infections.

3. Describe how cholesteatomas, glomus tumors, and otosclerosis are similar in their effect on hearing.

4. Describe the mechanisms used by bacterial biofilms to reduce their susceptibility to antibiotic treatment.

❧ REFERENCES ❧

Chole, R. A., & Faddis, B. T. (2002). Evidence for microbial biofilms in cholesteatomas. *Archives of Otolaryngology—Head and Neck Surgery, 128,* 1129–1133.

Chole, R. A., & Faddis, B. T. (2003). Anatomic evidence for microbial biofilms in tonsillar tissues: A possible mechanism to explain chronicity. *Archives of Otolaryngology—Head and Neck Surgery, 129,* 634–636.

Forest, J. A., Jackson, C. G., & McGrew, B. M. (2001) Long-term control of surgically treated glomus tympanicum tumors. *Otology & Neurotology, 22,* 232–236.

Holt, J. J. (2003). Cholesteatoma and otosclerosis: Two slowly progressive causes of hearing loss treatable through corrective surgery. *Clinical Medicine & Research, 1,* 151–154.

Kazahaya, K., & Potsic, W. P. (2004). Congenital cholesteatoma. *Current Opinion in Otolaryngology & Head and Neck Surgery, 12,* 398–403.

Lowenheim, H., Koerbel, A., Ebner, F. H., Kumagami, H., Ernemann, U., & Tatagiba, M. (2006). Differentiating imaging findings in primary and secondary tumors of the jugular foramen. *Neurosurgery Reviews, 29,* 1–11.

Mencher, G. T., Gerber, S. E., & McCombe, A. (Eds.). (1997). *Audiology and auditory dysfunction.* Needham Heights, MA: Allyn & Bacon.

Post, J. C., Stoodley, P., Hall-Stoodley, L., & Ehrlich, G. D. (2004). The role of biofilms in otolaryngologic infections. *Current Opinion in Otolaryngology & Head and Neck Surgery, 12,* 185–190.

Rash, E. M. (2004). Recognize cholesteatomas early. *Nurse Practitioner, 29,* 24–27.

Roland, P. S., Marple, B. F., & Meyerhoff, W. L. (Eds.). (1997). *Hearing loss.* New York: Thieme Press.

Chapter

18

Noise-Induced Hearing Loss

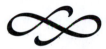

William W. Clark, Ph.D.
Director, Program in Audiology and Communication Sciences
Washington University School of Medicine
St. Louis, Missouri

The descriptions of normal mammalian hearing provided in Chapters 6 through 15 emphasize the remarkable sensitivity of the ear. Young, normal human listeners can detect pressure variations as small as 0.00002 Pascals. But our ears are also quite resilient. We can detect "microscopic" pressure variations and also receive sound-pressure variations more than a million times larger without experiencing damage. If your sense of touch extended over a similar range, you would be able to feel the weight of a feather placed on your hand and also sustain the weight of a large pickup truck without experiencing pain or injury.

But when an ear is exposed to too much sound, it can be injured or break. If the damage is significant, the patient will experience a "noise-induced" hearing loss. At one time or another, nearly every person has experienced a hearing loss caused by excessive noise exposure. Attending a rock concert or a sporting event often includes enough sound to cause small hearing losses, but these losses usually recover after a few minutes or a few hours. Symptoms of these "temporary" losses include a feeling of fullness or pressure in the ear, sensation of speech as "muffled," and often, tinnitus. Exposures to more intense noise and for longer periods can cause permanent losses of hearing. Individuals who are employed in noisy occupations, who enjoy noisy recreational activities such as hunting or target shooting, or who listen to amplified music at maximum volume levels for prolonged periods are at risk for sustaining a significant sensorineural hearing loss caused by noise exposure.

This chapter reviews the basic characteristics of temporary and permanent hearing losses caused by exposure to noise. This chapter also describes **acoustic trauma,** as well as the important role of one type of leisure noise: firing guns, which contributes significantly to permanent hearing loss in humans. This chapter emphasizes the clinical presentation of hearing loss and identifies factors that will help the audiologist determine whether noise should be considered as a possible cause. (For a complete description of the cellular mechanisms of noise-induced hearing loss (NIHL), see the review by Henderson and colleagues [Henderson, Hu, Bielefeld, & Nicotera, 2007]).

HISTORICAL PERSPECTIVE

That noise can interfere with the quality of life has been known for centuries. In fact, an early community noise ordinance restricted chariot riding in Rome to daylight hours because the noise of the metal wheels on the cobblestone streets annoyed the residents at night. Another ordinance, dating to about 600 BC, banned roosters from a wealthy Italian town because the residents liked to sleep late. But the fact that noise exposure could cause significant permanent hearing loss was not generally recognized until the 1700s, when it was noted that individuals who worked as smiths, hammering copper into vases and bowls, lost their hearing at an early age because of the excessive noise (*ex continuo illo strepitu, aures male affici* ["the ears are injured by that perpetual din"]; Ramazzini, 1700; Franco, 1999). In the 1800s, the term *boilermakers' deafness* was used to characterize hearing losses experienced by blacksmiths and those in the boiler industry who engaged in hammering metal throughout the workday. One of the earliest studies was conducted by Haberman (1890), who studied anatomic changes in the inner ears of a boilermaker who had been run down by a train he did not hear approaching.

The industrial revolution of the late 1800s created additional sources of loud noise exposure for workers. This was due to the development of power, first by steam and later by electricity, to increase machinery productivity. An unfortunate by-product of power is noise associated with the manufacturing process. Coincident with the start of industrial revolution was a new understanding of the structure of the inner ear, sparked by Corti's description of the organ that now bears his name (Corti, 1851), and important theories of hearing such as those proposed by von Helmholtz (1863). Although much progress was made in our understanding of how the ear worked over the next century, little progress was made in our understanding about how the ear and hearing were damaged by noise (Hawkins and Schacht, 2005).

The major impetus for concern about hearing loss caused by excessive exposure to noise came during and at the end of World War II. Although the effects of blast injury on the hearing of soldiers had been previously reported, equipment for generating and quantifying noise exposure in the laboratory was not available until the late 1920s and early 1930s. By the start of World War II, the U.S. government recognized that intense sound was a probable hazard and a possible offensive weapon and commissioned a series of studies through the National Defense Research Committee (Davis, 1991). Although the offensive weapon work remains classified, Hallowell Davis and his colleagues published a classic study in 1950 of the effects of intense pure-tone exposures on human ears (Davis, Morgan, Hawkins, Galambos, & Smith, 1950). The need for providing assessment and rehabilitation of soldiers returning from combat with NIHL played a key role in the establishment of audiology as a profession in the late 1940s (Katz, 2002).

Efforts to regulate occupational noise in the United States began with the military in the mid 1950s (United States Air Force, 1956), and they were followed by regulations promulgated in 1970 under the Occupational Safety and Health Act, which established the Occupational Safety and Health Administration and charged it with the responsibility to protect the safety and health of a large segment of the U.S. workforce (Occupational Safety and Health Administration [OHSA], 1983; National Institute for Occupational Safety and Health [NIOSH], 1998). These regulations stimulated a number of experimental studies designed to quantify the effects of excessive exposure, particularly occupational exposure, on hearing.

Concern about the potential for leisure also increased during the same period, spurred, undoubtedly, by the increasing popularity of rock music and rock concerts; the development of the personal stereo and MP3 players (Clark, 1991b; Fligor & Cox, 2004); and the need to understand the relative contributions of leisure noise, occupational noise, and presbycusis to the total hearing loss experienced by an individual who continues to work and play in noise as he or she grows older (Axelsson, 1996).

TEMPORARY THRESHOLD SHIFTS

Like every other system in the human body, ears can become fatigued if they are called on to work too hard or too long. It may be surprising to learn that even rather low levels of sound, if listened to continuously, can reduce slightly one's ability to hear. Even the sound of your instructor's voice, at about 70- to 75-dB sound pressure level (SPL) in a typical classroom, can cause a slight decrease in hearing after a 1-hour lecture. When the sound is turned off, fortunately, the ear can recover completely, usually within a few hours. Because the ear is so easily fatigued by even moderate levels of exposure, it is probably fair to say that most of us spend a portion of our day with a slight hearing loss, even though it is not noticeable. The term **threshold shift** is used to describe a change in hearing sensitivity, usually toward poorer hearing, and it is measured in decibels. Because the student's hearing in our example recovered completely within a few hours after the exposure, this shift would be called a **temporary threshold shift (TTS).**

Exposures to higher levels of sound cause more severe TTSs, and if the shift is large enough, you will be able to notice it. Most of you have had an experience similar to the following: You drive home on noisy freeway in noisy traffic after a busy day, playing the radio at a fairly loud, but comfortable listening level. You park the car in the garage and retire for a quiet, restful night. The next morning you start your car, and the radio is so loud it startles you, even though it is playing at the same level as it was when you drove home. Why does it sound so much louder in the morning? Even though you did not notice it, you had experienced a TTS while driving home. And most likely, you did not notice that you had been turning up the volume on the radio periodically during your trip to maintain a constant loudness level. Fatigued, your ears heard the sound of the radio as comfortably loud in the evening, but rested, they perceived the sound as extremely loud, even though it was the same volume. Figure 18-1 presents a graph showing the general relations among exposure level, duration, and the amount of TTS.

This hypothetical chart provides a useful summary of the major relations between exposure level and duration and the growth of TTS in humans. It was designed to describe the worst-case scenario in which the noise exposure was concentrated in the frequency region where the ear is most sensitive

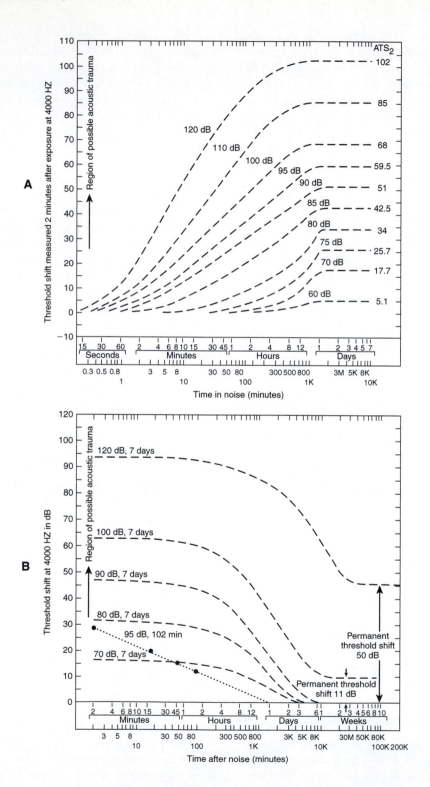

(2,800–4,000 Hz), and thresholds were measured at 4,000 Hz. Figure 18-1A shows the growth of TTS during exposure to continuous noise. The parameter is the A-weighted sound level. For all exposure levels, thresholds begin to decline after exposure durations of minutes to hours, continue to decline for about 12 to 24 hours, and then stabilize at flat, or asymptotic, levels as the exposure continues. The level of the stabilized threshold shift is called **asymptotic threshold shift (ATS).**

As you would expect, the more severe exposures cause TTS to start earlier, to grow more rapidly than exposures at lower levels, and to produce larger ATS. For exposures less than 85-dB SPL, it takes several hours for TTS to begin to accumulate to measurable values. In contrast, exposure at 120-dB SPL for even 5 minutes will cause more than 30 dB of TTS.

Another "take-home" message from this graph is that ATS is always lower than the exposure level; that is, noise exposures cannot cause ATS that exceeds the SPL of the noise. Finally, this refers to the worst-case scenario. If the offending noise is concentrated at frequencies where the human ear is less sensitive, one would expect a lower ATS value. Consider an exposure to a band of noise centered at 250 Hz. Because the ear is about 20 dB less sensitive at 250 Hz than it is at 4,000 Hz, the "effective" exposure would be the SPL of the exposure, reduced by 20 dB. Reading from the graph, a sound of 100-dB SPL at 250 Hz would effectively be 80 dB, and would produce an ATS of 34 dB.

The concept of ATS is intriguing. Taken at face value, it suggests that during noise exposure the ear reaches a new, and less sensitive, steady-state condition in which the degenerative and restorative processes are equal. If an individual with ATS is taken away from the noise, hearing sensitivity returns toward pre-exposure conditions.

Typical patterns of recovery of ATS after noise exposure are shown in Figure 18-1B. For low levels of exposure, exposures of short duration, or both, threshold recovers approximately linearly in log time and is complete by 1 day after exposure (see Figure 18-1B, dotted line). For more severe exposures, TTS is larger and recovery is delayed, but it is usually complete within about a week. If the noise exposure is severe, thresholds do not recover completely; that is, the subject sustains a persistent or **permanent threshold shift (PTS)** (Clark, 1991a). PTSs caused by noise exposure are referring to as **"NIPTS" (noise-induced permanent threshold shifts)** in the literature that deals with noise exposure regulations (American National Standards Institute, 1996; NIOSH, 1998).

The symptoms of TTS include tinnitus, a sensation of fullness or pressure in the ear, and perception of speech as sound "dull" or "muffled" (Clark & Bohne, 1999). Most people have experienced some or all of these symptoms after listening to loud music, either live or over headphones, engaging in noisy activities such as shooting firearms, or attending sporting events (Clark, 1992). Fortunately, like TTS itself, the symptoms usually subside within about a day.

For exposures that produce large TTSs, the maximum shift is observed a half-octave greater than the exposure frequency; TTSs observed after less severe exposures that produce only small TTS tend to show their maxima at the exposure frequency. Although the "half-octave" shift has been known since the publication of Davis and colleagues' classic study (Davis et al., 1950), the explanation for why it occurs had to await advances in the understanding of cochlear mechanics. At lower sound stimulation levels, the response of the basilar membrane is the combination of the passive mechanics and the active processes of the outer hair

FIGURE 18-1 Hypothetical growth and recovery curves for hearing loss caused by exposure to a band of noise placed at the region of maximum sensitivity for human ears for 7 days. The parameter is the sound pressure level (SPL) of the noise. (A) Thresholds measured during noise. (B) Recovery functions after termination of the noise. (Reprinted with permission from Miller, J. D. (1974). Effects of noise on people. *Journal of the Acoustical Society of America, 56 (3)*, 729–64. Copyright 1974, American Institute of Physics.)

cell (OHC) complex. Exposures that produce only small TTSs are attributed to damage to the active feedback mechanism of the OHCs. In contrast, high-level exposures eliminate the active process entirely, and the cochlear response is determined solely by the passive mechanics (Fridberger, Zheng, Parthasarathi, Ren, & Nuttal, 2002; Ruggero, Rich, & Recio, 1996). The passive mechanical response is maximal a half-octave greater than the exposure frequency (Bies, 1996). As the hearing sensitivity recovers, the maximum threshold shift moves back toward the exposure frequency.

PERMANENT THRESHOLD SHIFTS

PTSs occur when TTS does not fully recover (as shown in Figure 18-1 for the two most severe exposures). Because the recovery of a threshold shift is always complete within a few weeks, PTS can be defined as any change in hearing sensitivity after noise exposure that persists for more than 4 weeks (Quaranta, Portalini, & Henderson, 1998). Unlike TTSs, PTS is most commonly seen in the frequency region of 3 to 6 kHz, regardless of the frequency content of the exposure (Clark & Bohne, 1999). Although the amount of PTS grows with increasing duration of exposure, it does not appear to exceed the ATS produced after the first day. That is, the ATS measured after 1 day of exposure to continuous noise appears to set an upper bound on the PTS that can result from the exposure, even after years of exposure (Bohne & Clark, 1982; Bohne, Clark, & Harding, 1994).

STUDIES OF OCCUPATIONAL NOISE EXPOSURE

Obviously, the most direct way to determine the hazardous effects of noise on people is to study individuals who are overexposed. But ethical considerations limit the types of experimental studies that can be conducted on human subjects. We simply cannot expose human subjects to sounds that might pose any risk for creating a permanent hearing loss! So how do we obtain information about human responses to excessive noise exposure? One way is to

study the hearing of groups of individuals who work in noisy industries, and to use the data to infer the risk for eventual permanent NIHL. Examples of comprehensive published studies of people exposed to noise include those by Lempert (Lempert & Henderson, 1973), Taylor (Taylor, Pearson, Mair, & Burns 1965), Passchier-Vermeer (1968), and Burns and Robinson (1970). One of the first things you will notice about these references is that they were all published more than three decades ago. The purpose of federal workplace noise regulations implemented in the United States and other developed countries in the late 1970s and early 1980s was to protect workers from hazardous occupational noise. This has been accomplished by reducing noise exposures and requiring workers to wear hearing protection when noise cannot be reduced or eliminated (e.g., Occupational Safety and Health Administration [OSHA], 1983). Successful implementation of the regulations theoretically eliminated excessive exposure for all workers and prevented any further scientific study of dose-response relationships between occupational noise exposure and related noise-induced hearing loss.

However, these previous studies have value; in fact, reports from the National Institute for Occupational Safety and Health (NIOSH, 1998; Prince, Stayner, Smith, & Gilbert, 1997; Prince, 2002; Prince, Gilbert, Smith, & Stayner, 2003) re-evaluated the "old" NIOSH data, using newer, more sophisticated statistical techniques. These newer analyses have helped researchers better understand how many people who work in noisy occupations are at risk for acquiring a significant hearing loss, over and above that caused by aging alone, because of their workplace noise exposure.

A review of the methods, findings, and conclusions of Taylor and colleagues' (1965) classic study of hearing in jute weavers in Dundee, Scotland, provides a "sound" summary for much of the current knowledge about NIHL from chronic exposure to continuous noise for a working lifetime. Taylor and colleagues surveyed the noise in 14 jute mills in Dundee, Scotland, and measured the hearing levels of employed and retired workers for various durations. All of the subjects were female workers, and length of service varied from less than 1 to 39 years. Another unusual characteristic of this survey is that the jute weaving process, and the resulting noise exposure, had not changed over a period of more than 50 years. It is rare, indeed, to find an industrial process that has not changed dramatically in 50 years, and a work environment where employees were exposed at essentially continuous noise throughout their workday. The noise levels were relatively constant at 99- to 102-dB SPL throughout the working day, and the spectrum was relatively flat.

Because some hearing loss was expected due to aging (presbycusis), Taylor and colleagues (1965) reported their data as the "median estimated noise-induced threshold shift," calculated as the difference, in decibels, between the median hearing levels of the jute weavers and hearing levels of an age-matched non-noise–exposed population obtained from a British standard. Their findings are reproduced in Figure 18-2. Separate graphs are shown for groups of workers exposed for different periods (ranging from <1 to 5–9 years in Figure 18-2A, and 5–9 to 35–39 years in Figure 18-2B).

When studying these data, remember that the graphs are not audiograms, they are threshold shift functions. In modern terminology, these functions would be called "noise-induced permanent threshold shifts," and would be labeled "NIPTS." Careful examination of the findings from this Taylor and colleagues' classic study (1965) will help the audiologist understand and remember important general points about NIPTS from occupational noise exposure.

The first salient point is that the losses appear first, and most often, for the 4-kHz test frequency. This occurred even though the noise from the textile mill was broadband and contained energy at all frequencies. For all exposure durations, the losses were greatest at 4 kHz. This audiometric characteristic is called a **4-kHz notch,** and it is commonly seen in patients with NIHL (McBride & Williams, 2001; Clark & Bohne, 1999). Keep in mind, though, that notches can and do occur in patients without a history of noise exposure; therefore, the "notch" should not be considered diagnostic and should not be called a "noise" notch.

A second characteristic is that the losses are larger at 4 kHz for workers with longer durations of exposure, but most of the growth occurs in the first 15 to 20 years. Keep in mind that the data in Figure 18-2 are the results of a cross-sectional study; that is, all the data were collected at one point in time. It is not known for certain whether the workers exposed for 35 to 39 years had hearing that was similar to workers exposed for shorter durations (e.g., 10–15 years) earlier in their careers when they had worked in the jute weaving industry for only that long; that is, data are for subjects at an earlier time point are not available, and the progression of hearing loss for each subject is not charted at different time points. But even with that limitation, the group data clearly show that the hearing losses increase rapidly for exposure durations of up to 15 to 20 years, but change less for longer durations or exposure.

A final important point from these data is that the progression of hearing loss at the lower frequencies (250 Hz to 2.0 kHz) is much slower and more linear than the losses at the high frequencies. Hearing losses in the low-frequency range also are less severe (NIPTS < 40 dB) than losses at 4.0 kHz, which can reach levels of 60 to 70 dB. As a result, patients with long histories of significant occupational noise exposures will exhibit marked hearing losses for the so-called noise frequencies, 3, 4, and 6 kHz, but will usually retain relatively good low-frequency hearing and will maintain relatively good speech discrimination.

Noise and Presbycusis

Because the data shown in Figure 18-2 are threshold shift functions, they can be converted back to the "original" audiograms by adding the presbycusis values for each group. The resultant audiograms for the groups are shown in Figure 18-3. These graphs, therefore, display the actual hearing levels of the subjects who participated in Taylor and colleagues' study (1965).

For the 35- to 39-year-old workers, with 15 to 19 years of exposure, the contribution of presbycusis is relatively small, and the composite audiogram

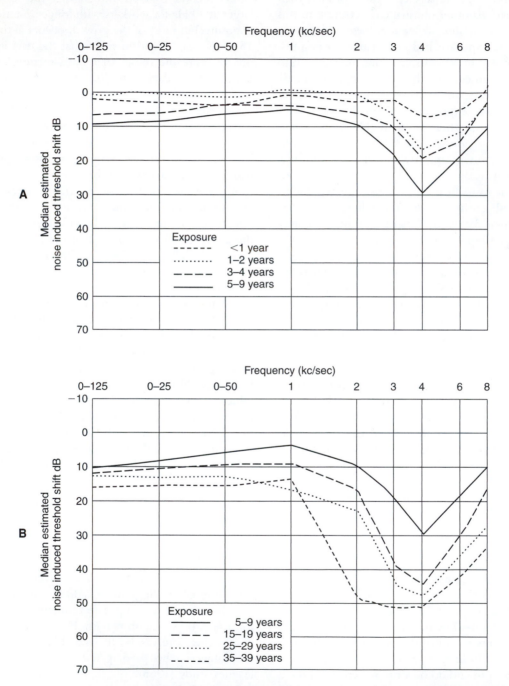

FIGURE 18-2   Median estimated noise-induced threshold shift for female workers exposed for 1 to 9 years (A) and 5 to 39 years working in the jute weaving industry in Dundee, Scotland. (Reprinted with permission from Taylor, W., Pearson, J., Mair, A., & Burns, W. (1965). Study of noise and hearing in jute weaving. *Journal of the Acoustical Society of America, 38,* 113–120. Copyright 1965 American Institute of Physics.)

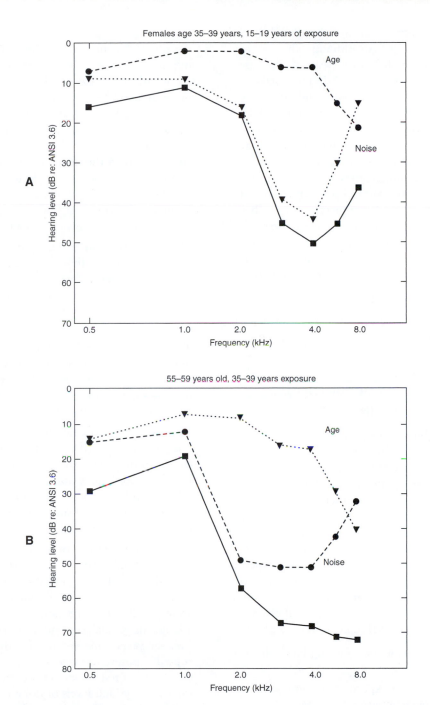

FIGURE 18-3 Combined influence of noise and age on the audiogram of a hypothetical female worker in Taylor and colleagues' study (1965). (A) Age 35 to 39 years, with 15 to 19 years of exposure to jute weaving noise; (B) age 55 to 59 years, with 35 to 39 years of exposure. Presbycusis thresholds (labeled "age") are derived from Annex B of American Standard ANSI S 3.44 (American National Standards Institute, 1996) and represent median threshold values for age-matched female subjects.

still displays the "notch" created by the NPTS function (see Figure 18-3A). Although the 55- to 59-year-old workers with 35 to 39 years of exposure to occupational noise had larger NIPTS functions, the contribution to the composite audiogram by presbycusis is much larger and swamps the NIPTS component. As a result, older workers may not display an audiometric notch, even though they may have been exposed to excessive occupational noise and may have had a "notch" in their audiogram for many years. This is important to keep in mind if you see older clients with significant presbycusis. Just because they do not have a notch in their audiogram, it does *not* mean that they have not sustained a NIHL. The converse statement is also true: Some patients will have notches in their audiograms even though they have not been exposed to noise. Therefore, the presence or absence of a "notch" cannot be used solely to diagnose NIHL (American Academy of Otolaryngology-Head and Neck Surgery Foundation, 1998).

CHARACTERISTICS OF OCCUPATIONAL NOISE-INDUCED HEARING LOSS

The American College of Occupational and Environmental Medicine has published a summary statement to help occupational physicians make a differential diagnosis of occupational noise exposure as a potential cause of a patient's hearing loss (American College of Occupational and Environmental Medicine, 2003). Although audiologists do not make medical diagnoses, it is certainly within the scope of practice of audiology to offer expert opinions about whether excessive exposure to workplace noise should be considered as a possible cause a patient's hearing loss. The principal characteristics of occupational NIHL are as follows:

- It is always sensorineural, affecting hair cells in the inner ear.

- Because most noise exposures are symmetric, the hearing loss is typically bilateral.

- Typically, the first sign of hearing loss from noise exposure is a "notching" of the audiogram at 3000, 4000, or 6000 Hz, with recovery at 8000 Hertz (Hz). The exact location of the notch depends on multiple factors, including the frequency of the damaging noise and the length of the ear canal. Therefore, in early noise induced hearing loss, the average hearing thresholds at 500, 1000, and 2000 Hz are better than the average at 3000, 4000, and 6000, and the hearing level at 8000 Hz is usually better than the deepest part of the "notch." This "notching" is in contrast to age-related hearing loss, which also produces high frequency hearing loss, but in a down-sloping pattern without recovery at 8000 Hz.

- Noise exposure alone usually does not produce a loss greater than 75 decibels (dB) in high frequencies and 40 dB in lower frequencies. However, individuals with superimposed age-related losses may have hearing threshold levels in excess of these values.

- The rate of hearing loss as a result of chronic noise exposure is greatest during the first 10–15 years of exposure, and decreases as the hearing threshold increases. This is in contrast to age-related loss, which accelerates over time.

- Most scientific evidence indicates that previously noise-exposed ears are not more sensitive to future noise exposure and that hearing loss from noise does not progress (in excess of what would be expected from the addition of age-related threshold shifts) once the exposure to noise is discontinued.

- In obtaining a history of noise exposure, the clinician should keep in mind that the risk of noise-induced hearing loss is considered to increase significantly with chronic exposures above 85 dBA for an 8-hour time-weighted average. In general, continuous noise exposure over the years is more damaging than interrupted exposure to noise, which permits the ear to have a rest period. However, short exposures to very high levels of noise in occupations, such as construction or firefighting, may produce significant loss, and measures to estimate the health effects of such intermittent noise are lacking. When the noise exposure

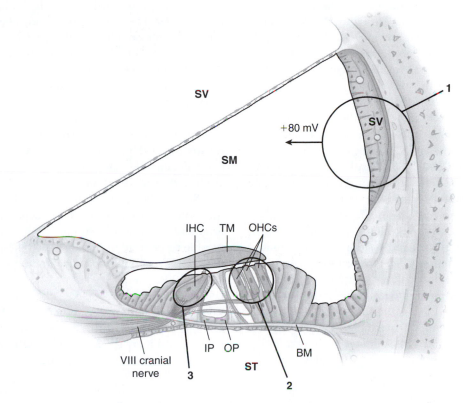

FIGURE 18-4 Schematic cross section of the cochlea showing the functional systems that work together to transduce sound into neural input. The lateral wall and stria vascularis (SV, 1) generate the endolymphatic potential, which powers the outer hair cell (OHC) cochlear amplifier (2). The amplified vibrations are transmitted to the inner hair cells (IHCs), which stimulate the afferent auditory nerve (3). These three systems represent points of vulnerability. BM, Basilar membrane; H, helicotrema; IP, inner pillar cells; OP, outer pillar cells; RM, Reissner's membrane; SM, scala media; ST, scala tympani; SV, stria vascularis; TM, tectorial membrane.

history indicates the use of hearing protective devices, the clinician should also keep in mind that the real world attenuation provided by hearing protectors may vary widely between individuals (American College of Occupational and Environmental Medicine, 2003, p. 579).

MECHANISMS OF NOISE-INDUCED HEARING LOSS

Although the effects of noise on hearing have been known for many years, we are still learning about the anatomic and physiologic changes that are asso-

ciated with NIHL. Although there has been much progress since the late 1990s, scientists are still just beginning to understand the complex processes that govern the functional and structural processes relating to temporary and permanent hearing losses caused by excessive exposure to noise.

It may be helpful to think again about the major systems that contribute to good hearing before trying to determine the agents responsible for hearing loss. These systems are identified in a schematic cross section of the cochlear duct shown in Figure 18-4.

Remember that the actual transducers are the inner hair cells (IHCs), passive mechanoreceptors that convert vibratory motion into electrical potentials. The rest of the "stuff" in Figure 18-4 should be considered as the "supporting" cast. They include cells that support the important architecture of the cochlear duct and protect the integrity of the fluid barriers between the three scalae: media, tympani, and vestibuli; the thin double layer of cells composing Reissner's membrane; and the cells composing the reticular lamina: the outer and inner pillar cells, Deiters', Hensen's and Claudius cells.

Chapters 9 and 10 explain how the macromechanics and micromechanics of the cochlea operate to control auditory sensitivity and frequency selectivity. In a general sense, the normal inner ear operates like a sensitive microphone and amplifier. This amplifier is powered by the **stria vascularis,** which is the **battery**—it creates and maintains a large positive endocochlear potential (EP) of about +90 mV by pumping potassium ions (K^+) into the scala media. The EP charges the OHCs and renders them motile through activation of mechanoelectric transduction channels in their apices (Patuzzi, 2002). The mechanical responses of the OHCs amplify low-level signals that are not strong enough to stimulate the IHCs directly; that is, their active and nonlinear responses can be considered as the cochlear amplifier (Davis, 1983; Kemp, 1978). As discussed in Chapter 13, the activity of the OHCs results in the production of distortion that can be recorded in the ear canal as otoacoustic emissions (OAEs). It is important to remember that OAEs are present throughout the dynamic range of hearing, but at stimulus levels greater about 50-dB SPL, the mechanical displacement of the basilar membrane "swamps" the OAE response. Thus, it is appropriate to consider OAEs as functionally significant only for relatively low-level signals, that is, less than 30- to 50-dB SPL.

The amplified vibrations are passively detected by the IHCs, and their discharge releases the neurotransmitter glutamate across the synaptic cleft to cause a discharge of the auditory nerve. Hearing loss, either temporary or permanent, might be caused by a disruption of functional capacity of any of these systems, or a combination of some or all of them. Currently, a full description of the pathophysical processes that explain temporary or permanent hearing loss is being actively studied in many laboratories (Henderson, Bielefeld, Harris & Hu, 2006; Henderson, Hu, Bielefeld, & Nicotera, 2007).

Scientists do know some things, however. Acoustic trauma (see later description) results when the incoming sound has sufficient strength to dislodge the organ of Corti from the basilar membrane. The mechanism is mechanical, and the damage is permanent and irreversible. The fluids intermix, and OHCs and IHCs, as well as supporting cells, degenerate and are replaced by scar tissue (Bohne & Rabbitt, 1983).

Sounds between about 90 and 140 dBA have the potential to produce PTS, depending on the level and duration of exposure. The cells most vulnerable to damage in ears that have significant PTSs are OHCs and IHCS. Damage in the basal turn usually includes complete loss of OHCs and IHCs in restricted regions (Bohne & Clark, 1982); in the apical turn, it is common to observe significant OHC loss but little IHC damage, even for long-duration exposures. Figure 18-5 is a photomicrograph of a normal organ of Corti and one with a discrete "wipeout" of all sensory and supporting cells.

Figure 18-5 is a "bird's-eye view" of the organ of Corti. The darkly stained fibers are the myelinated nerve fibers. The single row of IHCs and three rows of OHCs, as well as the inner and outer pillar cells, can also be discerned. Figure 18-5A shows a normal organ of Corti, and Figure 18-5B presents an ear that has been exposed to a noise that caused a PTS. Note that the OHCs, IHCs, and pillar cells have degenerated in a narrow region, and they have been replaced by a thin layer of squamous epithelial tissue. In summary, individuals with significant PTS will most likely have regions of total cell loss in the basal turn of the cochlea and accompanying high-frequency hearing losses. Because the OHCs are the generators of OAEs, loss or reduction of functional capacity of OHCs is accompanied by reduction or elimination of transient and distortion product OAEs (Zurek, Clark, & Kim, 1982; Shera, 2004). In fact, tests of OAEs have been proposed as early indicators of NIHL in industrial or military environments (e.g., Marshall & Heller, 1998; Miller, Marshall, Heller, & Hughes, 2006).

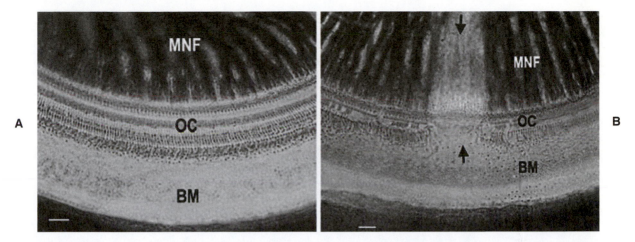

FIGURE 18-5 Photomicrographs of the 4-kHz region of the organ of Corti in a non–noise-exposed control and a noise-exposed animal. (A) This view shows the organ of Corti (OC) as it is attached to the basilar membrane (BM). Its sensory cells are innervated by the peripheral processes of the primary auditory neurons (MNF). (B) After excessive noise exposure, a portion of the organ of Corti has degenerated and has been replaced by squamous epithelial tissue. The nerve fibers have also disappeared, and there is spotty loss of sensory and supporting cells adjacent to the lesion.

The mechanisms underlying TTS and the relation between TTS and PTS remain unclear, although they are being actively pursued. Several attractive candidates, or "likely suspects," may be responsible or partially responsible for TTS. It would be expected that high levels of sound might affect the stria vascularis. If the oxygen supply to the stria was compromised, or if the OHCs consumed too much current, one would expect the endolymphatic potential to decline; that is, the battery would discharge. Reducing the EP would result in poorer transduction and might lead to TTS. Although acute swelling of the stria vascularis has been observed after exposure to high–level sound that produces TTS (Hawkins, 1971; Wang, Hirose, & Liberman, 2002), EP shifts do not appear to be related to the TTS (Hirose & Liberman, 2003).

It is known that noise exposure can disrupt the stereocilia of the OHCs. Broken tip links, fused stereocilia, and other changes can lead to a loss of structural integrity of the cells (Tsuprun, Schachern, Cureoglu, & Paparella, 2003). Patuzzi (1998, 2002) has shown that the mechanoelectric transduction channels at the apical end of the stereocilia can be inactivated by TTS-producing

noise, and that the time course of reactivation of the channel is closely correlated with recovery of TTS. Finally, Bohne and colleagues (Nordmann, Bohne, & Harding, 2000) have shown that pillar cells are buckled and the tips of the OHC stereocilia are temporarily detached from the tectorial membrane during TTS.

Excessive exposure to noise can also lead to swelling and rupture of the terminals of the afferent auditory nerve fibers that innervate the IHCs. The neurotransmitter is glutamate, and excessive stimulation can lead to an overstimulation of the glutamate receptors on the postsynaptic cells, resulting in TTSs or PTSs (Puel, D'Aldin, Saffiende, Eybalin, & Pujol, 1996).

ACOUSTIC TRAUMA

A brief exposure of sufficient intensity can stretch the basilar membrane beyond its elastic limits and damage it mechanically. Although the term *acoustic trauma* is sometimes used generally to describe damage to the ear or hearing caused by noise exposure, audiologists should reserve the term to identify noise exposures that produce an immediate injury

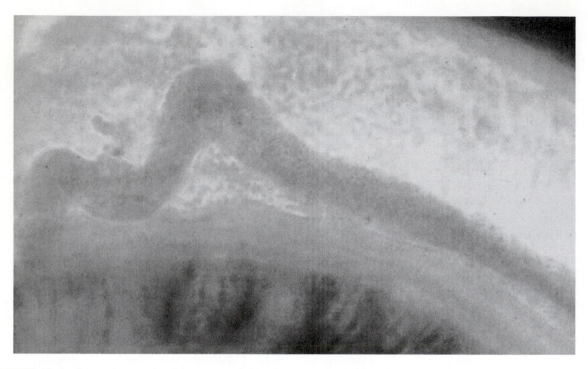

FIGURE 18-6 Photomicrograph of the organ of Corti in an animal that has sustained an acoustic trauma. Note that the organ of Corti has become detached from the basilar membrane and is "corkscrewing" up into the scala media. (Courtesy Barbara Bohne, Ph.D.)

to the ear and subsequent permanent hearing loss of sudden onset. The endolymph and perilymph within the cochlea differ in their ionic concentrations, and they are kept separate by cell barriers, as well as active processes in the normal ear (see Chapter 8 for discussion). If the barriers are broken, the fluids can intermix, which makes a "poison" for the outer and IHCs. The hair cells swell, then rupture and die. They do not regenerate, but are replaced by a layer of scar tissue (squamous epithelial tissue). Figure 18-6 is a photomicrograph of an inner ear that has sustained acoustic trauma.

Figure 18-6 shows an animal subject just after an exposure that produced an acoustic trauma. Note that the organ of Corti has been dislodged from the basilar membrane and is coiling upward in a "corkscrew" fashion. Within a few days after the exposure, all the sensory and supporting cells in this region of the cochlea degenerated, and the region

was covered with a single layer of squamous epithelia. The region of the cochlea most sensitive to acoustic trauma is the basal turn of the cochlea; acoustic trauma rarely, if ever, affects the apical half of the inner ear. The susceptibility of the basal half of the cochlea undoubtedly reflects the transfer characteristics of the outer and middle ear, as well as the spectral spread of the short-duration sounds that are capable of causing trauma.

So what are the characteristics of sounds that make them capable of producing an acoustic trauma? First, the exposure needs to be above a so-called **critical level;** that is, the signal must contain enough energy to stretch the basilar membrane/organ of Corti complex beyond its elastic limits. The critical level varies somewhat among individuals and among species, but in humans, it exceeds 140-dB peak SPL, which is the basis of current and recommended limits imposed by occupational noise regulations (OSHA, 1983; NIOSH, 1998). Second, the exposures are **impulsive,** rather than **continuous.** That is, they are usually of an extremely short duration, on the order of microseconds to just a few milliseconds. Third, the **rise time** of the signal appears to be related to the hazard it creates. One important predictor of the hazard from impulsive exposure is how rapidly the sound pressure increases from ambient to peak levels (Price & Kalb, 1991). Conceptually, the faster the rise time of the acoustic stimulus, the more the "torque" that would be applied to the basilar membrane and the larger its displacement. Sounds with rapid rise times and high peak SPLs are also particularly damaging to the sensory cells of the cochlea because they are too brief to elicit physiologically normal protective functions. For example, an impulsive sound at levels greater than 140-dB peak SPL would definitely elicit the acoustic reflex. But the latency of the reflex, on the order of 25 milliseconds at best, is far too slow to effect any attenuation of a sound passing through the middle ear on its way to the cochlea. Similarly, central inhibitory mechanisms, such as sound-activated inhibition mediated through the efferent olivocochlear system, are simply too slow and cannot protect the cochlea from a single, rapid insult.

What kinds of sounds in the environment are capable of producing acoustic trauma? Practically, the power required for producing overpressures of 140 dB or more limits acoustic trauma to explosive events—the detonation of a firecracker near the ear, for example, or the report of large-caliber firearms. In industry, workers can be exposed to high levels of impact noise, such as sounds produced by hammering on a metal surface, but impact noise exposures seldom reach levels greater than 140-dB peak SPL.

A relatively modern source of impulsive noise is that produced by the rapid deployment of automobile airbags. The rapid expansion of the bag inside a closed vehicle can produce impulsive noises greater than 170-dB peak SPL, and there are reports in the literature documenting acoustic trauma from airbag deployment (Price & Kalb 1999; Yaremchuk, & Dobie, 2001; Chao & Pomerantz, 2004). Airbags designed to protect occupants from crashes to the side of the vehicle, often mounted in the seat or on the headliner of the vehicle, present two additional hazards to the ear. First, they must deploy more quickly than the front airbags because the point of impact is much closer to the passengers in the vehicle, and the shorter rise time increases the risk for acoustic injury. Second, because the bag contacts the side of the head, the bag can "slap" the ear, trapping and compressing a column of air inside the ear canal and rupturing the tympanic membrane.

Because explosions and other impulsive noise events are rare, opportunities to study the pathologic effects of acoustic trauma are limited. Much of what is known comes from studies conducted on military personnel engaged in combat training or from animal subjects. Unfortunately, since the turn of the millennium, there has been an increase in the number of military operations and terrorist attacks worldwide that have included the detonation of explosives. Individuals near the attacks who survive commonly experience blast trauma, which is a severe form of acoustic trauma. For example, Mrena, Paakkonen, Back, Pirvola, and Ylikoski (2004) report the audiometric findings from a group of 29 people who experienced ear trauma after a suicide bomber detonated explosives inside a mall in Finland, killing 7 people and injuring 160. Eight of the patients situated near the site of the detonation had ruptured tympanic membranes, and more than half of the subjects reported hearing loss and tinnitus. Although these extremely intense exposures can cause significant other physical injuries, including pneumothorax and petechial hemorrhages, it is likely that the rupture of the tympanic membrane actually protects the cochlea from further insult, by reducing energy transfer to the footplate of the stapes.

Individuals also can be injured by detonation of firecrackers near the ear, and audiologists and otologists occasionally treat patients after these events. Reported cases in the literature include an infant riding in the backseat of a passing automobile who sustained a profound hearing loss after someone threw a lighted firecracker through the open window (Brookhouser, Worthington, & Kelly, 1992), and particularly Ward and Glorig's (1961) older description of hearing loss in a college student caused by the

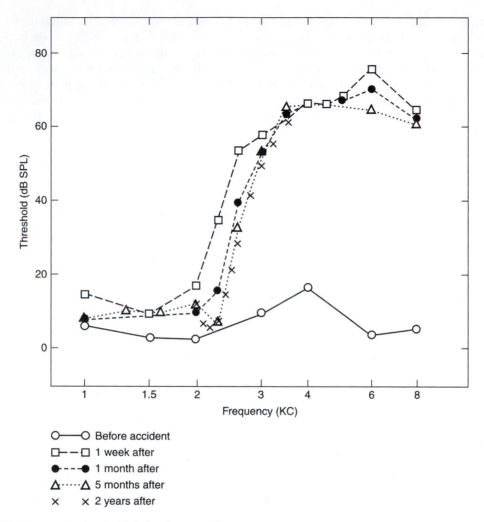

FIGURE 18-7   Permanent threshold shifts after a single exposure to a firecracker 15 inches from the right ear of a college student. KC, Kilocycles per second (kilohertz); SPL, sound pressure level. (Adapted from Ward and Glorig, 1961.)

detonation of a firecracker within about 15 inches of his right ear. Figure 18-7 reproduces a graph depicting the threshold shift experienced by the student described in Ward and Glorig's report.

Before the accident, the student had been participating in a hearing study, and a record of his audiometric thresholds was available. Figure 18-7 shows the student's threshold shifts for frequencies between 1 and 8 kHz. Before the exposure, thresholds were normal across the frequency range tested. Threshold shifts were determined by subtracting the subject's

thresholds before the accident from the measured thresholds. One week after the discharge, thresholds were elevated by 50 to 75 dB at frequencies Greater than 2 kHz. The exposure produced no substantive hearing losses below 2 kHz. Subsequent audiometric tests conducted over a 2-year period after the accident indicated no substantive recovery at any frequency. The pattern of the hearing loss observed in Figure 18-7 provides a helpful reminder to the audiologist of the principal characteristics of acoustic trauma.

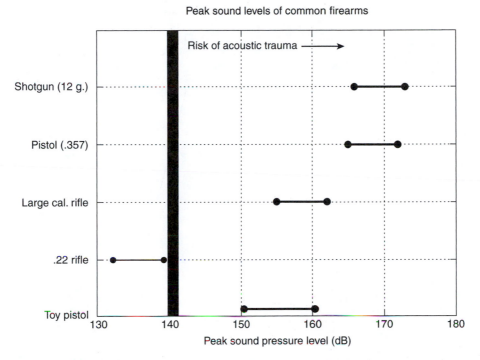

FIGURE 18-8 Peak sound pressure levels of firearms, measured at the ear of the shooter. (Adapted from Odess, 1973; personal measures by the author.)

First, the exposure must exceed a peak SPL of 140 dB. Although measures of the exposure to the college student were not included in Ward and Glorig's (1961) report, it can be estimated using the tools provided in Chapter 2. Firecrackers have been reported to produce peak SPLs in excess of 160 dB at a distance of 2 meters (Smoorenburg, 1993). To estimate the exposure at 15 inches, one can invoke the inverse square law, which leads to the conclusion that the student was exposed to a level that exceeded 175-dB peak SPL.

Second, even though the energy in the exposure was spread across a large frequency spectrum because of its short duration, the hearing loss was limited to the high frequencies, above 2.0 kHz. Like most hearing losses caused by noise exposure, this student's audiogram displayed a sloping high-frequency loss, with a characteristic "notch" pattern, meaning that the threshold at 8 kHz was better than the threshold at 6 kHz. Also note the abrupt slope

of the loss, that is, the steepness of the threshold shift between 2.0 and 4.0 kHz.

Third, unlike hearing losses caused by exposure to continuous noise at lower levels, the injury is instantaneous and permanent. Recovery of hearing after the incident rarely occurs.

Impulsive Noise from Hunting and Target Shooting

If explosions are so rare in the workplace or in the real world, why should the audiologist even care about acoustic trauma? The answer is that there is another source of impulsive noise that creates a risk for millions of people in the United States. That source is the noise associated with the sports of hunting and target shooting. Figure 18-8 presents a chart of reported peak SPLs produced by commonly used firearms, measured at the ear of the shooter.

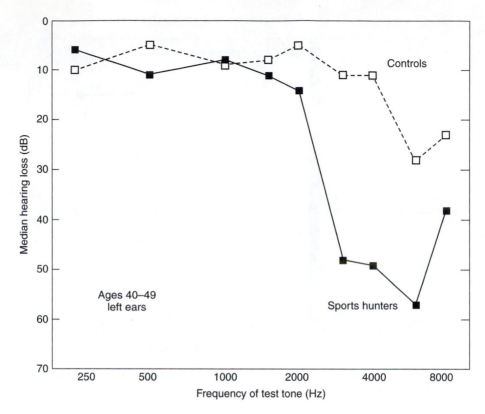

FIGURE 18-9 Median hearing loss in frequent sports shooters and age-matched control subjects. (Adapted from Taylor and Williams, 1966.)

Of these common firearms, only the smaller caliber .22 rifles did not exceed 140-dB peak SPL. Large-caliber rifles, shotguns, and pistols all produce peak exposures that can exceed 170-dB peak SPL. It should not be surprising that clinical reports documenting hearing loss after exposure to shooting can be found in the literature dating back to the 1800s (Toynbee, 1860). Although a review of the individual studies is beyond the scope of this chapter, several general features of acoustic trauma should be kept in mind during the audiometric examination of a patient. Following are several key points about acoustic trauma from sport shooting:

1. Firearms can cause acoustic trauma. Most firearms produce impulsive levels to the unprotected ear that exceed safe levels of exposure to

impulse noise (Clark, 1992; Odess, 1973). In a study of hearing loss caused by shooting, Johnson and Riffle (1982) found worse hearing in male shooters versus nonshooters, but no differences for female subjects. They attributed the difference to that female shooters typically shot guns of small caliber, whereas male shooters tended to use larger caliber firearms. One early study of hearing levels of age- and sex-matched shooters and control subjects (Taylor & Williams, 1966) compared the hearing levels of 103 sports hunters with 21 physicians who were not exposed to shooting noise. For all age-groups, sports hunters were found to have significantly worse hearing than the control group for all frequencies from 3 to 8 kHz; in addition, hearing levels in the left ear were significantly worse than the right ear. Figure

18-9 shows the median hearing levels for the left ears of the 40- to 49-year-olds hunters and control subjects. Although both groups show a "notch" in the audiogram at 6.0 kHz, the mean hearing levels of the shooters at 3, 4, and 6 kHz were about 35 dB worse than the control subjects.

2. Virtually all studies of hearing losses in groups of shooters show an asymmetric pattern of hearing loss, with the thresholds for the ear contralateral to the firearm poorer than the ipsilateral ear by about 15 dB for high-frequency (3–8 kHz) stimuli and up to 30 dB for frequent shooters. This is because the head creates an acoustic shadow to the ear closest to the gun; a shooter firing a rifle from the right shoulder will tip his head to the right sighting the gun, exposing the left ear more prominently to the source of noise, which comes from the end of the barrel.

3. Many of your patients have a shooting history. Surveys of hunting and target shooting among industrial workers indicate that at least 50% of male workers occasionally engage in shooting activities (see Clark, 1991b, for review). A cross-sectional cohort study of recreational firearm use in the residents of Beaver Dam, Wisconsin (Nondahl, Cruickshanks, Wiley, Klein, Klein, & Tweed, 2000), found a positive history for hunting and target shooting in 75% of the male and 11% of the female residents. These numbers are consistent with reports indicating that more than 70 million Americans own more than 258 million guns (National Research Council, 2005). The National Research Council figures include only the "reported" ownership statistics; the actual number may be far higher.

4. Workers in noisy industries who engage in sport shooting may develop additional hearing losses caused by gunfire noise over whatever loss they may sustain because of occupational exposures.

↝ SUMMARY ↜

Exposure to excessive noise at work or during recreational activities is a major cause of NIHL in the United States. Exposures at low levels or for relatively brief periods cause only temporary hearing losses. These losses, often accompanied by symptoms of fullness, tinnitus, or muffled speech sounds, recover completely within minutes or hours. At greater levels, and for much longer periods, noise can cause permanent hearing losses. These losses begin in the 4-kHz region, and with continued exposure, they grow over approximately the first decade, then stabilize. Although noise does not cause complete deafness, it can and does contribute significantly to the hearing problems of people in the United States as they age and sustain additional losses because of presbycusis.

Particularly hazardous are exposures to extremely intense sounds, such as the report of a large-caliber firearm, which can cause acoustic trauma. Millions of people in the United States who own and shoot guns are at risk for acoustic trauma, unless they take steps to protect their ears during shooting activities.

The good news is that NIHL is entirely preventable by avoiding excessive exposure to hazardous noise when possible and wearing hearing protection when necessary. Counseling patients who may be at risk for NIHL is a key responsibility of the audiologist, and this chapter was developed to provide useful tools to accomplish that goal.

❧KEY TERMS❧

Audiometric notch
(4-kHz notch)
Acoustic trauma
Asymptotic threshold
shift (ATS)
Battery

Continuous noise
Critical level
Impulsive noise
NIPTS (noise-induced
permanent thresh-
old shifts)

Permanent threshold
shift (PTS)
Rise time
Stria vascularis

Temporary threshold
shift (TTS)
Threshold shift

❧STUDY QUESTIONS❧

1. Why isn't more known about permanent hearing loss in humans?

2. Identify three regions of the cochlea that are vulnerable to excessive noise exposure.

3. How does acoustic trauma differ from NIHL?

4. How are studies of NIHL and the field of audiology related?

5. Is hearing loss caused by shooting a more important problem in the United States than occupational noise exposure or presbycusis? Explain your answer.

❧REFERENCES❧

American Academy of Otolaryngology-Head and Neck Surgery Foundation. (1998). *Evaluation of people reporting hearing loss.* Subcommittee on the Medical Aspects of Noise, American Academy of Otolaryngology-Head and Neck Surgery Foundation, Alexandria, VA.

American College of Occupational and Environmental Medicine. (2003). Noise-induced hearing loss. *Journal of Occupational and Environmental Medicine, 45,* 579–581.

American National Standards Institute, Inc. [ANSI]. (1996). *American National Standard: Determination of occupational noise exposure and estimation of noise-induced hearing impairment* (ANSI S3.44-1996). New York: American National Standards Institute, Inc.

Axelsson, A. (1996). Recreational exposure to noise and its effects. *Noise Control Engineering Journal, 44*(3), 127–134.

Bies, D. A. (1996). The half-octave temporary threshold shift. *Journal of the Acoustical Society of America, 100*(4), 2786.

Bohne, B. A., & Clark, W. W. (1982). Growth of hearing loss and cochlear lesion with increasing duration of noise exposure. In R. P. Hammernik, D. Henderson, & R. Salvi (Eds.), *New perspectives on noise-induced hearing loss* (pp. 283–302). New York: Raven Press.

Bohne, B. A., Clark, W. W., & Harding, G. (1994). *Hearing loss and cochlear damage after a working lifetime of noise.* Abstracts of the 17th Midwinter Meeting of the Association for Research in Otolaryngology. St. Petersburg Beach, FL, February 8–14, 1994.

Bohne, B. A., & Rabbitt, K. D. (1983). Holes in the reticular lamina after noise exposure: Implications for continued damage in the organ of Corti. *Hearing Research, 11,* 41–53.

Brookhouser, P. E., Worthington, D. W., & Kelly, W. J. (1992). Noise-induced hearing-loss in children. *Laryngoscope, 102*(6), 645–655.

Burns, W., & Robinson, D. W. (1970). *Hearing and noise in industry.* London: Her Majesty's Stationary Office.

Chao, N., & Pomerantz, W. J. (2004). Acute hearing loss after airbag deployment. *Pediatric Emergency Care, 20,* 683–686.

Clark, W. W. (1991a). Recent studies of temporary threshold shift (TTS) and permanent threshold shift (PTS) in animals. *Journal of the American Acoustical Society of America, 90,* 155–163.

Clark, W. W. (1991b). Noise exposure and hearing loss from leisure-time activities: A review. *The Journal of the Acoustical Society of America, 90,* 175–181.

Clark, W. W. (1992). Hearing: The effects of noise. *Otolaryngology-Head and Neck Surgery, 106,* 669–676.

Clark, W. W., & Bohne B. A. (1999). Effects of noise on hearing. *Journal of the American Medical Association, 281,* 1658–1659.

Corti, A. (1851). Recherches sur l'orane de Corti de l'ouie des mammiferes. *Zeitschrift für Wissenschartliche Zoologie, 3,* 100–106.

Davis, H. (1983). An active process in cochlear mechanics. *Hearing Research, 9,* 79–90.

Davis, H. (1991). *The professional memoirs of Hallowell Davis.* St. Louis, MO: Central Institute for the Deaf.

Davis, H., Morgan, C. T., Hawkins, J. E., Jr., Galambos, R., & Smith, F. W. (1950). Temporary deafness following exposure to loud tones and noise. *Acta Oto-Laryngologica Supplement, 88,* 1–57.

Fligor, B., & Cox, L. (2004). Output levels of commercially available portable compact disc players and the potential risk to hearing. *Ear & Hearing, 25*(6), 513–527.

Franco, G. (1999). Ramazzini and workers' health. *Lancet, 354,* 858–861.

Fridberger, A., Zheng, J., Parthasarathi, A., Ren, T., & Nuttall, A. (2002). Loud sound-induced changes in cochlear mechanics. *Journal of Neurophysiology, 88,* 2341–2347.

Habermann, J. (1890). Uber die Schwerhorigkeit der Kesselschmiede. *Arch Ohrenheilk 30,* 1–25.

Hawkins, J. E., Jr. (1971). The role of vasoconstriction in noise-induced hearing loss. *Annals of Otology, Rhinology, and Otolaryngology, 80,* 903–913.

Hawkins, J. E., & Schacht, J. (2005). Sketches of otohistory Part 10: Noise-induced hearing loss. *Audiology Neurotology, 10,* 305–309.

Helmholtz, H., von. (1863). *Die Lehre von den Tonempfundungen: als physiologische Grundlage fur die Theorie der Musik.* Friedrich Vieweg & Sohn.

Henderson, D., Bielefeld, E., Harris, K., & Hu, B. (2006). The role of oxidative stress in nose-induced hearing loss. *Ear & Hearing, 27,* 1–19.

Henderson, D., Hu, B., Bielefeld, E., & Nicotera, T. (2007). Cellular mechanisms of noise-induced hearing loss. In K. Campbell (Ed.), *Pharmacology and ototoxicity for audiologists* (pp. 216–229). Clifton Park, NY: Thomson Delmar Learning.

Hirose, K., & Liberman, M. C. (2003). Lateral wall histopathology and endocochlear potential in the noise-damaged mouse cochlea. *Journal of the Association for Research in Otolaryngology, 4,* 339–352.

Johnson, D. L, & Riffle, C. (1982). Effects of gunfire on hearing level for selected individuals of the Inter-Industry Noise Study. *Journal of the Acoustical Society of America, 72,* 1311–1314.

Katz, J. (2002). Clinical audiology. In J. Katz (Ed.), *Handbook of clinical audiology* (5th ed., pp. 4–5). Philadelphia: Lippincott Williams & Wilkins.

Kemp, D. T. (1978). Stimulated acoustic emissions from within the human auditory system. *Journal of the Acoustical Society of America, 64,* 1386–1391.

Lempert, B. L., & Henderson, T. L. (1973). *Occupational noise and hearing 1968 to 1972: A NIOSH study.* Cincinnati, OH: U.S. Department of Health, Education, and Welfare, Public Health Service, Center for Disease Control, National Institute for Occupational Safety and Health, Division of Laboratories and Criteria Development.

Marshall, A., & Heller, L. M. (1998). Transient-evoked otoacoustic emissions as a measure of noise-induced threshold shift. *Journal of Speech Language and Hearing Research, 41*(6), 1319–1334.

McBride, D. I., & Williams, S. (2001). Audiometric notch as a sign of noise induced hearing loss. *Occupational and Environmental Medicine, 58,* 46–51.

Miller, J. A. L., Marshall, L., Heller, L. M., & Hughes, L. M. (2006). Low-level otoacoustic emissions may predict susceptibility to noise-induced hearing loss. *Journal of the Acoustical Society of America, 120*(1), 280–296.

Miller, J. D. (1974). Effects of noise on people. *Journal of the Acoustical Society of America, 56*(3), 729–764.

Mrena, R., Paakkonen, R., Back, L., Pirvola, U., & Ylikoski, J. (2004). Otologic consequences of blast exposure: A Finnish case study of a shopping mall bomb explosion. *Acta Oto-Laryngologica, 124*(8), 946–952.

National Research Council. (2005). *Firearms and violence: A critical review.* Washington, DC: National Academies Press.

National Institute for Occupational Safety and Health [NIOSH]. (1998). *Criteria for a recommended standard. Occupational exposure to noise. Revised criteria.* U. S. (DHHS Publication No. 98-126). Cincinnati, OH: NIOSH.

Nondahl, D. M., Cruickshanks, K. J., Wiley, T. L., Klein, R., Klein, B. E. K., & Tweed, T. S. (2000). *Archives of Family Medicine, 9,* 352–357.

Nordmann, A. S., Bohne, B. A., & Harding, G. W. (2000). Histopathological differences between temporary and permanent threshold shift. *Hearing Research, 139,* 13–30.

Occupational Safety and Health Administration [OSHA]. (1983). *Occupational noise exposure: Hearing conservation amendment; final rule.* Occupational Safety and Health Administration, 29 C.F.R. 1910.95; 48 Fed. Reg. 9738-9785.

Odess, J. S. (1973). Acoustic trauma of sportsman hunter due to gun firing. *Laryngoscope, 82,* 1971–1989.

Passchier-Vermeer, W. (1968). *Hearing loss due to exposure to steady-state broadband noise* (Report No. 35 and Supplement to Report No. 35). Bilthoven, The Netherlands: Institute for Public Health Engineering.

Patuzzi, R. (1998). Exponential onset and recovery of temporary threshold shift after loud sound: Evidence for long-term inactivation of mechano-electrical transduction channels. *Hearing Research, 125,* 17–38.

Patuzzi, R. (2002). Non-linear aspects of outer hair cell transduction and the temporary threshold shifts after acoustic trauma. *Audiology and Neuro-Otology, 7*(1), 17–20.

Price, G. R., & Kalb, J. T. (1999). Auditory hazard from airbag noise exposure. *Journal of the Acoustical Society of America, 106,* 2629–2637.

Prince, M. M. (2002). Distribution of risk factors for hearing loss: Implications for evaluating risk of occupational noise-induced hearing loss. *Journal of Acoustical Society of America, 112,* 557–567.

Prince, M. M., Gilbert, S. J., Smith, R. J., & Stayner, L. T. (2003). Evaluation of the risk of noise-induced hearing loss among unscreened male industrial workers. *Journal of the Acoustical Society of America, 113*(2), 871–880.

Prince, M. M., Stayner, L. T., Smith, R. J., & Gilbert, S. J. (1997). A reexamination of risk estimates from the NIOSH Occupational Noise and Hearing Survey (ONHS). *Journal of the Acoustical Society of America, 101,* 950–963.

Puel, J. L., D'aldin, C. G., Saffiende S., Eybalin, M., & Pujol, R. (1996). Excitotoxicity and plasticity of IHC-auditory nerve contributes to both temporary and permanent threshold shift. In A. Axelsson, H. M. Borchgrevink, R. P. Hamernik, P.-A. Hellstrom, D. Henderson, & R. J. Salvi (Eds.). *Scientific basis of noise-induced hearing loss* (pp. 36–42). New York: Thieme.

Quaranta, A., Portalini, P., & Henderson, D. (1998). Temporary and permanent threshold shift: An overview. *Scandinavian Audiology, 27*(Suppl 48), 75–86.

Ramazzini, B. (1700). *De morbis artifactum.* In W. C. Wright (Trans.), *Arch-lycei moderatoribus, mutinae* (p. 437). New York: Hafner Pub. Co., 1964.

Ruggero, M. A., Rich, N. C., & Recio A. (1996). The effect of intense acoustic stimulation on basilar-membrane vibrations. *Auditory Neuroscience, 2,* 329–345.

Shera, C. A. (2004). Mechanisms of mammalian otoacoustic emission and their implications for the clinical utility of otoacoustic emissions. *Ear & Hearing, 25*(2), 86–97.

Smoorenburg, G. F. (1993). Risk of noise-induced hearing-loss following exposure to Chinese Firecrackers. *Audiology, 32*(6), 333–343.

Taylor, G. D., & Williams, E. (1966). Acoustic trauma in the sports hunter. *The Laryngoscope, 76,* 863–879.

Taylor, W., Pearson, J., Mair, A. & Burns, W. (1965). Study of noise and hearing in jute weaving. *Journal of the Acoustical Society of America, 38,* 113–120.

Toynbee, J. (1860). *The diseases of the ear: their nature, diagnosis, and treatment.* London: John Churchill.

Tsuprun, V., Schachern, P. A., Cureoglu, S., & Paparella, M. (2003). Structure of the stereocilia side links and morphology of auditory hair bundle in relation to noise exposure in the chinchilla. *Journal of Neurocytology, 32,* 1117–1128.

United States Air Force. (1956). *Hazardous noise exposure.* Washington, DC: U.S. Air Force, Office of the Surgeon General, AF Regulation 160-3.

Ward, W. D., & Glorig, A. (1961). A case of firecracker-induced hearing loss. *Laryngoscope, 71,* 1590–1596.

Wang, Y., Hirose, K., & Liberman, M. C. (2002). Dynamics of noise-induced cellular injury and repair in the mouse cochlea. *Journal of the Association for Research in Otolaryngology, 3,* 248–268.

Yaremchuk, K., & Dobie, R. A. (2001). Otologic injuries from airbag deployment. *Otolaryngology-Head and Neck Surgery, 125*(3), 130–134.

Zurek, P. M., Clark, W. W., & Kim, D. O. (1982). The behavior of acoustic distortion products in the ear canals of chinchillas with normal or damaged cochleas. *Journal of the Acoustical Society of America, 72,* 774–781.

↵SUGGESTED READING ↝

Ahroon, W. A., & Hamernik, R. P. (1999). Noise-induced hearing loss in the noise-toughened auditory system. *Hearing Research, 129,* 101–110.

Attias, J., Sapir, S., Bresloff, I., Reshef-Haran, I., & Ising, H. (2004). Reduction in noise-induced temporary threshold shift in humans following oral magnesium intake. *Clinical Otolaryngology, 29,* 635–641.

Borg, E., & Engstrom, B. (1989). Noise level, inner hair cell damage, audiometric features, and equal-energy hypothesis. *Journal of the Acoustical Society of America, 85,* 1776–1782.

Brink, L. L., Talbott, E. O., Burks, J. A., & Palmer, C. V. (2002). Changes over time in audiometric thresholds in a group of automobile stamping and assembly workers with a hearing conservation program. *American Industrial Hygiene Association, 63,* 482–487.

Canlon, B., Fransson, A., & Viberg, A. (1999). Medial olivocochlear efferent terminals are protected by sound conditioning. *Brain Research, 850,* 253–260.

Chan, P. C., Ho, K. H., Kan, K. K., Stuhmiller, J. H., & Mayorga, M. A. (2001). Evaluation of impulse noise criteria using human volunteer data. *Journal of the Acoustical Society of America, 110,* 1967–1975.

Cho, Y., Gong, T. W., Kanicki, A, Altschuler, R. A., & Lomax, M. I. (2004). Noise overstimulation induces immediate early genes in the rat cochlea. *Molecular Brain Research, 130,* 134–148.

Cruickshanks, K. J., Klein, R., Klein, B. E. K., Wiley, T. L., Nondahl, D. M., & Tweed, T. S. (1998). Cigarette smoking and hearing loss: The Epidemiology of Hearing Loss Study. *Journal of the American Medical Association, 279,* 1715–1719.

Eddins, A. C., Zuskov, M., & Salvi, R. (1999). Changes in distortion product otoacoustic emissions during prolonged noise exposure. *Hearing Research, 127,* 119–128.

Gratton, M. A., Smyth, B. J., Schulte, B. A., & Vincent, D. A., Jr. (1995). Na, K-ATPase activity decreases in the cochlear lateral wall of quiet-aged gerbils. *Hearing Research, 83,* 43–50.

Hamernik, R. P., & Ahroon, W. A. (1988). Threshold recovery functions following impulse noise trauma. *Journal of the Acoustical Society of America, 84,* 941–950.

Hamernik, R. P., Ahroon, W. A., Jock, B. M., & Bennett, J. A. (1998). Noise-induced threshold shift dynamics measured with distortion-product otoacoustic emissions and auditory evoked potentials in chinchillas with inner hair cell deficient cochleas. *Hearing Research, 118,* 73–82.

Heinrich, U.-R., & Feltens, R. (2006). Mechanisms underlying noise-induced hearing loss. *Drug Discovery Today: Disease Mechanisms, 3,* 131–135.

Le Prell, C. G., Yagi, M., Kawamoto, K., Beyer, L. A., Atkin, G., Raphael, Y., et al. (2004). Chronic excitotoxicity in the guinea pig cochlea induces temporary functional deficits without disrupting otoacoustic emissions. *Journal of the Acoustical Society of America, 116*(2), 1044–1056.

Van Laer, L., Carlsson, P., Ottschytsch, N., Bondeson, M. L., Konings, A., Vandevelde, A., et al. The contribution of genes involved in potassium-recycling in the inner ear to noise-induced hearing loss. *Human Mutation, 27*(8), 786–795.

Chapter

19

Ototoxin-Induced Hearing Loss

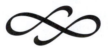

Leonard P. Rybak, M.D., Ph.D.
Professor of Surgery, Division of Otolaryngology
Southern Illinois University School of Medicine
Springfield, Illinois

Ototoxicity is the capacity of a drug or chemical agent to cause damage to the structure or function of the inner ear. These compounds may affect hearing, balance, or a combination of both. Many agents can cause ototoxicity. This chapter deals with some of the more common drugs that can cause hearing loss and injury to the cochlea. These drugs include the **aminoglycoside antibiotics,** the anticancer drugs (cisplatin and carboplatin), salicylates, quinine, and the erythromycins. The effects on the cochlea and vestibular portions of the inner ear observed in animals including proposed mechanisms are described and compared with the adverse actions in humans.

AMINOGLYCOSIDE ANTIBIOTICS

The aminoglycoside antibiotics are important drugs that were developed to fight tuberculosis and other bacterial infections. The first drugs of this class were streptomycin and dihydrostreptomycin. During the initial clinical evaluation of these drugs, it was discovered that they could damage the kidneys and the inner ear. Since that time, a number of new aminoglycosides have been developed. Dihydrostreptomycin was taken off the market. Other members of this group of antibiotics include neomycin, kanamycin, gentamicin, tobramycin, amikacin, netilmicin, and sisomicin. Neomycin, amikacin, and kanamycin appear to be more toxic to the cochlea than to the vestibular system. Streptomycin and gentamicin appear to selectively damage the vestibular system, although hearing loss can occur. The most severe organ toxicity caused by these agents targets the kidney. The toxic effects of these agents on the kidney and the inner ear tend to occur with chronic treatment. Ototoxicity tends to become apparent only after days or weeks of treatment. The overall incidence of aminoglycoside cochleotoxicity is estimated to be about 20%, whereas vestibulotoxicity may occur in 15% of patients treated (Forge & Schacht, 2000).

Animal Studies

The pathology of aminoglycoside ototoxicity appears to be well represented in animal studies. Both in animal and in human temporal bone histopathologic studies, the cochlear or the vestibular hair cells, or both, serve as the primary targets for aminoglycoside injury. In the organ of Corti, the outer hair cells in the basal turn of the cochlea are the first to be damaged (Figure 19-1).

Inner hair cells appear to be more resistant than outer hair cells. The reason for this difference could lie in the differential concentration of the reducing compound, **glutathione,** in the cells of the cochlea. Animal studies have shown that the outer hair cells of the basal turn contain the lowest concentration of this compound (Sha, Taylor, Forge, & Schacht, 2001).

Experimental animals may show depression of the cochlear microphonic potential and increased compound action potential thresholds after aminoglycoside administration (see Chapters 10 and 11). Otoacoustic emissions (OAEs) can be used for non-invasive monitoring of ototoxicity of aminoglycosides in animals or in humans (see Chapter 13). The stria vascularis may become thinner because of losses of marginal cells (Hawkins, 1973). These late effects of aminoglycosides may contribute to the overall clinical manifestation of ototoxicity (Forge & Schacht, 2000). The mechanisms of ototoxicity of aminoglycosides appear to be the following scheme, developed from animal studies. The aminoglycoside combines with iron in the hair cell to form a complex. This complex activates oxygen to make extremely reactive molecules called **free radicals.** These reactive forms of oxygen (also called reactive oxygen species or ROS) can then react with various molecules in the cell to damage the membrane and other cellular components. This can indirectly trigger a process of programmed cell death (Forge & Schacht, 2000). In experimental animals, the administration of drugs that chelate with iron may prevent the formation of the aminoglycoside-iron complex. Antioxidant molecules can also protect

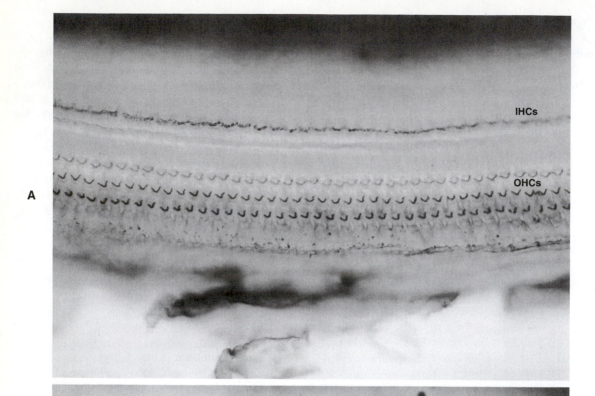

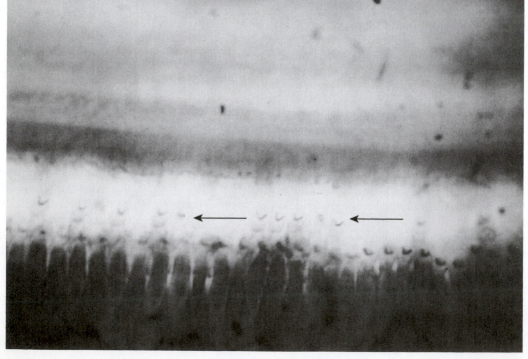

against aminoglycoside ototoxicity, and thus prevent damage by reactive oxygen species. Recent studies have also demonstrated that salicylate attenuated gentamicin-induced hearing loss in guinea pigs (Sha & Schacht, 1999). Salicylate is both a **scavenger** of free radicals and an iron chelator. This means it could protect against gentamicin ototoxicity by inactivating ROS, or by binding free iron, thus slowing the generation of ROS. It will be interesting to see whether large-scale clinical trials confirm the protective effect of salicylates such as aspirin against the ototoxic effects of aminoglycosides.

Clinical Studies

As the drug treatment is prolonged, the damage may spread to the more apical regions. This pattern is reflected in the audiometric findings (Figure 19-2), in which the high frequencies are the first to be affected in the patient (Fausti, Rappaport, Schecter, Frey, War, & Brummett, 1984).

Progressive destruction of spiral ganglion cells has been described in animal studies, as well as in human temporal bone histopathology reports (Johnsson, Hawkins, Kingsley, Black, & Matz, 1981). A recent study of human temporal bones removed from patients with aminoglycoside ototoxicity demonstrated that, in some patients, the spiral ganglion cells can be injured directly by aminoglycoside antibiotics. Some segments of the cochlea had normal-appearing hair cells accompanied by reduction in the spiral ganglion cell numbers. Thus, in some cases, the hearing loss may result from degeneration of either the spiral ganglion cells or the hair cells (Hinojosa, Nelson, Lerner, Redleaf, & Schramm, 2001). As mentioned earlier, the high-frequency hearing loss occurs first. High-frequency audiometry may detect hearing loss before it becomes clinically detectable (Fausti et al., 1984). Later, hearing loss may progress to lower frequencies to include the impor-

tant speech range, resulting in a permanent loss of communication ability. A hearing loss of 20 dB at two or more adjacent test frequencies should be documented to accept the diagnosis of drug-induced hearing loss, after excluding other causes.

Changes in the level of distortion product otoacoustic emissions may precede changes in other physiologic measures of cochlear function (Brown, McDowell, & Forge, 1989) (see Chapter 13). OAEs have been used clinically to monitor auditory function in patients with cystic fibrosis being treated chronically with aminoglycoside antibiotics for pulmonary infections. A recent publication contends that evoked OAEs are a sensitive and reliable indicator of subtle inner ear dysfunction and are more sensitive than pure-tone audiometry for monitoring cochlear function of patients with cystic fibrosis during treatment with aminoglycosides (Stavroulaki et al., 2002). Distortion product OAEs seem preferable to transiently evoked OAEs because they can be measured over a broader frequency range with more sensitive frequency-specific responses.

Monitoring of serum levels of aminoglycosides is a routine clinical practice. Blood levels are drawn at the time of peak and **trough** concentration. An association has been made between mean trough levels of aminoglycosides and ototoxicity (Lerner et al., 1981). These levels are measured just before the next dose of aminoglycoside injection.

Various risk factors have been investigated to determine whether they contribute to a greater incidence of ototoxicity in patients being treated with aminoglycosides. Bacteria in the bloodstream, fever, and liver and kidney dysfunction have been reported to be significant risk factors associated with ototoxicity in patients treated with aminoglycosides in prospective, double-blind clinical trials of gentamicin, tobramycin, and amikacin (Moore, Smith, & Lietman, 1984). Combined administration of two

FIGURE 19-1 Surface preparations of the basal turn of the chinchilla cochlea, showing pathologic lesions caused by kanamycin. (A) Normal cochlea shows intact stereocilia on the single row of inner hair cells (IHCs) and the three rows of V-shaped outer hair cells (OHCs). (B) Kanamycin-treated cochlea shows extensive destruction of outer hair cells. Only occasional remaining V-shaped stereocilia can be seen (arrows).

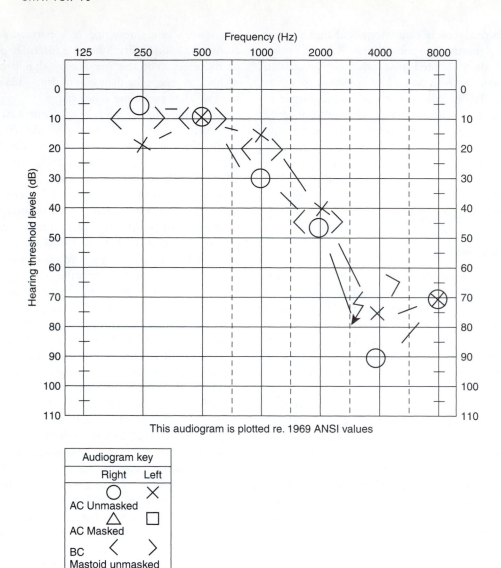

FIGURE 19-2 Audiogram obtained from a patient with gentamicin ototoxicity. Note the symmetric, severe, high-frequency sensorineural hearing loss.

ototoxic drugs may result in enhanced ototoxicity. For example, ethacrynic acid, a **loop diuretic,** was found to enhance the ototoxicity of aminoglycosides in patients with **uremia** (Mathog & Klein, 1969). These findings have been confirmed in ani-mal studies (West, Brummett, & Hines, 1973). A mutation of the mitochondrial RNA may result in a dramatic increase in the sensitivity of patients to even a single dose of aminoglycoside antibiotic. This mutation follows a maternal inheritance pattern

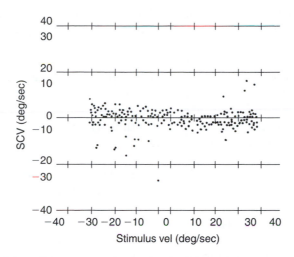

Test: VOR
Stim: 0.05 Hz sinusoidal
30.00 deg/sec

	Gain	Mean	Stdev
Lft:	0.02	0.52	3.29
Rht:	0.00	0.09	6.27

FIGURE 19-3 Vestibulo-ocular reflex response obtained with rotational chair testing in a patient who experienced severe gentamicin vestibular ototoxicity. This patient has severe bilateral vestibular loss, as indicated by the minimal gains and negligible slow component velocity (SCV) of nystagmus with rotations regardless of the velocity of the stimulus.

and has been described in Chinese, Arab-Israeli, Japanese, and North American families (Prezant et al., 1993). It has been stated that 17% of patients with aminoglycoside-induced hearing loss may have this mutation (Forge & Schacht, 2000). For some unknown reason, only cochlear sensitivity to aminoglycoside ototoxicity is seen in these patients, but no enhancement of vestibular ototoxicity has been seen (Forge & Schacht, 2000).

Vestibular Toxicity of Aminoglycosides

Animal studies of the vestibular system show that the hair cell damage begins in the apex of the cristae and in the striolar regions of the maculae (Lindemann, 1969) (see Chapter 16). Hair cell loss then extends to the periphery of the vestibular sensory epithelium, where the type I hair cells are first affected (Wersall, Lundquist, & Bjorkroth, 1969). Vestibular injury from aminoglycosides may be manifested in the patient by severe unsteadiness.

This becomes worse in an environment with reduced visual cues, such as in the dark. Vestibular testing can be difficult to perform in critically ill patients. **Caloric tests** primarily help to demonstrate unilateral vestibular damage, although with severe vestibular toxicity, there may be a reduced caloric response bilaterally. **Rotational chair testing** (Figure 19-3) and **dynamic posturography** may not be universally available. In recent years, gentamicin has been used to intentionally ablate vestibular function in patients with Ménière's disease.

ANTINEOPLASTIC AGENTS
Cisplatin

Cisplatin is a potent anticancer agent that is used to treat a variety of malignant tumors. These tumors include: cancers of the ovary, testes, and bladder; certain lung tumors, and squamous cell carcinomas of the head and neck. Severe side effects tend to limit the ability to adequately treat some patients.

Such unwanted effects include nausea and vomiting, **neurotoxicity,** damage to the kidneys, and hearing loss.

Experimental Studies in Animals   Animal studies have demonstrated that the outer hair cells of the basal turn of the cochlea are the most vulnerable to injury after cisplatin administration (Figure 19-4). The stria vascularis is also susceptible to injury, particularly after high-dose cisplatin treatment (Meech, Campbell, Hughes, & Rybak, 1998). The exact cellular mechanisms of cisplatin ototoxicity are not completely defined. However, the injury to the cells of the inner ear may be related to the production of reactive oxygen molecules in the inner ear by cisplatin (Rybak, Husain, Morris, Whitworth, & Somani, 2000). In tissue culture of rat organ of Corti, reactive oxygen molecules have been demonstrated after exposure to cisplatin (Kopke et al., 1997). These reactive molecules may then trigger the death of outer hair cells by activating enzymes that kill the cells (Deravajan et al., 2002). The outer hair cells of the basal turn of the cochlea may be more vulnerable because they contain a smaller concentration of the antioxidant molecule glutathione, which would otherwise protect the cells against injury by reactive oxygen molecules (Sha & Schacht, 2001).

Clinical Studies   Although the **nephrotoxicity** can be reduced by hydration and other treatments, less success has been reported in prevention of hearing loss. Children appear to be more susceptible to hearing loss than adults (McHaney, Thibadoux, Hayes, & Green, 1983). Hearing loss tends to be permanent and affects both ears symmetrically. The hearing loss incidence is highly variable and appears to be related to dose, age of the patient, and other

factors, such as noise exposure (Bokemeyer et al., 1998). Although the high frequencies are typically affected first, hearing impairment may extend into the middle-frequency range when doses in excess of 100 mg/M^2 are used. When ultrahigh-frequency audiometric testing is used, as many as 100% of patients receiving high-dose cisplatin (150–225 mg/M^2) may demonstrate some degree of hearing loss. Ototoxic reactions appear to be more likely in patients with low serum **albumin** and those with **anemia** (Kopelman et al., 1988).

In children undergoing chemotherapy with cisplatin, screening tests using OAEs were reported to show good correlation with pure-tone audiometry in the presence of normal middle ears. In this group, 90% experienced sensorineural hearing loss at 8 kHz. Increased risk for hearing loss was correlated inversely with age at first treatment with cisplatin and was directly related to the number of cycles and the cumulative dose of cisplatin given to these children (Allen, Tiu, Koike, Ritchey, Kurs-Lasky, & Wax, 1998). The ototoxicity of cisplatin is reportedly enhanced by **cranial** irradiation (Granowetter, Rosenstock, & Packer, 1983).

Other risk factors have been identified in a group of patients with testicular cancer. Permanent ototoxicity was identified in 20% of patients treated with a standard dose of cisplatin. However, a history of previous noise exposure tripled the probability of hearing loss. More than half of those who received higher doses of cisplatin (>400 mg/M^2) experienced permanent loss of hearing. In this study, risk factors for cisplatin hearing loss included: (1) high cumulative dose of cisplatin; (2) history of noise exposure; (3) high dose of vincristine, which by itself causes reversible hearing loss (Bokemeyer et al., 1998).

Symptoms that may alert the health care professional to the possibility of hearing loss in patients

FIGURE 19-4   Scanning electron micrographs of the surface of the organ of Corti from the basal turn of the rat cochlea. (A) Normal rat cochlea shows intact W-shaped stereocilia on the three rows of outer hair cells and a linear array of stereocilia on the single row of inner hair cells. (B) Cochlea of a rat with severe cisplatin ototoxicity. The stereocilia of the inner hair cells are well preserved, but most of the outer hair cells are destroyed. Only a few remaining hair cells with intact stereocilia remain. The clear region between inner and outer hair cells is occupied by heads of pillar cells.

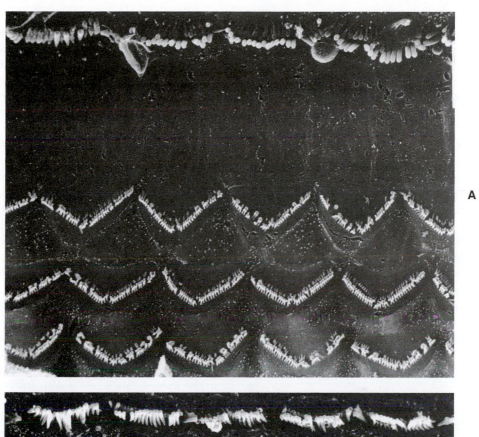

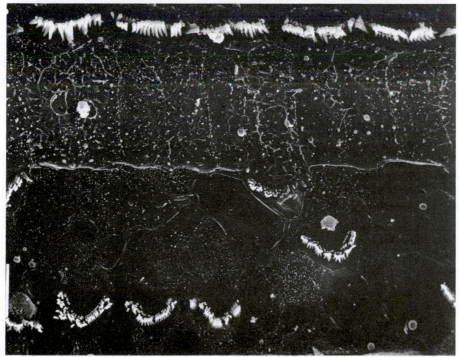

receiving cisplatin include: ear pain, subjective complaint of hearing loss, and tinnitus. Tinnitus has been reported in 2% to 36% of patients receiving cisplatin. This may be transient, lasting a few hours or days, or it may be permanent. Studies of the inner ear of temporal bones removed from patients at autopsy have been conducted. The cochlea of a 9-year-old child with a brain tumor who suffered hearing loss from cisplatin was found to have degeneration of the outer hair cells in the lower turns of the cochlea, the spiral ganglia, and the cochlear nerve. The vestibular ganglion cells and the vestibular nerve were normal (Strauss, et al., 1983). Another study examined the inner ear tissues of five patients who experienced cisplatin ototoxicity. Scanning electron microscopy showed large, fused stereocilia of the outer hair cells with damage to the cuticular plate (Wright & Schaefer, 1982). In a study of human temporal bones removed from patients treated with cisplatin, irradiation, or a combination of both treatments, the spiral ganglion cells and inner and outer hair cells were decreased in number and the stria vascularis were found to be degenerated (Hoistad et al., 1998).

Carboplatin

Carboplatin is a newer analog of cisplatin that was introduced into clinical trials in 1981. It was found to be less nephrotoxic than cisplatin, and preliminary reports suggested that carboplatin was less ototoxic than cisplatin. Bone-marrow suppression has been the primary dose-limiting toxicity of carboplatin. The latter toxic effect can be overcome by the use of autologous stem-cell rescue combined with the use of **hematopoietic** growth factors. This has permitted oncologists to use higher doses of carboplatin to improve its antitumor efficacy.

Animal Studies Carboplatin appears to be unique in its ototoxic effects. In the chinchilla, the inner hair cells are preferentially damaged (Wake, Takeno, Ibrahim, & Harrison, 1994). Less is known about the exact mechanism of carboplatin ototoxicity than is the case for cisplatin.

Clinical Studies Unfortunately, carboplatin may be more ototoxic than initially appreciated. Nine of 11 children with **neuroblastoma** treated with high-dose carboplatin experienced hearing losses in the speech frequencies. The hearing losses were sufficiently severe that hearing aids were recommended (Parsons et al., 1998). Notably, these children had all received previous cisplatin treatment. In addition, several patients had also received aminoglycoside antibiotics. Thus, carboplatin appears to be quite ototoxic, especially in children who have been previously exposed to treatment with cisplatin or other ototoxic agents and in patients with brain tumors who undergo opening of the blood–brain barrier with mannitol before carboplatin administration. In the latter group, 79% of patients experienced hearing loss (Neuwelt et al., 1998).

LOOP DIURETICS

The loop diuretics are so named because they exert their therapeutic effects through their action on the **loop of Henle** of the kidney. By acting on this part of the kidney, they cause a dramatic increase in the output of urine. These drugs are used to treat congestive heart failure in infants and adults, to treat high blood pressure, to remove excess fluid from the lungs in newborns with immature lungs, and to assist in the management of edema from liver or kidney failure. Ototoxicity has been reported with most of these compounds.

Animal Studies

Studies in experimental animals and a few human temporal bone histopathologic reports show that the primary target of loop diuretics is the stria vascularis. Animal studies have shown extensive edema of the stria vascularis (Figure 19-5) in conjunction with loss of auditory function (Rybak, 1993).

More recent studies in the chinchilla have suggested that the ototoxicity of ethacrynic acid may be mediated through impaired blood flow in the lateral wall of the cochlea. In these experiments, the blood vessels supplying the modiolus, spiral lamina, and vestibular end organs appeared normal. In contrast, the

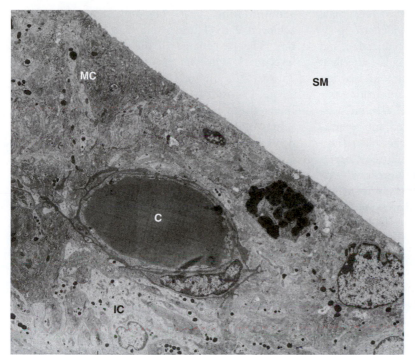

A

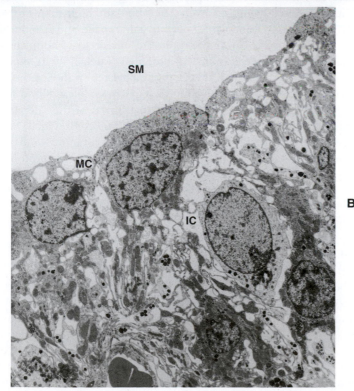

B

FIGURE 19-5 Transmission electron micrograph of the stria vascularis from the chinchilla. (A) Normal stria shows compact arrangement of the cells. There are no fluid spaces between cells. (B) After treatment with furosemide, fluid spaces appear between the cells. Such changes correlate with marked loss of auditory function, with a marked diminution of the endocochlear potential and a substantial increase of compound action potential thresholds. C, Capillary (densely packed with red blood cells); IC, intermediate cells; MC, marginal cells; SM, scala media.

vessels supplying the lateral wall of the cochlea (spiral ligament and stria vascularis) showed evidence of poor flow at 2 minutes after ethacrynic acid injection, and the vessels appeared to be devoid of red blood cells at 30 minutes after injection. The compound action potential, cochlear microphonics, and summating potential all declined without recovery after the microcirculatory changes in the lateral wall vessels, and reperfusion was delayed in the stria vascularis arterioles relative to other blood vessels in the lateral wall (see Chapter 10). Such ischemia followed by reperfusion could generate large quantities of reactive oxygen species, which could cause structural and functional damage to the inner ear (Ding, McFadden, Woo, & Salvi, 2002).

Clinical Studies   Ethacrynic acid was soon discovered to cause hearing loss after it was introduced into clinical medicine in the 1960s. Numerous cases of transient and even permanent deafness have been reported. Permanent, profound mid- and high-frequency sensorineural hearing loss has been reported in a kidney transplant patient who was treated with ethacrynic acid. This patient was rehabilitated with hearing aids (Rybak, 1988). Some outer hair cell loss in the basal turn has been also reported in temporal bone studies of patients with ethacrynic acid ototoxicity (Matz, 1976). Furosemide has also been found to cause temporary and some permanent cases of hearing loss. Permanent hearing loss has been reported in adults and in high-risk premature infants treated with furosemide (Brown, Watchko, & Sabo, 1991). Bumetanide, a more potent chemically related diuretic, has been reported to cause a much smaller incidence of hearing loss (Tuzel, 1981).

SALICYLATES

Salicylates such as aspirin have been used for many years to treat headache, mild-to-moderate pain, and arthritis. Salicylates have been known to be ototoxic for many years. They are widely known to cause tinnitus and hearing loss, which is usually temporary.

Animal Studies

In animal experiments, it has been shown that salicylates quickly enter the perilymph after systemic administration, and the peak concentration is achieved 2 to 4 hours after intraperitoneal injection. The percentage of the corresponding blood level reached in the perilymph can be as high as 25% to 33% (Juhn, Rybak, & Jung, 1985; Silverstein, Bernstein, & Davies, 1967; Boettcher, Bancroft, & Salvi, 1990). The relation between serum and perilymph concentration of salicylate has been described as nearly linear in chinchillas (Boettcher et al., 1990) and in rats (Jastreboff & Sasaki, 1986). Chinchillas receiving 450 mg/kg salicylate intraperitoneally were found to have serum levels of 25 to 50 mg/dL. At this level, animals were found to have an average evoked response threshold increase of 30 dB, primarily at the higher frequencies (Boettcher et al., 1990). Guinea pigs that were administered the same dose of salicylate were found to have increased spontaneous activity of inferior colliculus neurons, which may represent a tinnitus-like phenomenon (Jastreboff & Sasaki, 1986).

Direct perfusion of sodium salicylate into the cochlea suppresses the compound action potential resulting from low- but not high-intensity sound stimuli in experimental animals, and it reduces the cochlear microphonic potential without changing the summating potential (Puel, Bobbin, & Fallon, 1990). The effects of salicylates on the inner ear may be mediated by changes in cochlear blood flow, as well as by changes in stiffness of the lateral membrane of outer hair cells (Lue & Brownell, 1999).

Histopathologic studies of animal and human temporal bones removed after salicylate ototoxicity have not shown any significant hair cell damage or injury to the stria vascularis (Deer & Hunter-Duvar, 1982; Bernstein & Weiss, 1967). Additional studies have failed to show any injury to the spiral ganglion or the myelin sheath of the eighth nerve (Falk, 1974).

Clinical Studies

Various studies have shown that hearing loss may be related to blood concentration of salicylates. Patients receiving aspirin have been shown to experience hearing losses of up to 30 dB when their serum concentrations of salicylate are between 20 and 50 mg/dL (Myers & Bernstein, 1965). However, more recent studies of human volunteers receiving aspirin have reported that hearing loss and tinnitus may occur at lower blood concentrations than those previously reported. Even at total salicylate concentrations of 11 mg/dL, the hearing loss at any frequency was 12 dB.

A linear relation appears to exist between hearing loss and free salicylate concentration (Day et al., 1989). Salicylates are tightly bound to serum proteins, and only a small percentage of serum concentration is unbound or free. The severity of tinnitus worsens as plasma salicylate concentrations increase to greater than 40 mg/dL, with a continuous increase in tinnitus over the range of plasma salicylate concentrations of 40 to 320 mg/dL.

Although site of lesion testing of patients with salicylate-induced hearing loss strongly suggests a cochlear pattern (McCabe & Day, 1965), the fact that salicylate-induced hearing loss is reversible correlates with lack of significant permanent damage to the cochlea.

QUININE AND RELATED DRUGS

Quinine is an alkaloid drug that has been used to treat malaria. It is also used to treat leg cramps. Quinine is a component in tonic beverages. Quinine is ototoxic. Hearing loss is part of a syndrome known as cinchonism, which is characterized by deafness, vertigo, tinnitus, headache, visual loss, and nausea.

Animal Studies

In guinea pigs, increasing concentrations of quinine in the blood correlated with a stepwise increment in auditory threshold shifts of up to 35 dB (Alvan, Karlsson, & Villen, 1989). Significant increases of the compound action potential threshold in guinea pigs after quinine administration was confirmed in a recent study. Furthermore, the compound action potential N1 response was broadened to the first click in a train of click stimuli (Ochi, Kinoshita, Kenmochi, Nishino, & Ohashi, 2003). In chinchillas, a single intramuscular injection of 150 mg/kg quinine caused a reversible 20-dB threshold shift in auditory brainstem response threshold. Similar threshold shifts were observed after local application

of quinine to the round window membrane (Lee, Heinrich, & Jung, 1992).

Perceptual tinnitus can be produced by quinine. A condition-suppression study of rats demonstrated that behavioral changes suggesting a dose-dependent tinnitus could be induced by quinine. This behavioral evidence of tinnitus could be blocked by the calcium–channel blocker nimodipine (Jastreboff, Brennan, & Sasaki et al., 1991). However, nimodipine did not alter the effects of quinine on the compound action potential (Ochi et al., 2003).

Clinical Studies

Transient hearing loss may appear within a few hours after starting high-dose treatment of malaria. After prolonged daily treatment, as many as 20% of patients may report hearing loss. The hearing loss is usually reversible and affects the high frequencies first. There may be a characteristic notch at 4 kHz. Speech discrimination scores may be less than 30% (Koegel, 1985). Some patients may have hearing loss in the conversational frequencies; if so, the hearing loss may be permanent (Miller, 1985).

Ultrahigh-frequency audiometry may detect hearing loss from quinine at an early stage. A series of 10 patients receiving quinine therapy for acute malaria was reported. Patients experienced high-tone loss of auditory acuity, which resolved after completion of therapy (Roche et al., 1990). The hearing impairment in humans (Alvan et al., 1991; Karlsson et al., 1990) was found to correlate with the plasma concentration of quinine.

ERYTHROMYCIN AND RELATED ANTIBIOTICS

Although erythromycin has been used in clinical medicine since the 1950s, the first case of ototoxicity attributed to erythromycin was not reported until 1973 (Mintz, Amir, Pinkhas, & de Vries, 1973). A number of cases of bilateral sensorineural hearing loss after high-dose oral or intravenous administration of this antibiotic have been reported. Most patients who sustain hearing loss are older adults and have liver or kidney failure or have been treated for Legionnaires' disease. Symptoms of ototoxicity include "blowing" tinnitus, subjective loss of hearing, and occasionally, vertigo. Others may describe symptoms of central nervous system dysfunction, such as confusion, fear, psychiatric symptoms (Umstead & Newman, 1986), visual changes, slurred speech, feeling of being drugged, or lack of control (Cohen & Weitz, 1981). Most cases of hearing loss and tinnitus have been temporary, and reversed within 6 to 14 days after cessation of erythromycin therapy (Swanson, Song Fine, Orloff, Chen, & Vin, 1992). However, permanent tinnitus despite recovery of hearing has been reported (Levin & Behrenth, 1986), and permanent hearing loss was reported in a woman who was treated with intravenous erythromycin for pneumonia (Dylewski, 1988). Hearing loss from erythromycin has been observed in patients who had received kidney or liver transplants. In the kidney transplant patients, hearing loss was confirmed audiometrically in 11 of 34 (32%) courses of intravenous erythromycin lactobionate treatment for pneumonia. The incidence rate was 53% in patients given 4 g of the drug daily compared with 16% in patients treated with 2 g daily. No difference was evident in the kidney or liver function between these groups of patients receiving the dosage regimens describe earlier. Prompt recognition of the problem and modification of therapy allowed for complete reversal of hearing losses in these patients (Vasquez, Maddux, Sanchez, & Pollak, 1993). Three patients who were liver transplant recipients experienced development of erythromycin ototoxicity. It was proposed that an interaction between the antibiotic and the antirejection drug cyclosporin might have resulted in hearing loss in these patients (Moral et al., 1994).

The following guidelines have been proposed to prevent erythromycin ototoxicity:

1. The daily dose of erythromycin should not exceed 1.5 g if the serum **creatinine** concentration is greater than 180 mol/L.

2. Pretreatment audiograms should be obtained, especially in older adult patients and in patients with kidney or liver insufficiency.

3. Caution should exercised when erythromycin is used in combination with other ototoxic drugs (Schweitzer & Olson, 1984).

Audiograms in patients with erythromycin ototoxicity can show a flat type of sensorineural hearing loss, although high-frequency loss has been reported. Auditory brainstem response testing in two patients with erythromycin ototoxicity demonstrated absence of waves I to III during treatment with erythromycin, when the patients had documented sensorineural hearing loss on audiograms and normalization of evoked response waveforms after stopping erythromycin therapy, with recovery of hearing (Sacristan et al., 1993).

ERYTHROMYCIN ANALOGUES

A newer antibiotic in the same class as erythromycin, azithromycin, has been associated with ototoxicity.

Animal Studies of Erythromycin Analogues

Guinea pigs that were administered azithromycin or a related drug, clarithromycin, demonstrated a reversible alteration of transiently evoked OAEs (Uzun, Koten, Adali, Yorulmaz, Yahiz, & Karasalihoglu, 2001). The mechanisms of ototoxicity of erythromycin and the related antibiotics azithromycin and clarithromycin currently are unknown.

Clinical Studies

Azithromycin ototoxicity was first reported in patients with acquired immunodeficiency syndrome who were receiving long-term treatment for disseminated *Mycobacterium avium* infections. Three patients reported hearing loss between 1 and 3 months into the course of therapy. Bilateral mild-to-moderate sensorineural hearing loss was documented, which resolved after cessation of treatment with this antibiotic within 2 to 4 weeks (Wallace, Miller, Nguyen, & Shields, 1994). In another series of similarly treated patients, 8 patients were reported to have ototoxicity. They received high-dose azithromycin (600 mg four times daily by mouth). Four patients had mild-to-moderate sensorineural hearing loss, and one had simply a change in acoustic reflex decay. Hearing recovered to normal within an average of 4.9 weeks in all patients who had a repeat audiogram (Tseng, Dolovich, & Salit, 1997).

A 47-year-old woman developed complete deafness after receiving 8 days of treatment with azithromycin (Bizjak, Haug, Schilz, Sarodia, & Dressing, 1999). A 39-year-old otherwise healthy woman experienced the sudden onset of bilateral tinnitus after initiation of azithromycin therapy for a urinary tract infection. She noticed the onset of tinnitus within 24 hours of taking the first daily dose (500 mg) of the standard 5-day course of the antibiotic. The patient stopped the drug after the second dose because of worsening tinnitus and subjective hearing loss. Audiometry results showed a moderate-to-severe high-frequency sensorineural hearing loss on the right and a mild-to-moderate high-frequency sensorineural hearing loss on the left. Speech discrimination scores were 92% on the right and 96% on the left. Repeat audiogram performed 12 months later showed no change in hearing thresholds, and the patient still reported bilateral tinnitus, although it was somewhat less severe (Ress & Gross, 2000). An additional two cases of reversible sensorineural hearing loss have been reported (Mamikoglu & Mamikoglu, 2001).

⌇SUMMARY⌇

Ototoxic drugs can cause clinical symptoms of hearing loss with or without balance disorders. Aminoglycoside antibiotics, such as gentamicin, and anticancer drugs, such as cisplatin or carboplatin, can cause a high incidence of permanent hearing loss. The outer hair cells in the basal turn of the cochlea appear to be the primary target for these drugs, resulting in permanent high frequency sensorineural hearing loss. Monitoring for hearing loss in patients treated with these drugs may show early onset of ototoxicity, particularly if high-frequency audiometry is used. Evoked OAEs may also be used as a screening tool. Blood levels of aminoglycosides can be monitored to keep the drug concentration in the therapeutic range and may help to reduce the likelihood of hearing loss. Vestibular toxicity from aminoglycosides is more difficult to predict and vestibular testing may not be possible in critically ill patients who cannot be moved to a testing area. Both aminoglycosides and cisplatin damage the kidneys, as well as the cochlea. The risks for hearing loss from cisplatin include high total dose, prior noise exposure, and combined treatment with vincristine. Carboplatin is also ototoxic, especially in patients who are being treated for brain tumors, especially with manipulation of the blood–brain barrier. Loop diuretics, such as furosemide, cause temporary or permanent hearing loss, especially in patients with poor kidney function. Salicylates, like aspirin, cause reversible tinnitus and temporary hearing loss that are related to the blood level of the drug. Erythromycin can cause hearing loss when given in high doses to patients with kidney or liver insufficiency. Contrary to most other ototoxins, which cause a high-frequency hearing loss, erythromycin usually causes a flat loss of hearing across frequencies. The mechanisms of hearing loss from erythromycin and its analogues, clarithromycin and azithromycin, are not known. It is important to be aware that various drugs can cause hearing loss, and that pretreatment and follow-up testing is important to detect drug-induced hearing loss.

⌇KEY TERMS⌇

Albumin
Aminoglycoside antibiotics
Anemia
Atrophy
Basal turn

Blood–brain barrier
Caloric testing
Cochlear microphonic potential
Compound action potential

Cranial
Creatinine
Crista
Distortion product otoacoustic emissions

Dynamic posturography
Free radicals
Glutathione
Hematopoietic
Intraperitoneal

Loop of Henle

Loop diuretics

Nephrotoxicity

Neuroblastoma

Neurotoxicity

Ototoxicity

Rotational chair

testing

Scavenger

Trough

Uremia

∿STUDY QUESTIONS∿

1. Describe the pattern of damage to cells in the cochlea caused by aminoglycoside antibiotics and cisplatin.

2. List two symptoms associated with salicylate-induced ototoxicity.

3. List two features of erythromycin ototoxicity.

4. Specify how loop diuretics act on the cochlea.

∿REFERENCES∿

Allen, G. C., Tiu, C., Koike, K., Ritchey, A. K., Kurs-Lasky, M., & Wax, M. (1998). Transient-evoked otoacoustic emissions in children after cisplatin chemotherapy. *Otolaryngology and Head and Neck Surgery, 118,* 584–588.

Alvan, G., Karlsson, K. K., Hellgren, U., et al. (1991). Hearing impairment related to plasma quinine concentration in healthy volunteers. *British Journal of Clinical Pharmacology, 31,* 409–412.

Alvan, G., Karlsson, K. K., & Villen, T. (1989). Reversible hearing impairment related to quinine blood concentrations in guinea pigs. *Life Sciences, 45,* 751–755.

Bernstein, J. M., & Weiss, A. D. (1967). Further observation on salicylate ototoxicity. *Journal of Laryngology and Otology, 81,* 915.

Bizjak, E. E., Haug, M. T. 3rd, Schilz, R. J., Sarodia, B. D., & Dressing, J. M. (1999). Intravenous azithromycin-induced ototoxicity. *Pharmacotherapy, 19,* 245–248.

Boettcher, F. A., Bancroft, B. R., & Salvi, R. J. (1990). Concentration of salicylate in serum and perilymph. *Archives of Otolaryngology & Head and Neck Surgery, 116,* 681.

Bokemeyer, C., Berger, C. C., Hartmann, J. T., Kollmansberger, C., Schmoll, H-J., Kuczyk, M. A., et al. (1998). Analysis of risk factors for cisplatin-induced ototoxicity in patients with testicular cancer. *British Journal of Cancer, 77,* 1355–1362.

Brown, A. M., McDowell, B., & Forge, A. (1989). Acoustic distortion products can be used to monitor the effects of chronic gentamicin treatment. *Hearing Research, 423,* 143–156.

Brown, D. R., Watchko, J. F., & Sabo, D. (1991). Neonatal sensorineural hearing loss associated with furosemide: A case control study, *Developmental Medicine and Child Neurology, 33,* 816–823.

Cohen, I. J., & Weitz, R. (1981). Psychiatric complications with erythromycin. *Drug Intelligence & Clinical Pharmacy, 15,* 388.

Day, R. O., Graham, G. G., Bieri, D., et al. (1989). Concentration-response relationships for salicylate-induced ototoxicity in normal volunteers. *British Journal of Clinical Pharmacology, 28,* 695–702.

Deer, B. C., & Hunter-Duvar, I. (1982). Salicylate ototoxicity in the chinchilla: A behavioral and electron microscope study. *Journal of Otolaryngology, 11,* 260.

Devarajan, P., Savoca, M., Castaneda, M. P., Park, M. S., Esteban-Cruciani, N., Kalinec, G., & Kalinec, F. (2002). Cisplatin-induced apoptosis in auditory cells: Role of death receptor and mitochondrial pathways. *Hearing Research, 174,* 45–54.

Ding, D., McFadden, S. L., Woo, J. M., & Salvi, R. J. (2002). Ethacrynic acid rapidly and selectively abolishes blood flow in vessels supplying the lateral wall of the cochlea. *Hearing Research, 173,* 1–9.

Dylewski, J. (1988). Irreversible sensorineural hearing loss due to erythromycin. *Canadian Medical Association Journal, 139,* 230.

Falk, S. A. (1974). Sodium salicylate. *Archives of Otolaryngology, 99,* 393.

Fausti, S. A., Rappaport, B. Z., Schechter, M. A., Frey, R. H., War, T. T., & Brummett, R. E. (1984). Detection of aminoglycoside ototoxicity by high frequency auditory evaluation: Selected case studies. *American Journal of Otolaryngology, 5,* 177–182.

Forge, A., & Schacht, J. (2000). Aminoglycoside antibiotics. *Audiology & Neuro-otology, 5,* 3–22.

Granowetter, L., Rosenstock, J. G., & Packer, R. J. (1983). Enhanced cisplatinum neurotoxicity in pediatric patients with brain tumors. *Journal of Neuro-oncology, 1,* 293.

Hawkins, J. E. (1973). Ototoxic mechanisms: A working hypothesis. *Audiology, 12,* 383–393.

Hinojosa, R., Nelson, E. G., Lerner, S. A., Redleaf, M. I., & Schramm, D. R. (2001). Aminoglycoside ototoxicity: A human temporal bone study. *Laryngoscope, 111,* 1797–1805.

Hoistad, D. L., Ondrey, F. G., Mutlu, C., Schachern, P. A., Paparella, M. M., & Adams, G. L. (1998). Histopathology of human temporal bone after cis-platinum, radiation or both. *Otolaryngology and Head and Neck Surgery, 118,* 825–832.

Jastreboff, P. J., Brennan, J. F., & Sasaki, C. T. (1991). Quinine-induced tinnitus in rats. *Archives of Otolaryngology & Head and Neck Surgery, 117,* 1162–1166.

Jastreboff, P. J., & Sasaki, C. T. (1986). Salicylate-induced changes in spontaneous activity of single units in the inferior colliculus of the guinea pig. *Journal of the Acoustical Society of America, 80,* 1384.

Johnsson, L. G., Hawkins, J. E., Kingsley, T. C., Black, F. O., & Matz, G. J. (1981). Aminoglycoside-induced cochlear pathology in man. *Acta Otolaryngologica Supplementum, 383,* 1–19.

Juhn, S. K., Rybak, L. P., & Jung, T. T. K. (1985). Transport characteristics of the blood-labyrinth barrier. In D. Drescher (Ed.), *Auditory biochemistry.* Springfield, IL: Charles C. Thomas.

Karlsson, K. K., Hellgren, U., Alvan, G., et al. (1990). Audiometry as a possible indicator of quinine concentration during treatment of malaria. *Transactions of the Royal Society of Tropical Medicine and Hygiene, 84,* 765–767.

Koegel, L., Jr. (1985). Ototoxicity: A contemporary review of aminoglycosides, loop diuretics, acetylsalicylic acid, quinine, erythromycin and cisplatinum. *American Journal of Otology, 6,* 190–199.

Kopelman, J., Budni, A. S., Sessions, R. B., Kramer, M. B., & Wong, G. Y. (1988). Ototoxicity of high-dose cisplatin by bolus administration in patients with advanced cancer and normal hearing. *Laryngoscope, 98,* 858–864.

Kopke, R. D., Liu, W., Gabaizadeh, R., Jacono, A., Feghali, J., Spray, D., Garcia, P., Steinman, H., Malgarange, B., Ruben, R. J., Rybak, L., & Van de Water, T. R. (1997). Use of organotypic cultures of Corti's organ to study the protective effects of antioxidant molecules on cisplatin-induced damage of auditory hair cells. *American Journal of Otology, 18,* 559–571.

Lee, C. S., Heinrich, J., & Jung, T. T. K. (1992). Quinine-induced ototoxicity: Alterations in cochlear blood flow. *Otolaryngology and Head and Neck Surgery, 233.*

Lerner, S. A., Seligsohn, R., Bhattacharya, I., Hinojosa, R., & Matz, G. (1981). Pharmacokinetics of gentamicin in the inner perilymph of man. In S. A. Lerner, G. J. Matz, & J. E. Hawkins, Jr. (Eds.), *Aminoglycoside ototoxicity* (pp. 357–381). Boston: Little, Brown.

Levin, G., & Behrenth, E. (1986). Irreversible ototoxic effect of erythromycin. *Scandinavian Audiology, 15,* 41.

Lindemann, H. H. (1969). Regional differences in sensitivity of the vestibular sensory epithelia to ototoxic drugs. *Acta Otolaryngologica, 67,* 177–189.

Lue, A. J. C., & Brownell, W. E. (1999). Salicylate induced changes in outer hair cell lateral wall stiffness. *Hearing Research, 135,* 163–168.

Mamikoglu, B., & Mamikoglu, O. (2001). Azithromycin ototoxicity. *Annals of Otology, Rhinology & Laryngology, 110,* 102.

Mathog, R. H., & Klein, W. J., Jr. (1969). Ototoxicity of ethacrynic acid and aminoglycoside antibiotics in uremia. *New England Journal of Medicine, 280,* 1223–1224.

Matz, G. J. (1976). The ototoxic effects of ethacrynic acid in man and animals. *Laryngoscope, 86,* 1065–1086.

McCabe, P. A., & Dey, F. L. (1965). The effect of aspirin upon auditory sensitivity. *Annals of Otology, Rhinology, and Otolaryngology, 74,* 312–325.

McHaney, V. A., Thibadoux, G., Hayes, F. A., & Green, A. A. (1983). Hearing loss in children receiving cisplatin chemotherapy. *Journal of Pediatrics, 102,* 314–317.

Meech, R. P., Campbell, K. C. M., Hughes, L. P., & Rybak, L. P. (1998). A semiquantitative analysis of the effects of cisplatin on the rat stria vascularis. *Hearing Research, 124,* 44–59.

Miller, J. J. (Ed.) (1985). Antimalarial drugs. *CRC handbook of ototoxicity* (pp. 9–15). Boca Raton, FL: CRC Press.

Mintz, U., Amir, J., Pinkhas, J., & de Vries, A. (1973). Transient perceptive deafness after erythromycin. *Journal of the American Medical Association, 225,* 1122–1123.

Moore, R. D., Smith, C. R., & Lietman, P. S. (1984). Risk factors of auditory toxicity in patients receiving aminoglycosides. *Journal of Infectious Diseases, 149,* 23–30.

Moral, A., Navala, M., Rimola, A., Garcia-Valdecasas, J. C., Grande, L., Visa, J., & Rodes, J. (1994). Erythromycin ototoxicity in liver transplant patients. *Transplant International, 7,* 62–64.

Myers, E. N., & Bernstein, J. M. (1965). Salicylate ototoxicity. *Archives of Otolaryngology, 82,* 483.

Neuwelt, E. A., Brummett, R. E., Doolittle, N. D., Muldoon, L. L., Kroll, R. A., Pagel, M. A., et al. (1998). First evidence of otoprotection against carboplatin-induced hearing loss with a two-compartment system in patients with central nervous system malignancy using sodium thiosulfate. *Journal of Pharmacology and Experimental Therapeutics, 286,* 77–84.

Ochi, K., Kinoshita, H., Kenmochi, M., Nishino, H., & Ohashi, T. (2003). Effects of nimodipine on quinine ototoxicity. *Annals of Otology, Rhinology & Laryngology, 112,* 163–168.

Parsons, S. K., Neault, M. W., Lehmann, L. E., Brennan, L. L., Eickhoff, C. E., Kretschman, C. S., et al. (1998). Severe ototoxicity following carboplatin-containing regimen for autologous marrow transplantation for neuroblastoma. *Bone Marrow Transplant, 22,* 669–674.

Prezant, T. R., Agapian, J. V., Bohlman, M. C., Bu, X., Oztas, S., Qiu, W. Q., Arnos, K. S., Cortopassi, G. A., Jaber, L., & Rotter, J. I. (1993). Mitochondrial ribosomal RNA mutation associated with both antibiotic-induced and non-syndromic deafness. *Nature Genetics, 4,* 289–294.

Puel, J-L., Bobbin, R. P., & Fallon, M. (1990). Salicylate, mefenamate, meclofenamate and quinine on cochlear potentials. *Otolaryngology and Head and Neck Surgery, 102,* 66.

Ress, B. D., & Gross, E. M. (2000). Irreversible sensorineural hearing loss as a result of azithromycin ototoxicity. A case report. *Annals of Otology, Rhinology & Laryngology, 109,* 435–437.

Roche, R. J., Simamut, K., Pukrittayakamee, S., et al. (1990). Quinine induces reversible high-tone hearing loss. *British Journal of Clinical Pharmacology, 29,* 780–782.

Rybak, L. P. (1988). Ototoxicity of ethacrynic acid (a persistent clinical problem). *Journal of Laryngology and Otology, 102,* 518–520.

Rybak, L. P. (1993). Ototoxicity of loop diuretics. *Otolaryngologic Clinics of North America, 26,* 829–844.

Rybak, L. P., Husain, K., Morris, C., Whitworth, C., & Somani, S. (2000). Effect of protective agents on cisplatin ototoxicity. *American Journal of Otology, 21,* 513–520.

Sacristan, J. A., De Cos, M. A., Soto, J., Zurbano, F., Pascual, J., Tasis, A., Valle, R., & De Pablos, C. (1993). Ototoxicity of erythromycin in man: Electrophysiologic approach. *American Journal of Otology, 14,* 186–188.

Schweitzer, V. G., & Olson, N. R. (1984). Ototoxic effect of erythromycin therapy. *Archives of Otolaryngology, 110,* 258.

Sha, S. H., & Schacht, J. (1999). Salicylate attenuates gentamicin-induced ototoxicity. *Laboratory Investigation, 79,* 807–813.

Sha, S-H., Taylor, R., Forge, A., & Schacht, J. (2001). Differential vulnerability of basal and apical hair cells based on intrinsic susceptibility to free radicals. *Hearing Research, 155,* 1–8.

Silverstein, H., Bernstein, J., & Davies, D. G. (1967). Salicylate ototoxicity: A biochemical and electrophysiological study. *Annals of Otology, Rhinology & Laryngology, 76,* 118.

Stavroulaki, P., Vossinakis, J. C., Dinopoulou, D., Doudounakis, S., Adamopoulos, G., & Apostopoulos, N. (2002). Otoacoustic emissions for monitoring aminoglycoside-induced ototoxicity in children with cystic fibrosis. *Archives of Otolaryngology & Head and Neck Surgery, 128,* 150–155.

Strauss, M., Towfighi, J., Lord, S., Lipton, A., Harvey, H. A., & Brown, B. (1983). Cisplatinum ototoxicity:

Clinical experience and temporal bone histopathology. *Laryngoscope, 93,* 1554–1559.

Swanson, D. J., Song Fine, M. J., Orloff, J. J., Chen, S.Y., Vin, S.W. (1992). Erythromycin ototoxicity: Prospective assessment with serum concentrations and audiograms in a study of patients with pneumonia. *American Journal of Medicine, 92,* 61–68.

Tseng, A. L., Dolovich, L., & Salit, I. E. (1997). Azithromycin-related ototoxicity in patients infected with human immunodeficiency virus. *Clinical Infectious Diseases, 24,* 77–78.

Tuzel, I. H. (1981). Comparison of adverse reactions to bumetanide and furosemide. *Journal of Clinical Pharmacology, 21,* 113–114.

Umstead, G. S., & Newman, K. H. (1986). Erythromycin ototoxicity and acute psychotic reaction seen in cancer patients with hepatic dysfunction. *Archives of Internal Medicine, 146,* 897.

Uzun, C., Koten, M., Adali, M. K.,Yorulmaz, F.,Yagiz, R., & Karasalihoglu, A. R. (2001). Reversible ototoxic effect of azithromycin and clarithromycin on transiently evoked otoacoustic emissions in guinea pigs. *Journal of Laryngology and Otology, 115,* 622–628.

Vasquez, E. M., Maddux, M. S., Sanchez, J., & Pollak, R. (1993). Clinically significant hearing loss in renal allograft recipients treated with intravenous erythromycin. *Archives of Internal Medicine, 153,* 879–882.

Wake, M.,Takeno, S., Ibrahim, D., & Harrison, R. (1994). Selective inner hair cell ototoxicity induced by carboplatin. *Laryngoscope, 104,* 488–493.

Wallace, M. R., Miller, L. K., Nguyen, M.T., Shields, A. R. (1994). Ototoxicity with azithromycin. *Lancet, 343,* 241.

Wersall, J., Lundquist, P-G., & Bjorkroth, B. (1969). Ototoxicity of gentamicin. *Journal of Infectious Diseases, 119,* 410–416.

West, B. A., Brummett, R. E., & Himes, D. L. (1973). Interaction of kanamycin and ethacrynic acid. *Archives of Otolaryngology, 98,* 32–37.

Wright, C. G., & Schaefer, S. D. (1982). Inner ear histopathology in patients treated with cisplatinum. *Laryngoscope, 92,* 1408–1413.

⌣SUGGESTED READING⌣

Wu, W-J., Sha, S-I I., & Schacht, J. (2002). Recent advances in understanding aminoglycoside ototoxicity and its prevention. *Audiology & Neuro-otology, 7,* 171–174.

Chapter
20

Genetic Aspects of Hearing Loss

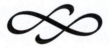

Kevin K. Ohlemiller, Ph.D.
Associate Professor of Otolaryngology
Washington University School of Medicine
St. Louis, Missouri

About half of *congenital* (i.e., present at birth) hearing loss results from genetic mutations. An unknown proportion of adult-onset hearing loss also has an explicitly genetic cause, or is strongly influenced by genetics. The ongoing revolution in molecular techniques and genetic manipulation virtually guarantees that audiologists will take part in discussions centered on diagnosing, managing, and eventually treating hearing loss associated with specific genetic defects. They will also find themselves helping families to understand the somewhat opaque language of genetics and geneticists. The primary goal of this chapter is not to catalogue specific mutations. In that regard, it would be out of date before it is published. Instead, the goal is to give audiologists the tools to understand the language of the medical literature, to become self-sufficient in keeping up with the expanding list of **genes,** and types of genes, that can affect hearing. We attempt to present a conceptual framework that is more than just a string of definitions. Certain mutations that are particularly illustrative or prevalent are discussed.

INCIDENCE VERSUS PREVALENCE OF GENETIC HEARING LOSS

When describing how frequently a particular health condition occurs, it is important to distinguish between *incidence* (frequency of occurrence among total births) and *prevalence* (frequency in a population of interest) (Shprintzen, 1997). The difference between these can be illustrated by considering the case of a genetic defect that is incompatible with survival. Whereas the incidence of the defect could be estimated from medical records, its prevalence among adults would be zero. The incidence of genetic prelingual deafness has been estimated at about 1 in 1,000, that is, roughly half of all cases (Van Laer, 2003). About 80% of these cases may be characterized as autosomal recessive, 15% as autosomal dominant, and a trace percentage (2–3%) as **X-linked.** While the prevalence of hearing impairment among adults in the United States and Europe is estimated to be about 3% (Bitner-Glindzicz, 2002), the prevalence of genetically related hearing

impairment among adults is unknown. Genetic contributions to congenital deafness are easier to estimate than those to adult-onset deafness. The reason is that environmental contributions at birth will often be attributable to known causes, such as maternal illness or drug exposure, permitting an estimate of genetic contributions as well. Later in life, environmental factors will be more difficult to isolate, and many gene–environment interactions remain to be discovered.

WHAT ARE GENES?

Genes are fundamentally blueprints to guide cells in the making of **proteins.** Proteins, in turn, are central to everything else cells do or make. They comprise many cellular structural components (e.g., actin, tubulin, collagen). They also serve as **enzymes,** or catalysts, speeding the cells' countless chemical reactions by more than 1 million-fold. This includes the reactions required to break down raw materials, generate energy, and synthesize lipids and new **DNA.** Among proteins' other important functions, they serve as transporters (e.g., hemoglobin, ferritin), signal mediators (e.g., ion channels, receptors), regulators of gene expression, and immune factors.

All proteins are strings of **amino acids** (so-named because they all possess a nitrogen-based "amino" group). These vary in the hydrophilic or hydrophobic ("water-loving" or "water-fearing") nature and in the sulfur/oxygen content of their "side chain." The amazing variation and versatility of proteins derives primarily from differences in how they combine the 20 different amino acids in sequences that may include as few as 1 or more than 1,000. The order and type of amino acids determines which segments of a protein will attract each other, and thereby how the entire protein chain will fold. Although most proteins undergo modification within the endoplasmic reticulum and Golgi apparatus (see Chapter 4), it is the coding sequence of each gene that determines the amino acid sequence, and thus the shape and major functional possibilities of any protein. This is a beautiful principle, allowing stunning variety and complexity to arise from a modest set of genetic codes and only

20 building blocks. Through a kind of "data compression," our genomic blueprint collection of about 30,000 genes codes for more than 90,000 proteins (Mattick, 2004). Until recently, scientists believed the gene-to-protein ratio was 1:1, and that our wonderful human complexity must come from having more genes than simpler organisms. In fact, *corn* has more genes than humans, and the basis of our apparent complexity may instead lie at the level of gene regulation (Ast, 2005).

Recall from Chapter 4 that genes and the **chromosomes** on which they reside are composed of deoxyribonucleic acid (DNA). The **transcription** ("reading") of each gene is mediated by a particular form of a related compound, **ribonucleic acid (RNA),** known as **messenger RNA (mRNA),** so named because it conveys structural information about proteins from the cell nucleus to synthesis machinery in the cytoplasm. The latter step, termed **translation,** occurs in conjunction with organelles called **ribosomes**. The code carried by mRNA molecules is *complementary* to the code of the source DNA (see later). DNA, RNA, and proteins all share the property of being polymers, that is, long chain molecules composed of repeated units. In the same way that proteins are strings of amino acids, DNA and RNA are strings of *nucleotides* and *nucleosides,* respectively. Collectively, DNA and RNA and their constituent building blocks are termed *nucleic acids.* The polymer nature of proteins and nucleic acids allows high "information density" and phenomenal diversity of function to arise from simple building blocks and minimal rules for their assembly.

TYPES OF GENES

Each of our 30,000 genes falls into one of four functional categories: structural, regulatory, transfer RNA (tRNA), and ribosomal RNA (rRNA) genes (Shprintzen, 1997).

Structural Genes

Structural genes code for proteins that conduct the typical functions described earlier, such as catalysis, and the makeup of cell structural components. The name, unfortunately, may seem to imply that these genes all code for cell structural elements, but it actually refers to the primary involvement of these genes with the structure of proteins that carry out the vast majority of cell functions.

Regulatory Genes

Regulatory genes determine when, and in what quantity, other genes are expressed. Consider that all of our cells possess the same genes. It thus cannot be the genetic content, but rather the *pattern of gene expression,* that distinguishes our countless cell types. It is furthermore the pattern of gene expression that determines overall body plan and the differentiation of tissue types during development. Indeed, the entire process of development beginning with the fertilized egg is "kick-started" by the presence in the egg cytoplasm of regulatory factors that determine which genes are expressed first. One prominent class of developmentally related regulatory genes is the *homeobox* (HOX) genes. These genes control major characteristics such as limb and organ formation, including the layout of sensory organs.

The significance of gene regulation cannot be overstated. Incredibly, although as little as 2% of the genome of mammals may be devoted to structural genes, more than half of the genome appears devoted to regulation of that 2% (Ast, 2005). Rather than the number of genes, what appears to "scale up" with the sophistication and complexity of animals is the proportion of the genome that is regulatory in nature. Regulatory genes may code for proteins that bind to segments of structural genes that either cause them to be expressed or inhibited. Among these are *transcription factors,* which are proteins that initiate the transcription of several genes serving a related function. Regulatory genes can also code for special forms of RNA that can bind either to DNA or to mRNA, and thus inhibit the expression of genes or production of their structural proteins (Mattick, 2004).

Transfer RNA and Ribosomal RNA Genes

Some genes code for RNA molecules whose purpose is not to be translated into an amino acid sequence. Instead, they govern the translation process itself. Transfer RNAs (tRNAs), which coincidentally fold to form a "T" shape, lie at the heart of translation, literally "translating" the mRNA coding sequence into an amino acid sequence. A specific tRNA molecule recognizes and binds each of the 20 amino acids on one end of the "T," and recognizes the mRNA code for that amino acid at the other end. Also essential to translation is rRNA, which combines with certain proteins to form the ribosomes. rRNA is the most abundant RNA in most cells and is transcribed at a specific location in the cell nucleus known as the *nucleolus.* Ribosomes move along an mRNA sequence and guide the matchup of tRNA with their appropriate mRNA codes. As the ribosome moves, the amino acid chain grows.

THE GENETIC CODE

For all its size, the composition of DNA is fairly simple: a string of four *bases* (adenine, thymine, cytosine, and guanine) in variable order. There are actually two strands of DNA, weakly bound together so that adenine on one strand always binds to thymine on the other, and cytosine on one strand always binds to guanine on the other (Figure 20-1). Thus, it is said that DNA is composed of two complementary strands, and one could recreate either strand from the other. Unlike DNA, mRNA does not form double strands. It also substitutes the base uracil for thymidine. Transcription of DNA into mRNA requires that the two DNA strands separate. With the help of enzymes, the code contained on one strand, the *template strand* (also called the *antisense strand*), is converted into the complementary code sequence in the mRNA (Figure 20-2). Except for the swapping of uracil for thymidine, the result is that the mRNA sequence ends up matching that of the remaining *coding strand* (or *sense strand*) of DNA.

The order of bases is highly specific. Every three bases form a *codon,* the code "word" for a particular amino acid (Table 20-1). Because there are 4 possible bases, and every 3 constitute a codon, this means that there are 64 possible "words" in the genetic code (4 × 4 × 4). All 64 are used, yet there are only 20 amino acids. What do the seemingly extra

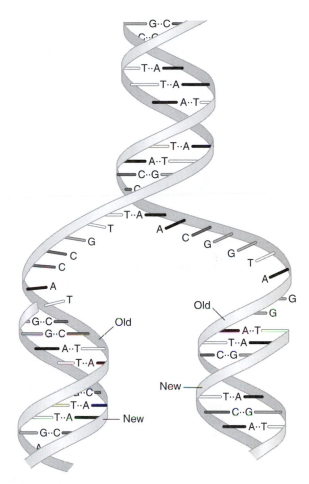

FIGURE 20-1 The DNA double helix with complementary bonding between adenine (A) and thymine (T), and guanine (G) and cytosine (C). Lower part of figure shows unwinding and synthesis of new DNA, as would occur in mitosis or meiosis. Each strand provides the sequence for a new complementary strand.

44 codons do? The genetic code is somewhat like the letters associated with the numbers on a telephone keypad. The numbers 2 to 9 are each linked to three letters, so that any number cannot specify a unique letter, nor can any number sequence specify a unique word. Yet, any word will specify a unique sequence of numbers (which is why companies will pay extra for easily remembered words that also convey their phone numbers). As shown in Table

DNA

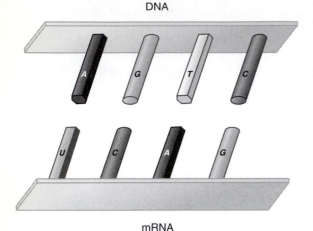

mRNA

FIGURE 20-2 Schematic transcription of a DNA sequence into its complementary messenger RNA (mRNA). Note that mRNA substitutes uracil (U) for thymine (T).

20-1, every 3-letter codon specifies a single amino acid, but 18 of the 20 amino acids can be specified by multiple codes. In addition, three codons are "stop" codons, signaling the end of a protein coding sequence and ending the transcription of a particular mRNA.

The nature of the genetic code is surprising in several ways. On first examination, it appears inefficient, perhaps with a "thrown together" quality. Indeed, it was "thrown together" in the trial-and-error experiment that is evolution. Yet, mathematical modeling has shown it to be more tolerant of errors than other codes that might have arisen (Freeland & Hurst, 2004). Note in Table 20-1 that the first two bases are generally sufficient to specify a particular amino acid. What the table does not show is that errors at the third position will often code for amino acids with similar properties, so that the function of the final protein product may be retained. In fact, errors in mRNA translation tend to occur at the third position, so that this may represent an evolutionary "fix" to the most common translation errors (Freeland & Hurst, 2004). Also remarkable is that essential aspects of the code are common to all organisms. The construction and function of our DNA is much

TABLE 20-1   Messenger RNA Codons and the Amino Acids for Which They Code

Codon Sequence	Amino Acid	Codon Sequence	Amino Acid
UUU	Phenylalanine	GAG	Glutamic acid
UUC	Phenylalanine	UGU	Cysteine
UUA	Leucine	UGC	Cysteine
UUG	Leucine	UGG	Tryptophan
CUU	Leucine	CGU	Arginine
CUC	Leucine	CGC	Arginine
CUA	Leucine	CGA	Arginine
CUG	Leucine	CGG	Arginine
AUU	Isoleucine	AGA	Arginine
AUC	Isoleucine	AGG	Arginine
AUA	Isoleucine	AGU	Serine
AUG	Methionine	AGC	Serine
GUU	Valine	UCU	Serine
GUC	Valine	UCC	Serine
GUA	Valine	UCA	Serine
GUG	Valine	UCG	Serine
UAU	Tyrosine	GGU	Glycine
UAC	Tyrosine	GGC	Glycine
UAA	Stop Codon	GGA	Glycine
UAG	Stop Codon	GGG	Glycine
UGA	Stop Codon	CCU	Proline
CAU	Histidine	CCC	Proline
CAC	Histidine	CCA	Proline
CAA	Glutamine	CCG	Proline
CAG	Glutamine	ACU	Threonine
AAU	Asparagine	ACC	Threonine
AAC	Asparagine	ACG	Threonine
AAA	Lysine	ACA	Threonine
AAG	Lysine	GCC	Alanine
GAU	Aspartic acid	GCA	Alanine
GAC	Aspartic acid	GCG	Alanine
GAA	Glutamic acid	GCU	Alanine

These are complementary to the DNA codons from which they are transcribed. Most amino acids can be encoded by more than one sequence (methionine and tryptophan are exceptions). Three codons are "stop" codons.

like that of insects, plants, fungi, bacteria, and corporate lobbyists. This strongly supports a common origin for all earthly life.

GENE STRUCTURE

Generally, the stretch of DNA we call a gene codes for one protein chain, and it may be alternatively referred to as a *cistron*. The ultimate protein product may not be functional alone, but only after forming a *multimer,* or cluster of proteins, to form a single functional unit. The proteins that comprise a multimer may be the same, somewhat similar, or completely different.

Most mRNA messages undergo a great deal of "editing" before they are translated. The parts of genes that code for proteins, called *exons,* are interrupted by noncoding sequences known as *introns.* These are removed from the mRNA in an editing process termed *splicing.* Initially believed to be an evolutionary quirk, or randomly inserted junk, introns hold one key to the versatility of the human genome (Ast, 2005). Introns contain regulatory base sequences that determine whether adjacent exons are to be included or spliced out of the final mRNA product. As a result, different exons may be removed in different cell types, or under different environmental circumstances, to yield proteins that differ slightly—or greatly—in shape and function. The alternate message forms are called *splice variants.* When different splice variants give rise to different versions of the same protein, the different versions are called *isoforms.* Different isoforms of a single protein may also arise from different genes, however. A typical cistron includes about three alternative splice variants (Ast, 2005). The average protein-encoding gene is 28,000 base pairs in length and comprises 8.8 exons interspersed with 7.8 introns.

Another possible gene structure that merits mention is one whereby a single mRNA message is cut, or "cleaved," into multiple messages coding for two or more proteins. Often the proteins are related in function and may become part of the same multimer. Such genes and mRNA are termed *polycistronic.*

CHROMOSOMES AS GENE LIBRARIES

If we had a collection of blueprints for making more than 90,000 different items and needed to be able to quickly access any one of them, we would need a well-organized library. If the blueprints were genes, then the chromosomes constitute a readily accessible library (despite actually being somewhat randomly organized). Within the human cell nucleus, each of the 46 chromosomes (22 pairs of **autosomes** and 1 pair of sex chromosomes [XX or XY]) is composed of a single roughly meter-long DNA molecule, tightly coiled around scaffold proteins. Each chromosome houses perhaps 1,500 genes. **Homologous** pairs of chromosomes (i.e., containing the same genes) include one contributed by each parent. Thus, for any autosomal gene, there are two copies. Female individuals also have two copies of genes on the X chromosome, while males have only one. The thick, banded structures that we may think of as chromosomes (Figure 20-3) can be observed only during **mitosis** and **meiosis,** when they are packaged for efficient transfer. The banding patterns obtained by Giemsa staining (thus the designation "G bands") are quite constant and reproducible, allowing each chromosome to be identified visually, as is done in a routine clinical technique known as *karyotyping.* A general region of a chromosome is typically stipulated by its location on the long arm (q) or short arm (p) (Figure 20-4) and its proximity to a particular staining band. This is not specific, given that adjacent bands might be millions of base pairs apart. The physical location of a gene on a chromosome is referred to as a **locus** (plural, loci).

Other than the Y chromosome, there is no "theme" to any chromosome. The tens of thousands of genes required to make a human are strewn randomly across the 22 autosomes and the X chromosome. Evolution appears to have favored the retention of useful genes, but not to have necessarily discouraged extra DNA or the migration of genes to new locations in the genome. The Y chromosome is an interesting exception,

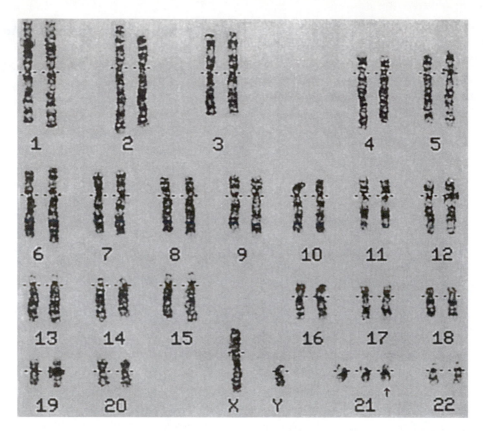

FIGURE 20-3   Karyotype of a normal male human includes 22 pairs of autosomes and 1 pair of sex chromosomes (X and Y). Banding patterns (G bands) reflect Giemsa staining and are highly reproducible.

apparently compressing the minimal set of genes that establish "maleness" (Note that there is no evidence for a "hogging the TV remote" locus.). The migration of genes involves large chunks of DNA. Nevertheless, comparison of human DNA with that of other mammals shows that many of the gene adjacencies are preserved, as if the human genome were cut into about 100 pieces and rearranged. Such regions of preserved gene order between species are called *syntenic.*

Not all genes in a cell reside on the nuclear chromosomes. Mitochondria, the organelles that produce most of the cell's energy, also house some of their own DNA (abbreviated mtDNA). Mitochondria are believed to have originated as separate organisms that invaded eukaryotic cells to form a mutually beneficial

relationship. The original mitochondrial genome may have included about 100 protein-, tRNA-, and rRNA-encoding genes, all but 37 of which have migrated over time to the nucleus (Fischel-Ghodsian, 2003). All of a person's mitochondria come from the egg (or *ovum*) and are inherited only from the mother. Most traits related to mitochondrial genes that have migrated to the nucleus are inherited in the same manner as other autosomal traits. Mitochondria present in the fertilized egg replicate (including their DNA) and are passed on to all cells of an organism. Over time, mitochondrial genes in adults undergo changes (mutations) that are passed on through replication, so that most cells end up with some degree of *heteroplasmy,* or genetic heterogeneity among their mitochondria.

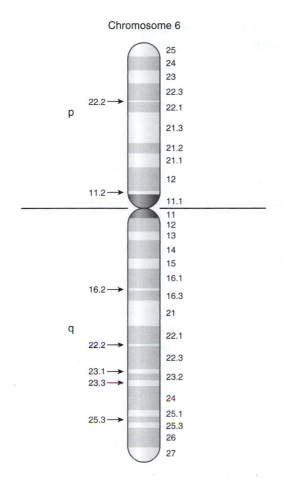

Chromosome 6

FIGURE 20-4 Schematic representation of normal human chromosome 6, showing characteristic G bands. p and q indicate *short* and *long* arms, respectively. These are also reproducible, so that a given locus is usually specified as to which arm it is on. (Adapted from Shprintzen, 1997.)

DNA INSTABILITY AND MUTATION

DNA is unstable. Virtually all human DNA is under constant assault from the environment; thus, repairs are constantly necessary to prevent the production of faulty proteins. The copying of DNA is also an error-prone process. Changes in the DNA code are termed *mutations* (see later). Mutations that occur as DNA is copied in meiosis, the sequence of cell divisions that give rise to make eggs and sperm, may

be inherited by any offspring. In addition, *somatic mutations* can arise early in development during the rapid period of cell mitosis (simple cell division). In that case, the effects of any mutation may be regionalized within the embryo.

Paradoxically, in the tendency of DNA toward mutation lies the keys to our diversity, our sophistication as a species, and many feared genetic diseases. Nucleic acids were probably among the earliest biomolecules produced by organic chemical reactions, and the first self-duplicating biomolecule. The capability of DNA and RNA to duplicate and recombine made them ideal to serve as the blueprints for building organisms. Yet, the error-prone nature of these processes has favored mutation, as well as the accumulation of "extra" DNA that formed the raw material of evolution. Over short periods—such as our lifetimes—we'd still prefer that our DNA remains as stable possible.

Are all mutations bad? *Mutation* simply means "change," and it is the nature of DNA to do so. The most common type of mutation is a single base change, or *substitution*. Let us consider the range of its possible effects. First, because only about 2% of the genome codes for protein, a substitution will most likely occur in a nontranscribed region (with potentially no effect) or a regulatory region. In the latter case, it may alter the amount of some protein that is made. If the substitution affects a protein-coding sequence, particularly if the substitution occurs within the first two base pairs of a codon, the result will probably be the insertion of a different amino acid (termed a *missense mutation*). Although proteins may be hundreds or thousands of amino acids long, not all amino acids contribute equally to function. Instead, there will be key locations in the chain that establish the overall shape, as well as critical locations for the reaction(s) or structural elements in which the protein is involved. DNA coding errors that result in amino acid substitutions at those sites will probably impair the function of the protein. Substitutions elsewhere may have little effect. Substitution may also give rise to an abnormal "stop" codon, leading the premature termination of an mRNA or eventual protein sequence (termed a *nonsense mutation*). These are typically degraded, and it is as if the protein were never made. These will typically be deleterious. Finally, some substitutions may shift the "reading frame" of some or all codons in the gene (hence they are *frameshift mutations*). This typically yields no mRNA, or one that is rapidly degraded. Not surprisingly, these also are usually harmful. Frameshifts are particularly likely in the event of another type of DNA copying error, wherein one or more extra bases are either added *(insertion errors)* or left out *(deletion errors)*.

As discussed earlier for base substitutions, insertions and deletions, the odds vastly favor that a mutation will be harmful, or at best, neutral. This is not really surprising. The genetic code humans carry is highly developed and specific. If we were to drop a fragile ceramic vase, the odds would greatly favor it breaking into many useless pieces. Just by chance, it might yield a potential bowl or soup spoon, but probably not. Yet suppose we could drop a million vases, or a billion vases. It is through the law of large numbers, the cumulative odds of unlikely events over ten thousands of years, that the potential benefits of mutations manifest themselves. Over such long periods, evolution and natural selection increase the prevalence of gene variants that yield benefits and reduce the prevalence of variants that are harmful, but they exert no pressure on variants that are neutral in their effect. The human genome is primarily a collection of random mutation "experiments" that produced benefit, or at least did no harm. Mutation is so relentless and pervasive that each person represents a virtually unique collection of gene variants, or **alleles,** across our genome. Sequence variations in some segment of DNA across a population are termed *polymorphisms*. Polymorphisms may confer health benefits (e.g., good vision, low hereditary risk for heart disease) or disease risk. Many physical features that distinguish individuals (e.g., shape of face, eye color, hair color) are the result of neutral polymorphisms, conferring no particular advantage. Because all polymorphisms began as mutations, we are all "mutants" in some way, and we think of the outward consequences of our genetic makeup simply as *traits*.

DUPLICATION AND RECOMBINATION ERRORS IN MEIOSIS

Errors in DNA duplication and **recombination** in the process of meiosis are responsible for most genetic diseases. During meiosis, 46 chromosomes in sperm and ovum are reduced to 23 (one of each pair), so that the egg will regain the normal complement on fertilization (Figure 20-5). This occurs because meiosis includes one DNA duplication phase but two division cycles. Mutations that arise during the DNA duplication stage will be passed on as newly arisen base sequences. Once sperm and ova are produced, their DNA remains susceptible to mutations that may be caused by environmental influences, including chemical mutagens and radiation. These mutations also will be passed on.

After the duplication phase, the homologous chromosomes (one from each parent) move into close apposition and randomly exchange stretches of base pairs in a process called *recombination* (see Figure 20-5). The alignment process itself is usually precise, so that homologous DNA sequences are swapped. The starting points of recombination are random, however. The swapping of base sequences can occur anywhere, although statistically, recombination typically will occur *between* gene coding sequences so that complete genes will tend to be exchanged.

Recombination of DNA in the process of sperm and egg production simply shuffles functional, viable DNA sequences passed on from the previous generation. Some form of recombination is virtually universal across all life-forms, and presumably developed because it is far more likely to create new possibilities and benefits than harm. However, errors can arise through faulty alignment of homologous chromosomes and improper separation after recombination. When these processes go awry, chromosomes can come away from recombination with large segments of extra DNA, backward DNA, or missing DNA. This situation is known as *chromosomal rearrangement* or *aneuploidy*, and as might be expected, it is usually catastrophic, because many genes may be affected.

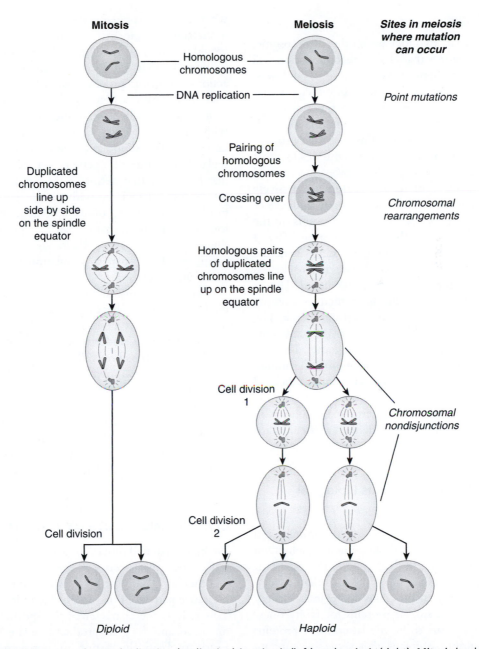

FIGURE 20-5 Schematic of DNA duplication (replication) in mitosis (left) and meiosis (right). Mitosis leads to daughter cells that are clones (exact DNA copies) of the original cell, and the normal (diploid) number of chromosomes is maintained. Meiosis allows for recombination of homologous chromosomes, leading to new DNA sequences. Errors in initial DNA copying stage lead to point mutations. Errors in separation of chromosomes after recombination lead to rearrangements (aneuploidy). Two sequential divisions after only one round of synthesis in meiosis lead to reduction of the normal chromosome number by half (haploid). Fertilization yields a diploid zygote.

Gene Linkage

The farther apart two loci are on the chromosome, the more likely it is that chance recombination will occur between them during meiosis. The lowest probability that this will occur is 0.5: Recombination will either occur or it will not, much like flipping a coin. Even multiple recombination sites between loci would not alter this probability (Imagine flipping multiple coins.). If we consider loci that are progressively closer together, however, we would see the probability of recombination progressively reduced to near zero. This is a direct consequence of the real physical connection between points on the same chromosome and the decreasing probability of recombination within small segments. Any time the probability of recombination between two loci is less than 0.5, they are said to be *linked*. This is spatial—not functional—linkage, which has nothing to do with what the genes in question encode. The particular alleles of linked genes carried by any individual will tend to be passed on together. The first gene "maps" were linkage maps, assembled through observation of which alleles tended to be inherited together. The first notions of distance along the chromosome were derived from recombination rates. One *centimorgan* (cM) is defined as the distance between loci that yields a 1% recombination rate.

Mutation "Hotspots" versus Biological Bottlenecks

If our genome codes for some 90,000 proteins and mutation is not an unusual phenomenon, why then are there not at least 90,000 genetic diseases? Is it because some genes are more unstable than others? Or is it because most processes and reactions allow for substitution of similar proteins for faulty ones? The answer appears to be the latter. Most proteins exist in multiple isoforms that serve overlapping functions. These may arise from editing of mRNA to include different introns (see earlier discussion), but often they are the product of completely different genes. Most of this functional redundancy presumably reflects the accumulation of extra gene copies over the course of evolution. Nevertheless,

whether any particular gene or protein will acquire interchangeable forms is a matter of chance. It would seem inevitable that there would remain bottlenecks, that is, important components and reactions requiring proteins for which there is no backup. Typically, when a genetic disease becomes well characterized, it is found that many people with the disease carry different mutations of the same gene. This supports the notion that it is the irreplaceable nature of a gene rather than any particular instability that defines a disease. It is true that for any gene associated with disease, certain mutations will be more common. Often, this will be found to arise from many cases being traceable to a single individual. This *founder effect* explains why members of an isolated population will carry the exact same mutation.

The notion of functional bottlenecks is particularly relevant to hearing. The cochlea contains many unique cell types, all of which perform some unique, if poorly understood, function. Moreover, our hearing is based on cellular specializations (e.g., stereocilia, tectorial membrane, molecules underlying outer hair cell motility) that appear nowhere else in the body. Such structures may never (or at least, not yet) become specified completely by genes that have functional "backups." Indeed, as deafness genes have been discovered, they disproportionately code for stereocilia and tectorial membrane components (see later).

CLASSIFYING TRAITS BY INHERITANCE

We have separated mutations according to the physical change that occurs at the level of base pairs. Another way to divide them is according to the inheritance pattern of the observable traits they cause. This reflects the character of the specific gene, the mutation, and the gene product (see later). It is necessary to clarify the distinction between the actual genetic makeup of an individual (**genotype**) and what would be observed (**phenotype**). Because one can be **homozygous** for a particular allele (both alleles the same) or **heterozygous** (two different alleles), the phenotype need not reflect the genotype.

Dominant and Recessive Traits

A trait is **dominant** if only one mutant allele is adequate to determine the phenotype. It is **recessive** if both alleles must include the mutation to affect the phenotype. For a dominant trait, it cannot be determined without testing whether an individual is heterozygous or homozygous, because heterozygotes do not present a separate phenotype. If one parent is heterozygous for a dominant allele and the other parent does not carry the allele, 50% of the children will be expected to carry the mutation and show the associated phenotype (Figure 20-6).

Several scenarios can give rise to a dominant trait. Sometimes a mutation in a gene encoding an enzyme does not merely inactivate the enzyme, but instead imparts the enzyme with a new function. The new function may be completely unrelated to the original function, and it may be either harmful or beneficial. Even one mutant allele coding for such an enzyme can cause a mutant phenotype. Alternatively, the gene may encode a protein that is normally inserted into a multimeric structure (such as a membrane channel). Faulty versions of one protein may be incorporated into the otherwise normal structure, rendering it nonfunctional. This will usually be deleterious.

Recessively inherited traits arise principally when an individual carries no functional copy of a gene and no compensatory genes or mechanisms cover the same function. For a recessive trait to be inherited, both parents must carry at least one allele for the trait. Parents will often be heterozygous, will not show the mutated phenotype, and are termed *carriers*. Assuming heterozygous parents, 25% of the children will be expected to carry both mutated alleles and show the phenotype (Figure 20-7).

Incomplete Dominance

Sometimes heterozygotes at a particular locus will show a phenotype that is intermediate between that of homozygotes for the mutated and nonmutated alleles. One way this can occur is when one normal copy of the gene cannot make enough of the product for the affected process to proceed normally. This is known as *haploinsufficiency*.

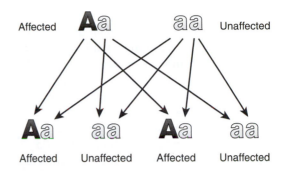

FIGURE 20-6 Autosomal dominant transmission of a trait *(A)*. Each parent carries two copies of the same gene, but one parent is heterozygous for the *A* allele. Half (50%) of the offspring are expected to be affected.

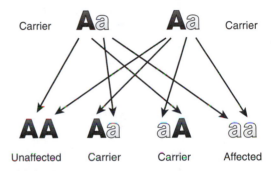

FIGURE 20-7 Autosomal recessive transmission of a trait *(a)*. In this scenario, each parent is heterozygous and is an unaffected carrier. One fourth (25%) of the offspring are expected to be homozygous for the *a* allele and to show the trait.

X-Linked Inheritance

Much more than the Y chromosome, the X chromosome contains genes that serve a broad range of functions and are vital for normal health. If an otherwise recessive mutation occurs on the X chromosome, female individuals will be unaffected, because they have another copy of the same gene. Male individuals, however, are *hemizygous* for genes on the X chromosome, meaning that they have only one copy. Male individuals will therefore show such traits as if they were dominant. X-linked traits are passed from mother to son.

Mitochondrial Inheritance

Mitochondrial inheritance is mentioned earlier in this chapter, but it is also included here to emphasize it as a distinct mode of inheritance. Mitochondrial genes are vital for cellular energy production. Mutations in the mitochondrial genome will typically be deleterious, but only for affected mitochondria and their replicative offspring. (Recall that mitochondria are replaced by simple division.) The phenotype of an individual will be affected only to the extent that critical cells carry mostly abnormal mitochondria. The scope of the effect will be most pronounced if the mother contributes abnormal mitochondrial genes to the egg, because these will be passed to all cells of the embryo after fertilization. Mitochondrial mutations can be passed from mother to both sons and daughters. Despite the universal need for an energy source among all cells, the effects of mitochondrial mutations appear to target particular tissues, including heart, skeletal muscle, and the cochlea.

VARIABILITY OF PHENOTYPE

Two individuals with mutations of the same gene often show somewhat different phenotypes. Unless the individuals are related, or come from the same isolated population, this will often be due to differences in the exact nature of the mutation itself. Changes in different base pairs will be expected to exert different effects on the functionality of the protein or gene product. Some changes might simply render a protein less than optimal, whereas others might make it totally nonfunctional. Mutations of regulatory genes may alter the amount of product that is made.

Even two people carrying exactly the same mutation can still exhibit different phenotypes. This will usually be due to the influence of *modifier genes.* Most traits do not follow simple inheritance rules (i.e., dominant, recessive, and so forth), but instead are strongly affected by multiple loci. Two people carrying the same mutation at one locus will nearly always possess different alleles of the modifier genes. These may partially compensate for some effects of mutation. Mutations and traits that are not readily modifiable are said to be highly **penetrant.**

Some mutations may exert their effects only in the presence of particular environmental triggers. In the case of genetically related, late-onset, or progressive hearing loss, exposure to ototoxic compounds or excessive noise may accelerate hearing loss or may be required for its initiation.

SYNDROMIC VERSUS NONSYNDROMIC GENETIC DISEASE

Some genetic defects can exert effects on multiple cell types or organs, causing multifaceted diseases known as **syndromes.** One way this can occur is through mutation of a single gene that is critical to the function of multiple tissues and cell types. More often, it involves disruption of many genes through chromosomal arrangement. Lying between these in scale are *contiguous gene syndromes,* which arise through loss or disruption of large segments of DNA, yet the alterations are too small to detect by karyotyping. Syndromes exhibit tremendous variability across individuals. The reasons for this are those described earlier (differences in mutation, different alleles of modifier genes), yet syndromes present the additional complication that each aspect of a syndrome (each affected tissue or organ) may have its own set of modifier genes. Thus, the broad presentation of any syndrome (degree of involvement of all affected tissues), may vary greatly, even for individuals with the same mutation. Because of their multifaceted phenotype, syndromes have been particularly amenable to characterization and linkage studies. Hearing loss has been listed as a component of more than 400 syndromes (Steel & Kros, 2001). These make up about 30% of all cases of genetic deafness (Bitner-Glindzicz, 2002).

IDENTIFYING GENETIC CAUSES OF DISEASE

Mutations of known or unknown genes that affect hearing will be diagnosed through a multistage process. The first requirements are recognition of the hearing loss itself and determination of other health problems that may indicate a syndrome. Environmental causes must be ruled out. The first step in genetic analysis typically involves *genetic mapping,* which is based on cosegregation of the deafness phenotype and known physical locations in the genome. There already exist many known deafness genes, with which the results of genetic mapping may be compared. This is called the *candidate gene* approach (Steel & Kimberling, 1995). Moreover, some well-characterized loci have already emerged as major causes of deafness. It may be advantageous to examine individuals with certain phenotypes for these mutations early in the characterization process.

If genetic mapping suggests a new mutation, it will be desirable ultimately to obtain the detailed gene sequence and nature of the mutation through a process of *physical mapping*. This has historically been an arduous process but will be greatly accelerated by the complete sequencing of the human and mouse genomes. Detailed knowledge of the sequence means that the gene product is also known, although not necessarily its function. However, the amino acid sequence can then be compared with vast computer databases of known proteins. Ideally, the ultimate result is the discovery of a new gene that impacts hearing via a known biochemical pathway.

Complementary Sequences as the Key to Mapping

Essentially all methods for isolating and tracking DNA rely on the binding of complementary sequences. A stretch of single-strand DNA with the base sequence T-A-G-C will bind to its complement A-T-C-G. If we wanted to know whether the T-A-G-C sequence was present in a DNA sample, we could synthesize many copies of the "probe" complementary sequence, "tag" them so that they could be measured or visualized, and add them to the sample. The mixture would then be heated to dissociate the two strands of the sample DNA. Binding of the labeled probe is then automatic. After any unbound probe is washed away, the presence of the target sequence is verified by measuring the amount of tag present. The tag may be radioactive, so that the measured radioactivity of the sample will indicate how much of the target is present, or it may be fluorescent, so that the intensity of fluorescence may be quantified. In reality, the target sequence sought will be hundreds or thousands of bases long. The probe may also be long, but only just long enough to provide binding that will be specific to the target sequence. The longer the probe, the fewer possible sequences that may be bound and labeled by accident.

The principle of complementary binding has found many uses. Even without knowing the location of a sequence of interest, a DNA sample can be probed to determine whether a particular mutation is present, or the presence of a mutation in a particular gene can be determined by how well the sample binds a normal sequence of that gene. Even single-base alterations can be detected by quantifying the strength of binding of the probe to the sample. Base mismatches will reduce the strength of binding, so that less heat is required to dissociate them. The more mismatches, the less heat required. Longer probes will increase the dissociation temperature.

Genetic Mapping

If a hearing loss is believed to be genetic, but there is no clear candidate gene, examining the inheritance pattern is the first step toward mapping. This method relies on the cosegregation of hearing loss and *genetic markers*. These are short DNA segments that are distributed at known locations roughly evenly throughout the genome, and that are known to be highly polymorphic. Within closely related groups, the sequence of any marker will be similar. A *pedigree* is assembled from as many closely related individuals as possible to form a linkage map, showing the pattern of transmission and establishing who is affected (Figure 20-8). DNA from the same population is then examined to determine which marker(s) cosegregates with the hearing loss. The marker(s) that show little or no recombination must be physically close to the mutated gene. How close? The distance depends on the number of subjects and samples that can be analyzed. More subjects and more linked markers provide better resolution. Isolated populations and consanguineous extended families are thus especially amenable to linkage analysis. The statistical significance of any indicated linkage is evaluated using the logarithm of odds ratio, or *LOD score* (Steel & Kimberling, 1996). LOD

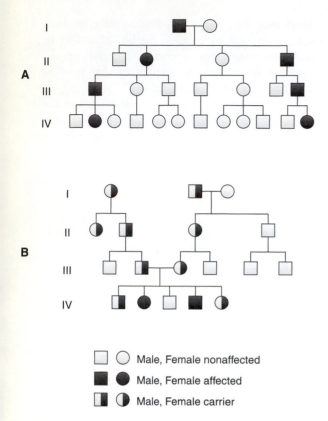

□ ○	Male, Female nonaffected
■ ●	Male, Female affected
◧ ◐	Male, Female carrier

FIGURE 20-8 Example pedigrees for autosomal dominant transmission of a trait (A) and autosomal recessive transmission (B). (A) Roughly half the offspring of affected individuals in each generation are affected. (B) Two families carrying the same trait intermarried in generation III. Among their five offspring in generation IV, two were carriers and two were affected.

scores of +3.00 or greater are taken to indicate significant linkage.

Physical Mapping

Genetic mapping in humans typically can localize a deafness gene only to within a few million base pairs, that is, a few centimorgans. That may be adequate when the indicated location reasonably matches a mutation known to affect hearing, so that a candidate gene approach can be applied. However, if there is no candidate gene, and a novel mutation is suspected, fine mapping and ultimately the

identification of the mutated sequence becomes the goal. This basically involves cutting the genome into progressively smaller pieces until a small fragment is found to contain the mutated sequence, followed by base-by-base sequencing of the fragment or comparison with an existing database. This process typically requires amplification of the sample, that is, making more copies for analysis. There are several methods for this. Some entail inserting the fragments into bacteria or yeast cells. When this is done appropriately, the DNA replication machinery of these organisms is fooled into copying the DNA of interest as they multiply. A powerful, cell-free method is the polymerase chain reaction, in which short sequences are mixed with DNA-building enzymes and single nucleotide bases to provide raw material. The mixture is then repeatedly heated and cooled. Each cycle doubles the amount of the desired sequence. This exponential growth allows tremendous amplification in a short time. All methods for copying DNA are collectively referred to as *cloning.* Cloned organisms, by extension, are those carrying the exact same DNA.

Hearing-Related Genes as Candidate Genes

At least hypothetically, another strategy for identifying candidate genes merits discussion. Suppose we knew all the genes that play a role in hearing. Couldn't we then simply compare all mutations against the sequence of those genes? That is possible, but there are too many caveats for it to have played a large role thus far. Because all cells of the body have the same DNA, yet there are many cell types, it is clearly the pattern of gene *expression* that differentiates cells. Gene expression can be tracked by isolating all the mRNA within a cell. Recall that these no longer match the original gene sequence, because all introns have been removed. Nevertheless, these can be *reverse transcribed* into the complementary DNA (cDNA) sequence and used to probe the genome for homologies within exons. Another ingenious trick has been to subtractively compare cDNA samples from different tissues. In this way, it has been possible to identify genes that are expressed only in the cochlea, and thus are particularly promising candidate deafness genes.

Cochlea-specific mRNAs can then be localized to particular cell types by *in situ hybridization,* in which fluorescently labeled tags are applied that bind to mRNAs of interest. The cells that express these mRNAs can then be visualized under a microscope. A frequent complication is that cells do not exist in one state only. Different mRNA profiles will be expressed in any cell as a function of development, stress condition, or disease state. Some genes that are critical during development are not expressed in the developing ear, but rather in adjacent tissues. Some important mRNAs may still exist at levels too low to be detected. Finally, although examining mRNA profiles in animals, especially mice, has provided valuable insights into human genetic deafness, the gene expression profile will not be identical. No perfect substitute for human mRNA expression profiles exists. Particularly given that mRNA rapidly degrades, this work has progressed slowly.

Value of Mouse Models in Gene Characterization

Our growing understanding of mouse hearing and deafness, and of the mouse genome, has greatly accelerated the search for human deafness genes. The mouse cochlea functions like the human cochlea. Moreover, when mice show genetic or environmental hearing loss, typically the same type of pathology is found as in the human cochlea. Inbred mouse strains, which result from at least 20 generations of brother × sister matings, are for all practical purposes clones. By working within a strain, variability of results due to uncontrolled genetic variance is essentially eliminated. The value of mice was first demonstrated in the discovery and evaluation of animals with spontaneous deafness mutations in large commercial colonies. Until recently, no large-scale national screening effort had been attempted, so most such discoveries were made because caretakers noticed unusual behaviors, such as circling. Many mutations that affect hearing also affect the vestibular system, so that most of the early models included defects in both systems. When such mice are discovered, they are carefully bred to reproduce the trait and determine its inheritance

pattern. Establishing pedigrees and performing genetic analysis can be done extremely efficiently in mice, because large numbers of offspring can be created and obscuring genetic variation can be minimized. Whereas the typical resolution limit of linkage analysis in humans is about 1.0 cM, in mice it can be as little as 0.1 cM. Several naturally occurring mouse deafness mutations have eventually been found to have human homologs. Simultaneous mapping and sequencing of the mouse and human genomes has promoted leap-frog–style gains, whereby new knowledge in one rapidly leads to new knowledge in the other.

The greatest value of mice for hearing research currently lies in scientists' ability to create mutations in candidate genes and evaluate the resulting phenotypes. The importance of a gene for cochlear development or function can be tested by making a *knockout* mouse, which carries two completely nonfunctional alleles. Whether more of a particular molecule is harmful or beneficial can be tested by making a *transgenic* mouse, which may carry several extra copies of a gene. Whether a particular allele of a human or mouse gene exerts a dominant effect can also be tested in this way. Especially when the gene in question codes for a protein fundamental for cell survival, knockout and transgenic mouse models will resemble their human counterparts. Often, differences are found, although these too are frequently informative. Regardless of whether a particular gene is thought to be involved in deafness, its function can be examined using these methods; therefore, knockout and transgenic models are an important tool for basic scientists. Sometimes the addition or inactivation of a gene is found to be lethal, or the experimental question addresses a particular stage of development. In such circumstances, conditional mutations may be engineered, wherein the mutation is activated only at certain times or in certain tissues.

NAMING CONVENTIONS FOR GENES

As human deafness loci are discovered, they are given names that are systematic but may appear opaque to nongeneticists. The most reasonable way to name any gene would be according to its function. However, that is essentially never known at the time of discovery. Basic scientists in genetics have—and often take—the opportunity to name new genes in humorous reference to the phenotype (e.g., *noggin, ether-a-go-go, wocko*) or something more whimsical. Mouse deafness genes usually have been given more or less meaningful names that also referred to the phenotype (e.g., *shaker, deafness, whirler, age-related hearing loss*), but these names generally have not followed any system. Syndromic human deafness genes are initially named for the syndrome (e.g., PDS [Pendred]; USH [Ushers]; BSND [Bartter]). The names of nonsyndromic human deafness genes always begin with "DFN," followed by a one character designation for the mode of inheritance ("A" for dominant; "B" for recessive) and a number, according to the order of mapping. Modifier genes are designated DFNM, followed by the order of mapping. When the function of a gene becomes known, it is renamed by consensus. Thus, when it was determined that DFNB1 coded for a particular form of membrane channel protein known as connexin, the gene was renamed *CX26*. As new alleles of a gene are discovered, they are designated by superscripts. One complexity in terminology is introduced by the fact that some alleles can lead to dominant inheritance, whereas other alleles of the same gene are recessive. Also, for some genes, different alleles can be associated with either syndromic or nonsyndromic deafness. Thus, a deafness gene often cannot be simply described as syndromic or nonsyndromic. Only particular alleles may be associated with a syndrome.

FUNCTIONAL CLASSIFICATION OF GENETIC DEAFNESS

Before considering specific deafness genes and mutations, it may be useful first to consider how these may generally affect the appearance and function of the cochlea. Despite the tremendous number of known mutations that impact hearing, these fall into a surprisingly small number of general patterns with regard to the cell types most affected (Steel, 1995).

Morphogenetic

During early development, certain genes are important for establishing the boundaries of the cochlear capsule and the membranous labyrinth. Mutations promoting *morphogenetic defects* will lead to wholesale disruption in the layout of the cochlea and its epithelia. In such cases, hearing is never normal, or never present. Morphogenetic defects often appear as part of a syndrome.

Neuroepithelial

Neuroepithelial defects include all abnormalities of the organ of Corti. They are progressive and degenerative in nature, and often principally involve hair cells. Hair cells may be present initially, but degenerate thereafter. Typically, hearing is never normal. Cochlear cells are interdependent, such that loss of one cell type can promote loss of another. Defects of supporting cells and even fibrocytes within the spiral ligament can promote hair cell loss. The degeneration pattern thus may not reliably indicate which cell type is directly impacted by mutation.

Cochleosaccular

Cochleosaccular defects involve an abnormal distribution of *melanocytes* during development. These cells, named for their production of *melanin,* migrate during development to specific regions of the embryo. Within the ear, they locate within the stria vascularis to become the strial intermediate cells. Melanocytes sometimes fail to migrate to the correct locations, although in a highly variable and unpredictable way. An affected individual may have one cochlea with an abnormal stria (thus monaural hearing loss), patchy depigmentation of hair and skin, plus one blue and one brown eye. This can occur because the cochlear stria, epidermis, and the iris of the eye are all developmentally related and contain melanocytes. In the affected ear, the stria is dystrophic, Reissner's membrane is collapsed onto the organ of Corti, and there is no endocochlear potential. Eventually, the organ of Corti degenerates. The saccule is also affected, probably because it relies on the cochlear duct for endolymph production. Note that cochleosaccular defects (also called *pigmentation defects*) are distinct from albinism, in which melanocytes are normal but produce no melanin and which is not associated with hearing loss.

MAJOR KNOWN DEAFNESS GENES

To stay current with the most recently discovered deafness genes, clinicians are urged to frequently seek out reviews within the audiologic and medical literature. Rather than attempt to present a comprehensive or current list, this section considers particularly instructive or prevalent mutations for which the gene product is known (Tekin, Amos, & Pandya, 2001; Bittner-Glindzicz, 2002; Van Laer et al., 2003; Freidman et al., 2003; Fischel-Ghodsian, 2003; Ohlemiller, Vogler, Daly, & Sands, 2001; Steel & Kros, 2001).

Connexin 26 (CX26/DNFA3/DFNB1)

The connexins are a family of membrane channels that directly connect cells electrically, effectively rendering them as continuous compartments for particles of certain size. During transduction, potassium flows into hair cells from scala media and out through their basolateral walls. This potassium could be "recycled," if it could be shuttled back to the stria vascularis. Moreover, if it remains in the extracellular space around the hair cells in sufficiently high concentrations, it is believed to be toxic to these cells. Accordingly, supporting cells in the organ of Corti appear connected by a junctional network that shuttles potassium to the spiral ligament. When defective subunits are incorporated, the operation of the channel is impaired and neuroepithelial degeneration results. Mutations in other potassium channel genes, including CX30, CX31, KCNQ4, KVLQT1, and KCNE1, may cause deafness through a similar mechanism. Different alleles of CX26 can cause either dominant or recessive and either syndromic or nonsyndromic deafness. Up to 50% of recessively inherited nonsyndromic deafness may be due to this gene. Specific screening for mutations of CX26 may therefore be appropriate when recessive genetic deafness of unknown origin is encountered.

Unconventional Myosins (MYO7A/USH1B; MYO15/DFNB3)

Myosins are proteins that generate motion, in combination with actin. Mutations in genes coding for at least two "unconventional" myosins (VIIA and XV) appear critical for hair cell stereocilia function and are associated with deafness. In the cochlea, neuroepithelial degeneration is observed. MYO7A is also expressed in the retina and has been found to underlie one of the more severe forms of Usher's syndrome.

Harmonin (USH1C/DFNB18)

Harmonin is a "PDZ domain" protein, meaning that it plays a key role in the organization of multimeric structures. Harmonin and MYO7A (see earlier) may play a role in stereocilia formation and function, which may explain why both are involved in forms of Usher's syndrome.

Cadherin 23 (CDH23/USH1D/DFNB12)

Cadherin 23 is one of a class of proteins (the cadherins) that mediates many cellular interactions from signaling to simple mechanical anchoring. Cadherin 23, or otocadherin, plays a currently little understood role in stereocilia formation and stabilization. In mice, the *ahl* allele (*Cdh23^{ahl}*) promotes both age-related hearing loss and noise injury. It is not clear whether there is an allele that has a similar effect in humans.

Pendred Syndrome (PDS/SLC26A4/DFNB4)

The hallmarks of Pendred syndrome are autosomal recessive congenital deafness and goiter. SLC26A4 (pendrin) is a chloride transporter expressed in the endolymphatic duct that may be involved in endolymph homeostasis. Some mutations in the gene encoding this protein lead to nonsyndromal fluctuating hearing loss with frequent vestibular involvement.

Transcription Factor POU4F3 (DFNA15)

POU4F3 appears to be required for hair cell survival. It was the first gene found to be associated with delayed onset progressive hearing loss. Neuroepithelial degeneration becomes sufficiently severe to cause hearing loss by about age 20.

Waardenburg's Syndrome (PAX3/WSI/WS3; SOX10/WS4)

Waardenburg's syndrome encompasses a diverse set of pathologies, all involving cochleosaccular (pigmentation) defects. Accordingly, the phenotype often includes abnormal pigmentation of skin, hair, and the iris of the eye. Mutations in transcription factors PAX3 and SOX10 account for at least three forms of this syndrome.

Mucopolysaccharidosis (MPSI/Hurler syndrome; MPSVII/Sly syndrome; MPSII/Hunter syndrome; MPSIV/ Morquio syndrome)

The mucopolysaccharidoses (MPSs) are a class of at least 11 autosomal recessive conditions that involve the inability to degrade extracellular matrix molecules known as *glycosaminoglycans* (GAGs). These mediate cell–cell adhesion and other interactions in many organs, including the cochlea. Each form of MPS entails mutation and dysfunction of an enzyme normally involved in the degradation of a particular GAG. Incompletely degraded GAGs build up within organelles called *lysosomes,* which normally serve to recycle damaged cellular components. Unable to complete the degradation cascade, lysosomes become engorged, cellular metabolic and mechanical properties are altered, and cell–cell adhesion is abnormal. All MPSs lead to early and progressive hearing loss that may be conductive or mixed sensorineural/conductive, although degeneration and sensory cell loss may never occur. The MPSs are syndromes and may also include enlargement of liver and spleen, skeletal abnormalities, impaired vision, mental retardation, and shortened life span.

COCH/DNFA9

Mutations in the *COCH* gene lead to late-onset, progressive neuroepithelial degeneration and vestibular defects. Symptoms may outwardly resemble Ménière's disease. The COCH protein is one of the extracellular matrix proteins that make up cochlear connective tissues such as the spiral ligament and may be the most abundant cochlear protein.

Alpha Tectorin (TECTA/DFNA8/DFNA12/DFNB21)

Alpha tectorin is one of the key constituent proteins of the tectorial membrane. Disruption of the *TECTA* gene leads to neuroepithelial degeneration.

Collagens (COL4A3, COL4A2, COL4A5/Alport syndrome; COL2A1, COL11A1, COL11A2/ Stickler syndrome/Marshal syndrome)

Collagens are a diverse set of proteins that make up most of the extracellular matrix, including spiral ligament, basilar membrane, tectorial membrane, and spiral limbus. Genetic abnormalities of collagen formation and degradation may promote sensorineural hearing loss without actual degeneration and cell loss, and thus depart somewhat from the more common neuroepithelial pattern.

Mitochondrial Ribosomal RNA 12S

The A1555G mutation in the mtRNA 12S gene has received much attention for the manner in which it operates. Because it is mitochondrial, the associated hearing loss is maternally inherited. In addition, the mutation renders the gene similar to bacterial rRNA; therefore, affected individuals may be particularly susceptible to aminoglycoside antibiotics.

ᴄ:SUMMARY:ᴐ

Although therapies to correct or prevent genetic hearing loss are not yet available, identifying the specific genetic defect causing deafness in a patient can provide a prognosis and assist its management. In cases of congenital deafness, identifying a genetic cause can help couples anticipate the likelihood that their other children may also be affected. Some mutations may promote primarily conductive hearing loss, and thus be more amenable to hearing aids, whereas some mutations that promote inner ear de-generation may be incompatible with cochlear implantation. Understanding the genetic causes of deafness can aid in determining the most appropriate course of treatment. Parents facing hearing loss in a child will often be overwhelmed by surrounding medical issues and the dense terminology of genetics. By keeping current on the genes and mechanisms of genetic deafness, and by serving as translators of the language of genetics, audiologists can help these parents plan and cope.

ᴄ:KEY TERMS:ᴐ

Allele	Gene	Mitosis	Ribosome
Amino acid	Genotype	mRNA	RNA
Autosomes	Heterozygous	Penetrance	Syndrome
Chromosome	Homology	Phenotype	Transcription
DNA	Homozygous	Protein	Translation
Dominant	Locus	Recessive	X-linkage
Enzyme	Meiosis	Recombination	

ᴄ:STUDY QUESTIONS:ᴐ

1. Describe the roles of DNA, mRNA, rRNA, and tRNA.

2. Define transcription and translation.

3. In addition to proteins, what else can genes code for?

4. Why might different base substitution mutations that lead to different amino acid substitutions yield different phenotypes?

5. What is the physical basis of gene linkage?

6. Describe the notion of how mechanistic "bottlenecks" may determine what genetic diseases humans experience.

7. Describe two ways a dominant trait may arise.

8. Why are traits determined by mtDNA maternally inherited?

9. Name two reasons why individuals with mutations in the same gene might show different phenotypes.

10. Contrast neuroepithelial and cochleosaccular pathologies.

⌁REFERENCES⌁

Ast, G. (2005). The alternative genome. *Scientific American, 292,* 58–65.

Bitner-Glindzicz, M. (2002). Hereditary deafness and phenotyping in humans. *British Medical Bulletin, 63,* 73–94.

Fischel-Ghodsian, N. (2003). Mitochondrial hearing loss. *Ear and Hearing, 24,* 303–313.

Freeland, S. J., & Hurst, L. D. (2004). Evolution encoded. *Scientific American, 290,* 84–91.

Friedman, T. B., Schultz, J. M., Ben-Josef, T., Pryor, S. P., Lagziel, A., Fisher, R. A., Wilcox, E. R., Riazuddin, S., Ahmed, Z. M., Belyantseva, I. A., & Griffith, A. J. (2003). Recent advances in the understanding of syndromic forms of hearing loss. *Ear and Hearing, 24,* 289–302.

Hayes, D., & Northern, J. L. (1996). *Infants and hearing.* San Diego: Singular Publishing.

Kelly, T. E. (1986). *Clinical genetics and genetic counseling.* Chicago, IL: Year Book Medical Publishing.

Mattick, J. S. (2004). The hidden genetic program of complex organisms. *Scientific American, 291,* 61–67.

Modell, B., & Modell, M. (1992). *Towards a healthy baby: Congenital disorders and the new genetics in primary health care.* London: Oxford University Press.

Ohlemiller, K. K., Vogler, C. A., Daly, T. M., & Sands, M. S. (2001). Preventing sensory loss in a mouse model of lysosomal storage disease. In: J. F. Willott (Ed.), *Handbook of mouse auditory research: From behavior to molecular biology* (pp. 581–601). New York: CRC Press.

Shprintzen, R. J. (1997). *Genetics, syndromes, and communication.* San Diego: Singular Publishing.

Steel, K. P. (1995). Inherited hearing defects in mice. *Annual Review of Genetics, 29,* 675–701.

Steel, K. P., & Kimberling, W. (1995). Approaches to understanding the molecular genetics of hearing and deafness. In T. Van De Water, A. N. Popper, & R. R. Fay (Eds.), *Clinical aspects of hearing* (pp. 10–40). New York: Springer.

Steel, K. P., & Kros, C. J. (2001). A genetic approach to understanding auditory function. *Nature Genetics, 27,* 143–149.

Tekin, M., Amos, K. S., & Pandya, A. (2001). Advances in hereditary deafness. *Lancet, 358,* 1082–1090.

Van Laer, L., Cryns, K., Smith, R. J. H., & Van Camp, G. (2003). Nonsyndromic hearing loss. *Ear and Hearing, 24,* 275–288.

⌁SUGGESTED READING⌁

Gorlin, R. J., Toriello, H. V., & Cohen, M. M. (1995). *Hereditary hearing loss and its syndromes.* New York: Oxford University Press.

Martini, A., Read, A., & Stephens, D. (Eds.). (1996). *Genetics and hearing impairment.* San Diego: Singular.

Schuknecht, H. F. (1993). *Pathology of the ear.* Philadelphia: Lea and Febiger.

Willott, J. F. (Ed.). (2001). *Handbook of mouse auditory research: From behavior to molecular biology.* New York: CRC Press.

Chapter

~:21:~

Age-Related Hearing Loss

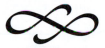

Kevin K. Ohlemiller, Ph.D.
Associate Professor of Otolaryngology
Washington University School of Medicine
St. Louis, Missouri

If we are privileged to live long enough, the outward signs of aging become our hard-earned, and dubious, reward. Many of the hallmarks of aging, such as gray hair and redistribution of body fat, are largely without health implications (although perhaps harmful to our vanity). Such large-scale changes, however, reflect fundamental cellular changes that eventually promote decline; thus, there is a fine line between "normal" aging and age-related health complications. At sufficiently advanced ages, there is little distinction. In the case of hearing and aging, the criteria for significant pathology are straightforward: Is hearing sensitivity affected? Is auditory perception, particularly speech perception, affected? And most importantly, is the quality of life reduced? For at least 40% of people

older than 65 years, and the majority of those older than 75, the answer to these questions is "Yes" (Figures 21-1 and 21-2). This proportion may be expected to grow as baby boomers age. Age-related hearing loss, or **presbycusis,** is the major form of hearing loss and the major neurodegenerative disease of aging. In coming years, it may preoccupy most audiologists. This chapter attempts to place presbycusis into the larger context of cellular aging and cell loss. Then the contribution of various cell types to hearing loss, focusing on the cochlea, is considered. Within the cochlea, changes in three separate structures or populations appear to have the most dramatic effect on hearing, and they form the basis for distinct classes of presbycusis, as proposed by H. Schuknecht (1964, 1974; Schuknecht & Gacek,

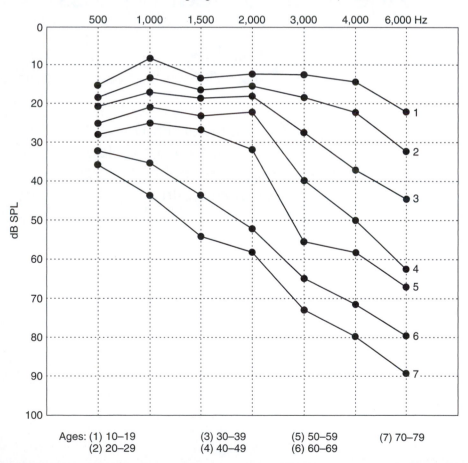

FIGURE 21-1 Median thresholds in decibels sound pressure level for men by age-group. (Adapted from Glorig et al., 1957.)

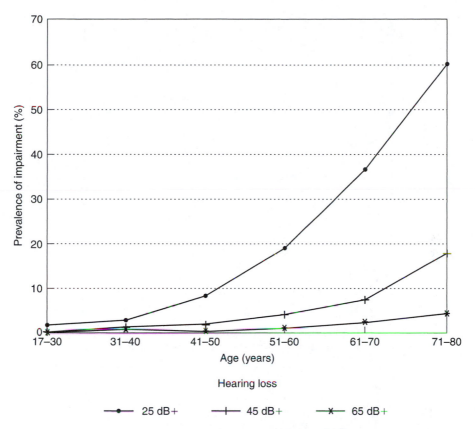

FIGURE 21-2 Prevalence of hearing loss versus age, taken from a study in Great Britain. Thresholds were averaged at 0.5, 1.0, 2.0, and 4.0 kHz for each subject. (Adapted from Davis, 1989.)

1993). These structures are hair cells and organ of Corti (the principal affected structures in **sensory presbycusis**), afferent neurons (the basis of **neural presbycusis**), and stria vascularis (the focus of **strial presbycusis**). Although changes in both pinna and middle ear are thought to contribute somewhat to presbycusis, their influence is probably dwarfed by changes in the cochlea. The definition of presbycusis is not limited to the periphery, however; therefore, essential aspects of **central presbycusis** also are considered in this chapter.

AGING AS A CELLULAR PROCESS

If any one of a host of critical cell types in the body, including muscle fibers, neurons, fibrocytes (which maintain connective tissue), and osteocytes (which maintain bone), were to be quantified, some degree of reduction with age would be found. This certainly applies to the cochlea, wherein progressive loss of neurons, hair cells, and other cell types is well documented (Figure 21-3). The outward signs of aging of any tissue may simply become apparent as constituent cells fall below some threshold, in terms of both number and functionality.

Intrinsic versus Extrinsic Aging Processes

Three widely recognized basic cellular mechanisms could lead to age-related cell loss in the cochlea and elsewhere: (1) progressive homeostatic imbalance, (2) **programmed aging,** and (3) limits on cell division. These mechanisms may act in the same cells, although the third mechanism will

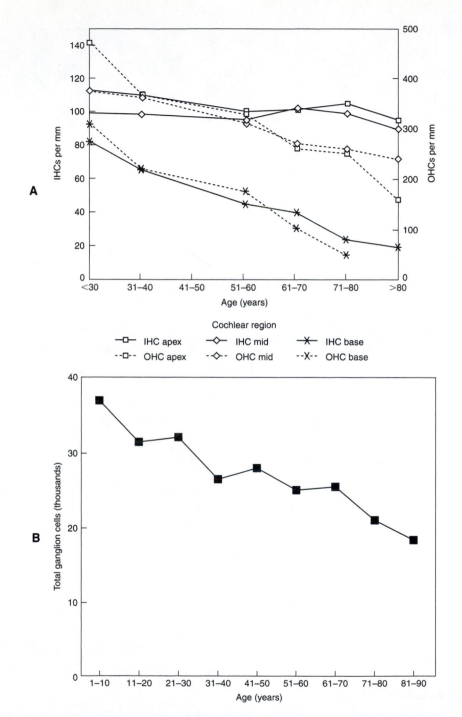

FIGURE 21-3 (A) Inner (IHC) and outer hair cell (OHC) density versus age in the basal, middle, and apical regions of the cochlea. Data were pooled across subjects of varying hearing ability. (Adapted from Bredberg, 1968.) (B) Total spiral ganglion cells versus age. (Adapted from Otte, et al., 1978.)

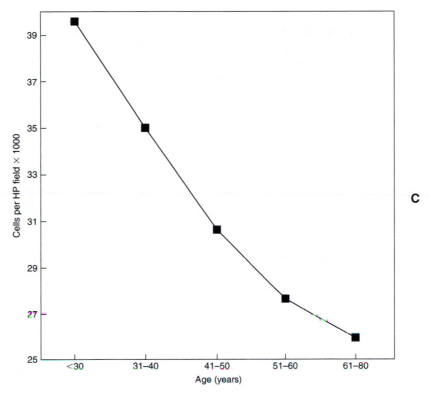

C

FIGURE 21-3, cont'd   (C) Density of fibrocytes in the cochlear spiral ligament versus age. Subjects had no known hearing impairment. (Adapted from Wright & Schuknecht, 1972.)

apply only to the minority of cells that continue to divide into adulthood. The first mechanism, pertaining to **homeostasis** (maintenance of an optimal internal state), particularly emphasizes environmental influences and gene-environment interactions, and it is probably most relevant to presbycusis. Progressive disruption of the ability of sensory cells to maintain homeostasis may magnify the impact of environmental stressors later in life, leading to an accumulation of cellular injury (e.g., Richardson and Holbrook, 1996).

If we could somehow eliminate all sources of stress and injury, could we stop the aging process? Such questions can really only be addressed in simple model organisms (such as fruit flies) or in cell culture, and in any event, disagreement remains on this point. Some evidence supports the notion that cells contain an intrinsic genetic program that shuts

down transcription of whole sets of genes over time, leading eventually to destabilization and death (see Seidman, Ahmad, & Bai, 2002). If this is the case, what serves as the "clock," telling cells when to launch the program? Casual observation reveals there can be no fixed life span for any cell type. Consider, for example, that humans and mice have significantly different life spans (~75 vs ~3 years); yet, near the end of their life spans, they show a similar cochlear pathology, including hair cell loss. Suppose the expected life for an uninjured outer hair cell were 65 years, regardless of species. We can readily see why a typical human might begin to lose hair cells after a few decades, but why would a mouse do so in less than 3 years? The cells and their immediate environment are essentially the same in humans and mice (and mice probably have a healthier lifestyle!). The major difference is that basal **metabolic rate** is much lower for large animals than for small animals. Any programmed aspect of aging must be normalized to an organism's metabolic rate, and rate of oxygen consumption (Barda, 2002). This suggests that such a program is driven by stress and injury generated as a by-product of metabolism, and it is unlikely to be completely intrinsic or automatic.

Among those cells that retain the capacity for **mitosis** (division) throughout the life of an organism, there are restrictions. Even under optimal conditions, any cell type appears to undergo only a fixed number of divisions. Such observations have led to theories of aging based on inherent limitations on the number of times chromosomes may be copied (see Seidman et al., 2002). This mechanism of aging appears most relevant to tissues that emphasize cell replacement over repair. Although it may have some applicability to cochlear aging, its meaning for actual age-related *hearing loss* is less clear (see later for further discussion).

Cellular Injury by Oxidative Stress

If much of aging is based on cellular injury, to what kind of injury are cells subject? Topping the list is **oxidative stress.** It is paradoxical that oxygen is the best friend and worst enemy of most living cells. The evolution of aerobic (oxygen-based) metabolism made it possible for cells to increase their energy consumption and their range of activities. Oxygen is useful precisely because of its ability to break down carbon-carbon and carbon-hydrogen chemical bonds, the types of bonds that form biomolecules. One can immediately see, however, why this might also present a problem. Cells use oxygen to break down raw materials to form their own constituents and to fuel energy production, but they must avoid being oxidized themselves. Inevitably, some oxidative attack on cellular DNA, proteins, and lipids does occur. In fact, it never stops, and it is exacerbated by nearly any type of environmental stress. The observation that most injury to cells appears to be oxidative lends prominence to the Free Radical Theory of Aging, first proposed by Harman (1956). This theory asserts that aging is basically progressive oxidation.

Metaphors that compare human aging with rusting are therefore partly correct (at least with regard to the basic chemistry of aging).

Aspects of the Free Radical Theory appear applicable to presbycusis. In the cochlea, oxidative stress is increased by noise, ototoxins, and ischemia (Evans & Halliwell, 1999; Kopke, Allen, Henderson, Hoffer, Frenz & Van De Water, 1999). The main targets of attack appear to be hair cells. This makes sense, in that oxidative injury will tend to occur at interfaces between the body and the environment, that is, at the point where energy in the environment is converted into excitation of sensory cells. As discussed in Chapter 10, hair cells convert mechanical energy to electrical excitation. This process inescapably exposes hair cells to mechanical trauma and metabolic stress.

Aerobic cells, including those in the cochlea, have evolved to fend off oxidative attack in several ways: First, key reactions involving oxygen are quarantined to a particular organelle, the **mitochondrion.** Inevitably, however, reactive oxygen-containing molecules (better known as **reactive oxygen species** [ROS]), "escape" the intended reactions and boundaries. Cells also reduce oxidative injury by producing or taking up **antioxidants,** which either catalyze reactions that remove ROS or serve as "decoys" for ROS. However, no amount of antioxidants appears able to eliminate oxidative injury. Within the cochlea, this has been reinforced by many experiments aimed at pharmacologically or genetically enhancing cochlear antioxidant defenses (Ohlemiller, 2003).

Mitochondrial Limits on Cell Maintenance

Cells possess a host of self-repair mechanisms. So why should injury accumulate? The limiting component may be the mitochondria (Sastre, Pallardo, De La Asuncion, & Vina, 2000). Unique among organelles, mitochondria house their own DNA. This DNA codes for many essential components of energy production, but it does not code for extensive protective or repair components. In addition, the packing of mitochondrial DNA does not offer the same degree of protection as that of nuclear DNA (DNA within the cell nucleus). Damage to mitochondrial DNA also means that new mitochondria will carry the same errors, because new mitochondria come from replication of the old. Finally, as stated earlier, reactions that are conducted in mitochondria create most of the cell's ROS. All of these factors may combine to promote the accumulation of DNA errors within individual mitochondria, so that overall energy production is reduced, and the function of the entire cell is impaired. This view of aging, known as the **mitochondrial clock theory** (see Seidman, 2000) is perhaps a corollary to the Free Radical Theory, because most of the injury presumably arises from oxidative stress. As in many tissues, accumulation of mitochondrial DNA mutations with age has been observed in the cochlea (Pickles, 2004). This accumulation can be reduced by both antioxidants and **caloric restriction** (Seidman, 2000), which primarily slows metabolism. Such evidence supports a role in presbycusis for cumulative mitochondrial damage through oxidative injury.

Limitations on Cell Repair and Replacement

Tissues that have sustained some degree of injury might fend off cell loss by replacement of constituent cells by mitosis, or cell division. Unfortunately, only a few cell types are normally replaced in adult mammals. Most neurons are not replaced, neither are cochlear hair cells nor most other specialized cells of the organ of Corti and stria vascularis. Such cells are referred to as **postmitotic.** This limitation places a premium on protective and repair capabilities, yet cochlear sensory cells do not appear ideally equipped in this regard. Histologic indications of age-related pathology of sensory cells include accumulation of **lipofuscin** (sometimes referred to as "age pigment"), which may indicate impaired protein degradation and recycling processes. Clumping of hair cell stereocilia and deformation of the cuticular plate can be seen, suggesting that nonfunctional hair cells can survive for some time (e.g., Scholtz, Kammen-Jolly, Felder, Hussl, Rask-Andersen, & Schrott-Fischer, 2001). Throughout the organ of Corti, cells with darkened nuclei and cytoplasm can be observed (e.g., Ohlemiller & Gagnon, 2004a). It is unclear which cells showing

these signs go on to die, or whether supporting cell pathology can promote hair cell loss.

Among those cochlear cells that can be replaced, restrictions exist. Many sensory cells are capable of replacement, including olfactory receptors, taste buds, mechanoreceptors in the skin, and even vestibular hair cells (Warchol, Lambert, Goldstein, Forge, & Corwin, 1993). Within the cochlea, however, cell replacement appears limited to fibrocytes of the lateral wall and some cells of the stria vascularis (e.g., Conlee, Gerrity, & Bennett, 1994; Dunaway, Mhaskar, Armour, Whitworth, & Rybak, 2003). Still, these decrease in number with age. Such cells are believed to serve a distributed function and are initially present in larger-than-needed numbers, so that modest losses may have little effect on hearing.

CLASSIFYING PRESBYCUSIS

Presbycusis is not a single entity, but many. How to subdivide presbycusis in a way that is diagnostically and prognostically meaningful has remained a debated issue. To understand the causes of presbycusis, and thereby promote its prevention and treatment, researchers and clinicians have taken the approach of subdividing it according to either possible cause or the pattern of cellular pathology.

Classifying Presbycusis by Cause

Attempts have been made to divide presbycusis into multiple environmentally linked components, plus a hypothetical "pure" aging component (see Willott, 1991). Environmental risk factors for presbycusis may include chronic noise exposure, ototoxic medications, occupational exposure to toxic gases and solvents, smoking, head trauma, increased blood lipid levels, hypertension, and cardiovascular disease (e.g., see Fransen, Lemkens, Van Laer, & Van Camp, 2003). All these may promote injury to sensory cells, either through direct trauma, metabolic stress, or ischemia-like effects, so that most presbycusis is viewed by some as mechanistically indistinguishable from other acquired hearing loss. According to this view, genetic factors that promote presbycusis will include those that cripple cellular defensive and repair processes. Some risk factors (e.g., cardiovascular disease, hypertension) reflect internal conditions, rather than environment per se. Yet, they may, in turn, reflect the interaction of environment (e.g., exercise, diet) and genetics (e.g., alleles that influence fat or cholesterol metabolism).

Because a "stress-free" environment cannot be achieved experimentally, the existence of a "pure" aging component in the cochlea is difficult to prove. Comparison of nonindustrial and industrial cultures (e.g., Rosen, Bergman, Plester, El Mofti, & Satti, 1962) suggests that most presbycusis is environmentally driven. Yet even remote, nonindustrial societies do not entirely escape presbycusis (Rosenhall & Pedersen, 1995), and a role for programmed aging in sensory cells cannot be ruled out. Intrinsic limits on the renewal of some cochlear tissues by cell replacement (described earlier) also qualify as an intrinsic aging mechanism. It is worth emphasizing, however, that the prevalence of presbycusis in the very old, although high (>60%), is not 100%. This argues that much of presbycusis is genetically and environmentally influenced, and thus should be preventable.

Classifying Presbycusis by Affected Cell Type

The currently dominant framework for classifying of presbycusis by appearance is that of H. Schuknecht, having been laid out in a series of articles written over 30 years, and in his classic book *Pathology of the Ear* (1974). In his observations of many temporal bones from aged individuals, Schuknecht suggested that age-related cochlear degeneration fits into distinct patterns, according to cell types or structures affected (Schuknecht, 1964, 1974; Schuknecht & Gacek, 1993). He believed that these patterns could also be linked to particular features of audiograms. Based on his observations, Schuknecht proposed that presbycusis comprises six categories: *sensory, neural, strial, cochlear conductive, mixed,* and *indeterminate.* To sharpen the boundaries between categories and assist diagnosis, he applied severity criteria, whereby a certain degree of cell loss was required for classification, based on comparison of cell counts and hearing

performance. Because it was recognized that all principle cell types of the cochlea show a reduction in number with age, the appearance of a particular form of presbycusis was taken to represent an *accelerated* loss of specific cells, beyond that normally associated with aging.

Sensory Presbycusis As defined for humans, sensory presbycusis refers to degeneration of the organ of Corti that extends at least 10 mm from the cochlear base, that is, into the region subserving speech perception (Figure 21-4). Pathology principally of the basal organ of Corti results in an audiogram that is abnormal only at the highest frequencies. Schuknecht believed that sensory presbycusis was the least common form, with an incidence estimated at less than 10% of all cases. As hair cells degenerate, secondary neuronal degeneration follows at the same location; therefore, some researchers have recommended the term *sensorineural* presbycusis for this category. Among primates at least (including humans), secondary neuronal degeneration may be quite delayed (with favorable implications for cochlear implants). Sensory presbycusis is particularly difficult to distinguish from injury caused by noise or ototoxins, because these exert their most obvious effects on the basal organ of Corti. Accordingly, it may be the form most closely associated with injury and may, in fact, be mechanistically and anatomically indistinguishable from noise or ototoxic injury. Most animal models applied to the study of presbycusis more closely approximate sensory presbycusis than any other form. Good animal models are important because they permit the study of particular pathologies in isolation, whereas most human temporal bones will show a confounding mix of pathologies. Animal models also permit direct tests of environmental and genetic influences.

Neural Presbycusis Neural presbycusis refers to loss of radial afferent neurons that project to inner hair cells (Figure 21-5). Schuknecht estimated the incidence of this form of presbycusis at 15% to 30% of all cases. Neural presbycusis refers to unusually rapid loss that becomes limiting for hearing. It does

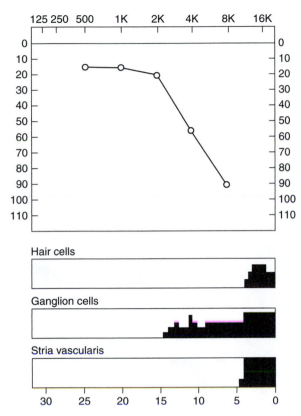

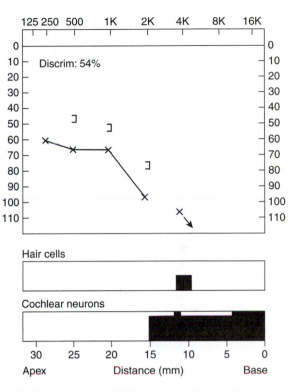

FIGURE 21-4 Sensory presbycusis as observed in a 70-year-old man. Diagnostic features are high-frequency hearing loss and basal hair cell loss (indicated by *black regions* in bottom graphs). Basal neuronal loss is probably secondary to hair cell loss. Minimal strial degeneration may not have affected hearing. (Reprinted by permission of the publisher from PATHOLOGY OF THE EAR by Harold F. Schuknecht, M.D., p. 390, Cambridge, Mass.: Harvard University Press, Copyright © 1974 by the President and Fellows of Harvard College.)

FIGURE 21-5 Neural presbycusis as observed in a 74-year-old patient. Diagnostic feature is loss of more than 50% of radial afferent neurons and impaired speech discrimination. Spatial pattern of loss does not account for reduced sensitivity at low frequencies, however. (Reprinted by permission of the publisher from PATHOLOGY OF THE EAR by Harold F. Schuknecht, M.D., p. 392, Cambridge, Mass.: Harvard University Press, Copyright © 1974 by the President and Fellows of Harvard College.)

not include loss that occurs secondary to loss of inner hair cells. According to Schuknecht, neuronal loss in human neural presbycusis is typically evenly distributed along the cochlear spiral. The severity criterion for this classification is a total loss of 50% or more, based on the extent that may lead to impaired word discrimination. Losses up to 50% may produce no clinical signs (Pauler, Schuknecht, & Thornton, 1986). Even more remarkable is that

changes in the audiogram may not occur before nearly 90% of neurons are lost! The fact that speech discrimination and threshold sensitivity are different in their imperviousness to neuronal loss suggests that redundancy of neurons is far more important for perception of complex stimuli than for simple detection. Nevertheless, it is highly fortunate for the operation of cochlear implants that loss of even half of all neurons appears to have modest consequences.

The existence of neural presbycusis as a disease of *aging* is controversial. Some have suggested it merely represents a delayed form of auditory neuropathy (Starr, Picton, & Kim, 2001). Candidate causes are many, but notably exclude either noise or ototoxins, neither of which seems able to produce a cochlear state resembling neural presbycusis. One theory incorporates the phenomenon of **excitotoxicity** (Pujol, Rebillard, Puel, Lenoir, Eybalin, & Recasens, 1991). Recall from earlier chapters that glutamate is accepted as the major neurotransmitter mediating communication between hair cells and afferent neurons. One characteristic of many glutamatergic synapses is that the release of too much glutamate can damage postsynaptic processes. Although this injury may be reversible, prolonged excitotoxic stress (perhaps caused by genetic alleles that impair neurotransmitter uptake or chronic hypoxia that promotes excess release) could lead to permanent loss of dendrites, and eventually entire neurons. In addition, observations in humans and animals indicate that some neuronal loss may follow subtle pathology of pillar cells and other supporting cells within the organ of Corti (Suzuka & Schuknecht, 1988; Ohlemiller & Gagnon, 2004b). Thus, some loss that would be superficially considered "primary" (because the hair cell targets are still present) may actually be secondary to little understood events in the organ of Corti. There may also be genetic influences on neural survival factors that predispose some individuals to neural loss.

Strial Presbycusis Strial presbycusis denotes hearing loss caused by degeneration of the stria vascularis, usually in the midcochlear to apical regions, with resulting reduction in the endocochlear potential (EP) (Figure 21-6). As discussed in Chapter 10, the stria-generated EP constitutes a significant portion of the driving force for hair cell receptor currents. Reduction of this driving force would be expected to cause increased hearing thresholds. Although the hearing loss may be "flat," the greatest threshold elevation often appears at high frequencies. This may reflect greater dependence on active mechanical processes in the cochlear base, relative to the apex. The cochlea is surprisingly tolerant to degenerative changes in the

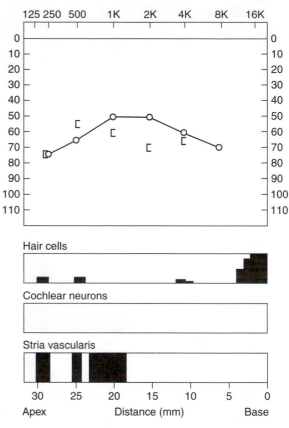

FIGURE 21-6 Strial presbycusis as observed in an 89-year-old man. Diagnostic features include relatively flat elevation of thresholds and loss of at least 30% of stria. (Reprinted by permission of the publisher from PATHOLOGY OF THE EAR by Harold F. Schuknecht, M.D., p. 396, Cambridge, Mass.: Harvard University Press, Copyright © 1974 by the President and Fellows of Harvard College.)

stria. Up to 30% to 40% of the stria may degenerate all along the cochlear spiral before changes in the audiogram occur (Schulte & Schmiedt, 1992). Schuknecht noted that strial presbycusis tends to occur earlier in life than other forms and shows a stronger familial component. Hence, it is particularly likely that there are genetic alleles that promote this form of presbycusis. Its incidence rate was estimated at 20% to 35% of all cases.

Age-related strial degeneration has been described in many human and animal studies, although most often in combination with other pathologic agents. One animal model, the Mongolian gerbil, may particularly suitably model strial presbycusis, in that age-related strial degeneration may drive most of the observed hearing loss (Schulte & Schmiedt, 1992; Spicer & Schulte, 2002). Initial pathologic factors include degeneration and thinning of the stria itself, followed by loss of fibrocytes in ligament. It is been noted in humans and animals that age-related strial degeneration is often accompanied by constriction or loss of local capillaries. The gerbil model supports this as a causative agent (Gratton, Schmiedt, & Schulte, 1996). The stria is highly metabolically active and is the most highly vascularized structure in the inner ear. This has led to the proposal that strial presbycusis is caused by a chronic ischemia-like condition. No link between strial degeneration and cardiovascular disease has been shown in humans, and no genes that predispose individuals to strial presbycusis have been identified. Just as for neural presbycusis, neither noise nor ototoxins appear to produce a cochlear state resembling strial presbycusis. Although sufficient doses of either factor can cause strial degeneration, the organ of Corti is more severely affected.

Cochlear Conductive Presbycusis Cochlear conductive presbycusis remains unproven. This classification was created to cover cases showing linearly descending audiograms (>50 dB decline overall) that appeared unexplained by clear degeneration (about 15–22% of cases). Schuknecht suggested that, in some individuals, subtle changes in the passive mechanical properties of the organ of Corti, basilar membrane, or adjacent spiral ligament may interfere with transduction, even without notable cell loss.

Mixed Presbycusis Mixed presbycusis was taken by Schuknecht to be present when two distinct types of degeneration were found and the shape of the audiogram was consistent with the sum of their effects. Schuknecht felt this applied in about 25% of cases.

Status of Schuknecht's Framework

Although Schuknecht was not the first to propose all the preceding categories, his synthesis remains the most comprehensive. However, Schuknecht's framework has many limitations. First, it was constrained by the problems often posed by human temporal bones. These are best interpreted in light of life history, yet health records often paint an incomplete picture of recreational and occupational noise and ototoxin exposure. Frequently, mediocre preservation of samples forced an emphasis on cell numbers rather than cell appearance for evaluation and classification. The framework had an *ad hoc* character, perhaps attempting to "shoehorn" cases into too few categories. Up to 25% of cases were considered **indeterminate,** showing no apparent relation between histopathology and the appearance of the audiogram. Many authors have expressed doubt regarding the diagnostic value of the shape of the audiogram (e.g., Chisolm, Willott, & Lister, 2003). Even if pathologies of different structures or cells independently contribute to the audiogram, many possible combinations may yield a particular shape. The framework is also incomplete. Details that did not appear to fit anywhere included occasional atrophy of Reissner's membrane, degeneration of spiral limbus, and loss of fibrocytes from the spiral ligament (Figures 21-7 and 21-8A).

Despite its deficiencies, the core assertion of Schuknecht's framework—*independent* pathology of organ of Corti, afferent neurons, and stria vascularis—has appealing clarifying power and testability. If each of these structures/cell types possesses distinct environmental and genetic risk factors for age-related degeneration, then identifying these risk factors is an important research goal. Although Schuknecht's scheme has been criticized, it has not been replaced or greatly refined since it was proposed. Observations in humans and animals have largely provided general support, yet few studies have been directed at testing its foundations. Studies seeking to relate specific environmental risk factors to

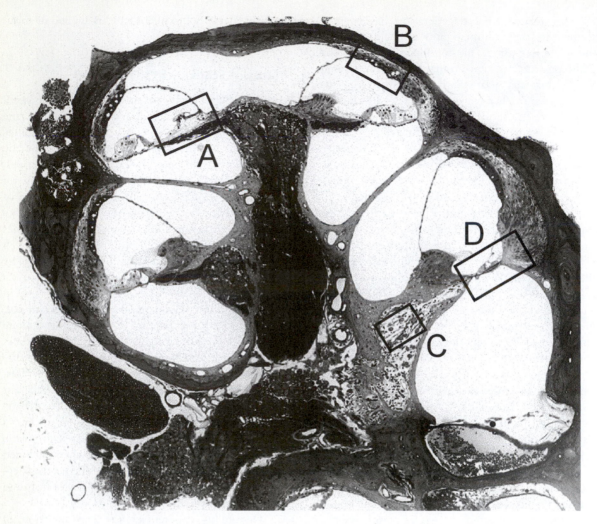

FIGURE 21-7 Midmodiolar section from a 14-month-old female C57BL/6 mouse cochlea illustrating most of the types of cell loss found across all types of presbycusis. These include hair cell loss, organ of Corti anomalies, neuronal loss (probably secondary to hair cell loss in this case), strial degeneration, and loss of fibrocytes in spiral ligament and limbus. (See Figure 21-8 for an expanded view of boxed areas.)The animal had almost no hearing but a normal endocochlear potential. C57BL/6 mice carry a gene *(Cdh23ahl)* that promotes sensory presbycusis-like pathology. Other pathology may be related to additional unknown genes.

audiograms or temporal bone histopathology have rarely attempted to link any risk factor with a particular form of presbycusis.

ROLE OF GENETICS IN PRESBYCUSIS

Currently, no genes have been identified that merit the term *presbycusis gene.* There are, however, clues

from work in animals as to how such genes might operate, particular with regard to sensory presbycusis. One prominent example is the *ahl* allele of the mouse otocadherin gene (*Cdh23,* thus the allele is *Cdh23ahl*) (see Figures 21-7 and 21-8). Otocadherin appears to play a role in establishing the integrity of the stereociliary bundle (Di Palma et al., 2001). The *ahl* allele promotes hair cell loss and pathology re-

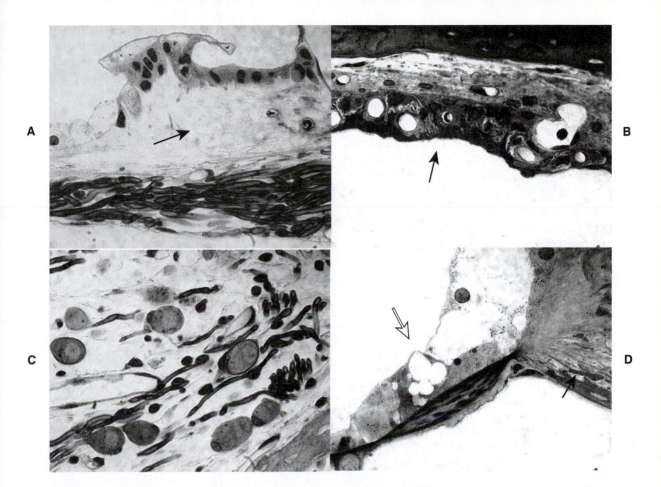

FIGURE 21-8 Enlarged view of boxed regions from Figure 21-7. (A) Loss of fibrocytes in apical spiral limbus *(arrow),* common in aging but with unknown implications for hearing. (B) Abnormal cell appearance in stria vascularis in the apical turn *(arrow).* (C) Loss of spiral ganglion cells and their projections to hair cells in the lower base. Much of this loss could be secondary to hair cell loss. (D) Hair cell loss and degeneration of the organ of Corti in the lower base *(white arrow).* *Black arrow* indicates loss of fibrocytes from the spiral ligament.

sembling *sensory* presbycusis. It also exacerbates noise injury (Davis, Newlander, Ling, Cortopassi, Kreig, & Erway, 2001), so that a mechanistic link between sensory presbycusis and noise injury is supported.

Many specific components of cellular repair and protective mechanisms are known. These include DNA repair enzymes, protein chaperones (which help stabilize key proteins), and antioxidant enzymes. If the function of these were impaired by genetic mutation, one prediction is that cells sub-

jected to even normal levels of environmental stress may over time sustain injury that presents as presbycusis. Not long ago, the only way to test mutations for their ability to promote pathology was to generate random mutations in animals using radiation or mutagenic compounds. Through genetic engineering, it is now routine to disable specific genes or add multiple copies of genes, typically in mice or rats. The effects on aging of the resulting up- or down-regulation of particular proteins or factors can then be examined explicitly. Recent work has shown that genetic impairment of antioxidant enzymes (proteins that promote chemical reactions that remove ROS) both hastens apparent aging and exacerbates noise injury (McFadden, Ding, Ohlemiller, & Salvi, 2001; Ohlemiller, McFadden, Ding, Lear, & Ho, 2000). This essentially offers proof of concept that presbycusis-promoting genes could include those involved in protection from oxidative stress. Research is certain to accelerate in this area, as the effects of other mutations are examined.

CENTRAL AUDITORY CONSEQUENCES OF PERIPHERAL DEGENERATION

Age-related changes in the peripheral and central auditory system take different forms and exert different effects on auditory perception. It is therefore important to distinguish between *direct* effects of aging on the auditory periphery and auditory central nervous system (ACNS), respectively, and the effects *peripheral pathology alone* on the function of the ACNS. First, we consider the latter. The most dramatic coding effects of peripheral pathology are expected to be increased thresholds, reduced dynamic range (through loss of nonlinear compression), and reduced frequency resolution. Both sensory and strial presbycusis would be expected to exert all three effects, through their impact on outer hair cell–mediated active processes (see Chapters 9 and 10). Elevated thresholds will, of course, impair detection. In addition, broadening of tuning and reduced dynamic range will distort the representation of the stimulus spectrum. Sound localization may also be impaired (McFadden & Willott, 1994). Neural presbycusis presents a different set of predictions. Because the organ of Corti may not be directly affected, threshold sensitivity, dynamic range, and frequency tuning of individual surviving afferent neurons may be normal (depending on whether the inner hair cell afferent synapse is functioning normally). Central auditory activity associated with detection tasks may be little altered. Recall from Chapter 11, however, that peripheral neural redundancy (many neurons having a broad range of sensitivities and dynamic ranges innervating any given hair cell) may be important for preservation of the stimulus spectrum. Neural presbycusis would reduce this useful redundancy, altering representation of the stimulus spectrum, and probably detection of signals in noise.

How are the physiology and "wiring" of the ACNS affected by peripheral degeneration? After loss of input, neurons in auditory brainstem centers close to the cochlea (in terms of the number of interposed synaptic connections) may show sluggish responses to any sound, elevated thresholds, and reduction in cell size (Frisina, 2001). Surprisingly, however, there is little overall cell loss. In mice with sensory presbycusis-like pathology, most neuronal loss appears confined to the cochlear nucleus. The brain is highly **plastic,** in that intercellular connections are readily modified by life experiences. Although central plasticity is not generally associated with the birth of many new cells, the capacity for forming and eliminating synapses presumably enhances the adaptability of the brain, even into advanced age. Studies have identified remapping of higher auditory centers after age-related loss of peripheral input (e.g., Willott, Aitkin, & McFaddin, 1993). High-CF neurons in primary auditory cortex may, after severe degeneration of the cochlear base, begin responding to lower frequencies. Higher sensory centers do not become isolated and inactive after peripheral pathology, but instead undergo a shift in the balance of excitatory and inhibitory inputs to become retuned. This retuning leads to the overrepresentation of those frequencies whose cochlear "drive" remains somewhat intact and does not confer any clear advantage. Nevertheless, it is possible that some accompanying features of this plasticity assist the brain in reducing the impact of cochlear degeneration and the resulting loss of information.

AGE-RELATED CENTRAL AUDITORY CHANGES

Evidence for "pure" age-related central auditory changes (those ostensibly not reflecting peripheral changes) has been uncovered in humans by comparing auditory perception in young subjects and older subjects showing minimal hearing loss. Among such older subjects, impaired perception of speech in noise has been reported (Frisina, 2001). This impairment may correlate with decreased temporal fidelity, as determined by gap detection experiments (e.g., Mazelova, Popelar, & Syka, 2003). These experiments measure the shortest detectable gap (silent period) in tones or noise. In the absence of anatomic assessment, impaired speech perception per se must be considered inconclusive evidence for a "pure" central effect. From the prior discussion, we know that "normal hearing" based on an audiogram may overlook extensive afferent neuronal loss as found in neural presbycusis, a peripheral condition that can also lead to impaired speech perception. On first consideration, the finding of reduced temporal fidelity in older subjects, a condition that has not generally been linked to peripheral neuronal loss, appears likely to have a purely central origin. However, recent experiments (Oxenham & Bacon, 2003) have shown that loss of compressive nonlinearity in the cochlea can affect performance on temporal tasks. A more compelling centrally mediated phenomenon, found in aging humans and animals (e.g., Jabobson, Kim,

Romney, Zhu, & Frisina, 2003), is reduction of contralateral suppression of distortion product otoacoustic emissions (DPOAEs). It is well known that the amplitude of DPOAEs can be reduced by the presentation of noise or tones to the opposite ear. This effect is presumably mediated by the cochlear medial efferent system, which provides negative feedback to outer hair cell–based amplification. Reduction of this effect in aging probably does reflect central changes. If, as some have proposed, the medial efferent system aids in the detection of signals in noise, changes in efferent function could partly explain age-related impairment of speech perception.

The anatomic changes that may underlie the perceptual changes just considered appear mostly characterized by modest but variable cell loss, reduction in synaptic density, and alterations in synaptic chemistry (Willott, 1991). Some of the more significant changes include reductions the number of cells that project from lower to higher centers. For example, in mice, the number of cells projecting from the cochlear nucleus and superior olivary complex to the inferior colliculus decreases with age (Frisina, 2001).

ᵔ SUMMARY ᵔ

Presbycusis is certain to require increasing attention from clinicians as the average age of Americans increases. Of the many facets of age-related cochlear degeneration that have been identified, the current prevailing notion is that degeneration of three major components (organ of Corti, stria vascularis, and afferent neurons) can account for most hearing loss that is diagnosed. A key component of Schuknecht's framework—and one that merits further examination in humans and animals—is the idea that these components can degenerate independently, and thus contribute independently to hearing loss. Different individuals may be at risk for losing their hearing principally because of changes in one of these components, according to their genetic

makeup, their environment, and the interplay between these. In the coming years, it will be important to identify risk factors for presbycusis and to inform and protect those individuals at risk for particular types of pathology. Some people may have a special need for hearing protection or should avoid noisy work environments altogether. Some may be especially at risk for hearing loss as a complication of hypertension or other cardiovascular disorders. Although prevention and treatment of presbycusis are not yet practical, pharmacologic approaches such as antioxidants, growth factors, or drugs that promote blood flow may prove effective. Audiologists may frequently help to identify patients who could benefit from particular strategies.

∿KEY TERMS∿

Antioxidant
Caloric restriction
Central presbycusis
Excitotoxicity
Homeostasis
Indeterminate
   presbycusis

Lipofuscin
Metabolic rate
Mitochondrion
Mitochondrial clock
   theory
Mitosis

Mixed presbycusis
Neural presbycusis
Oxidative stress
Plasticity
Postmitotic
Presbycusis

Programmed aging
Reactive oxygen
   species
Sensory presbycusis
Strial presbycusis

∿STUDY QUESTIONS∿

1. Describe the link between basal metabolic rate and mitochondrial injury.

2. Why might oxygen be said to be both friend and enemy of aerobic cells?

3. Name and characterize five major types of cochlear presbycusis that Schuknecht described.

4. Characterize the relation between hearing loss and loss of (1) hair cells, (2) afferent neurons, (3) strial cells, and (4) ligament fibrocytes.

5. Name some problems with the use of audiograms to diagnose particular forms of presbycusis.

6. Why might impaired speech perception in noise despite a normal audiogram *not* be diagnostic of a "pure" central aging effect?

∿REFERENCES∿

Barda, G. (2002). Rate of generation of oxidative stress-related damage and animal longevity. *Free Radical Biology and Medicine, 33,* 1167–1172.

Bredberg, G. (1968). Cellular pattern and nerve supply of the human organ of Corti. *Acta Otolaryngologica Supplementum, 236,* 1–135.

Chisolm, T. H., Willott, J. F., & Lister, J. J. (2003). The aging auditory system: Anatomic and physiologic changes and implications for rehabilitation. *International Journal of Audiology, 42,* 2S3–2S10.

Conlee, J. W., Gerrity, L. C., & Bennett, M. L. (1994). Ongoing proliferation of melanocytes in the stria vascularis of adult guinea pigs. *Hearing Research, 79,* 115–122.

Davis, A. C. (1989). The prevalence of hearing impairment and reported hearing disability among adults in Great Britain. *International Journal of Epidemiology, 18,* 901–907.

Davis, R. R., Newlander, J. K., Ling, X.-B., Cortopassi, G. A., Kreig, E. F., & Erway, L. C. (2001). Genetic basis for susceptibility to noise-induced hearing loss in mice. *Hearing Research, 155,* 82–90.

Di Palma, F., Holme, R. H., Bryda, E. C., Belyantseva, I. A., Pellegrino, R., Kachar, B., Steel, K. P., & Noben-Trauth, K. (2001). Mutations in *Cdh23,* encoding a new type of cadherin, cause stereocilia disorganization in waltzer, the mouse model for Usher syndrome type 1D. *Nature Genetics, 27,* 103–107.

Dunaway, G., Mhaskar, Y., Armour, G., Whitworth, C., & Rybak, L. P. (2003). Migration of cochlear lateral wall cells. *Hearing Research, 177,* 1–11.

Evans, P., & Halliwell, B. (1999). Free radicals and hearing: Cause, consequence and criteria. *Annals of the New York Academy of Science, 884,* 19–40.

Fransen, E., Lemkens, N., Van Laer, L., & Van Camp, G. (2003). Age-related hearing impairment (ARHI):

Environmental risk factors and genetic prospects. *Experimental Gerontology, 38,* 353–359.

Frisina, R. D. (2001). Possible neurochemical and neuroanatomical bases of age-related hearing loss—presbycusis. *Seminars in Hearing, 22,* 213–225.

Glorig, A., Wheeler D., Quiggle R., Grings W., & Summerfeld, A. (1957). *1954 Wisconsin state fair hearing survey—Statistical treatment of clinical and audiometric data.* San Francisco, CA: American Academy of Ophthalmology and Otolaryngology [Monograph].

Gratton, M. A., Schmiedt, R. A., & Schulte, B. A. (1996). Age-related decreases in endocochlear potential are associated with vascular abnormalities in the stria vascularis. *Hearing Research, 102,* 181–190.

Harman, D. (1956). Aging: A theory based on free radical and radiation chemistry. *Journal of Gerontology, 11,* 98–300.

Jacobson, M., Kim, S., Romney, J., Zhu, X., & Frisina, R. D. (2003). Contralateral suppression of distortion-product otoacoustic emissions declines with age: A comparison of findings in CBA mice with human listeners. *The Laryngoscope, 113,* 1707–1713.

Kopke, R., Allen, K. A., Henderson, D., Hoffer, M., Frenz, D., & Van De Water, T. (1999). A radical demise: Toxins and trauma share common pathways in hair cell death. *Annals of the New York Academy of Sciences, 884,* 171–191.

Mazelova, J., Popelar, J., & Syka, J. (2003). Auditory function in presbycusis: Peripheral vs. central changes. *Experimental Gerontology, 38,* 87–94.

McFadden, S. L., Ding, D.-L., Ohlemiller, K. K., & Salvi, R. J. (2001). The role of superoxide dismutase in age-related and noise-induced hearing loss: Clues from Sod1 knockout mice. In J. F. Willott (Ed.), *Handbook of mouse auditory research: From behavior to molecular biology* (pp. 489–504). New York: CRC Press.

McFadden, S. L., & Willott, J. F. (1994). Responses of inferior colliculus neurons in C57BL/6J mice with and without sensorineural hearing loss: Effects of changing the azimuthal location of an unmasked pure-tone stimulus. *Hearing Research, 78,* 115–131.

Ohlemiller, K. K. (2003). Oxidative cochlear injury and the limitations of antioxidant therapy. *Seminars in Hearing, 24,* 123–133.

Ohlemiller, K. K., & Gagnon, P. M. (2004a). Apical-to-basal gradients in age-related cochlear degeneration and their relationship to 'primary' loss of cochlear neurons. *Journal of Comparative Neurology, 479,* 103–116.

Ohlemiller, K. K., & Gagnon, P. M. (2004b). Cellular correlates of progressive hearing loss in 129S6/SvEv mice. *Journal of Comparative Neurology, 469,* 377–390.

Ohlemiller, K. K., McFadden, S. L., Ding, D.-L., Lear, P. M., & Ho, Y.-S. (2000). Targeted mutation of the gene for cellular glutathione peroxidase (*Gpx1*) increases noise-induced hearing loss in mice. *Journal of the Association for Research in Otolaryngology, 1,* 243–254.

Otte, J., Schuknecht H. F., & Kerr A. G. (1978). Ganglion cell populations in normal and pathological human cochleae: Implications for cochlear implantation. *Laryngoscope, 38,* 1231–1246.

Oxenham, A. J., & Bacon, S. P. (2003). Cochlear compression: Perceptual measures and implications for normal and impaired hearing. *Ear and Hearing, 24,* 352–366.

Pauler, M., Schuknecht, H. F., & Thornton, A. R. (1986). Correlative studies of cochlear neuronal loss with speech discrimination and pure-tone thresholds. *Archives of Otolaryngology, 243,* 200–206.

Pickles, J. O. (2004). Mutation in mitochondrial DNA as a cause of presbyacusis. *Audiology & Neuro-otology, 9,* 23–33.

Pujol, R., Rebillard, G., Puel, J.-L., Lenoir, M., Eybalin, M., & Recasens, M. (1991). Glutamate neurotoxicity in the cochlea: A possible consequence of ischaemic or anoxic conditions occurring in ageing. *Acta Otolaryngology (Stockh), 476*(Suppl), 32–36.

Richardson, A., & Holbrook, N. J. (1996). Aging and the cellular response to stress: Reduction in the heat shock response. In N. J. Holbrook, G. R. Martin, & R. A. Lockshin (Eds.), *Cellular aging and death* (pp. 67–80). New York: Wiley-Liss.

Rosen, S., Bergman, M., Plester, D., El Mofti, A., & Satti, M. (1962). Presbycusis study of a relatively noise-free population in the Sudan. *Annals of Otology, Rhinology, and Otolaryngology, 71,* 727–742.

Rosenhall, U., & Pedersen, K. E. (1995). Presbycusis and occupational hearing loss. *Occupational Medicine: State of the Art Reviews, 10,* 593–607.

Sastre, J., Pallardo, F. V., De La Asuncion, J. G., & Vina, J. (2000). Mitochondria, oxidative stress and aging. *Free Radical Research, 32,* 189–198.

Scholtz, A. W., Kammen-Jolly, K., Felder, E., Hussl, B., Rask-Andersen, H., & Schrott-Fischer, A. (2001). Selective aspects of human pathology in high-tone hearing loss of the aging inner ear. *Hearing Research, 157,* 77–86.

Schuknecht, H. F. (1964). Further observations on the pathology of presbycusis. *Archives of Otolaryngology, 80,* 369–382.

Schuknecht, H. F. (1974). *Pathology of the ear.* Cambridge, MA: Harvard University Press.

Schuknecht, H. F., & Gacek, M. R. (1993). Cochlear pathology in presbycusis. *Annals of Otology, Rhinology, and Otolaryngology, 102,* 1–16.

Schulte, B. A., & Schmiedt, R. A. (1992). Lateral wall Na,K-ATPase and endocochlear potentials decline with age in quiet-reared gerbils. *Hearing Research, 61,* 35–46.

Seidman, M. D. (2000). Effects of dietary restriction and antioxidants on presbycusis. *The Laryngoscope, 110,* 727–738.

Seidman, M. D., Ahmad, N., & Bai, U. (2002). Molecular mechanisms of age-related hearing loss. *Ageing Research Reviews, 1,* 331–343.

Spicer, S. S., & Schulte, B. A. (2002). Spiral ligament pathology in quiet-aged gerbils. *Hearing Research, 172,* 172–185.

Starr, A., Picton, T. W., & Kim, R. (2001). Pathophysiology of auditory neuropathy. In Y. Sininger & A. Starr (Eds.), *Auditory neuropathy: A new perspective on hearing disorders* (pp. 67–81). San Diego: Singular.

Suzuka, Y., & Schuknecht, H. F. (1988). Retrograde cochlear neuronal degeneration in human subjects. *Acta Otolaryngologica Supplementum, 450,* 2–20.

Warchol, M. E., Lambert, P. R., Goldstein, B. J., Forge, A., & Corwin, J. T. (1993). Regenerative proliferation in inner ear sensory epithelia from adult guinea pigs and humans. *Science, 259,* 1619–1622.

Willott, J. F. (1991). *Aging and the auditory system: Anatomy, physiology, and psychophysics.* San Diego: Singular Publishing Group.

Willott, J. F., Aitkin, L. M., & McFaddin, S. L. (1993). Plasticity of auditory cortex associated with sensorineural hearing loss in adult C57BL/6J mice. *Journal of Comparative Neurology, 329,* 402–411.

Wright, C. G., & Schuknecht, H. F. (1972). Atrophy of the spiral ligament. *Archives of Otolaryngology, 96,* 16–21.

∿SUGGESTED READING∿

Hull, R. H. (1995). *Hearing in aging.* San Diego: Singular Publishing Group.

Maurer, J. F., & Rupp, R. R. (1979). *Hearing and aging.* New York: Grune and Stratton.

Chapter

22

Potential Therapies for Hearing Loss:
Preventing Hair Cell Death
and Promoting Hair Cell Regeneration

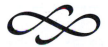

Mark E. Warchol, Ph.D.
Professor of Otolaryngology
Washington University School of Medicine
St. Louis, Missouri

Sensory hair cells in the human ear are produced during the first trimester of embryonic development. As discussed in previous chapters, hair cells can be lost later in life as a consequence of noise exposure, treatment with ototoxic drugs, inner ear infections, or simply as a result of normal aging. Because the mature cochlea appears to have no ability to produce new hair cells, the loss of cochlear hair cells leads to permanent deficits in hearing. This unfortunate situation applies only to the ears of mammals; the ears of nonmammalian vertebrates (fish, amphibians, reptiles, and birds) possess a remarkable ability to regenerate sensory hair cells. Studies of hair cell **regeneration** in these nonmammalian species have raised the hope that it might be possible to induce similar forms of regeneration in the human ear. For this goal to be realized, however, we need to understand the basic biology of the regenerative process. Such studies are at the forefront of efforts to restore hearing through biological repair. Similarly, our understanding of how hair cells die after exposure to noise or ototoxic drugs has expanded rapidly in recent years. A key insight to emerge from such studies is that, rather than just dying passively, hair cells appear to die by an active "suicidal" process. A more complete understanding of this death process should lead to the development of clinical methods

for preventing the loss of sensory cells from the cochlea and vestibular organs. This chapter examines some emerging methods for preventing and treating sensorineural hearing loss, by rescuing hair cells after injury or by inducing hair cell regeneration.

PROGRAMMED CELL DEATH (APOPTOSIS)

Until recently, the study of cell death had focused on the role of death during normal embryonic development. The developing brain, for example, initially produces an excess number of neurons. Many of these neurons then die during later development, so that the correct neural circuitry of the brain is "sculpted" by eliminating inappropriate or nonessential nerve cells. A similar form of cell death occurs during the formation of the hands and feet. In the early embryo, the newly formed digits of the hands and feet are connected together by sheets of epithelial cells. These cells are genetically programmed to die later in development, resulting in free (rather than webbed) fingers and toes. But despite the acknowledged importance of cell death during development, the biological mechanisms remained obscure. An important breakthrough came from basic biological studies of the nematode worm *Caenorhabditis elegans* (see Box 22-1). These studies indicated that cell death

---

BOX 22-1   Cell Death in *Caenorhabditis elegans*

It might seem unlikely that the study of an animal as simple as the nematode worm *Caenorhabditis elegans* might lead to insights that have transformed many fields of medicine. Investigations of the biology of this animal have occupied hundreds of biologists since the late 1970s and have been particularly valuable in understanding the causes of cell death. The mature worm is only ~1 mm in length and is composed of *exactly* 959 cells. Because of the simplicity of the worm (at least when compared with higher organisms), it has been possible to identify and trace the development of each of the animal's 959 cells. Surprisingly, a detailed examination of the embryonic development of *C. elegans* demonstrated that the immature worm contains 1,090 cells. Thus, it appears that the embryo produces 131 "extra" cells, which are then programmed to die during development. Later work

identified several genes that are necessary for cell death to occur. If one of those genes is damaged, the mutant worm develops into maturity with 1,090 cells. This was the first demonstration that cell death might be under the direct control of specific genes. Soon after, it was discovered that a nearly identical gene was present in humans, and that mutation to that gene resulted in a type of lymphoma. This finding suggested that the process of programmed cell death is similar in animals as different as nematodes and humans. It has also stimulated a huge effort toward the identification of the mechanisms of cell death. One measure of the importance of this research is that the scientists who initiated the studies of cell death in the nematode received the Nobel Prize for Medicine in 2002.

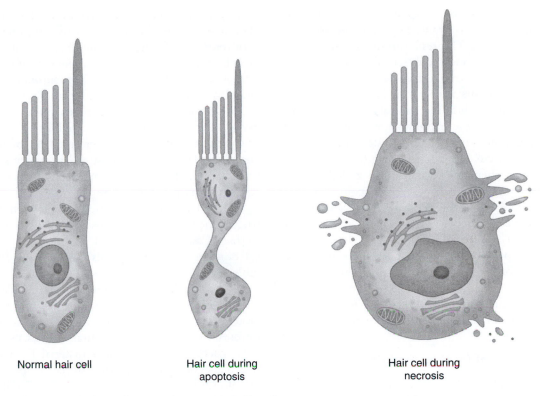

Normal hair cell   Hair cell during apoptosis   Hair cell during necrosis

FIGURE 22-1   Morphology of apoptotic versus necrotic cells.

in the embryo was under tight genetic control, and that several specific genes are necessary for cell death to occur. As a result, it became evident that cells do not die passively. Instead, they activate a biochemical "program" that leads to death via a precise sequence of events. This active death process has been called *programmed cell death* or **apoptosis.**

In recent years, it has become apparent that programmed cell death is not limited to embryonic development, but that it also occurs in many regions of the adult body, both in normal tissues and in response to pathology or injury. Cells in some organ systems, such as the lungs, skin, and gut, exhibit a pattern of normal turnover and replacement. At any given time, a certain number of cells in those tissues undergo apoptosis and are then replaced by new cells created via cell division (i.e., *mitosis*). It is critical that these two processes of cell death and cell production be balanced, so that the number of

new cells produced is exactly matched by the number of cells that die. Unregulated cell addition without a corresponding level of cell death underlies many types of cancers. Thus, cell death is not necessarily a pathologic phenomenon. Instead, normal levels of cell death are necessary to maintain many tissues in a healthy state.

The process of programmed cell death or apoptosis should be distinguished from another form of cell death known as **necrosis** (Figure 22-1). Cells undergoing either apoptosis or necrosis exhibit certain highly stereotyped changes in their appearance. Apoptotic cells shrink and their nuclei become dense and punctate. Their membranes, however, remain intact, so that the contents of the cell are not released into the external environment. Such cells also undergo chemical changes on their surfaces that cause them to be engulfed ("phagocytosed") by neighboring cells. In contrast, necrotic cells typically swell and develop openings in their membranes, allowing the cell's contents to be released into the extracellular space. This results in the recruitment of white blood cells and the onset of inflammation. A key feature of necrosis is that it is a passive process that usually occurs after a cell has experienced a massive injury, such as mechanical trauma. Necrosis does not require the expression of new genes and the production of new proteins. Instead, necrosis occurs when a cell is no longer able to maintain its structure; it then quickly falls apart and dies. Detailed studies of hair cell injury after acoustic trauma or treatment with ototoxic drugs have yielded evidence for both apoptosis and necrosis in the inner ear. Most of the loss of hair cells from the inner ear appears to occur via apoptosis, but there is also some evidence for necrosis of cochlear hair cells after severe acoustic trauma. Because apoptosis appears to be the most common death pathway in the ear, its mechanisms are examined in detail here.

Mechanisms of Programmed Cell Death

Cells respond to injury or stress in their external environment by altering their internal biochemistry. One early cellular response to stress is the formation of increased levels of reactive oxygen species (ROS) (see Chapter 21). As noted previously, ROS production in the inner ear has been implicated in age-related hair cell death. The presence of increased levels of ROS within cells appears to activate certain proteins that convey a signal from the cell's cytoplasm into the nucleus (Figure 22-2). Once activated, these proteins can initiate the expression of genes that are required for cell death. The identities of many of these genes are currently unknown, but it has been established that blocking the expression of new genes and the synthesis of new proteins will prevent cell death.

The next step in the cell death process involves changes in the cell's mitochondria. Mitochondria are small organelles within cells that are responsible for the production of energy that powers all of the cell's biochemical processes. A key chemical in this energy production process is cytochrome c. In healthy cells, cytochrome c is confined to mitochondria. During the cell death process, however, small pores are formed in mitochondria, allowing cytochrome to leak out into the interior of the cell (the *cytoplasm*). The presence of cytochrome c in the cytoplasm occurs only during pathologic events and is interpreted by the cell's biochemical machinery as a "death signal." The susceptibility of cells to this process is related to their numbers of mitochondria. Hair cells, like most other sensory receptors, have high levels of metabolic activity and contain many mitochondria.

The release of cytochrome c from mitochondria triggers the activation of a class of proteins known as caspases. Caspases are the final "executioners" in the cell death process. Healthy cells contain many caspase molecules in their inactivated ("proactive") state. Once activated, caspases function like molecular scissors—they diffuse throughout a cell and cut its proteins into small fragments. In this way, activated caspases destroy the cell's structural proteins, its metabolic machinery, and its genetic material. During the final phases of the death process, the cell's DNA is cut up into short (~120 base pair) segments. The entire cell death process can proceed quickly. In many cases, the elapsed time between exposure to a noxious stimulus and the final phase of the death process is about 1 to 2 hours.

Programmed Cell Death in the Inner Ear

Hair cells in the ears of human embryos are produced at about the 8th to 10th week of gestation. After birth, many hair cells are capable, at least in principle, of surviving for an entire human life span. Many 80-year-old adults, for example, have reasonably good hearing, and those individuals "hear" with 80-year-old hair cells. A similar pattern of cell production and longevity is observed in most regions of the brain. Neurons are produced in the embryonic brain, and many survive for an entire lifetime. Nevertheless, most people experience some loss of sensory hair cells (and neurons) during the aging process. Hair cells can also be lost after exposure to noise or ototoxic drugs. How do these

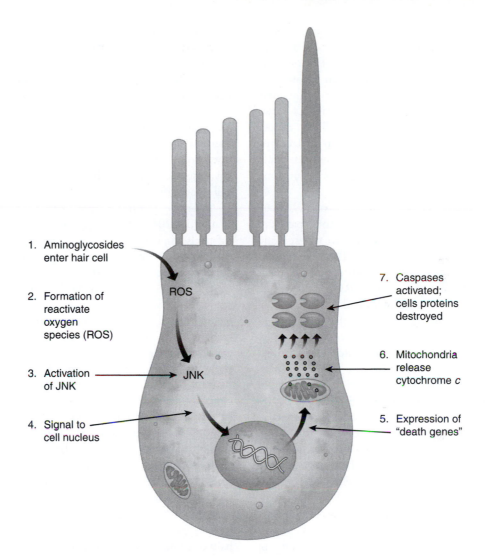

1. Aminoglycosides enter hair cell
2. Formation of reactivate oxygen species (ROS)
3. Activation of JNK
4. Signal to cell nucleus
5. Expression of "death genes"
6. Mitochondria release cytochrome *c*
7. Caspases activated; cells proteins destroyed

FIGURE 22-2 (See Color Plate) Programmed cell death pathway in hair cells. JNK, c-Jun N-terminal kinase; ROS, reactive oxygen species.

hair cells die? A great deal of recent evidence indicates that much of the loss of hair cells that occurs after acoustic trauma or administration of ototoxic drugs occurs via apoptosis. Hair cell death after noise or drug exposure exhibits many of the defining features of apoptosis, including release of cytochrome *c* from mitochondria, activation of caspases, degradation of intracellular proteins and DNA, and the presence of small, fragmented nuclei.

Methods for Preventing Cell Death

The discovery that cell death is brought about by a metabolically active process has raised the possibility that this death pathway might be blocked by pharmacologic intervention. Drugs that block the activity of cell death signaling molecules, the synthesis of new proteins, the release of cytochrome *c* from hair cell mitochondria, and the activation of caspases currently are being developed. Some of these drugs have been shown in laboratory experiments to inhibit the death of hair after exposure to aminoglycoside antibiotics. Although the ototoxic effects of aminoglycosides have been known for more than 50 years, those drugs are still widely used, particularly in developing countries. The usefulness of aminoglycosides (as well as cancer chemotherapy agents such as cisplatin and carboplatin) would be greatly enhanced if methods could be devised to prevent those drugs from damaging hearing and balance function.

Ideally, it would be preferable to block cell death as early as possible in the apoptotic pathway, so as to minimize internal damage to the cell and changes in the cell's physiology. For this reason, many studies have focused on protecting hair cells by reducing the accumulation of ROS. This can be accomplished by either blocking the formation of ROS or by neutralizing ROS after they are formed. Aminoglycoside antibiotics are actively taken up by hair cells; once inside, they generate ROS through chemical reactions that involve free iron molecules. It has been suggested that binding free iron might prevent hair cell death. Surprisingly, this can be accomplished by treatment with salicylate (aspirin). Early clinical trials have suggested that moderate-to-high doses of aspirin can reduce the ototoxic effects of aminoglycosides, but much additional work needs to be conducted before salicylates can be used as a preventive for ototoxicity. In addition to blocking the formation of ROS, it also appears reasonable that neutralizing ROS activity might reduce or prevent ototoxicity. ROS can neutralized by treatment with so-called antioxidants or *free radical scavengers*. These include dietary supplements such as vitamins C and E, as well as many more potent antioxidants. To date, the results of some animal studies have suggested that treatment with antioxidants may slightly reduce cisplatin ototoxicity, but it is clear that simply administering large doses of vitamins is not sufficient to rescue hair cells from the toxic effects of aminoglycosides or cisplatin.

Cell death can also be blocked in the mid stages of the apoptotic process. One crucial signal in hair cell death is the activation of a protein known as c-Jun N-terminal kinase (commonly abbreviated as JNK). Activation of JNK has also been implicated in the death of neurons in conditions such as Parkinson's disease and amyotrophic lateral sclerosis (ALS). Because JNK appears to be involved in the death of both neurons and sensory receptor cells, much effort has been directed toward developing drugs that will selectively block JNK activation. So far, studies conducted in animal models have suggested that inhibiting JNK can prevent hair cell death after acoustic trauma or aminoglycoside treatment (e.g., Pirvola et al., 2000; Matsui, Gale, & Warchol, 2004). These drugs are currently in clinical trials for other neurologic conditions, and they may also be applied toward preventing sensory deficits in the near future.

Finally, cell death can be blocked at its terminal stages, by inhibiting the activity of caspases. Several chemicals have been shown to bind to the caspase molecule and interfere with its ability to cleave proteins. Laboratory studies indicate that such drugs are capable of blocking the death of many types of cells. In particular, a number of recent studies indicate that treatment with these so-called caspase inhibitors can prevent the death of hair cells after exposure to aminoglycosides. Because caspase inhibitors act relatively late in the cell death pathway, it is possible that hair cells will still suffer permanent damage before caspases are blocked. Nevertheless, laboratory data suggest that hair cells that are rescued by caspase inhibition can survive even after the drug treatments have been halted. In addition, the rescued hair cells appear to retain the ability to function as sensory receptors (e.g., Matsui et al., 2003). This is encouraging, but long-term systemic treatment with caspase-inhibiting drugs would pose potential problems. Normal ongoing cell death is necessary in many parts of the body; therefore, much additional research is necessary before methods for preventing ototoxicity can enter clinical practice. Given the dramatic increase in our understanding of the mechanisms of cell death, it appears likely that the coming decade will bring new methods for preventing sensory cell death in the inner ear.

BOX 22-2 Postembryonic Growth of the Inner Ear

Study of the inner ears of nonmammalian vertebrates (fish, amphibians, reptiles, and birds) has yielded numerous insights into the mechanisms of growth and repair in the mammalian ear. One notable feature of the nonmammalian ear is the ability to produce hair cells after embryonic development. The vestibular organs of some animals (e.g., fish and frogs) are constantly increasing in size, mainly by the concentric addition of new hair cells at the borders of the sensory epithelia. Given enough time, some of these sensory organs can grow quite large. In fact, the vestibular maculae in some species of sharks contain more than 1,000,000 hair cells. A somewhat different pattern of postembryonic hair cell production is observed in the inner ears of birds. The avian cochlea and vestibular organs do not increase in size during mature life, and the numbers of hair cells in those organs remains constant. If existing hair cells are killed, however, the avian ear is capable of quickly producing replacement hair cells. As noted earlier, these new hair cells arise from the division of supporting cells. The ears of fish and amphibians can also regenerate hair cells, mainly through the proliferation of supporting cells. Thus, a strong correlation exists between the ability of supporting cells to proliferate and the ability to regenerate hair cells. Unfortunately, the ability of supporting cells to proliferate is limited in the vestibular organs of mammals and appears to be nonexistent in the organ of Corti. It is unclear why the potential for hair cell replacement in the mammalian ear is so restricted, at least when compared with these other species.

HAIR CELL REGENERATION

The embryonic development of the mammalian inner ear has been the subject of intense study for more than a half century, and many of the basic features of cochlear development have been described (see Chapter 6). It is known, for example, that sensory hair cells arise from the division of specialized precursor cells within the embryonic ear. Once the correct number of hair cells is produced, these precursor cells stop dividing. This production of sensory cells in the embryo is limited to a relatively short period. That fact, combined with the common observation that sensorineural hearing loss is almost always a permanent condition, led to the assumption that the mature inner ear was incapable of replacing hair cells after injury. This assumption was initially challenged by the demonstration that the ears of cold-blooded vertebrates such as fish and frogs are capable of producing many new hair cells during mature life. In those species, many parts of the body continue to growth throughout life. As part of this growth process, new hair cells are continuously added to the sensory organs of the inner ear, resulting in increased size and sensitivity (Box 22-2). These studies were influential, because they convinced researchers that the production of hair cells was not *necessarily* limited to embryos. The observations also raised the possibility that such species might be able to produce new hair cells after injury from sound exposure or ototoxic insult.

Subsequent work showed that the ears of most nonmammalian vertebrates are able to regenerate hair cells after injury. This includes species whose ears normally grow and add new hair cells during mature life (e.g., fish and amphibians), as well as birds, whose ears do not increase in size after maturity. The most dramatic example of hair cell regeneration is observed in the avian cochlea after noise damage. Exposing chickens (or other bird species) to 120 dB sound pressure level (SPL) for 24 to 48 hours results in a large hair cell lesion in a portion of the cochlea. Surprisingly, however, if we were to examine the injured cochlea about a month after the noise exposure, we would find that the damaged area has been completely repopulated by new hair cells. In fact, new hair cells appear as early as 3 days after injury, and full recovery is observed after 2 to 3 weeks (Cotanche, 1987). Subsequent studies showed that this recovery of hair cells is paralleled by the recovery of hearing thresholds, indicating that the newly produced hair cells are functional and can transmit

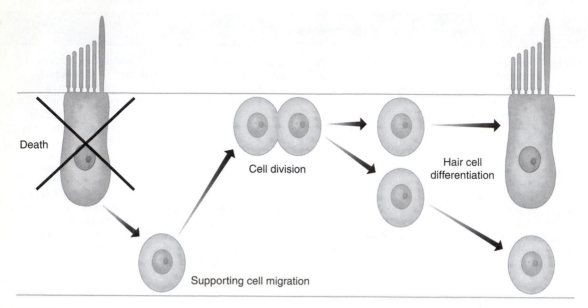

FIGURE 22-3   Regeneration via renewed cell proliferation.

information to the auditory nerve. A similar pattern of hair cell recovery is observed in the avian vestibular organs, after injury by exposure to aminoglycoside antibiotics.

Sources of Replacement Hair Cells

How can the mature ear produce new hair cells after injury? Most studies have focused on the role of supporting cells in the regenerative process. In the avian ear, the death of hair cells causes nearby supporting cells to undergo cell division, leading to the production of new cells (Corwin & Cotanche, 1988; Ryals & Rubel, 1988). Some of these new cells then differentiate as replacement hair cells, whereas others go on to become supporting cells (Figure 22-3). This mechanism of repair via the production of new cells is similar to the process of wound healing in the skin. Like wound repair, regeneration in the ear begins quickly after injury. Supporting cells in the avian ear first begin to divide about 12 to 16 hours after the loss of hair cells. This cell division continues for several days; once a full population of replacement hair cells is formed, supporting **cell proliferation** stops and the ear returns to its normal state.

Production of replacement hair cells by renewed cell division appears to underlie the majority of sensory regeneration that occurs in the avian cochlea and vestibular organs, and it has also been demonstrated in the ears of fish and amphibians. There is, however, evidence for other repair mechanisms in the vertebrate ear. It has been suggested that supporting cells may be able to change directly into hair cells, without first undergoing cell division. In addition, a closer examination of ototoxic injury has shown that many hair cells may not actually die after treatment with aminoglycosides. Instead, a sizable fraction of hair cells appear to survive ototoxic insult, albeit in a damaged state. Such hair cells typically lose their stereocilia bundles, as well as other cellular structures that are necessary for sensory function, but recent evidence suggests that hair cells are capable of regrowing these structures. Research on hair cell repair is at an early stage, and it is not known whether hair cells in the mammalian cochlea can lose and regrow stereocilia bundles. Nevertheless, a complete understanding of the basic biological mechanisms of this repair process may lead to development of methods for stimulating the growth of stereocilia in the human ear.

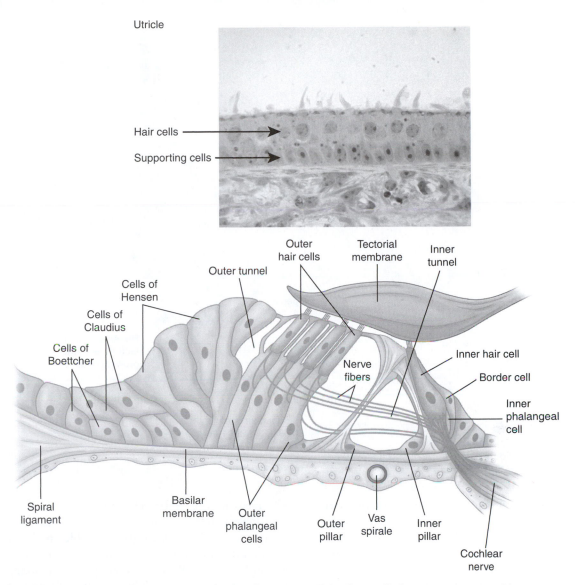

FIGURE 22-4 (See Color Plate) Morphology of supporting cells in the vestibular organs versus cochlea.

Hair Cell Regeneration in the Mammalian Ear

The clear demonstration of hair cell regeneration in the ears of birds has prompted a re-examination of the evidence (or lack thereof) for hair cell regeneration in the mammalian ear. For several reasons, most studies have focused on the mammalian vestibular organs, rather than the cochlea. The anatomy of the vestibular organs in mammals closely resembles the anatomy of those organs in birds; therefore, it is reasonable to expect that mammals might retain some ability to regenerate vestibular hair cells. In fact, supporting cells in the mammalian vestibular organs have been shown to proliferate in response to hair cell injury (Forge, Li, Corwin, & Nevill, 1993; Warchol, Lambert, Goldstein, Forge, & Corwin,

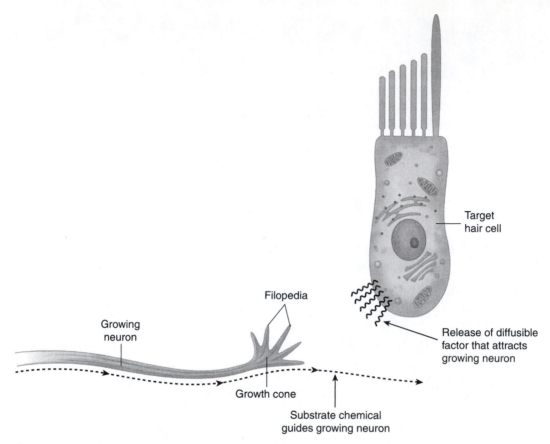

FIGURE 22-5   Guidance cues for growing auditory neurons.

1993). It is crucial to note, however, that the number of dividing cells observed in the mammalian utricle is about 100-fold less than in the avian ear under comparable conditions. This disparity almost certainly accounts for the large difference in the regenerative abilities of the avian and mammalian ears.

Although cells in the vestibular organs of mammals possess a modest ability to proliferate after hair cell injury, current data indicate that the mammalian organ of Corti does not retain any capacity for regeneration. The reasons for this lack of regenerative ability are unknown, but it should be noted that the cellular anatomy of the mammalian cochlea is quite different from the hearing organs of nonmammals (Figure 22-4). It may be that the complex structure of the supporting cells in the organ of Corti (Deiters'

cells, Hensen's cells, Pilar cells, among others) is incompatible with the ability to proliferate. The cellular complexity of the mammalian cochlea probably underlies the uniquely mammalian ability to hear at high frequencies (>8–10,000 Hz), and it is tempting to speculate that the inability of the mammalian cochlea to regenerate is part of an evolutionary trade-off that led to the development of sensitive high-frequency hearing.

Rewiring the Ear: Regeneration of Auditory Neurons and the Recovery of Hearing

The spiral ganglion cells of the auditory nerve transmit information from the cochlea to the auditory areas of the brainstem. When hair cells are lost after cochlear damage, the synaptic connections between hair cells and spiral ganglion neurons are broken. These synapses must be re-formed for hearing to return after hair cell regeneration. In addition, the frequency-place code of the cochlea will be restored only if afferent neurons are able to contact hair cells at the appropriately tuned locations in the cochlea. It is not known how this is accomplished, but regenerating neurons possess unique structures that participate in the navigation process. One characteristic of growing neurons is the presence of a specialized structure called a *growth cone* (Figure 22-5). The growth cone is located at the growing tip of the neuron and contains a number of finger-like processes (filopodia). During neuronal growth, the filopodia actively explore the immediate surroundings of the nerve cell. Depending on the particular chemicals that they encounter, filopodia can steer the growing neuron in a particular direction or can cause the neuron to stop growing altogether. Filopodia respond to two general classes of **guidance** cues: the chemical composition of the surface that the neuron is growing on (so-called substrate cues) and soluble chemicals that are secreted from a particular target. Substrate molecules can act as tracks or trails that guide growing neurons to a particular location. Filopodia are also able to sense the concentration of secreted chemicals and can steer neurons either toward or away from the source of such chemicals. These methods of guiding growing nerve cells are quite general; they appear to account for the precise growth and connectivity of the entire nervous system during embryonic development.

The specific cues that guide the growth of neurons in the ear, either during embryonic development or during regeneration, are not known. It does appear, however, that both substrate-bound and diffusible cues are involved. Certain substrate molecules that are known to interact with growing neurons (e.g., laminin and tenascin) are present in the developing cochlea and are mainly found in the space that joins the spiral ganglion to the organ of Corti. It is likely that these molecules help to guide the growth of afferent neurons toward hair cells. Hair cells also produce and secrete chemicals that are known to at-

tract growing neurons; thus, the proper growth and targeting of auditory neurons probably involves several distinct guidance cues. Identification of these cues is of great interest, because knowledge of how cochlear neurons grow may lead to development of methods for improving the interface between cochlear implants and the auditory nerve.

Prospects for Sensory Regeneration in the Human Ear

What do these studies of regeneration in the ears of animals tell us about the potential for regeneration in the human ear? First, the studies clearly show that the production of hair cells is not limited to embryos, but can also occur in mature animals. Also, because replacement hair cells are produced by the division of supporting cells, the ability of supporting cells to proliferate is a key determinant of regenerative ability. Currently, a single study has shown that supporting cells in the human utricle can proliferate in a similar fashion to the vestibular organs of other mammals (Warchol et al., 1993). This result offers hope that methods can be developed that will increase regenerative proliferation in the human ear. Finally, it should be emphasized that there is currently no evidence for spontaneous regeneration of the mature cochleae of mammals. This is still an active area of research, and a further understanding of how cell division in the cochlea is regulated may lead to methods for inducing hair cell replacement in the human organ of Corti.

Therapeutic Promise of Stem Cells

Another approach to biological repair of the inner ear involves the use of embryonic or adult **stem cells.** Stem cells are a unique class of cell that can continue to divide and produce new cells of many different types of tissues. The mature human body contains more than 200 distinct cell phenotypes (e.g., skin cells, muscle cells, neurons, various types of white blood cells, and so forth). True *totipotent* stem cells (stem cells that can produce any cell or tissue type) are probably limited to early-stage embryos. The attainment of such cells for therapeutic purposes is currently fraught with a number of technical and ethical problems. Notably, however, many tissues of the mature body apparently contain *pluripotent* or *multipotent* stem cells that can produce a more limited range of cell types. For example, stem cells isolated from the bone marrow (which normally produces blood cells) may also be able to produce nerve cells under the proper conditions. Although it is possible that the vestibular organs of mammals contain a small number of resident stem cells (e.g., Li, Roblin, Lu, & Heller, 2003), it appears unlikely that any stem-cell population is present in the mature cochlea.

Given the likely absence of stem cells in the cochlea, it has been suggested that stem cells might be transplanted into the damaged ear. Stem-cell transplantation into the brain currently is being tested in the treatment of several degenerative conditions, such as Parkinson's disease. Once stem cells are introduced into the mature ear, it is hoped that they would migrate to the appropriate locations and differentiate into new hair cells or spiral ganglion neurons. For this reason, it is of great interest to understand the factors that influence the differentiation of stem cells, and many current studies are attempting to identify biological molecules that will cause stem cells to become hair cells. A solution to this problem will almost certainly be aided by studies of the early embryology of the inner ear. Once the specific molecules that induce ear formation in the embryo are identified, scientists should be able to use these same signals to instruct stem cells to become hair cells and sensory neurons. Stem cells could then be isolated from adult tissues (such as from the blood or skin) and instructed to become hair cell precursors. These cells could then be transplanted into the cochlea. Because the cells could be obtained from the bone marrow or skin of a person who will ultimately receive the transplant, there would be no problems of tissue compatibility or immune rejection. This scenario remains speculative. In the short term, the most likely application for stem-cell technology is in the production of new auditory neurons, which might be used to enhance the performance of cochlear implants.

ᨠSUMMARYᨠ

It is now well established that much of the death of hair cells that occurs after acoustic trauma or ototoxicity is mediated by the metabolically active process of apoptosis. In addition, many of the crucial signaling events required for apoptotic death have been characterized, and it has been shown that blocking these events (via treatment with certain drugs) can prevent cells from dying. Taken together, these findings offer hope for the development of methods to prevent hair cell death after sound exposure or treatment with ototoxic drugs. Other work has shown that the ears of all nonmammalian vertebrates (fish, amphibians, reptiles, and birds) can regenerate sensory hair cells after injury. Unfortunately, the mammalian cochlea is not capable of this type of repair; therefore, the loss of hair cells (together with the resulting hearing loss) is permanent. Nevertheless, it is hoped that a detailed understanding of the cellular mechanisms of repair processes in the nonmammalian ear will lead to the development of methods for the induction of similar types of regeneration in the human inner ear.

ᨠKEY TERMSᨠ

Apoptosis	Necrosis	Regeneration	Stem cell
Cell proliferation	Neuronal guidance		

ᴄ≀STUDY QUESTIONS≀ᴄ

1. What are some key differences between cell death that occurs via apoptosis versus necrosis?

2. The ears of most nonmammalian vertebrates (e.g., fish, frogs, birds, among others) can regenerate hair cells after ototoxic injury. How are these new hair cells actually produced?

3. The mammalian ear has a limited capacity for regeneration. What is one key limitation on the regenerative ability of the mammalian cochlea?

4. Name two signals or guidance cues that growing auditory neurons (spiral ganglion cells) could potentially use to navigate to their correct hair cell targets?

5. How might stem cells be used in the treatment of hearing and balance disorders?

ᴄ≀REFERENCES≀ᴄ

Corwin, J. T., & Cotanche, D. A. (1988). Regeneration of sensory hair cells after acoustic trauma. *Science, 240,* 1772–1774.

Cotanche, D. A. (1987). Regeneration of hair cell stereocilia bundles in the chick cochlea following severe acoustic trauma. *Hearing Research, 30,* 181–196.

Forge, A., Li, L., Corwin, J. T., & Nevill, G. (1993). Ultrastructural evidence for hair cell regeneration in the mammalian inner ear. *Science, 259,* 1616–1619.

Li, H., Roblin, G., Lu, H., & Heller, S. (2003). Generation of hair cells by stepwise differentiation of embryonic stem cells. *Proceedings of the National Academy of Sciences USA, 100,* 13495–13500.

Matsui, J. I., Haque, A., Huss, D., Messana, E. P., Alosi, J. A., Roberson, D. W., Cotanche., D. A., Dickman, J. D., & Warchol M.E. (2003). Caspase inhibitors promote vestibular hair cell function and survival following aminoglycoside treatment *in vivo. Journal of Neuroscience, 23,* 6111–6122.

Matsui, J. I., Gale, J. E., & Warchol, M. E. (2004). Critical signaling events in the aminoglycoside-induced death of sensory hair cells. *Journal of Neurobiology, 61,* 250–266.

Pirvola, U., Xing-Qun, L., Virkkala, J., Saarma, M., Murakata, C., Camoratto, A. M., Walton, K. M., & Ylikoski, J. (2000). Rescue of hearing, auditory hair cells, and neurons by CEP-1347/KT7515, an inhibitor of c-Jun N-terminal kinase activation. *Journal of Neuroscience, 20,* 43–50.

Ryals, B. M., & Rubel, E. W. (1988). Hair cell regeneration after acoustic trauma in adult coturnix quail. *Science, 240,* 1774–1776.

Warchol, M. E., Lambert, P. R., Goldstein, B. J., Forge, A., & Corwin, J. T. (1993). Regenerative proliferation in inner ear sensory epithelia from adult guinea pigs and humans. *Science, 259,* 1619–1622.

ᴄ≀SUGGESTED READING≀ᴄ

Raff, M. (1999). Cell suicide for beginners. *Nature, 396,* 119–122.

Forge, A., & Schacht, J. (2000). Aminoglycoside antibiotics. *Audiology and Neuro-Otology, 5,* 3–22.

Nicholson, D. W. (2000). From bench to clinic with apoptosis-based therapeutic agents. *Nature, 407,* 810–816.

Warchol, M. E. (2001). Regeneration of cochlear hair cells. In A. F. Jahn & J. Santos-Sacchi (Eds.), *Physiology of the ear* (pp. 241–256). San Diego: Singular Publishing.

Appendix: Study Questions and Answers

Chapter 1: Introduction

1. What is an audiologist and what does an audiologist do?

   Answer: The audiologist is the primary hearing care practitioner who assesses the nature and extent of the hearing or balance disorders; fits assistive devices, including hearing aids and cochlear implants; provides rehabilitative services, and conducts specialized testing.

2. Why does an audiologist need a sound background in the basic and applied sciences?

   Answer: A sound understanding of the scientific foundation of the practice of audiology is necessary for developing a thorough understanding of the current methods used in the profession and for developing new tests, tools, and rehabilitative techniques in the future. Audiologists with solid scientific backgrounds are also well suited for guiding the work of basic scientists toward clinically relevant issues.

3. What is meant by the term *translational research*? How is it relevant to audiology?

   Answer: Translational research refers to the process of converting "bench science" to clinical practice. Audiologists are the conduit between the basic science studies and the application of knowledge gained from these studies for patient use. They are valuable to consumers because their skills and experience can maximize the quality of life for the person with hearing loss, and they are also valuable to basic scientists because they can guide the direction of research toward better clinical interventions.

4. Identify two ways the normal ear can expand the dynamic range of hearing.

   Answer: (1) Motility of outer hair cells, evidenced by the presence of otoacoustic emissions, amplifies the response of the inner hair cells for soft sounds, expanding the dynamic range by about 30 dB. (2) The acoustic reflex and efferent inhibition both attenuate input for very high level sounds, keeping the inner hair cell from being overstimulated by signals greater than about 100 dB SPL.

5. Name three areas of the scope of practice of audiology that have been introduced since the early 1970s.

   Answer: Cochlear implants, digital hearing aids, balance assessment, tympanometry, auditory brainstem response (ABR), and otoacoustic emissions (OAEs).

Chapter 2: Basic Acoustics and Noise

1. Audiologists often use the term *dynamic range* to express the boundary conditions of human hearing. In the frequency domain, the range is 20 Hz to about 20,000 Hz; in the intensity domain, the range is from about 0 to about 120 dB SPL. In linear terms, which of the ranges, frequency or intensity, is larger, and by how much?

   Answer: The intensity dynamic range. It extends from 0 dB SPL, which is 10^{-12} watts/meter^2, to 120 dB SPL, which is 1 watt/meter^2. In intensity units, the ratio is 1 trillion to 1. In contrast, the frequency range is only 1,000 to 1. If we tried to draw the audiogram on a sheet of paper in linear units, and if we made the horizontal axis 10 inches wide to represent 20 Hz to 20,000 Hz linearly, and set the vertical axis to represent the same interval, the vertical axis would have to be 157,828 miles high. No wonder we need to invoke the laws of decibels in audiology.

2. Explain how noise berms positioned alongside highways reduce complaints from nearby residents.

   Answer: Noise berms do block some sound from entering adjacent neighborhoods. Because the barrier interrupts the direct path from the source (highway traffic) and the receiver (people enjoying the quiet of their property), sound must travel a greater distance and is attenuated slightly. High-frequency sounds are attenuated better than low-frequency sounds because their wavelength is short with respect to the size of the barrier and they travel in straight paths.

3. Why do sound level meters incorporate an A-weighted filter network?

   Answer: The purpose is to simulate the human response to sound, rather than to determine the total sound pressure level.

4. A rock band produces an average sound pressure level of 100 dBA measured at the ear of a listener 200 feet from the stage. Assuming no reflection of the sound by the ground or other objects, what would the level be at the listener's ear if he or she moved to a distance of 50 feet from the stage?

   Answer: 112 dBA. According to the inverse square law, the sound level would increase by 6 dB for each halving of the distance from the source.

Chapter 3: Filters and Spectra

1. Why should an audiologist care about spectral processing and filtering?

   Answer: The ear is a spectral analyzer and a filter. To understand normal and disordered hearing, the audiologist must have a good basic command of the acoustic principles that govern the detection of sounds by the ear. Furthermore, devices that are used to assist individuals with hearing loss change the acoustic characteristics of the sound entering the cochlear or the auditory nerve, and a complete understanding of the effects of those changes is necessary to design appropriate hearing aids or cochlear implants and to select the appropriate intervention strategy.

2. What differentiates "white" noise from "pink" noise?

   Answer: White noise contains equal energy per cycle, and pink noise contains equal energy per octave. Pink noise is generally more useful for audiologists because octave or $\frac{1}{3}$ octave bands of pink noise have the same sound pressure level.

3. What are the lower and upper cutoff frequencies of a $\frac{1}{3}$ octave band of noise centered at 8.0 kHz?

   Answer: A $\frac{1}{3}$ octave band of noise centered at 8.0 kHz (f_c) would have a lower cutoff frequency (f_l) $\frac{1}{6}$ octave below fc and an upper cutoff frequency (fu) $\frac{1}{6}$ octave above 1.0 kHz. Therefore, the lower cutoff frequency is:

   $$f_l = 2^{-\frac{1}{6}} * fc$$
   $$= 0.89 * 8,000$$
   $$= 7,127 \text{ Hz}$$

and the upper cutoff frequency is:

$$f_u = 2^{1/6} * fc$$
$$= 1.122 * 8,000$$
$$= 8,980 \text{ Hz}$$

You can check your math by using the formula to calculate the center frequency: the square root of the lower cutoff times the upper cutoff.

4. Three filters are designed for use in an automobile stereo. All three filters have Q_{3dB} values of 4.0 but different CFs. Do they have the same bandwidth?

Answer: No. Because the Q value is a ratio, the most one could say about these filters is that their bandwidths are proportional to their center frequencies.

5. Assume a complex signal is made up of three sinusoids: 500, 3,000, and 8,000 Hz. Explain how each of these signals would be affected by the acoustic effects of the outer and middle ears.

Answer: 500 Hz: This sinusoid is below the resonant frequency of the ear canal and is within the passband of the middle ear (see Figure 3-9). Therefore, it would pass to the stapes relatively unscathed.

3,000 Hz: This signal would be amplified by the resonance of the external canal by perhaps 15–20 dB, but is about 1½ octaves above the cutoff frequency of the middle ear. Therefore, it would be attenuated by about 15 dB by the middle ear. The result is that it would appear at the stapes at just about the same level (but phase delayed) as it came into the external ear.

8,000 Hz: This component would not be amplified by the external canal because it is far above the resonant frequency, and it is 3 octaves above the cutoff frequency for the middle ear. As shown in Figure 3-9, this signal would be attenuated by about 35 dB at the stapes.

Chapter 4: Essentials of Cell Structure and Function: An Introduction to Cell Biology

1. Draw a diagram of a living cell. Label the important organelles.

   Answer: See Figure 4-4.

2. List four components of the membrane system. Discuss how these components communicate with one another.

   Answer: The four components of the membrane system of most cells would include the nuclear envelope, endoplasmic reticulum, Golgi complex, and plasma membrane. Remember these components are functionally and often physically connected. The physical connection between the nuclear envelope and the endoplasmic reticulum helps to ensure that ribosomes will find mRNA molecules as they pass through the pores in the nuclear envelope. Manufactured proteins can then be inserted into the lumen of the endoplasmic reticulum for further modification. They are then transported via free vesicles to the cis face of the Golgi and properly folded and packaged as they move from cis to medial to trans Golgi compartments, where they are marked for delivery to specific sites within the cell. Often they will be delivered to the plasma membrane for excretion outside the cell.

3. List the three types of cytoskeletal elements and the important functions of each.

   Answer: The three major classes of cytoskeletal elements are microtubules, intermediate filaments, and actin filaments. Microtubules are important for cell division, cell polarization, intracellular transport, and ciliary motion. The tough, nonlabile intermediate filaments are important for mechanical strength. Actin filaments are necessary for proper cell motility, mechanical strength, and phagocytosis. They are also crucial for maintaining the necessary interaction between the cytoskeleton and the plasma membrane.

4. Research an organ found in the human body (your choice). Identify several different types of cells and tissues found in that organ. Consider how the different cells or tissues must interact to ensure proper organ function.

   Answer: Example 1: The small intestine contains smooth muscle for peristalsis, mucous secreting goblet cells, an epithelium specialized for absorption, blood and lymphatic vessels, and connective tissue.

   Example 2: Bone tissue is predominantly a hard connective tissue. It also contains a vascular network and a rather dispersed collection of bone cells called osteocytes. Other cells that produce bone, called osteoblasts, and cells that erode bone, called osteoclasts, may also be present. Bone tissue is usually encased in a richly vascular covering called periosteum.

Chapter 5: Introduction to Neurons and Synapses

1. How does a nerve cell maintain its resting potential?

   Answer: The cell contains specialized ion-selective channels across its membrane. Some of those channels include an active transport mechanism that consumes energy and pumps potassium ions out of the cell and sodium ions into it. The active pump works against the concentration gradient and creates a net charge difference across the membrane, producing a potential difference, or voltage gradient of about 50 mV between the inside and outside of most neurons.

2. What is the biological advantage of myelination of nerve fibers, and how does it work?

   Answer: The biological advantage is an increase in conduction velocity along a neuron. Myelin insulates the nerve fiber, allowing the propagating action potential to "skip" along the nodes of Ranvier, rather than traversing the entire length of the cell membrane.

3. What are the four functional zones of neurons, and how do they differ from each other?

   Answer: (1) Input zone (dendritic), (2) action zone (cell body), (3) transmission zone (axon), and (4) transmission zone (boutons and synapse).

4. What would happen to the membrane potential of a neuron if the active pump was poisoned?

   Answer: The cell would not be able to maintain its internal resting potential.

5. Describe the process by which synaptic vesicles are created and released into the synaptic cleft.

   Answer: Synaptic vesicles, the carriers of neurotransmitter, are assembled in the cell body and transported by intracellular mechanisms to the synaptic zone. In the synaptic zone they are filled with neurotransmitter chemicals. They coalesce along the cell wall, and, stimulated by the depolarization associated with the action potential, they move across the cell wall and burst on the outside of the cell, releasing a small packet of neurotransmitter into the synaptic cleft.

Chapter 6: Development of the Ear

1. How does the inner ear form during embryogenesis?

   Answer: The inner ear begins to form a little after 3 weeks gestation and is complete before the end of the third trimester. In the embryo, the inner ear develops before the middle and external ears. The inner ear originates as epidermal placodes (thickenings or discs) that appear on either side of the head at the level of the future hindbrain. The otic placode then develops into an otocyst or otic vesicle, a structure that has highly differentiated, sharply defined tissue borders. The otocyst gives rise to the hearing (cochlea) and vestibular (saccule, utricle, and semicircular canals) organs. Morphogenesis transforms the otocyst into the three dimensional shape of the inner ear, a labyrinth of ducts and recesses. The morphogenesis of the ear is accomplished in a series of interdependent steps that include patterning, growing, and sculpting and is governed by a set of patterning genes that include zinc finger proteins such as GATA3, members of the bone morphogenic proteins (BMP), FGF, homeodomain transcription factors (*Hox*), and *Pax* transcription factors (Figure 8-2). The cochlear duct forms from the separation of scala vestibuli by the vestibular (Reissner's) membrane and from the scala tympani by the basilar membrane. The lateral wall of the cochlear duct remains attached to the surrounding cartilage by the spiral ligament, whereas its medial portion is connected to and partly supported by a long cartilaginous process, the modiolus, the future axis of the bony cochlea (see Figure 8-1).

2. Describe the formation of hair cells and hair cell innervation.

Answer: Null mutation studies show that in addition to *Math1,* POU domain transcription factor *Brn3.1/3c,* as well as other transcription factors such as *Notch, Delta* and *Jagged,* are essential for hair cell development. Intracellular receptors for retinoic acid (Rxr and Rar) and thyroid hormone (TRα and TRβ) are also implicated in controlling cochlear differentiation and, especially, hair cell number. Initially epithelial cells of the cochlear duct are alike. With further development, however, epithelial cells of the cochlear duct separate into an inner ridge and an outer ridge. The inner ridge forms the future spiral limbus and associated structures. The outer ridge forms the future sensory epithelium (organ of Corti), where it differentiates into one row of inner and at least three rows of outer hair cells. An acellular, gelatinous substance, the tectorial membrane, attaches to the spiral limbus and eventually extends to the outer hair cells, where their stereocilia tips insert.

3. Give the primary events and structures during the formation of the middle and external ears.

Answer: The middle ear derives from the first pharyngeal pouch and extends as a tubotympanic recess. During gestational week 5, the distal part of the recess widens and gives rise to a primitive tympanic cavity, and the mesoderm between the two canals forms the tympanic membrane. The middle-ear ossicles develop from the cartilage of the first and second pharyngeal arches. The endodermal epithelial lining of the primitive tympanic cavity then extends along the wall of the newly developing space. The tympanic cavity is now at least twice as large as before. When the ossicles are entirely free of surrounding mesenchyme, the endodermal epithelium connects them in a mesentery-like fashion to the wall of the cavity. The external ear pinna, or auricle, also forms from tissues of the first and second pharyngeal arches. During the sixth gestational week, six tissue swellings termed *auricular hillocks* become apparent. The pinna originates on the embryonic neck below the lower jaw, and then as the mandible develops, the external ear moves relatively higher with a vertical orientation. By gestational week 9, each of the auricular hillocks has formed a distinctive portion of the definitive external ear. The outer (external) auditory meatus develops from the dorsal portion of the first pharyngeal cleft. The outer meatus develops around week 5 when it extends inward toward the pharynx. In the seventh month (trimester 3) this plug dissolves, and the epithelial lining of the floor of the meatus participates in forming the tympanic membrane (eardrum).

4. When is the fetus capable of responding to sounds?

Answer: It is likely that by the middle of prenatal life, definitely by 26–29 gestational weeks, the fetus can hear and respond to sounds. Myelination of the auditory pathway commences after the onset of hearing. Moreover, during trimester 3, the fetus is capable of discriminating between different frequencies and between speech stimuli. Fetal hearing, which occurs in a fluid environment, is via bone conduction.

5. What are the typical causes of congenital deafness?

Answer: Most types of congenital deafness are usually associated with deaf-mutism and are caused by genetic factors. In many cases, the genes involved in congenital deafness have been identified. Recessive inheritance is the most common cause of congenital deafness. Congenital deafness may be caused by abnormal development of the membranous and bony labyrinths or by the abnormal formation of the middle ear ossicles and eardrum. In extreme cases, the tympanic cavity and external meatus are absent. Congenital deafness may also be caused by environmental factors that interfere with normal development of the internal and middle ears. For example, a rubella viral infection during the seventh or eighth week of development can cause severe damage to the organ of Corti and result in sensorineural deafness. It has also been suggested that poliomyelitis, erythroblastosis fetalis, diabetes, hypothyroidism, and toxoplasmosis can cause congenital deafness.

Chapter 7: Structural and Functional Anatomy of the Outer and Middle Ear

1. Discuss how the external ear can aid in auditory perception. Does this differ for low- and high-frequency sounds? Explain why.

Answer: The external ear and head can alter the phase characteristics and amplitude of incoming sound stimuli. These changes are known as the transfer function and are frequency dependent. Briefly, low-frequency (long wavelength) sounds can wrap around the head and the brain can localize that sound in space by interpreting the difference in the time of arrival of the signal to each ear. High-frequency stimuli of shorter wavelength are baffled or reduced in amplitude at the offside ear, which enables the brain to localize these

sounds using differences in intensity at each ear. The external ear, primarily the concha and external auditory meatus, can also enhance the amplitude of certain frequencies through a property called *resonance*. Resonance is particularly effective at frequencies between 2 and 7 kHz.

2. Define resonance. Tell what frequencies are enhanced by the specific resonance capabilities of the outer ear. Why are these frequencies important for human hearing?

Answer: Resonance is the state of a system in which an enhanced vibration is produced by an incoming stimulus when the frequency of that stimulus matches the natural vibration frequency of the system. The external ear resonates to enhance signals in the frequency range of human speech, approximately 2 to 7 kHz.

3. What is the acoustic middle ear reflex? What is the likely functional significance of such a reflex?

Answer: The acoustic middle ear reflex is a reflexive contraction of the stapedius muscle initiated by a loud noise. The threshold of the reflex is about 85 dB and serves to compress amplitudes of signals louder than threshold. This may have protective functions or serve to reduce the masking of high-frequency signals by low frequencies.

4. How does the middle ear prevent airborne sound waves from being reflected as they hit the tympanic membrane?

Answer: The primary task of the middle ear structures is to match the impedance of an airborne sound stimulus to the fluid-filled compartments of the cochlea. It does this through various mechanisms that serve to increase the force applied to the oval window through the stapes.

5. Discuss the three different mechanisms the middle ear uses to match the impedance of air in the external ear canal to the fluids of the inner ear. Which of these mechanisms is the

most important? What would be the result if impedance was not matched?

Answer: Three different mechanisms are used to increase the force applied by a stimulus on the tympanic membrane as it is transmitted to the oval window membrane. The most important of these is the area ratio between the TM and oval window, resulting in a 17-fold increase in pressure. The flexible nature of the TM contributes another two-fold increase, and the lever action of the ossicles, the lever applied to the head of the stapes being shorter than the one attached to the TM, contributes another 1.3-fold increase.

Chapter 8: Cochlear Anatomy

1. Describe the gross structure of the inner ear and how it relates to the middle ear.

   Answer: The inner ear lies within the petrous portion of the temporal bone, medial to the middle ear. There are two openings from the middle ear into the inner ear: the oval window into which the footplate of the stapes fits and the round window closed by the round window membrane. The oval window opens into perilymphatic space of the vestibule, whereas the round window is located at the termination of scala tympani. The cochlea, the hearing portion of the inner ear, consists of three fluid channels spiraling around the central canal of spongy bone termed the modiolus.

2. Describe the three fluid compartments and their boundaries and the two fluids of the cochlea.

   Answer: The fluid channels of cochlea that are filled with perilymph are scala vestibuli and scala tympani. Scala media is located between the other two scalae. Reissner's membrane separates scala vestibuli from scala media and the basilar membrane separates scala tympani from scala media. Scalae vestibuli and tympani are in communication with each other at the cochlear apex through the heli-

cotrema. Perilymph contains a high concentration of sodium ions and a low concentration of potassium ions and is similar in ionic composition to cerebrospinal fluid. Endolymph contains a high concentration of potassium ions and a low concentration of sodium ions and is similar in ionic composition to intracellular fluid.

3. Describe the cochlear duct and its boundaries. What is special about its boundaries?

   Answer: The cochlear duct (also called the endolymphatic space) is bounded by the inner layer of Reissner's membrane, the marginal cells of the stria vascularis, the reticular lamina of the organ of Corti, the interdental cells of the limbus and apical surfaces of inner sulcus, and Claudius' cells. The cells forming the boundary of the endolymphatic space are joined at their apical edges to neighboring cells by tight junctions. The cochlear duct is filled with endolymph. Because the reticular lamina forms one boundary of the endolymphatic space, the fluid spaces in the organ of Corti (i.e., tunnel, Nuel) do not contain endolymph but a fluid similar to perilymph.

4. Name the cells of the organ of Corti. Describe their relation to one another as well as to the basilar membrane and TM.

   Answer: The organ of Corti contains sensory and supporting cells. There is a single row of inner hair cells and three rows of outer hair cells in mammalian cochleas. There are two general classes of supporting cells in the organ of Corti: cells containing parallel bundles of microtubules (pillar and Deiters' cells) and cells without microtubules (inner phalangeal and Hensen's cells). The hair cells are located in the superior half of the organ of Corti, whereas the inner and outer pillar cells, Deiters' cells, and inner phalangeal cells extend from the reticular lamina of the organ of Corti to the superior surface of the basilar membrane. Stereocilia (similar to elongated microvilli) extend from the apical surface of each hair cell into the endolymphatic space.

The tips of the tallest stereocilia on each outer hair cell project into the inferior surface of the tectorial membrane. The tips of the tallest stereocilia on the inner hair cells abut the lateral side of Hensen's stripe on the tectorial membrane.

5. Describe the afferent innervation of the IHC and the OHCs. How does it differ?

Answer: Each inner hair cell receives synaptic terminals from 10–20 Type I spiral ganglion cells. The peripheral processes of the Type I ganglion cells enter the organ of Corti through the habenulae perforata and run radially to the nearest inner hair cell. Each outer hair cell receives synaptic terminals from multiple (but an unknown number) Type II spiral ganglion cells. The peripheral process of each Type II ganglion cell enters the organ of Corti through a habenula perforata, turns in a basal direction, runs in the inner spiral bundle, crosses the tunnel, and enters an outer spiral bundle before synapsing on 6–60 outer hair cells in one or more rows.

Chapter 9: Macromechanics: Basilar Membrane Responses

1. What mechanical features of the basilar membrane (BM)/organ of Corti complex allow it to respond maximally in different places to signals of different frequencies?

Answer: Its mass and stiffness, with the apex being more massive and the base being stiffer and less massive.

2. What is the difference between a nonlinear process in transduction and an active process? How does each contribute to frequency tuning on the BM?

Answer: A **nonlinear** process means the output of the system is not a linear function of the input. It has been known for many years that the ear is nonlinear at very high signal levels, and this helps to "compress" the input on the basilar membrane. An **active** process,

on the other hand, means that energy is being added to the incoming signal by internal sources, and the result is an amplification of BM responses for low-level signals. The net result is an amplification of low-level stimuli and the compression of high-level stimuli, allowing the BM to respond over a large dynamic range of input signals. Therefore, the BM response is both nonlinear and active.

3. What observation from the field of psychoacoustics led to the hypothesis that the ear was nonlinear at low sound pressure levels?

Answer: The finding that subjects with normal hearing ability could hear combination tones at very low sound levels wth special testing techniques, first reported by Goldstein.

4. What paradoxical finding has been reported in numerous studies of normal and disordered hearing?

Answer: The finding that the damaged ear behaves linearly, that is without distortion, and that the normal ear behaves nonlinearly, that is with distortion.

5. What does the term "negative damping" mean in terms of basilar membrane responses to sounds?

Answer: It means that the BM response includes additional energy from internal sources (i.e., the outer hair cells), in addition to the energy in the acoustic signal delivered through the stapes.

Chapter 10: Micromechanics: Transduction and Hair Cell Function

1. Explain how basilar membrane motion in one direction can cause stereocilia motion in an orthogonal direction.

Answer: The rotation points of the basilar membrane and tectorial membrane are displaced (osseous spiral lamina versus spiral limbus). Vertical motion of both leads to sheering motion between the tectorial membrane (into which the OHC stereocilia insert) and the reticular lamina (where the stereocilia are rooted).

2. How does the nonlinearity of the stereocilia transducer channels cause the DC component of the receptor potential?

    Answer: The stereociliary transducer is asymmetric, in that a given bundle displacement in the depolarizing direction leads to greater changes than the same displacement in the hyperpolarizing direction. On average, the hair cell is depolarized by sound. This average change of the stimulus is the DC component of the receptor potential.

3. Explain why potassium currents flow through hair cells.

    Answer: Hair cells have a high concentration of potassium, similar to scala media, but a lower voltage ($\sim +80$–90 mV for the endocochlear potential vs ~ -40 mV for a typical hair cell at rest). Therefore, potassium moves into the hair cell as it moves down its electrical gradient. In contrast to hair cells, the fluid in scala tympani (and the organ of Corti surrounding the hair cells) is low in potassium. Potassium thus moves down its concentration gradient as it moves out through channels in the basolateral membrane.

4. Describe the two types of mechanical feedback by OHCs that could form the basis of the cochlear amplifier.

    Answer: Outer hair cells are known to change their length in response to changes in membrane voltage. This somatic motility may enhance the motion of the basilar membrane and be important for the cochlear amplifier. Also, because stereocilia bundle position is linked to channel opening, stereocilia transducer channels can produce force on the hair bundle as the channels open and close. The bundle may thereby push on the tectorial membrane, forcing the organ of Corti downward in a highly phase-dependent manner.

5. Compare the frequency tuning and input-output relations of the IHC AC and DC potentials with similar measures for the basilar membrane.

    Answer: Generally, the AC and DC components of the IHC receptor potential behave similarly as a function of frequency and intensity, although the DC component may have a higher threshold and be somewhat smaller. The frequency and intensity behavior of the IHC and basilar membrane overall are expected to be similar for a given location.

Chapter 11: Cochlear Afferent Neuronal Function

1. Describe the typical innervation pattern of radial afferent neurons. How many hair cells does one neuron typically contact? How many neurons typically contact a single IHC?

    Answer: Each radial afferent neuron typically contacts one or a few closely spaced inner hair cells. Each inner hair cell typically forms synaptic contacts with 20 afferent dendrites.

2. What distinguishes low-SR neurons by their thresholds? The shape of their rate-intensity curve? How is this thought to be relevant to perception?

    Answer: Low-SR neurons tend to have higher thresholds than their high-SR counterparts. They also may have intensity curves that show shallower slopes and sloping saturation, and thus possess a wider dynamic range. They may greatly extend the dynamic range of the neuronal population overall and establish the wide dynamic range of our perceptual abilities.

3. Describe how the IHC/afferent neuronal synapse is asymmetric and nonlinear.

    Answer: When the hair cell is at rest, the neuron spikes at its spontaneous rate, so the probability that a spike will occur at any time is greater than zero for most neurons. Large hair cell depolarizations have an essentially 100% probability of yielding a spike, and no higher probability is possible. By contrast, even small hyperpolarizations will greatly reduce spike probability to near zero. Therefore, spike probability can only follow small hair cell voltage changes and saturates more abruptly in the hyperpolarizing direction than in the depolarizing direction.

4. Describe the relation between the IHC DC response and afferent spike rate. How might synaptic nonlinearity enhance this?

   Answer: The inner hair cell DC response primarily determines the average spike rate. The asymmetric nonlinearity of the synapse superimposes an additional DC component, which may somewhat further increase the average spike rate.

5. How does the AC component of the IHC receptor potential cause neural phase-locking? Why does it decline at high frequencies?

   Answer: The AC component of the inner hair cell receptor potential is the basis of neural phase-locking. Phase-locking declines at high frequencies because the AC component of the hair cell response is filtered out by the capacitance of the hair cell membrane.

6. Why is it said that an apparent gap exists between the dynamic range of auditory neurons and our perceptual abilities? How is it probably resolved?

   Answer: At any frequency, the dynamic range of the auditory system exceeds 120 dB, whereas that of most neurons is typically only 20–30 dB. Variation in neuronal thresholds by SR and sloping saturation in low-SR neurons may greatly extend the dynamic range of small groups of neurons tuned to the same frequency, closing the apparent gap.

7. What is the relation between spike rate adaptation and forward masking?

   Answer: Spike rate adaptation appears as a decrease in firing rate during a stimulus and a pronounced decrease in firing rate when a stimulus is turned off. The latter is typically below a neuron's SR. During the post-stimulus period when firing rate is decreased, any new

stimulus will elicit a relatively decreased response. Reduction in response caused by a previous stimulus is known as forward masking and has a perceptual counterpart.

8. Why might we say that the synapse appears designed to emphasize changes in the acoustic environment?

   Answer: Spike rate adaptation (see answer to question 7) originates at the afferent synapse. It has the effect of emphasizing both the beginning and end of a stimulus.

9. How do neuronal frequency tuning curves change with increasing CF? What is the apparent relation between tuning curve tip width and critical bands? Is this more relevant to the notion of frequency *discrimination* or *resolution*?

   Answer: The relative bandwidth of frequency tuning curves decreases with increasing CF and is associated with an increase in Q_{10}. Tuning curve tip bandwidth roughly mirrors the width of perceptual critical bands. These may be thought of as independent frequency channels and are most relevant to the issue of frequency resolution.

10. Compare and contrast spike rate and synchrony suppression. How might these influence perception?

    Answer: Spike rate suppression is usually found only at the margins of rate tuning curves. It appears to reduce spectral contrast. Synchrony suppression is a reduction in phase-locking to a CF probe tone. It can be found anywhere in the tuning curve and may coincide with an overall increase in firing rate. If spectral shape can be encoded by phase-locking, synchrony suppression may enhance spectral contrast.

11. What are some possible limitations of rate-place coding?

    Answer: The notion of rate-place coding presumes that the goal of firing patterns across neurons is to create a spatial activity pattern that mirrors the spectral shape of the stimulus. Rate saturation and rate suppression in most neurons cause broadening of spectral peaks at high stimulus levels, apparently degrading the representation of spectral shape.

12. How might characteristics of onset responses and the rate-intensity behavior of low-SR neurons help preserve rate-place coding?

    Answer: When low-SR neurons are included in the spatial activity pattern (see answer to question 11), spectral shape is preserved. Onset responses have wider dynamic ranges than do steady-state responses and also show better preservation of spectral shape.

13. What is the compound action potential? What is the relation between N_1 of the CAP and Wave I of the ABR?

    Answer: The compound action potential occurs at the onset of a stimulus and consists of two negative-going peaks (N_1 and N_2). For low stimulus levels, N_1 represents the synchronous response of neurons tuned to the stimulus frequency. It is analogous to Wave I of the ABR.

Chapter 12: Cochlear Efferent Anatomy and Function

1. Where are the cell bodies of medial and lateral olivocochlear neurons located?

   Answer: Olivocochlear neurons have cell bodies located in the superior olivary complex that spans the hindbrain and pons. Medial olivocochlear neurons are found in medial and ventral portions of the periolivary nuclei, whereas lateral olivocochlear neurons are found in or near the lateral superior olive.

2. Olivocochlear axons travel across or in which cranial nerves (tracts)?

   Answer: Olivocochlear axons bundle together before crossing through the genu of the facial nerve tract and then exit the brainstem, traveling in the vestibular nerve before crossing into the cochlear nerve.

3. What are the crossed and uncrossed projections of olivocochlear axons?

Answer: Lateral olivocochlear neurons project mostly to the ipsilateral cochlea via uncrossed bundles, whereas medial olivocochlear neurons project mostly to the contralateral cochlea via crossed bundles.

4. How do medial and lateral olivocochlear neurons differ with respect to their terminations?

   Answer: Medial olivocochlear axons project to outer hair cells, whereas lateral olivocochlear neurons project to the dendrites of spiral ganglion fibers just below the inner hair cells.

5. What are the primary neurotransmitters used by olivocochlear neurons?

   Answer: Acetylcholine and GABA are the major neurotransmitters.

6. When the olivocochlear system is stimulated, what are the effects on the periphery?

   Answer: Increase in cochlear potential thresholds, reduction in the CAP amplitude, reduction in the afferent fibers discharge rate.

7. How does the medial olivocochlear reflex differ from the middle-ear-muscle acoustic reflex?

   Answer: The medial olivocochlear reflex has a low threshold for activation (10–20 dB above hearing level), is maximally responsive to mid- to high-frequency stimuli, and is mediated by modulation of outer hair cell function.

8. What role does the olivocochlear system play in masking noise?

   Answer: The medial olivocochlear reflex decreases the effects of excitatory masking. In the presence of continuous noise and a transient signal, the medial olivocochlear reflex decreases the steady response to noise by auditory nerve fibers, thereby increasing the response to a transient signal.

Chapter 13: Otoacoustic Emissions

1. Describe OAEs.

   Answer: Otoacoustic emissions are echoes within the ear canal that are generated from distortions within the cochlea. They have a latency of roughly 6–7 msec.

2. How are OAEs classified, and what stimuli are used to generate OAEs?

Answer: Otoacoustic emissions may be classified as either spontaneous (no sound stimulation) or evoked (after sound stimulation) echoes. Evoked OAEs are classically subdivided into transient evoked OAEs (TEOAEs) obtained in response to brief stimulus such as clicks or tone bursts, distortion product OAEs (DPOAEs) produced in response to pairs of pure tones, and stimulus frequency OAEs (SFOAEs) generated in response to continuous tonal stimulus.

3. How do OAEs originate? Provide evidence to support your argument.

Answer: Otoacoustic emissions are a by-product of what is called the "cochlear amplifier." They are generated because of nonlinear disturbances along the cochlear partition and produce "reverse" fluid motions that lead to vibrations of the oval window, ossicles, and eardrum. Otoacoustic emissions are sensitive indicators of the functional state of cochlear amplification and are only present when the cochlear amplifier is present and working. The cochlear amplifier and OAEs are similarly vulnerable to drugs, noise, and hypoxia. Because the outer hair cells are responsible, at least in part, for generation of the cochlear amplification, they are also believed to play a major role in the generation of OAEs.

4. What are the clinical advantages of OAE testing over more traditional audiologic tests?

Answer: Advantages of OAEs over traditional audiologic techniques include objectivity, efficiency, noninvasive, and sensitivity. Otoacoustic emissions are absent in ears that exhibit partial or complete hearing loss and are very sensitive to cochlear pathology. They are particularly well suited for subjects such as infants who are difficult to test and for field-testing at schools and industrial sites.

5. How does stimulation of the olivocochlear system affect OAEs?

Answer: Otoacoustic emissions are suppressed following presentation of sound stimuli to the same, opposite, or both ears. Suppression of OAEs is consistent with olivocochlear efferent effects and is believed to be mediated through the modulation of outer hair cell motility.

Chapter 14: Neuroanatomy of the Auditory System

1. What are the major lobes of the cerebral hemispheres?

Answer: The four major lobes of the brain are named for the bones of the skull that overlie them: frontal, parietal, temporal, and occipital.

2. What are the borders of the parietal lobe?

Answer: The parietal lobe resides between the frontal and occipital lobes and on top of the temporal lobe. The parietal lobe most notably receives somatic (body and skin) sensory information.

3. Describe the formation of the CNS.

Answer: The central nervous system is derived from a dorsally located, thickened plate of ectoderm, known as the neural plate, which first appears late in the third week of fetal life. This dorsal plate ectoderm eventually grows to form a neural groove, which is bounded on each side by an elevated neural fold that ultimately fuses to form the neural tube. First, the ectoderm in the dorsal midline of the embryo thickens forming the neural plate. After the neural plate enlarges dorsally, the neural groove forms the neural tube and overlying ectoderm. The neural tube differentiates into the brain and the spinal cord. By the time that the neural tube closes, three primary brain vesicles are evident from which the brain develops.

4. At the pons-medulla border, what sensory and motor information is present?

Answer: At the pons-medulla border, primary auditory and vestibular fibers from the inner ear enter the brainstem and facial motor fibers and olivocochlear fibers exit the brain stem.

5. Describe the pathway for sound localization in the brainstem.

Answer: Two prominent nuclei within the superior olivary complex are the lateral superior olive and the medial superior olive. The medial superior olive is more sensitive to interaural timing differences, whereas the lateral superior olive is more sensitive to interaural intensity differences. From the superior olivary complex, third-order neurons ascend in the lateral lemniscus.

6. Describe the cortical areas associated with the speech/language pathway.

Answer: Broca's area, Wernicke's area, and the primary auditory cortex comprise the major regions of the cerebral hemispheres specialized for speech and language. Broca's area is found in the inferior frontal gyrus. It is concerned mostly with the motor mechanisms associated with speech formulation. Wernicke's area is the major language association area and is located in the caudal region of the temporal lobe, adjacent to the auditory cortex.

Chapter 15: Functional Organization of the Auditory Central Nervous System

1. Defend the following claim: "We don't hear the world as it really is."

Answer: The auditory information processed by our brain is provided by the cochlea, which is a band-pass filter. In addition, lower brain centers suppress some information after extracting cues for functions such as localization and speech perception.

2. What is meant by multidimensional tuning?

Answer: Auditory neurons may be tuned for many features in addition to frequency, including stimulus rise/fall times, duration, AM rate, and FM rate.

3. What kinds of maps are well supported in the ACNS? What others have been proposed?

Answer: The most prominent mapping theme in the ACNS is organization by frequency. Maps within some structures for AM rate, sound source location, and pitch have been proposed.

4. What types of response properties and neuronal abilities change as one ascends the hierarchy within the ACNS?

Answer: The tails of frequency tuning curves are removed by lateral inhibition, so that tuning remains sharp high stimulus levels. Neurons acquire binaural response properties. Tuning for complex stimulus features duration, AM/FM rate) and combination sensitivity arise. All these appear essentially "complete" at the level of the inferior colliculus, however, and do not clearly become more refined at higher levels. Temporal following ability is progressively reduced at higher levels.

5. Explain the term *parallel-hierarchical* as it applies to the ACNS.

Answer: Acoustic information is recombined at each level in the ACNS to produce new selectivities and new functions. At each level, however, there are subdivisions within each auditory center and multiple centers operating in parallel.

6. How have observations of combination-sensitive neurons supported notions about the involvement of specialized neurons in perception?

Answer: We identify complex auditory stimuli such as speech using several cues, some of which seem to require comparisons of distinct components in both spectral and temporal domains. Combination sensitive neurons seem ideal for such tasks. Their demonstration in bats and primates supports the idea that they could play a role.

7. Contrast the general response property neurons in lemniscal and nonlemniscal pathways.

Answer: Lemniscal pathways are clearly tonotopically organized. Neurons in lemniscal centers are generally sharply frequency tuned and show minimal habituation. Nonlemniscal pathways show little or no tonotopy. Neurons in nonlemniscal centers are often poorly tuned. They may habituate readily and show preferences for dynamic or complex stimuli. They also tend to show more robust plasticity than lemniscal neurons.

8. Where do binaural interactions first arise within the ACNS? Contrast the general principles that underlie the operation of the centers that carry out analysis of interaural time and level differences.

   Answer: Binaural interactions first arise in the superior olivary complex. The medial superior olive carries out comparisons of interaural phase and time-of-arrival and receives predominantly low-frequency projections. The lateral superior olive carries out comparisons of interaural intensity and receives predominantly high-frequency projections.

9. Describe the duplex theory of sound localization and relate the operation of the medial superior olivary complex to the Jeffress model.

   Answer: The use of low- and high-frequency information, respectively, for interaural time and intensity comparisons follows from physical acoustics. Low frequencies have longer wavelengths, so that phase differences between the two ears can be detected. Low frequencies show little head-shadow effect, however, so they are not suitable for interaural intensity comparisons. The opposite characteristics apply to high frequencies, which are associated with short wavelengths and prominent shadow effects. Interaural time comparisons suggest the need for a neural architecture that matches frequency-specific inputs from the two ears over a wide range of interaural delays. Jeffress recognized that the distance across the head itself could provide a spatial delay line, which could be exploited and extended by brain centers.

10. What kinds of evidence might be brought to bear on questions regarding the function of a particular cortical area in hearing?

    Answer: A neural "candidate" to fulfill a particular type of sound analysis would be expected to have tuning properties suitable to that function. Lesion studies would be further expected to indicate that the structure in which the neuron is located is necessary to the function. Functional imaging studies (MEG, PET, fMRI) should show that the region of interest is active when the function is carried out in awake, behaving subjects.

Chapter 16: Vestibular System Function: From Physiology to Pathology

1. During surgery to remove an acoustic neuroma, the VIIIth nerve on the left side of the head is transected. What effects would you expect to see immediately? What long-term problems might the patient have?

   Answer: The patient would experience a profound hearing loss on that side. In addition, because he/she would lose immediately the spontaneous activity of the neurons that were transected on the affected side, the neurons of the vestibular nuclei receive a higher firing rate from the neurons on the intact side, which would be interpreted as a head turn away from the ear with the lesion. Eventually, the system would adjust to a new "set" point, but function might still be diminished.

2. You are administering a caloric test. When warm water is introduced in the right ear, what direction and type of nystagmus would you expect in a normal patient? If a labyrinthine lesion on the right ear is present, how would the nystagmus differ for right and left ear irrigations of warm water?

   Answer: In a normal patient, one would expect to see a horizontal nystagmus that beats to the right. If the right ear is affected, one would expect to see an asymmetric response, with the affected side showing a weaker nystagmus.

3. A patient is presented during ENT rounds with symptoms including unsteadiness when standing in the dark, nausea, dizziness, and nystagmus. CT and magnetic resonance imaging scans were unremarkable. The patient has been undergoing a lengthy treatment for tuberculosis with aminoglycosides. How would the vestibular system be affected?

Answer: The symptoms are most likely linked to the treatment with aminoglycosides. The effects are usually similar in both ears; there are usually no asymmetries found. However, the patients may report headache, nausea, vomiting, vertigo, and nystagmus.

4. Outline the VOR for a common horizontal rotational head movement. What are the neural pathways involved and what type of eye movement response will occur?

Answer: The reflex is initiated by head movement. If the head is moved to the left, the neurons from the left horizontal semicircular canal are depolarized and increase their firing rate. At the same time, neurons from the right horizontal canal are hyperpolarized and decrease their firing rate. Neurons in the left vestibular nuclei that receive projections directly from the left canal and from the right canal via commissural fibers are activated and send a signal across the midline to motor neurons in the right abducens nucleus. These neurons excite the lateral rectus muscle of the right eye, causing a movement of that eye toward the right. At the same time, interneurons in the right abducens nucleus project back across the midline to the motor neurons in the oculomotor nucleus, which excite the medial rectus muscle of the left eye, also moving it to the right. The result is a conjugate eye movement to the right that is compensatory, that is, it maintains a steady visual field when the head is turned.

5. Describe three ways one can measure eye movement in patients. What are the disadvantages of each?

Answer: (1) Electronystagmography involves measuring the electrical potential difference between the front and back of the eye using surface electrodes. The disadvantage is that only horizontal and vertical movements can be tracked. (2) Ocular videography uses an infrared camera mounted in goggles, and the images are decoded by computer. A disadvantage is that this system cannot track fast movements. (3) Magnetic search-coil technology is a modern technique that uses coils embedded in a contact lens that is worn by the patient. A disadvantage is that these tests must be completed in a magnetic field, requiring somewhat sophisticated technology.

Chapter 17: Pathology of the Middle Ear

1. Name and describe the common symptoms associated with ear disease.

Answer: The symptoms most commonly associated with ear disease are hearing loss, otalgia (ear pain), otorrhea (drainage from the ear), tinnitus (ringing in the ears), and vertigo (inappropriate sensation of body movement such as spinning).

2. Explain why children are more susceptible than adults to ear infections.

Answer: The Eustachian tube, which is responsible for draining secretions (fluid) from the middle ear, is more horizontally positioned in children than adults, making drainage more difficult. This positioning and the wider lumen of the tube in children also gives bacteria from the nasopharynx easier access to the middle ear. Blockage of the tube due to the irritation caused by second-hand smoke and chlorine in pool water can also prevent normal drainage of the middle ear.

3. Describe how cholesteatomas, glomus tumors, and otosclerosis are similar in their effect on hearing.

   Answer: All three of these disease states are capable of producing a profound conductive hearing loss. Otosclerosis typically reduces conduction by reducing the normal mobility of the ossicular chain, most commonly by freezing the stapes footplate in the oval window. Glomus tumors and cholesteatomas also cause conductive losses by filling the middle ear space, especially if they contact the tympanic membrane and ossicular chain. Pressure and the production of inflammatory molecules eventually lead to erosion of bony structures.

4. Describe the mechanisms used by bacterial biofilms to reduce their susceptibility to antibiotic treatment.

   Answer: Bacteria in biofilms change their phenotype to reduce their susceptibility to antibiotics. These changes may include a reduced expression of certain receptors and reduced protein synthesis and mitotic activities. The physical structure of the biofilm itself, as well as the polysaccharide matrix, also acts as a barrier to the penetration of antibiotics.

Chapter 18: Noise-Induced Hearing Loss

1. Why isn't more known about permanent hearing loss in humans?

   Answer: Because it is unethical to expose humans to noises that may cause permanent injury, it is difficult to study the relation among exposure, hearing loss, and damage to the inner ear. An additional challenge is that workplace noise regulations, if enforced, limit the amounts of noise to which workers can be exposed without wearing hearing protection.

2. Identify three regions of the cochlea that are vulnerable to excessive noise exposure.

Answer: (1) The stria vascularis, the source of the "power" for the endolymphatic potential displays temporary and permanent changes after noise. (2) The outer hair cell complex, which provides the active amplification at low levels, can be damaged (swollen, tip link breakage, etc) or destroyed completely. (3) The inner hair cells and the afferent nerve fibers can show the effects of excitotoxicity.

3. How does acoustic trauma differ from NIHL?

   Answer: Acoustic trauma is caused by brief exposures to extremely intense sounds such as the detonation of a firecracker near the ear or the report of a large caliber firearm. It is limited to exposures that exceed peak sound pressure levels of 140 dB. The damage is mechanical, instantaneous, and is accompanied by irreversible permanent hearing loss. In contrast, chronic NIHL grows slowly over months and years of repeated exposure and is related to dysfunction and damage to the delicately balanced homeostatic mechanisms maintaining cochlear function.

4. How are studies of NIHL and the field of audiology related?

   Answer: The major impetus for the development of audiology came from two sources: individuals who sustained hearing loss from working in noisy industries, such as boilermakers and coppersmiths, and soldiers returning from combat during World War II. Both created "casualties": people who needed rehabilitation and assistive technology to overcome their hearing losses.

5. Is hearing loss due to shooting a more important problem in the United States than occupational noise exposure or presbycusis? Explain your answer.

   Answer: From the other chapters of this book, you have learned that about 9 million Americans work in potentially hazardous occupational noise environments. On the other hand, 70 million Americans own more than

250 million guns! An additional factor is that the occupational noise environment is regulated by the federal government, and many individuals who must work in noise participate in hearing conservation programs, receiving annual audiograms and wearing hearing protection in environments with noise that exceeds daily levels of 90 dBA. So of the two, shooting seems to be more important, simply because more people are potentially affected.

This is a bit of a trick question because, as you know from the chapter on presbycusis, nearly everyone suffers from age-related hearing loss later in life. So the way to think about this question is that the effects of presbycusis visit everyone eventually, but they are exacerbated by NIHL either from workplace noise or from hunting/target shooting. As experts on hearing protection, audiologists can help their patients understand this very important relation and counsel people who work or play in noise to limit their exposures and to wear hearing protection around loud noise, so they may have a better chance to hear their grandchildren.

Chapter 19: Ototoxin-Induced Hearing Loss

1. Describe the pattern of damage to cells in the cochlea caused by aminoglycoside antibiotics and cisplatin.

   Answer: These agents cause permanent loss of outer hair cells in the basal turn of the cochlea.

2. List two symptoms associated with salicylate-induced ototoxicity.

   Answer: Reversible hearing loss and tinnitus.

3. List two features of erythromycin ototoxicity.

   Answer: Hearing loss in patients with kidney or liver disease.

4. Specify how loop diuretics act on the cochlea.

   Answer: They cause edema in the stria vascularis, leading to hearing loss

Chapter 20: Genetic Aspects of Hearing Loss

1. Describe the roles of DNA, mRNA, rRNA, and tRNA.

   Answer: DNA and the genes it contains serve as the blueprint for all cellular protein production. mRNA is transcribed from DNA and conveys the instructions for protein amino acid sequences from the cell nucleus to ribosomes in the cytoplasm. rRNAs are special RNAs that partly comprise ribosomes. Each tRNA bonds to both mRNA and a specific amino acid. Thus, tRNAs carry out the actual translation of the genetic code into an amino acid sequence. It is the sequence of amino acids that determines what a protein can do.

2. Define transcription and translation.

   Answer: Transcription is the process of creating an mRNA that is complementary to the DNA template strand. Translation is the conversion of the nucleic acid base sequence of mRNA into an amino acid sequence by tRNA.

3. In addition to proteins, what else can genes code for?

   Answer: In addition to structural genes, which code for most proteins, there are also regulatory genes that control transcription and genes that code directly for tRNA and rRNA.

4. Why might different base substitution mutations that lead to different amino acid substitutions yield different phenotypes?

   Answer: Some base substitutions (particular in those in the third codon position) may lead to the inclusion of an amino acid with similar properties to the one originally encoded. Such substitutions may have little effect on protein function. Alternatively, some substitutions may cause a very different amino acid to be inserted at a given position in a protein, but the position may be noncritical, so that protein function is not altered.

5. What is the physical basis of gene linkage?

    Answer: The physical basis of gene linkage is simply proximity on a chromosome and in the DNA sequence. Recombination is random and is less likely to occur between two bases when they are close together.

6. Describe the notion of how mechanistic "bottlenecks" may determine what genetic diseases humans experience.

    Answer: Mutation of DNA and genes is random, as is duplication of genes over evolutionary time. Duplication of entire genes or introns during evolution has given rise to multiple variants of many proteins. Some cells may express more than one of these and may be able to use one variant to replace another that is defective through mutation. Just by chance, however, many genes and proteins have not acquired "backups." Mutations in these genes may give rise to disease. This may be more likely in the case of structures that are highly cell specific, such as stereocilia.

7. Describe two ways a dominant trait may arise.

    Answer: Some mutations may alter a protein such that it takes on an entirely new function. If the function has an associated phenotype, just one copy of the mutation may be adequate for the phenotype to be evident. Also, a mutation may lead to a defective form of a protein that is nevertheless inserted into a multimeric structure, so that the entire structure does not function properly. A single copy of the mutation may similarly lead to an apparent phenotype.

8. Why are traits determined by mtDNA maternally inherited?

    Answer: Essentially, all the mitochondria of the fertilized egg (zygote) come from the egg, and thus from the mother. Mitochondria and their DNA reside in the cytoplasm, not the cell nucleus.

9. Name two reasons that individuals with mutations in the same gene might show different phenotypes.

    Answer: Two people may have different mutations of the same gene, with different functional consequences. They may also carry different alleles of modifier genes.

10. Contrast neuroepithelial and cochleosaccular pathologies.

    Answer: Neuroepithelial degeneration involves the organ of Corti and its neuronal supply. It may arise through mutations within any of the cells of the organ. It may also occur secondarily to mutations within cells outside the organ of Corti, including spiral ligament. Cochleosaccular degeneration involves abnormal developmental migration or function of pigmented cells, including intermediate cells of the stria vascularis. This can lead to abnormal composition of cochlear endolymph and loss of the endocochlear potential. Scala media may collapse, and secondary degeneration of the organ of Corti may occur.

Chapter 21: Age-Related Hearing Loss

1. Describe the link between basal metabolic rate and mitochondrial injury.

    Answer: Mitochondria lie at the heart of oxidative metabolism, which produces reactive oxygen species as a toxic by-product. Therefore, a higher metabolic rate exposes mitochondria to greater injury, including cumulative damage to mitochondrial DNA.

2. Why might oxygen be said to be both friend and enemy of aerobic cells?

    Answer: Oxygen is a corrosive molecule that promotes the breakdown of other molecules, especially biomolecules composed of carbon and hydrogen. Cells use oxygen to break down large biomolecules that serve as fuel and raw material for synthesizing cell components. In the process, cells risk being oxidized themselves.

3. Name and characterize five major types of cochlear presbycusis that Schuknecht described.

Answer: (1) Sensory presbycusis principally involves degeneration of organ of Corti. (2) Neural presbycusis involves primary loss of afferent neurons. (3) Strial presbycusis refers to strial degeneration and reduction in the endo-cochlear potential. (4) Cochlear conductive presbycusis hypothetically involves alterations in the passive mechanical properties of the basilar membrane and other moving structures, without explicit cell loss or degeneration. (5) Mixed presbycusis refers to some combination of the other four, potentially from independent causes, making independent contributions to the audiogram.

4. Characterize the relation between hearing loss and loss of (1) hair cells, (2) afferent neurons, (3) strial cells, and (4) ligament fibrocytes.

   Answer: At any cochlear location, even minor loss of either type of hair cell would be expected to reduce sensitivity and (for outer hair cells) dynamic range and sharp frequency tuning. Loss of most neurons at the same location may have little effect on sensitivity, but may impair detection of signals in noise. Widespread loss of strial cells (perhaps up to 40%) and ligament fibrocytes may have little effect on hearing.

5. Name some problems with the use of audiograms to diagnose particular forms of presbycusis.

   Answer: Contrary to Schuknecht's assertions, the shape of the audiogram may be a poor diagnostic tool because a particular audiogram shape could arise from many combinations from organ of Corti, stria vascularis, and neuronal pathology. A normal audiogram may hide moderate-to-severe afferent neuronal loss.

6. Why might impaired speech perception in noise despite a normal audiogram not be diagnostic of a "pure" central aging effect?

   Answer: Peripheral afferent neuronal loss, which an audiogram might miss, could impair speech perception.

Chapter 22: Potential Therapies for Hearing Loss: Preventing Hair Cell Death and Promoting Hair Cell Regeneration

1. What are some key differences between cell death that occurs via *apoptosis* vs. *necrosis*?

   Answer: Death via apoptosis is a metabolically active process that requires new gene expression, new protein synthesis, changes in mitochondria, and activation of specific "executor" proteins (caspases). Notably, apoptotic death can be prevented by treatment with certain drugs that block the progression of any of these steps. In contrast, necrosis is a (mostly) passive death process that results from massive structural injury to a cell. At present, there are no methods for reversing or preventing death via necrosis.

2. The ears of most nonmammalian vertebrates (e.g., fish, frogs, birds, among others) can regenerate hair cells after ototoxic injury. How are these new hair cells actually produced?

   Answer: Most regenerated hair cells are produced by renewed cell division. Specifically, injury to the sensory epithelium triggers the division among nearby supporting cells. The progeny of these dividing cells can then differentiate as replacement hair cells and supporting cells.

3. The mammalian ear has a very limited capacity for regeneration. What is one key limitation on the regenerative ability of the mammalian cochlea?

   Answer: In contrast to ears of nonmammals (see Question 2), supporting cells in the mammalian cochlea are not capable of dividing. Thus, the mammalian cochlea lacks the ability to produce new hair cells in response to injury.

4. Name two signals or guidance cues that growing auditory neurons (spiral ganglion cells) could potentially use to navigate to their correct hair cell targets.

Answer: Hair cells appear to release diffusible chemicals that attract growing neurons. Specifically, the filopodia of growing neurons can "sense" the concentration of these chemicals, which then guides them to sensory hair cells. Guidance to hair cells may also be achieved by the presence of specific molecules that are bound to surfaces on which the neurons grow, guiding them to their appropriate targets.

5. How might stem cells be used in the treatment of hearing and balance disorders?

Answer: Stem cells may potentially be induced to become hair cells and/or afferent (spiral ganglion or vestibular) neurons, which might then be surgically introduced into the inner ear.

Glossary

Abducens nucleus The sixth cranial nucleus located in the pons. It is composed of oculomotor neurons that project through the sixth cranial nerve to innervate the lateral rectus muscle of the eye. Other abducens neurons decussate (cross over) the midline to terminate on cells in the oculomotor nucleus (III cranial nucleus) that control the medial rectus muscle of the other eye.

Absolutely refractory period The period just after a neuron fires, during which it cannot fire again, no matter what the stimulus.

AC/DC An engineering term specifying whether a signal contains rapid (AC, or alternating current) or slow fluctuations (DC, or direct current). Cochlear hair cell electrical responses to sound generally contain both AC and DC components. In inner hair cells, these are largely responsible for changes in neuronal spike timing and rate, respectively.

Acetylcholine A primary, usually excitatory, neurotransmitter made of acetate and choline and whose effects can be mimicked by nicotine and muscarine.

Acoustic intensity Power through area in Watts per meter squared (W/m^2).

Acoustic middle ear reflex Sound-induced contraction of the stapedius muscle that results in amplitude compression of stimuli above a typical threshold of about 85-dB hearing level.

Acoustic reflex Mediated through the fifth and seventh cranial nerves, causes contraction of the stapedius and tensor tympani muscles of the middle ear, which alters its impedance and reduces sound transmission by up to 20 dB for intense sound input.

Acoustic stria Ascending auditory pathways from the cochlear nuclei.

Acoustic trauma Damage to the cochlea and hearing loss caused by exposure to high-level, short-duration sounds, such as explosions or the report of large-caliber firearms.

Actin filament The smallest of the cytoskeletal elements. Actin filaments are necessary for cell motility, division, and muscle contraction.

Action potential (spike) Reversal of the membrane potential of a neuron from negative to positive lasting a few milliseconds.

Active process (cochlear amplifier) (Cochlea) The biologically active component of the basilar membrane response to sound that adds energy, counteracting inherent damping.

Adenosine triphosphate (ATP) An active protein that supplies energy to the cell by breaking down; the source of energy for cellular activities. ATP is derived from the process of respiration, which occurs on the mitochondria inner membrane.

Afferent neuron Conducts information toward the brain from the periphery.

Albumin Protein that is present in the blood; it is synthesized in the liver.

Allele A particular form of a gene. It may differ from other forms by as little as a single base pair. Any gene may have countless alleles across a population, some of which may confer advantages, whereas others may have disadvantages or promote disease.

Amino acids Twenty special carboxylic acids containing an amino (NH^{3+}) side chain that form the structural basis of proteins.

Aminoglycoside antibiotics Class of antibiotics used to treat tuberculosis and infections caused by gram-negative bacteria, such as *Pseudomonas.*

Analog coding Representation of a signal in terms of its actual values, recorded continuously (see Digital coding).

Anemia Reduction or deficiency in the concentration of red blood cells in the circulation.

Antihelix The inner ridge of the external ear or auricle, just medial to the helix.

Antimasking Increasing the response to a tone in the presence of noise or other tones.

Antioxidant Any compound or molecule that reduces the reactivity of reactive oxygen species, thus protecting a cell or tissue.

Antitragus A small bump opposite the tragus that lies on the posteroinferior edge of the opening to the external auditory meatus.

Aperiodic waveform Waveform whose amplitude function is not periodic.

Apoptosis (programmed cell death, or PCD) A biologically active form of cell death requiring new protein synthesis and activation of caspase family proteins. Present data suggest that the majority of hair cell death after acoustic trauma or ototoxic exposure occurs by this process.

Area 41 Primary auditory cortex, consisting of a portion of the anterior and posterior temporal gyri and receiving auditory (geniculotemporal) radiations from the medial geniculate to the transverse temporal gyrus on the temporal cortex of the same side.

Area 42 An auditory association area (Wernicke's area) adjacent to area 41 on parts of the posterior transverse and superior temporal gyri.

Association cortex Area of the neocortex that receives either sensory or motor information via a primary cortical area.

Asymmetric nonlinearity A type of nonlinear system wherein the instantaneous relation between input and output is a different type of nonlinearity for positive changes than for negative changes. The relation between stereocilia deflection and hair cell membrane potential is of this type.

Asymptotic threshold shift (ATS) The limit of temporary threshold shifts in the presence of continuing noise exposure. Threshold shifts grow for 8 to 24 hours of exposure and then stabilize at asymptotic levels.

Atrophy Shrinkage in size of cells or tissue compartment, or both.

Au.D. Doctor of Audiology graduate degree, now offered by more than 70 programs in the United States.

Audiology A branch of science that is devoted to the study of hearing and balance, and their disorders.

Audiometric notch (4 kHz notch) An audiometric pattern commonly observed in patients with noise-induced hearing losses (NIHL). Hearing thresholds at 3, 4, or 6 kHz are worse than corresponding thresholds for lower frequency (500 Hz, 1 kHz, 2 kHz) or higher frequency (8 kHz) tones. Notches are not uniquely associated with NIHL, because some individuals without a history of excessive noise exposure exhibit them.

Auricle The part of the external ear that projects outward from the head; also called *pinna.*

Autonomic nervous system A portion of the nervous system that controls "automatic" activities, such as heartbeat, breathing, and digestion, through reflex arcs.

Autosomes The 22 pairs of chromosomes that do not directly determine sex or sex-related features.

A-weighting filter A filter inserted in a sound level meter to adjust the response according to human hearing.

Axon A long projection from a nerve cell that conducts electrical impulses away from the cell body toward the telodendria.

Axon hillock The "action zone" of a cell body, including the soma, and the root that sprouts the axon.

Bacterial biofilm Colonies of bacteria that can cooperatively change between active and sessile forms to enhance resistance to antibiotics and other environmental influences. Such biofilms are now thought to provide the mechanism for many chronic bacterial infections, including those of the middle ear.

Band-pass filter Allows only a restricted band of frequencies to pass through unattenuated.

Band-reject filter Stops a restricted band of frequencies from passing through.

Basal turn (lower turn) of the cochlea Portion of the cochlea that encodes higher frequency sounds.

Basilar membrane Fibroelastic membrane that extends between the osseous spiral lamina and spiral ligament.

Battery Refers to the active ionic pumps in the stria vascularis that create the +80 mV endolymphatic potential.

Best frequency The frequency of a sound stimulus that yields the largest response, or a response at the lowest intensity. "Response" could be the response of the basilar membrane, hair cell, or neuron.

Binaural Input from two ears.

Blood–brain barrier The physiologic properties of the blood vessels in the brain that limit the transfer of substances from the blood to the brain.

BM (basilar membrane) response The mechanical response of the basilar membrane.

Brainstem The diencephalons, composed of the midbrain, pons, and medulla.

Broca's speech area A region of the frontal lobe that is involved in the motor planning for speech and is associated with Broca's (motor) aphasia when damaged.

Caloric restriction Consumption of ~10% fewer calories than the typical diet would provide. Caloric restriction over years effectively promotes longevity and decreased age-related illness.

Caloric testing Evaluation of vestibular function using warm and cool water or air to stimulate eye movements (nystagmus).

Cell proliferation During this process, a cell duplicates its DNA and creates two complete sets of chromosomes. Each set of chromosomes then migrates to opposite sides of the cell and the cell divides into two "daughter" cells. The process of cell division is tightly regulated in most tissues of mature animals. Regenerated hair cells in the ears of nonmammalian vertebrates are created by the proliferation of remaining supporting cells.

Central nervous system The portion of the nervous system encased by the skull and the spinal column. It includes the cerebrum, brainstem, cerebellum, and the spinal cord.

Central presbycusis Age-related hearing loss or changes in perception caused principally by pathology within the central auditory system. Some changes in temporal acuity and some binaural interactions such as contralateral suppression of distortion product otoacoustic emissions may have a central basis.

Cerebellum A part of the rhombencephalon concerned with movement control.

Cerebral hemispheres The two sides of the cerebrum.

Cerebrum The telencephalon, largest part of the forebrain.

Characteristic frequency (best frequency) The frequency of a sound stimulus that yields the largest response, or a response at the lowest intensity. "Response" could be the response of the basilar membrane, hair cell, or neuron.

Characteristic impedance The opposition to movement created by the density and elasticity of the medium.

Cholesteatoma A tumor-like collection of keratinizing squamous epithelium that starts on the tympanic membrane and extends into the middle ear cavity, mastoid, or both, resulting in impaired conduction and erosion of adjacent bony structures.

Cholinergic Having to do with acetylcholine activity or responses.

Chromosome A single DNA molecule that may be longer than a meter and contains thousands of genes.

Cochlea (plural: cochleae or cochleas) Hearing portion of the inner ear of mammals.

Cochlear amplifier (active process) (Cochlea) The biologically active component of the basilar membrane response to sound that adds energy, counteracting inherent damping.

Cochlear duct Triangular-shaped space filled with endolymph. Its walls include Reissner's membrane, the stria vascularis, and the superior surfaces of the epithelial cells covering the basilar membrane.

Cochlear echo Subaudible sounds recorded from the external ear canal.

Cochlear microphonic (CM) An alternating current (AC) gross potential generated by large numbers of cochlear hair cells (see AC/DC), reflecting the AC component of the receptor potential. The CM follows the stimulus frequency.

Cochlear nuclei An auditory nuclear complex located on the dorsolateral medulla that receives afferent input via the eighth cranial nerve.

Cochleotopy A topographic representation of the cochlea superimposed on a structure within the brain.

Combination sensitivity Facilitative response of a neuron to combinations of discrete elements of a complex stimulus.

Complex waves Signals that are not composed of a single sinusoid.

Compound action potential A gross neural response measured by an extracellular electrode placed near the cochlea (typically on the eardrum or round window) at the start of a stimulus. It is based on the tendency for the initial spike (and to some extent the second spike) of all responding neurons to be somewhat synchronous. It usually includes two negative peaks dubbed N1 and N2.

Compound threshold shift (CTS) Threshold elevation measured before recovery is complete. Includes a temporary (TTS) and permanent (PTS) component.

Compression/saturation A feature of some nonlinear systems whereby large inputs are truncated and the output is less than a simple multiple of the input ($y < Ax$ for large y). The basilar membrane, hair cells, and cochlear neurons all show this effect for loud stimuli.

Compressive (or saturating) nonlinearity A type of nonlinear system wherein the growth of the output (y) per unit of input (x) is less than linear ($y = Ax$ for small x; $y < Ax$ for large x). The input-output relations of basilar membrane, hair cells, and neurons are of this type.

Concha The conical portion of the external ear leading directly into the external auditory meatus or ear canal.

Concentration gradient An electrochemical imbalance created by an active process that pumps ions across a barrier against the diffusion gradient.

Conductive presbycusis (sensory conductive presbycusis) Hypothetical form of age-related hearing loss taken to involve changes in passive mechanics without notable degeneration.

Continuous noise Noise with level variations that occur at durations of 1 second or less.

Contralateral Opposite side.

Core/belt/parabelt Loose functional division of sensory cortex implying higher levels of processing in a serial fashion. A core region receives relatively unprocessed information, then passes processed information to surrounding belt areas where information may be combined from other sensory modalities, motor information, or information about motivation/effect. Belt areas then project in parallel to parabelt areas, where yet more integrative processing may occur.

Cranial Pertaining to the brain or the skull.

Creatinine Substance present in the blood circulation that is excreted in the urine. Its concentration is inversely proportional to kidney function.

Crista The receptor epithelium of the semicircular canals that contains hair cells, support cells, and vestibular afferent nerve fibers.

Critical band In psychoacoustics, the minimum frequency separation of two narrow band stimuli whereby the two are processed independently without mutual suppression. Mechanistically related to the frequency tuning curve, and tuning curve bandwidths and critical bands show similar trends with increasing stimulus frequency.

Critical level Level of a sound exposure above which the cochlea can be damaged mechanically.

Cupula A gelatinous, fluid-tight partition that extends from the crista to the top of the ampullary wall. Hair cell stereocilia are embedded in the cupula and are displaced with cupula motion.

Cytoskeleton The system of structural support elements in the cell that provides mechanical stability, as well as movement.

Damping Reduction in amplitude of a signal produced by frictional resistance.

DART The four things sound can do when it encounters a barrier: diffract, absorb, reflect, transmit.

Decibel (dB) A logarithmic shorthand to express sound pressure or intensity levels.

Decussation Crossing of the midline by ascending or descending pathways.

Deiters' cell One of the major supporting cells of the organ of Corti that contains an intracellular bundle of microtubules extending from the base to the phalangeal process. The base of each outer hair cell is supported by one Deiters' cell.

Dendrite The input zone of a nerve fiber.

Dendritic arborization Dendritic extensions often resembling a tree that allow neurons to receive input from many cells.

Depolarization A decrease in the electrical potential across a cell membrane, caused by the cell becoming less negatively charged.

Diencephalon A region of the embryonic brainstem that gives rise to the thalamus and hypothalamus.

Differential recording A physiologic recording method based on two electrodes that sample different regions of an experimental preparation, the region of interest (active electrode), and a spatially remote region that is not expected to generate a response to the stimulus (reference electrode). A differential amplifier subtracts the signal recorded by the reference electrode from that recorded by the active electrode, and amplifies the difference. This has the effect of selectively amplifying only the signal of interest and suppressing random and biologically generated noise.

Differentiation Modification of embryonic tissues or cells from a generalized form into a specialized form.

Digital coding Representation of a signal as a binary digit (bit) that is either high or low at any moment. In the brain, real-world stimuli are coded digitally for the presence or absence of spikes. Each spike can be considered to be a momentary "high" bit value (see Analog coding).

Distortion Alteration of a signal by a nonlinear sytem, such that the output contains frequencies not present at the input.

Distortion product otoacoustic emissions (DPOAEs) Tone signals (distortion products) that are generated in response to the presentation of two simultaneous tone stimuli.

Dizziness A nonspecific term that generally denotes some form of spatial disorientation such as faintness or light-headedness and may or may not involve feelings of movement.

DNA Deoxyribonucleic acid, the molecular basis of genes and chromosomes, and the "blueprint" for all proteins made by a cell. It is composed of a sequence of four types of small nucleic acids (adenine, thymidine, guanine, and cytosine). Exists primarily in the form of two complementary strands loosely bound together.

Dominant A trait that can be observed even if only one copy of the gene responsible is present.

DP-gram A plot of the level of the distortion product otoacoustic emission (DPOAE) versus primary frequency.

Duplex theory A theory of binaural sound localization relying on detection of stimulus phase differences at low frequencies and differences in spectrum at high frequencies.

Dynamic posturography A system to evaluate balance using a computer-controlled movable platform with a movable visual surround.

Dynamic range The range of inputs to a system that yield different output values. Growth need not be linear.

Dysplasia Medically abnormal development or growth of a part of the body, for example, an organ, bone, or cell, including the total absence of such a part.

Ear lobe The lowermost portion of the auricle, not supported by cartilage.

Ectoderm Outermost of the three germ layers of the developing embryo, the other two being the mesoderm and the endoderm.

Effective quiet The maximum level of "background" sound that will not impede recovery from a temporary threshold shift; about 80 dB for humans.

Efferent neuron Conduct information away from the brain toward the periphery.

Effusion Filling of a space with fluid. In otitis media, the middle ear may fill with lymphatic fluid, giving rise to otitis media with effusion.

Electrochemical gradient A combination of both electrical and chemical gradients that cause ions to move from one compartment to another. Potassium in the inner ear flows in a loop, driven partly by electrical gradients across the hair cell membrane and partly because of potassium gradients across the hair cell membrane.

Endocochlear potential The electrical potential within cochlear scala media that serves to generate part of the electrochemical gradient that drives ion currents through hair cells.

Endoderm Innermost of the three germ layers of the developing embryo, the other two being the mesoderm and the endoderm.

Endolymph The fluid that fills the cochlear duct or endolymphatic space. It contains a high concentration of potassium ions and a low concentration of sodium ions, similar to intracellular fluid.

Endolymphatic space Cochlear duct. The endolymphatic space has a positive potential of 80 to 100 mV relative to the perilymphatic spaces.

Endoplasmic reticulum A portion of the membrane system that receives newly assembled proteins, modifies them, and packages them for transport to the Golgi apparatus.

Enzyme A protein that catalyzes (greatly speeds up) a biochemical reaction without being consumed or altered by the reaction.

Eustachian tube A tube that runs from the middle ear to the nasopharynx to allow pressure equilibration of the middle ear cavity.

Excitatory masking Noise band that contains frequencies and levels to which an auditory nerve fiber is sensitive, and thereby reduces the response of the fiber to those frequencies.

Excitotoxicity Toxicity associated with prolonged and excessive release of glutamate by hair cells in the cochlea or presynaptic neurons in the brain. Injury to postsynaptic cells may be reversible or permanent.

External auditory meatus The external ear canal; it runs from the concha to the tympanic membrane.

External ear That portion of the ear that is peripheral to the tympanic membrane, consisting of the auricle and external auditory meatus.

Extrapyramidal system A neural network in the central nervous system that controls motor movement.

Facilitation An increase in the response of a neuron by presentation of two stimuli, or two elements of a complex stimulus. Facilitation must be multiplicative; that is, the response to the combined stimulus must be more than the sum of responses to the individual components.

Fast Fourier transform (FFT) Method used with computers to extract Fourier transforms from discrete observations.

Feedback loop A feature of any system whereby the output is "fed back" to the input to either increase the output signal amplitude (positive feedback) or decrease the output signal amplitude (negative feedback).

Filter Any device that modifies the spectrum of its input and passes only a portion of the input to the output.

Fissure A deep recess in the surface of the brain. Fissures demark the boundaries between the various lobes of the cortex.

Forebrain The rostral portion of the developing brain that will become the cerebral cortex; also called the prosencephalon.

Forward masking Masking of the response of an auditory neuron to a probe by a prior stimulus.

Fourier transform A mathematical formula that can be used to describe the response of a physical system from the time domain to the frequency domain.

Free radicals Atoms, molecules, or ions that contain one or more unpaired electrons. They are often highly reactive with cell components, and thus destructive and toxic.

Free radical scavenger A molecule or compound that reduces (inactivates) free radicals.

Frequency Number of periodic repetitions (or cycles) per second, typically expressed in Hertz (Hz).

Frequency discrimination The ability to detect frequency differences between two nonsimultaneous narrowband stimuli.

Frequency resolution The ability to detect and perceive two simultaneous narrowband stimuli as separate stimuli.

Frequency tuning curve The relation between sound frequency and the lowest intensity at any frequency that yields a defined "criterion" response from the basilar membrane, hair cell, or neuron.

Frontal lobe The most anterior lobes of the brain; involved in the planning and execution of behavior.

Fundamental The lowest frequency component of a complex signal.

Gamma-aminobutyric acid (GABA) A primary neurotransmitter that has mostly inhibitory effects and is derived from glutamic acid.

Gap junction A connection between two cells that allows ions to flow from one cell to the other. It can be selective for particular ions or nonselective.

Gene A sequence of DNA coding for a single protein product. May include several proteins that interact to perform a single function.

Genotype The particular alleles carried by an individual on both chromosomes.

Gestation Carrying of an embryo or fetus inside the female.

Glia or glial cell A major cell type in nervous system that provides nutrients to neurons.

Glomus tumor A slow-growing true neoplasm (tumor) derived from oxygen pressure-sensing baroreceptors. They can arise from different sites within the temporal bone including the middle ear (globus tympanicum) or jugular vein (globus jugulare). Symptoms commonly include hearing loss and pulsating tinnitus.

Glutamate An amino acid thought to be the primary excitatory neurotransmitter in sensory systems, including the inner ear.

Glutathione A peptide or protein containing three amino acids that is important for inactivation of free radicals.

Golgi apparatus The final segment of the membrane system that performs final modifications to new proteins and packages them for delivery to the plasma membrane.

Gray matter The portion of the brain that includes nerve cells and is responsible for information processing.

Gross potential Electrical potentials recorded from large numbers of cells at the same time using a large extracellular (typically subcutaneous, round window, or intracochlear) electrode. Wave I of the auditory brain response, N1 of the compound action potential, cochlear microphonic, and summating potential are examples.

Gyrus A ridge on the surface of the cortex, usually located between two grooves, or sulci.

Habenula perforata (plural: habenulae perforata) Hole in basilar membrane below the inner hair cell through which nerve fibers enter and leave the organ of Corti.

Hair cell Cell misnamed for its sensory "hairs" (stereocilia) that transduces mechanical displacement of the organ of Corti/basilar membrane, cupula, or otolith into neural impulses.

Helicotrema A semilunar opening at the cochlear apex through which scala vestibuli and scala tympani communicate with each other.

Helix The outermost C-shaped ridge of the auricle.

Hematopoietic Pertaining to the bone marrow or blood-forming tissues.

Hensen's cell Cuboidal to columnar supporting cell of the organ of Corti that is located lateral to the third rows of outer hair cells and Deiters' cells. This cell contains no bundles of microtubules.

Hensen's stripe Darkly stained protuberance on the inferior surface of the tectorial membrane. The tallest stereocilia of the inner hair cells abut the lateral side of Hensen's stripe.

Heterozygous The state of having different alleles of a gene on homologous chromosomes where the gene is located.

High-pass filter Allows high frequencies to pass through unattenuated.

Hillock Small embryonic tissue hill or mound.

Hindbrain The most caudal portion of the developing brain; responsible for the medulla oblongata and the cerebellum.

Homeostasis Derived from Greek roots meaning "keep the same." Maintenance by any cell of an invariant internal state suitable for survival.

Homeostatic mechanism Serves to maintain the internal environment of tissues or cells at constant levels.

Homology When genes in different species or on different chromosomes are determined to be the same gene, serving the same purpose.

Homozygous The state of having the same allele of a gene on both homologous chromosomes where the gene is located.

Hyperpolarization An increase in the electrical potential across a cell membrane, caused by the cell becoming more negatively charged.

Hyper-recruitment A characteristic of some patients with sensorineural hearing loss who show abnormal sensitivity to loud sounds.

Impedance Resistance to movement or progress. The impedance of water is much greater than the impedance of air.

Impulsive noise Short duration, high-level noise, such as that produced by the explosion of a firecracker.

Incus The second or middle of the three auditory ossicles.

Indeterminate presbycusis Age-related hearing loss whose cellular basis cannot be determined from standard light microscopic evaluation.

Inertia The tendency to persist in the absence of external influences. Specifically, in physics, it is the tendency of a body to maintain its state of uniform motion unless acted on by an external force.

Inferior colliculus A nucleus in the midbrain from which all ascending auditory signals project to the thalamus.

Infrasound Sounds that are below the frequencies that can be detected by humans (i.e., <20 Hz).

Inhibitory postsynaptic potential (IPSP)/ excitatory postsynaptic potential (EPSP) Changes in resting membrane potential of a neuron caused by the action of neurotransmitters. They are either depolarizing (EPSP, serving to increase excitability) or hyperpolarizing (IPSP, serving to decrease excitability).

Intensity curve The relation between sound intensity in decibels and the spike rate of a responding auditory neuron.

Intensity response curve (input-output [I/O] curve) The relation between stimulus intensity and the spike rate of any neuron, or receptor potential amplitude of any receptor (hair) cell. In the cochlea, I/O curves typically show a rising portion and a flat (saturated) portion, and are said to be monotonic. Within the brain, they may rise and then fall with increasing stimulus intensity, and thus are nonmonotonic.

Intermediate filament An intermediate-sized element of the cytoskeleton primarily responsible for mechanical stability of the cell.

Internal auditory meatus The bony canal that transmits the auditory and vestibular nerves from the inner ear to the brainstem. Opening on the medial side of the temporal bone that transmits both the facial and vestibulocochlear nerves, as well as the blood supply to the inner ear.

Interneuron The majority of the estimated 10 billion neurons in the nervous system. They connect one neuron to another within a structure.

Interval histogram A neural spike counting scheme designed to discover order in the timing of spikes relative to the immediately previous spike. Bins typically a few microseconds in duration are aligned so that bin "0" starts immediately after any spike to obtain an interval histogram. The minimum interspike interval is expected to reflect the absolute refractory period. Histogram peaks (based on bin height) occurring at longer intervals would be expected to fall at multiples of the stimulus period if phase-locking is occurring.

Intraperitoneal Within a body compartment that contains the internal organs of digestion, the stomach, and intestines.

Inverse Fourier transform The Fourier transform used to extract the time function from the frequency function.

Inverse square law The acoustic intensity decreases by the inverse square of the distance from the source, or 6 dB per doubling, and a nonreflective field.

Ipsilateral Same side.

Irradiation Treatment with radiation, usually for cancer, using sources such as cobalt.

Iso-level curve The spike rate of an auditory neuron as a sound stimulus is swept across a wide frequency range with the intensity held constant.

Iso-response curve Essentially the same as a frequency tuning curve, but may examine a wider range of responses, that is, both near-threshold and suprathreshold responses. By choosing a range of fixed response criteria, a family of nested curves may be obtained for the basilar membrane, hair cell, or neuron.

Jeffress model A physical model for the localization of low-frequency stimuli whereby binaural phase analysis is conducted by central neurons that receive delayed inputs from one ear. Such a delay may, in theory, be based simply on additional length of axons crossing the midline, but in reality, it appears to involve synaptic mechanisms and to occur within both the medial superior olive and inferior colliculus.

Laser velocimetry A sensitive, noninvasive technique used for measuring basilar membrane motion.

Lateral efferent system Olivocochlear efferent neurons that reside in lateral regions of the superior olivary complex within the brainstem.

Lateral inhibition Sharpening of tuning (to frequency or any other sound parameter) in a neuron by inhibitory connections from neurons tuned to slightly different values of the parameter. For example, frequency tuning in a neuron tuned to 10 kHz might be sharpened by inhibition from neurons tuned just above and below 10 kHz.

Lateral lemniscus One of several small auditory relay nuclei ventral to the inferior colliculus.

Lateral superior olive Mid- to high-frequency binaural processing nucleus in the lateral regions of the superior olivary complex within the brainstem. A nuclear aggregate within the superior olivary complex involved in processing interaural intensity differences.

Lemniscal/nonlemniscal Separation of ascending auditory information according to whether it passes through the lateral lemniscus. Connections through the lemniscus are taken to provide more basic acoustic analysis and less integrative/complex analysis.

Limbus (limbic lobe) A mound of connective tissue on the superior lip of the osseous spiral lamina. It serves as the medial attachment of the tectorial membrane.

Lipid bilayer The spontaneous arrangement of lipid molecules into a double layer that is hydrophobic interiorly and hydrophilic on the outside.

Lipofuscin (age pigment) Dark-appearing accumulation of undegraded cellular waste products that may signal and possibly promote progressive impairment of cell and tissue function.

Locus A physical location on a chromosome holding a gene of interest.

Loop diuretics Drugs that increase the excretion of water and electrolytes by the kidney by acting on the loop of Henle.

Loop of Henle A thin, hair-pin–shaped portion of the kidney unit that controls a large portion of salt and water reabsorption.

Loudness recruitment A characteristic of individuals with sensorineural hearing losses who often have difficulty perceiving soft sounds, but louder sounds are perceived almost normally.

Low-pass filter Allows low frequencies to pass through unattenuated.

Macromechanics Large-scale movements of entire structures in the inner ear, such as the basilar membrane or whole organ of Corti.

Macula The receptor epithelium of the otolith organs (utricle and saccule) that contains hair cells, support cells, and vestibular afferent nerve fibers.

Malleus The first of the auditory ossicles, it is embedding in the tympanic membrane and articulates with the incus.

Map Organization of processing in the brain according to a known principle, such as frequency, space, or body surface.

Masker A sound that masks (suppresses) the response to a probe stimulus. The response that is suppressed may be electrical or behavioral.

Masking Decreasing the response to a tone by the addition of a noise or other tones.

Medial efferent system Olivocochlear neurons that reside mostly in medial and ventral regions of the superior olivary complex within the brainstem.

Medial geniculate An auditory relay nucleus within the thalamus that passes information between the inferior colliculus and the auditory cortex.

Medial longitudinal fasciculus A major fiber tract running along the midline of the brainstem. Descending fibers of the medial vestibulospinal tract and ascending fibers from the vestibular nuclei to the oculomotor nuclei run through the medial longitudinal fasciculus.

Medial superior olive A nuclear aggregate within the superior olivary complex involved in processing interaural time (phasic) differences.

Medial vestibulospinal tract A tract of descending fibers from vestibular nuclei neurons that project to the cervical spinal cord for head, neck, and postural control.

Medulla The part of the hindbrain caudal to the pons and ventral to the cerebellum.

Meiosis Reduction division for the purpose of generating germ cells, such that the number of chromosomes is reduced to one from each homologous pair.

Membrane voltage The voltage difference across the outer membrane of any cell.

Ménière's disease An inner ear disorder characterized by episodic vertigo, roaring tinnitus, low-frequency hearing loss, and aural fullness.

Meninges Three membranes (dura, arachnoid, and pia) that cover the surface of the brain.

Mesenchymal Embryonic tissue formed from elongated mesenchyme cells.

Mesencephalon Refers to the embryonic midbrain and is one of three basic subdivisions of the embryonic brain encephalon.

Metabolic rate The rate of energy expenditure and consumption of resources by a cell or an organism.

Metathetic continuum A continuum that changes in quality as one goes up the scale, like frequency.

Metencephalon The metencephalon is the region of the embryonic brain that causes the pons and cerebellum.

Micromechanics Small-scale movements of inner ear structures, such as stereocilia motion or hair cell motility.

Microtubule The largest of the cytoskeletal elements, microtubules play significant roles in cell division, polarization, and trafficking within the cell.

Midbrain One of the three divisions of the developing brain.

Mitochondrial clock theory A theory of cell aging whereby a significant fraction of mitochondria contain damaged DNA and exhibit impaired function. Even when these mitochondria are replaced by daughter organelles through repeated division, the new mitochondria carry mutations and are also impaired. Oxidative metabolism thus becomes progressively less efficient over time, and overall cell viability decreases.

Mitochondrion The organelle responsible for energy production in the form of ATP.

Mitosis Division of any cell into two identical cells.

Mixed presbycusis Age-related hearing loss meeting criteria for more than one of the generally recognized forms (sensory, neural, strial).

Modiolus Central core of spongy bone about which turn the spiral canals of the cochlea. It contains afferent and efferent nerve fibers of the cochlea.

Morphogenesis The processes that control the organized spatial distribution of cells that arises during embryonic development and that cause the characteristic forms of tissues and organs.

Mössbauer technique A technique for measuring basilar membrane motion, involving the emission of a radioactive particle placed on the basilar membrane.

Motion sickness The experience of nausea or vomiting when riding in an airplane, automobile, or amusement park ride.

Motor neuron An efferent neuron that controls movement.

mRNA Messenger RNA (ribonucleic acid); the form of RNA used to copy a DNA "blueprint" for making a protein and carry the information to the ribosome.

Multipolar neurons Neurons that have more than two processes.

Myelin or myelin sheath Fatty insulation around some neurons. The myelin sheath insulates the axon along most of its length, prevents the diffusion of ions across the cell wall, and speeds up neural transmission.

Necrosis A passive form of cell death characterized by swelling of the dying cell and rupturing of the membrane. Necrosis does not require metabolically active processes within the dying cell (e.g., synthesis of new proteins) and typically evokes an inflammatory response in injured tissues. Unlike apoptosis, necrotic cell death cannot be easily blocked by pharmacologic inhibitors.

Negative damping The effect of a negative resistance on the damping of a mechanical system, which creates amplification of the input.

Nephrotoxicity Toxic damage to the kidney.

Neural presbycusis Age-related hearing loss characterized by primary degeneration of spiral ganglion cells, that is, while their inner hair cell targets are still present. More than half may be lost before speech perception is affected, and up to 90% may be lost before thresholds in quiet are affected.

Neural tube Primitive embryonic central nervous system, consisting of a tube of neural ectoderm.

Neuroblastoma Tumor that usually occurs in childhood and may arise in the adrenal gland.

Neuron The basic building block of the nervous system.

Neuronal guidance The nervous system is composed of many billions of neurons, which are all "wired together" in a precise fashion. This network of neurons is created during embryonic development, and immature neurons use a variety of chemical signals to direct their growth. In the developing inner ear, afferent and efferent neurons grow toward their correct hair cell targets and establish synaptic contacts. Numerous chemical signaling molecules are thought to act as guidance cues in this process.

Neuropeptides Small, protein-like, amino acid sequences that cause neuromodulatory effects.

Neurotoxicity Toxic damage to nerve cells or their extensions.

Neurotransmitter Chemical substances synthesized by a neuron and released into the synaptic space by activation of the neuron. Neurotransmitters can be either excitatory or inhibitory.

Node of Ranvier Segmented, nonmyelinated areas interspersed along the myelin sheaths of some neurons.

Noise (1) Any sound or signal that is aperiodic (acoustics); (2) any signal that interferes with the quality or detection of another signal (engineering); (3) any signal that is unwanted (psychoacoustics); and (4) any sound that can negatively affect the physiologic or psychological well-being of an individual.

Noise-induced hearing loss (NIHL) Hearing loss caused by continuous or intermittent exposure to loud sounds.

Noise-induced permanent threshold shift (NIPTS) Permanent threshold shift caused by exposure to noise.

Nucleolus A prominent figure within the nucleus. The nucleolus manufactures ribosomes.

Nucleus (cell) The most prominent cell organelle, the nucleus houses the genetic material that is common to all the cells of a given organism.

Nucleus (neuronal architecture) An agglomeration of neural cell bodies within the brain. Its counterpart in the periphery is a ganglion.

Nuel spaces Fluid spaces within the organ of Corti that surround the bodies of the outer hair cells.

Nystagmus A rhythmic oscillation of the eyes in either the horizontal, vertical, or torsional directions.

Occipital lobe The most posterior lobe of the brain; responsible for visual processing.

Octave Frequency ratio of 2:1.

Oculomotor nucleus Third cranial nucleus located in the midbrain. It contains oculomotor neurons that innervate the medial rectus, superior rectus, inferior rectus, and inferior oblique muscles of the eye.

Ohm's acoustic law States that any periodic signal may be represented by a series of sinusoids with appropriate amplitudes and starting phases.

Olivocochlear pathway Collective term for efferent auditory neurons located in ventral and lateral regions of the superior olivary complex that project to the organ of Corti within the cochlea.

Ontogenetic development A process of normal development that describes how the human cellular structure and organization becomes more complex and interconnected as the body develops.

Organ of Corti Hearing organ in mammals.

Oscillopsia The sensation that objects are moving in a oscillating fashion when viewed.

Osseous spiral lamina Double layer of thin bone projecting from the modiolus. The peripheral processes of the spiral ganglion cells traverse the osseous spiral lamina on the way to the organ of Corti.

Ossicles The three tiny bones of the middle ear, the malleus, incus, and stapes.

Otalgia Ear pain that may be caused by local inflammation or referred to the ear by disease in another region such as the teeth or temporomandibular joint.

Otic placode Thickening of the surface ectodermal tissue in the area that will become the inner ear.

Otitis externa Inflammation of the external ear canal.

Otitis media Inflammation of the middle ear cavity that may be accompanied by the accumulation of fluid and resultant pressure against the tympanic membrane. Specific cases range from acute to chronic and may be excruciatingly painful or completely asymptomatic.

Otoacoustic emission (OAE) Sounds generated by the nonlinear activity of the outer hair cells of the cochlea that can be recorded in the ear canal.

Otoconia Biomineral particles made of calcium carbonate that lie in the otolith vestibular receptor organs.

Otocyst Invagination of the otic placode that forms a hollow vesicle.

Otolith Inertial receptor organ of the vestibular system that transduces linear accelerations from head motion.

Otorrhea A fluid discharge from the ear that may consist of purulent material due to infection and resultant rupture of the tympanic membrane or cerebrospinal fluid.

Otosclerosis A progressive growth of new spongy bone, particularly about the base of the stapes, that results in impaired ossicular movement.

Ototoxicity Toxic damage to hearing or balance caused by drugs.

Oxidative stress An imbalance in the redox state of any cell such that key structures and components (lipids, proteins, DNA) become oxidized and dysfunctional.

Parasympathetic system A division of the autonomic nervous system that maintains heart rate and respiratory, metabolic, and digestive functions under normal conditions.

Parietal lobe A lobe of the brain located above the temporal lobe, behind the frontal lobe, and in front of the occipital lobe; responsible for the integration of sensory information.

Penetrance The tendency of a particular genotype to be exhibited in the phenotype. Will depend on the dominant/recessive character of the allele, as well as the ability of other genes to affect the same trait.

Perilymph Fluid that fills scala vestibuli and tympani in the cochlea. It contains a high concentration of sodium ions and a low concentration of potassium ions and is similar to cerebrospinal fluid.

Period In any periodic signal, the amount of time to complete one cycle.

Period histogram (phase histogram or "folded" histogram) Similar to the poststimulus time histogram (PSTH), except for how time bins are aligned. For a PSTH, the time represented by any bin is referenced to stimulus onset (i.e., bin "0" starts at stimulus onset). For a period histogram, bins typically a few microseconds in duration are aligned with reference to a specific stimulus phase, and the overall time scale is "folded" over one stimulus period. Thus, for a 1-kHz tone, the maximum time on the x-axis would be 1 millisecond. The presence of a peak in a period histogram indicates phase-locking of spikes, and a flat histogram indicates no phase-locking.

Periodic waveform Signal that repeats itself in time.

Periolivary A collection of neurons that reside outside of any distinctive nuclear grouping within the superior olivary complex of the brainstem.

Peripheral nervous system The portion of the nervous system that is outside the skull and spinal column, including the cranial and spinal nerves.

Permanent threshold shift (PTS) Shift in hearing threshold that does not recover.

Permissible Exposure Limit The maximum daily allowable dose of noise, as specified by the Occupational Health and Safety Administration (OSHA) and other federal agencies.

Pharyngeal arches Embryonic gill-like structures in the neck region that cause bony structures necessary for phonation and hearing.

Phase The angular relation between a signal and its starting point or between two contemporaneous sinusoidal signals, measured in degrees or radians.

Phase-locking Representation of a sound stimulus for the precise timing (i.e., at a particular stimulus phase) of action potentials of an auditory neuron. In mammals, phase-locking generally only occurs for frequencies less than ~5 kHz and is negligible in the central auditory system above the brainstem. Sounds at high intensities near the best (characteristic) frequency generally yield the clearest phase-locking.

Phenotype The outward physical characteristics associated with a particular genotype.

Pillar cell One of the major supporting cells in the organ of Corti that contains an intracellular bundle of microtubules extending from the base to the head of the cell. Inner pillar cells are adjacent to the inner hair cells and have a thin head plate that covers the outer pillar heads. Outer pillar cells are adjacent to the first row of outer hair cells.

Pink noise Noise containing equal energy per octave.

Place coding Stimulus coding by auditory neurons principally in terms of place of innervation along the cochlear spiral.

Plasma membrane A selectively permeable, lipid bilayer that surrounds the cell, separating the intracellular and extracellular environments.

Plasticity (neuronal) The ability of neuronal connections and circuits to alter the number or strength of interconnections, serving an adaptive purpose. The purpose may be learning or compensation for damage.

Pons The part of the rostral hindbrain that lies ventral to the cerebellum and in between the midbrain and medulla.

Postmitotic A state achieved by cells that have ceased dividing. The fact that sensory cells such as mammalian cochlear hair cells are postmitotic places a premium on repair of these cells. Once gone, they are not replaced.

Poststimulus time histogram (PSTH) A counting method used to measure neural spike rate responses to stimuli. To obtain a PSTH, the time after a stimulus is turned on is divided into short (typically millisecond) intervals (bins) and each spike is added to a specific bin, depending on when it occurs relative to stimulus onset. After many stimulus presentations, the number of spikes in each bin (bin height) provides a graphic and quantitative indication of how spike probability varies for any neuron as a function of time. Using bin height, bin duration, and the number of stimulus presentations, spike rate in spikes per second can be computed for any bin.

Precentral gyrus A gyrus just anterior to the central sulcus in the frontal lobe that is a primary motor area.

Primary cortical area Area of the neocortex that directly either receives information from ascending sensory pathways or gives rise to motor information via descending motor pathways.

Programmed aging A concept of cellular aging as a genetic program that may be completely intrinsic or triggered by environmental events.

Prosencephalon Refers to the embryonic forebrain and is one of three basic subdivisions of the embryonic brain encephalon.

Protein A string of amino acids (anywhere from one to hundreds) that performs some biological function such as catalysis or the makeup of a cell structural component.

Prothetic continuum A continuum that contains a single attribute, but "more" is present as one goes up the scale. Sound pressure level is an example.

Pyramidal system A motor system that carries corticospinal axons from primary motor areas to motor neurons.

Q (of filter) The ratio of the center frequency of a filter, divided by the bandwidth.

Q_{10dB}/Q_{40dB} Conventions for quantifying the sharpness of tuning of auditory hair cells and neurons. To obtain these, the characteristic frequency is divided by the bandwidth of the frequency tuning curve at 10 or 40 dB above the threshold. These measures are loosely based on the broader engineering concept of the Q-value of a filter.

Quanta Discrete "packets" of neurotransmitter released by a hair cell (or other presynaptic cell) onto a neuron at a synaptic junction.

Quarter wavelength rule The resonant frequency of an open tube resonator is the frequency with a wavelength that is four times the length of the tube.

Radial afferent (type I) Afferent neurons that connect directly from inner hair cells. They comprise 90% to 95% of the afferent innervation from the cochlea.

Rate adaptation The tendency for spike rate and spike probability to decrease over time for a steady stimulus (e.g., a long tone). Spike rate generally decreases (as indicated by poststimulus time histogram) within a few milliseconds after a suprathreshold tone is turned on and settles over a few tens of milliseconds into an approximate steady-state firing rate that is lower than the initial firing rate. The implication of rate adaptation for coding is that the response of any cochlear neuron to a tone depends on its activity level the moment before.

Rate response Representation of a sound stimulus for the rate of action potentials of an auditory neuron. Sounds at high intensities near the best (characteristic) frequency generally yield the highest firing rates.

Rate suppression The ability of a stimulus to reduce the response of an auditory neuron (in terms of firing rate) to a probe tone presented near the characteristic frequency. Frequency/intensity combinations that yield rate suppression typically fall just outside the tip of the frequency tuning curve and just below the tail.

Rate-place code Stimulus coding by auditory neurons for place of innervation along the cochlear spiral and spike rate. Those neurons tuned to the energy peaks of any narrowband or broadband stimulus are expected to be most responsive, so that a spatial profile of spike rates should somewhat resemble the frequency spectrum of the stimulus (log scale). In reality, this is approximated only at low stimulus levels caused by rate saturation and suppression.

Receptor A specialized neuron that converts external signals, such as light, sound, physical pressure, or heat into neural signals.

Receptor potential (RP) The electrical response of a receptor cell to a stimulus. The hair cell receptor potential elicited by a toneburst will typically resemble the waveform of the tone (the AC component of the RP) but will also include an offset (the DC component).

Recessive A trait that can be observed only if both chromosomes where the gene resides hold the allele causing the trait.

Recombination At meiosis (process of germ cell production), alignment of homologous chromosomes and random swapping of segments so that new alleles from each parent come to lie within the same chromosome and are passed on together.

Rectus muscles Four of the six oculomotor muscles of the eye.

Refractory period The period after a neuronal action potential during which either no spike can occur (absolute refractory period) or is less likely to occur (relative refractory period). These are based on the time needed for voltage-gated sodium channels to reactivate after a spike.

Regeneration Re-formation of a particular structure or organ within the adult body. In adult humans, some portions of the nervous system are capable of regenerating (e.g., the olfactory sensory epithelia in the nose), but most cannot be repaired or replaced after injury.

Reissner's membrane The membrane that separates the cochlear duct from scala vestibuli.

Relatively refractory period Period of time after the absolutely refractory period, but before the neuron's resting potential is restored. During this time, the neuron can fire, but because it is hyperpolarized, more stimulation is needed.

Resonance A vibration of enhanced amplitude that is caused by a stimulus frequency that matches the best or resonant frequency of the system through which it is being transmitted.

Resting potential Voltage potential between the inside and outside of a cell, measured when it is in a resting state.

Reticular formation A region of the brainstem ventral to the cerebral aqueduct and fourth ventricle.

Reticular lamina Surface of the organ of Corti that faces the endolymphatic space. It is made up of the apical surfaces of the hair cells, the head plate of the inner pillar cells and phalangeal processes of the inner phalangeal cells, outer pillar cells, and Deiters' cells, all of which are joined at their luminal edges by tight junctions.

Rhombencephalon Refers to the embryonic hindbrain and is one of three basic subdivisions of the embryonic brain encephalon.

Ribosome The smallest cell organelle, responsible for assembling new proteins from free amino acids using a messenger RNA template.

Rise time Time over which a noise increases from ambient level to a percentage of its maximum level.

RNA (ribonucleic acid) The biochemical basis of several types of molecules involved in gene transcription and translation (messenger, transfer, and ribosomal RNA). Like DNA, it is composed of four types of nucleic acids adenine, cytosine, guanine, but substitutes uracil for thymidine. Unlike DNA it primarily exists as a single strand.

Rosenthal's canal Spiral canal located at the periphery of the modiolus that contains the bodies of the spiral ganglion cells.

Rotational chair testing A method for testing balance function using a chair that rotates in the horizontal plane.

Saccule An otolith vestibular receptor organ that lies nearly vertical in the sagittal head plane.

Saltatory conduction A transmission mode that allows action potential to "jump" from node to node, greatly increasing conduction velocity.

Saturating nonlinearity Term describing the nonlinear response of the basilar membrane to incoming sounds, meaning that the gain decreases with increasing stimulus intensity.

Scala (plural: scalae) (Media) Endolymph-filled fluid channel in the cochlea between scalae vestibuli and tympani. (Tympani) Perilymph-filled channel that is located inferior to the basilar membrane and closed off at the cochlear base by the round window membrane. (Vestibuli) Perilymph-filled channel that is located superior to Reissner's membrane.

Scavenger A molecule or chemical that neutralizes reactive oxygen species.

Semicircular canals Vestibular receptor organs that transduce rotational head motion.

Semipermeable membrane A membrane that is not permeable to all molecules. Although many ions can pass through it, they may do so to different degrees, and large molecules cannot pass at all.

Sensory presbycusis Age-related hearing loss characterized by degeneration of the organ of Corti.

Serum The watery portion of blood remaining after removal of red blood cells and clotting factors.

Sex-linked inheritance The phenotypic expression of an allele that is dependent on the sex of the individual and is directly tied to the sex chromosomes.

Sloping saturation A feature of the intensity response curve of (typically) an auditory neuron whereby the rising portion of the curve has a shallow slope and the saturated portion continues rising without becoming completely flat. This is usually observed for high-threshold neurons with low spontaneous firing rates. Such curves indicate a wide dynamic range, in that a wide range of intensities are associated with unique response amplitudes.

Sodium–potassium ATPase Protein that acts as a mechanical motor, pushing potassium (K^+) ions out of the cell and transmitting sodium (Na^+) ions into it. The "fuel" for the motor comes from the breakdown of the ATP protein into two components, ADP and P, which release energy into the pump.

Soma The cell body of a neuron housing most organelles, including the nucleus.

Somatic motility Changes in the length of outer hair cells in response to sound. May be the basis of the "cochlear amplifier."

Somatic nervous system A portion of the nervous system that is largely responsible for modulating the action of the skeletal (somatic) muscles involved in the voluntary control of speech and volitional movements.

Sound Particle disturbance in an elastic medium.

Sound pressure Pressure variations, produced by acoustic power (Newtons per meter squared [N/m^2]).

Sound pressure level (SPL) The value, in decibels, that a measured sound differs from a reference value that reflects the threshold of human hearing.

Spectrum Description of how energy is distributed across frequency.

Speed of sound In air, 340 m/sec, dependent on elasticity, density, and temperature.

Spike latency The time between a sound stimulus and the first action potential it elicits in an auditory neuron. Contributors to latency include stimulus rise/fall time, speaker delay, basilar membrane travel time, synaptic delay, and whether the neuron is primary or within the brain.

Spike probability The probability that a given neuron will exhibit an action potential at any moment.

Spike rate The rate at which action potentials occur in a neuron.

Spinal cord The part of the central nervous system lying within the vertebral column.

Spinovestibular fibers Afferent fibers that arise throughout the spinal tract and project to the medial and lateral vestibular nuclei.

Spiral afferent Afferent fibers that connect to many OHCs; comprise 5% to 10% of afferent neurons on the cochlear nerve.

Spiral ganglion cells Primary auditory neurons whose bodies are located in Rosenthal's canal.

Spiral ligament Thickened periosteal lining of the bony cochlea located lateral to the stria vascularis.

Spontaneous firing rate (SR) The rate of action potentials exhibited by most auditory neurons (and most central neurons) in the absence of any sound stimulus. In the cochlea, SRs may range from 0 to 120 spikes/sec. For any given neuron, the SR is fairly constant.

Spontaneous otoacoustic emissions (SOAEs) Continuous frequency responses with narrow bandwidths near 1 Hz that occur in the absence of any sound stimulation.

Stapedius A tiny muscle in the middle ear cavity that when contracted can stiffen the ossicular chain, specifically by limiting the movement of the stapes in the oval window. This muscle is involved in the acoustic middle ear reflex.

Stapedius muscle See Acoustic reflex.

Stapes The third of the auditory ossicles; its footplate is embedded in the oval window of the vestibule of the inner ear.

Stem cell A specialized type of cell found in early-stage embryos and in some mature tissues that is capable of repeated divisions. After a stem cell divides, one daughter cell can become another cell type (e.g., blood cell, liver cell, and so forth), whereas the other daughter cell retains the identity of a stem cell.

Stereocilia (singular: stereocilium) Elongated microvilli on the apical surface of the inner and outer hair cells.

Stiffness–limited system Stiffness is the resistance of an elastic body to deflection by an applied force. In such noncompliant systems, stiffness governs vibration responses.

Stria vascularis A vascular strip of tissue forming the lateral wall of the cochlear duct. Its cells are responsible for maintaining the ionic concentrations in endolymph and for generating the positive potential within the cochlear duct or endolymphatic space.

Strial presbycusis Age-related hearing loss characterized by degeneration of the stria vascularis and a decrease in the endocochlear potential (EP). Up to 40% of stria may degenerate before the EP decreases from its normal value near 90 mV.

Striola A region of the otolith macula that contains a high concentration of type I hair cells and dense otoconia. Much of the imaginary reversal line of hair cell polarity runs through the striola.

Sulcus A ridge on the surface of the cortex that separates the two gyri.

Summating potential (SP) Positive or negative direct current (DC) gross potential generated by large numbers of cochlear hair cells (see AC/DC), reflecting the DC component of the receptor potential. The sign $(+/-)$ depends on both the recording location and the stimulus.

Superior olivary complex A complex of auditory nuclei in the caudal pons and rostral medulla that receives and processes bilateral afferent input and sends signals to the inferior colliculi.

Superposition The instantaneous amplitude of a complex signal is the sum of the amplitudes of the sinusoidal signals that make it up.

Suppression (Cochlea) Reduction of the response of basilar membrane, hair cell, or neuron to a stimulus near the best (or characteristic) frequency by a second sound stimulus.

Suppression area Stimulus frequency/intensity combinations that reduce the basilar membrane, hair cell, or neural response to a probe tone, usually presented near threshold at the best (or characteristic) frequency. Suppression areas usually are most prominent on the flanks of the "tip" of the frequency tuning curve.

Suppressive masking Lower frequency noise band that reduces a high-frequency auditory nerve fiber response.

Sympathetic system A division of the autonomic nervous system involved in fight-or-flight situations.

Synapse The connection between neurons.

Synaptic cleft At a synapse, the space between the presynaptic and postsynaptic cell membrane.

Synchrony suppression Disruption of phase-locking of an auditory neuron to a tone by a second tone. It will be manifest as a redistribution of spikes in the phase histogram as spikes become phase-locked to the second tone. The overall firing rate may actually increase.

Syndrome A genetic disease that has multiple features.

Tectorial membrane An acellular gelatinous structure that extends over the superior surface of the organ of Corti. The tips of the tallest outer hair cell stereocilia are embedded in it.

Telodendria Arborization of nerve fibers at the end of the axon in the direction away from the cell body.

Temporal coding Stimulus coding by auditory neurons in terms of the timing of spikes, rather than the rate of spikes. May refer to encoding of stimulus phase (for tones less than ~5kHz) or the timing of amplitude modulations in the stimulus.

Temporal lobe Located on the sides of the cerebrum, below the Sylvian fissure. Responsible for processing of auditory information, including speech.

Temporary threshold shift A transient increase in hearing threshold.

Temporary threshold shift (TTS) Change in hearing that recovers completely within a period of a few hours to a few days.

Tensor tympani A tiny muscle in the inner ear cavity that when contracted can stiffen the ossicular chain and put tension on the tympanic membrane via the manubrium of the malleus.

Terminal bouton "Button" at the terminal ends of neurons packed with neurotransmitters, released when the neuron is activated.

Thalamus The dorsal part of the diencephalon highly interconnected with the cerebral cortex.

Tight junctions Junctions between cells that prevent ions from flowing through the surrounding space. Scala medium is largely sealed to ion influx or outflow by tight junctions between the cells that line it.

Tinnitus The perception of sound or ringing in the ear without an obvious physical cause; also called *phantom auditory perception*. May sound like whistling or clicking, and may be pulsatile or continuous in nature.

Tonic/phasic The character of a response of a neuron to an ongoing stimulus. Tonic firing is sustained firing (a feature of all cochlear neurons). Phasic firing is transient, often occurring only at stimulus onset (e.g., many cortical neurons).

Tonotopic organization A topographic map organized by frequency.

Topographical map The systematic organization within a sensory system or structure by a sensory quality.

Tragus A small tubercle or bump on the anterior side of the external auditory canal.

Transcription Conversion of the DNA code into a complementary messenger RNA sequence as part of the process of making a protein.

Transduction (General) Conversion of one type of energy to another (e.g., a microphone). (Inner ear) The point in the inner ear cascade where mechanical energy is converted to electrical energy (usually refers to the stereociliary bundle).

Transfer function Quantitative description of changes in phase and amplitude of sound stimuli between the source and the tympanic membrane, due predominantly to the head and outer ear.

Transient otoacoustic emissions (TEOAEs) Complex acoustic responses (frequency dispersive waveforms) that can be recorded in the ear canal after a short-duration stimulus such as a click or tone burst.

Translation Conversion of messenger RNA coding for a particular protein into its correct amino acid sequence by a ribosome.

Translational research Research that is conducted in basic science laboratories and developed into clinical practice.

Trapezoid body Region where auditory nerve fibers from the cochlear nuclei cross to the opposite side of the brainstem.

Traveling wave A wave that is moving and has a disturbance that varies both with time and with distance.

Trimester Roughly a 12-week period of gestation for a human fetus.

Trough (pharmacokinetics) The minimal concentration of a drug present in the blood just before administration of the next dose.

Tuning curve tip/tail Two general regions of a frequency tuning curve obtained for a healthy basilar membrane, hair cell, or neuron. The tail is a broad, flat region below the "best" or characteristic frequency (CF). The tip is the narrowly tuned to the CF. Tip and tail regions are most prominent for high-CF neurons.

Tympanic membrane The eardrum, a thin membrane of tissue that isolates the middle ear from the external ear and allows transfer of an airborne sound wave to the mechanical motion of the ossicles.

Type I and II hair cells Specialized mechanoreceptor cells of the vestibular system.

Ultrasound Sounds that are above the frequencies that can be detected by humans (i.e., >20 kHz).

Unipolar/bipolar neurons Neurons that have a single bifurcating process that comes off the cell soma.

Uremia A condition caused in patients caused by accumulation of poisonous by-products that build up in the blood and the body because of kidney failure.

Utricle An otolith vestibular receptor organ that lies nearly horizontal in the head.

Vertigo A sensation of irregular or spinning movement of oneself or surrounding objects.

Vestibular evoked myogenic potentials (VEMP) These potentials detect the sensitivity of the otolith organs to sound. Specifically, the saccule is sensitive to loud clicks, typically 95-dB hearing level or louder. Electrodes can be placed on the neck muscles, such as the sternocleidomastoid, with the patient sitting. The vestibulocollic response (VCR), the portion of vestibulospinal reflex primarily responsible for neck stabilization, can be monitored by recording electromyogenic potentials.

Vestibular ganglion Nerve cell bodies that transmit information from the vestibular part of the inner ear to the brain.

Vestibular nuclei Four major groups of cells in the medulla and pons that process information related to motion and spatial orientation.

Vestibulocochlear nerve The eighth cranial nerve that carries fibers innervating the vestibular and cochlear receptor organs.

Vestibulospinal fibers Descending fibers arising from vestibular nuclei neurons that terminate on spinal motor neurons throughout the cord.

Waveform Description of the amplitude of a signal in the time domain.

Wavelength The distance between two identical points on a periodic signal.

Wernicke's area An area on the superior surface of the temporal lobe associated with Wernicke's aphasia when damaged.

White matter The portion of the brain that carries myelinated nerve fibers and carries information between nuclei and receptors.

White noise Noise containing equal energy per cycle.

Wide dynamic range compression A feature of many digital hearing aids that provides differential amplification and compression of soft and loud sounds.

X-linkage Linkage of a genetic trait to a particular sequence on the X chromosome. The trait may appear dominant in male individuals because of the lack of any compensation by the Y chromosome.

Zonula occludens (plural: zonulae occludens) Tight junction that is formed by the fusion of the outer protein layers at the apical ends of adjacent epithelial cells.

Zwislocki coupler A 6.0-cm^3 metal cavity with the same impedance characteristics as the human ear.

Index

Page numbers followed by "f" denote figures; "t" denotes tables; "b" denotes boxes.